MITRAL VALVE:
Floppy Mitral Valve,
Mitral Valve Prolapse,
Mitral Valvular Regurgitation
Second Revised Edition

Edited by
Harisios Boudoulas, MD, PhD
Professor of Internal Medicine and Pharmacy
Division of Cardiology
The Ohio State University
Columbus, Ohio

and

Charles F. Wooley, MD
Emeritus Professor of Internal Medicine
College of Medicine and Public Health
The Ohio State University
Columbus, Ohio

Futura Publishing Company, Inc.
Armonk, NY

Library of Congress Cataloging-in-Publication Data

Mitral valve : floppy mitral valve, mitral valve prolapse, mitral valvular regurgitation/
edited by Harisios Boudoulas and Charles F. Wooley.—2nd rev. ed.
    p. ; cm.
    Includes bibliographical references and index.
    ISBN 0-87993-448-4 (alk. paper)
    1. Mitral valve—Displacement.   I. Boudoulas, Harisios.   II. Wooley, Charles F.
    [DNLM: 1. Mitral Valve Prolapse.   2. Mitral Valve Insufficiency. WG 262 M6827 2000]
    RC685.V2 M573 2000
    616.1'25—dc21

                                                                                    99-058262

Copyright © 2000
Futura Publishing Company, Inc.

Published by
Futura Publishing Company
135 Bedford Road
Armonk, New York 10504

LC#: 99-058262
ISBN#: 0-87993-448-4

To Students of Medicine

γηράσκω δ' αἰεὶ πολλὰ διδασκόμενος.
As I grow older, I always learn many new things.

Solon 640-556 BC

Acknowledgments

We are grateful for the presence and support of Olga Boudoulas and Mary Lucia Wooley.

We are pleased to acknowledge the professional wisdom and support of our colleagues in the Division of Cardiology and the Department of Internal Medicine, The Ohio State University, College of Medicine and Public Health.

Support was provided by the Overstreet Cardiovascular Teaching and Research Laboratory and the Columbus Foundation, Columbus, Ohio.

The many contributions of Elizabeth A. Sparks, MS, RN, our research associate, are deeply appreciated.

Dennis Mathias, graphic artist, created the cover design, and the graphics in the chapters originated at The Ohio State University.

The secretarial assistance of Dawn Serafinin was most valuable.

Linda Shaw, our editor at Futura, provided professional guidance each step of the way.

Steven E. Korn, Chairman of the Board, Futura Publishing Company, Inc., is a friend and trusted advisor for which we are grateful.

Harisios Boudoulas, MD, PhD
Charles F. Wooley, MD

The Cover

Front
Left panel: Close-up view of a portion of a floppy mitral valve with mitral valve prolapse showing distinct interchordal hooding of the mitral leaflet tissue. (From Edwards JE, Circulation 1971;93:606–612.)
Upper right: Floppy mitral valve viewed from the atrial aspect.
Middle panel: Orthostatis auscultatory phenomena are shown schematically. S1 = first heart sound; C = systolic click; S2 = second heart sound.
Lower right: Left ventriculogram: AL and PL, anterior and posterior mitral valve leaflets, respectively. Asterisks (*) indicate prolapsing scallops of the posterior mitral valve leaflet.

Back
Upper panel: Floppy mitral valve with mitral valve prolapse (arrows) by M-mode (upper left), two-dimensional (upper right), transesophageal (lower left), and three-dimensional echocardiogram (lower right).
Lower panel: Spectral Doppler recording from a patient with floppy mitral valve, mitral valve prolapse, and severe mitral valvular regurgitation (arrows). LV = left ventricle; LA = left atrium; RV = right ventricle; Ao = Aorta.

The Editors

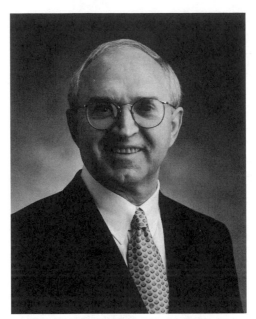

Dr. Harisios Boudoulas

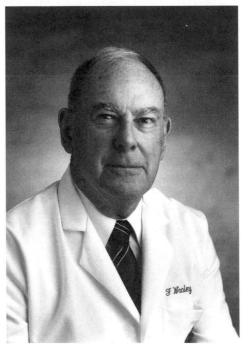

Dr. Charles F. Wooley

Contributors

Robert H. Anderson, BSc, MD
Joseph Levy Foundation Professor of Paediatric Cardiac Morphology, Cardiac Unit, Institute of Child Health, University College London, United Kingdom

Annalisa Angelini, MD
Associate Professor of Cardiovascular Pathology, Institute of Pathological Anatomy, University of Padua, Padua, Italy

Peter B. Baker, MD
Professor of Clinical Pathology, Department of Pathology, College of Medicine and Public Health, The Ohio State University, Columbus, Ohio, USA

Anton E. Becker, MD
Professor of Cardiovascular Pathology, Department of Cardiovascular Pathology, Academic Medical Center, University of Amsterdam, Amsterdam, The Netherlands

Bernard Bénichou, MD, PhD
Laboratory of Genetics, INSERM U533, Nantes University Medical Center, Nantes, France

Harisios Boudoulas, MD, PhD
Professor of Internal Medicine and Pharmacy, Division of Cardiology, The Ohio State University, Columbus, Ohio, USA

Lawrence H. Cohn, MD
Professor of Surgery, Harvard Medical School; Chief, Division of Cardiac Surgery, Brigham and Women's Hospital, Boston, Massachusetts, USA

David G. Criley
Director of Animation and Multimedia, Armus Corporation, Burlingame, California, USA

John Michael Criley, MD
Professor of Medicine and Radiological Sciences, UCLA School of Medicine, Saint John's Cardiovascular Research Center, Torrance, California, USA

Michael J. Davies, MD
British Heart Foundation, Professor of Pathology, Department of Histopathology, St. George Hospital Medical School, London, United Kingdom

Mary Elizabeth Fontana, MD
Associate Professor of Internal Medicine, Division of Cardiology, College of Medicine and Public Health, The Ohio State University, Columbus, Ohio, USA

Derek Gibson, MD
Reader in Cardiology, Royal Brompton Hospital, London, United Kingdom

Robert L. Hamlin, DVM, PhD, DACVIM
(Cardiology/Internal Medicine)
Professor, Department of Veterinary Biosciences, College of Veterinary Medicine, The Ohio State University, Columbus, Ohio, USA

Siew Yen Ho, PhD
Reader in Cardiac Morphology, Department of Paediatrics, National Heart and Lung Institute, Imperial College of Science, Technology and Medicine, London, United Kingdom

Susan L. Koletar, MD
Professor of Clinical Internal Medicine, Division of Infectious Diseases, College of Medicine and Public Health, The Ohio State University, Columbus, Ohio, USA

Albert J. Kolibash, MD
Associate Professor of Internal Medicine, Division of Cardiology, College of Medicine and Public Health, The Ohio State University, Columbus, Ohio, USA

Florence Kyndt, PhD
Pharmacist, Laboratory of Genetics, INSERM U533, Nantes University Medical Center, Nantes, France

Hervé Le Marec, MD, PhD
Professor of Medicine, Department of Cardiology, Nantes University Medical Center, Nantes, France

Robert C. Little, MD
Emeritus Professor of Physiology and Medicine, Emeritus Chairman, Department of Physiology, Medical College of Georgia, Augusta, Georgia, USA

William C. Little, MD
Chief, Division of Cardiology, Professor of Internal Medicine, Bowman Gray School of Medicine, Wake Forest University School of Medicine, Winston-Salem, North Carolina, USA

Michael J. Malkowski, MD
Director of Echocardiography, Heritage Valley Health System, Beaver, Pennsylvania, USA

Natesa G. Pandian, MD
Associate Professor of Medicine and Radiology, Tufts University School of Medicine, Director, Cardiovascular Imaging and Hemodynamic Laboratory, New England Medical Center, Boston, Massachusetts, USA

Anthony C. Pearson, MD
Associate Professor of Medicine, Division of Cardiology, College of Medicine and Public Health, The Ohio State University, Columbus, Ohio, USA

Ross M. Reul, MD
Resident in Surgery, Brigham and Women's Hospital, Boston, Massachusetts, USA

Jos R.T.C. Roelandt, MD
Head, Division of Cardiology, Professor of Cardiology, Thoraxcenter, Academic Hospital, Rotterdam, The Netherlands

Tsuguya Sakamoto, MD, FJCC, FACC
Editor-in-Chief, Journal of Cardiology, Tokyo, Japan

Stephen F. Schaal, MD
Professor of Internal Medicine, Division of Cardiology, College of Medicine and Public Health, The Ohio State University, Columbus, Ohio, USA

Jean-Jacques Schott, PhD
Senior Scientist, Laboratory of Genetics, INSERM U533, Nantes University Medical Center, Nantes, France

Andrew P. Slivka, MD
Associate Professor of Neurology, Division of Cerebrovascular Diseases, Department of Neurology, College of Medicine and Public Health, The Ohio State University, Columbus, Ohio, USA

Elizabeth A. Sparks, MS, RN
Research Associate, Division of Cardiology, College of Medicine and Public Health, The Ohio State University, Columbus, Ohio, USA

Gaetano Thiene, MD
Professor of Cardiovascular Pathology, Institute of Pathological Anatomy, University of Padua, Padua, Italy

Jean-Noël Trochu, MD
Associate Professor of Cardiology, Department of Cardiology, Nantes University Medical Center, Nantes, France

Elizabeth T. Walz, MD
Stroke Director, Mt. Carmel Medical Center, Columbus, Ohio

Charles F. Wooley, MD
Professor Emeritus, Internal Medicine, Division of Cardiology, College of Medicine and Public Health, The Ohio State University, Columbus, Ohio, USA

Jiefen Yao, MD
Erasmus University Rotterdam, Thoraxcenter, Academic Hospital, Rotterdam, The Netherlands

Introduction

Recognition of the broad pathologic spectrum of the floppy mitral valve (FMV) has been a major factor in the renaissance of interest in mitral valve function and disease. The clinical expressions associated with the FMV per se, with prolapse of the FMV, i.e., mitral valve prolapse (MVP), and the unique forms of mitral valvular regurgitation (MVR) resulting from the FMV/MVP dynamics are equally diverse. Thus, new perspectives about the etiology and pathogenesis of mitral valve disease based on the FMV/MVP/MVR triad continue to appear in the cardiovascular literature, challenging conventional wisdom.

Our initial studies at The Ohio State University in the early 1960s involved patients with apical systolic clicks and apical mid- and late systolic murmurs. Earlier clinical dogma had classified these unusual heart sounds and murmurs as extracardiac events. Using dynamic phonocardiography to extend our auscultatory observations in the early 1960s, we soon realized, as did many of our colleagues that the clinical dogma was incorrect.

Many of our colleagues at home and abroad were addressing the various facets of the FMV/MVP/MVR mosaic, albeit approaching the problem from different vantage points. It soon became apparent that this dynamic auscultatory complex was associated with dynamic cardiovascular phenomena, clinical expressions of a complex entity. Thus, new methods would be required for accurate assessment. This was at a time when classic auscultatory tenets were being reinterpreted in light of new methods of cardiac catheterization, angiography, and surgery, and traditional cardiac diagnostic certainties were being reconsidered. Postural auscultation, postural phonocardiography, intracardiac phonocardiography, cardiac catheterization, left ventricular cineangiography, and postural angiography were important steps in providing clinical, auscultatory, and hemodynamic coherence during this time period.

Terminology and Nosology

There are several ways to approach the FMV/MVP/MVR triad. Using both chronological and contemporary approaches reveals a great deal about how physicians learn about disease. The ever-changing technology of each particular era contributes to bursts of intellectual activity, followed by diastolic pauses of surprising lengths, when astute observations and concepts either did not reach threshold, or were buried and lost. These diastolic pauses were then followed by systolic periods of rediscovery, clarification, and progress.

The chronological approach begins with our 19th century predecessors who interpreted cardiovascular physical diagnosis against a background of late-stage disease and the end-of-life cardiac pathology, then moving forward to the middle of the 20th century. By this time the technology of the chest radiograph, cardiac fluoroscopy, and the electrocardiograph had been applied to the study of valvular heart disease, and cardiology and cardiac surgery were established specialties. The yield from this chronology is quite remarkable as we have the benefit of thoughtful observations and descriptions by some illustrious forebears along with the transmitted sense of excitement that accompanied their discoveries.

The more contemporary and futuristic approach is embodied in a global Medline search, keeping in mind the temporal limitations in this type of inquiry, i.e., that all knowledge did not begin in the 1960s. There are times, however, when the medical literature functions as a barometer, providing a graphic representation of clinicians' concerns with glimpses of the future. For example, using *mitral valve prolapse* or *floppy mitral valve* as the keywords in a Medline Pub-Med search from 1966 to 1998 yields approximately 3,600 citations.

A graph of the Medline citations retrieved, plotted against time provides an interesting temporal perspective (Fig. 1). Citation analysis obviously has intrinsic limitations unless the content of the paper has been read and analyzed. However, as a barometer of issues perplexing or stimulating clinicians, reviewing the literature by topic reveals patterns of content and highlights certain verities, while bearing witness to the destruction of certain straw men. Although in general the half-life of an individual paper may be quite short, the FMV/MVP/MVR literature contains a wealth of valuable information that forms a solid base or platform extending into the 21st century.

Beyond the numerical and temporal aspects of literature citation, the detailed analysis of the content of the reports reveals striking changes, reflecting maturation in clinical thought. We have moved on from the time when "prolapse" of the mitral valve was the central, or only, issue in many clinical studies. This was during the period when MVP diagnosis based on M-mode echo criteria was dissociated from the established FMV morphology, and the clinical auscultatory complex ignored or belittled. Similarly, the well-defined FMV pathologic-angiographic correlates were misplaced or forgotten. The gradual return to FMV morphology as the central core issue is well documented in the literature of the 1980s and 1990s, and reflects the more precise imaging criteria with appropriate clinical correlates.

During this time period, refinements in 2-D echo, Doppler, transesophageal echo (TEE), 3-D echo, and magnetic resonance imaging (MRI)

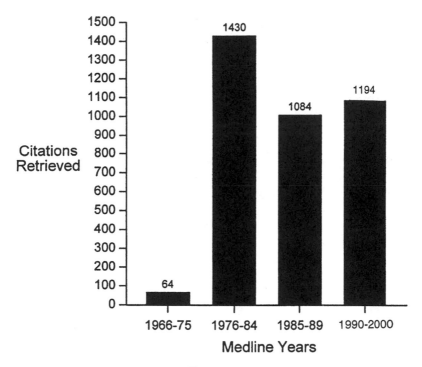

Mitral Valve Prolapse
Medline Search (National Library of Medicine)

Figure 1.

criteria were reconciled with established FMV morphology, while intra-operative TEE became an integral part of FMV surgical repair. In fact, it is during this time period that serial use of sophisticated imaging techniques and the introduction of new methods of surgical repair became part of the natural history of the FMV/ MVP /MVR triad.

Clinical awareness of the frequency and severity of FMV infective endocarditis, electrophysiological evaluation of the mechanisms of arrhythmias associated with the FMV/ MVP /MVR triad, the connective tissue syndrome etiologic and overlap issues, and the impact of surgical implications of mitral valve repair all became universal concerns during this time.

The analysis of MVR with echo Doppler color flow studies, definition of MVR jet characteristics, MVR volume and fraction, and the assessment of left atrial and left ventricular function introduced new terminology that replaced less precise clinical descriptors. Overall, the appraisal of the literature chronology and content reflects this rational approach to the central FMV core issues.

An unexpected result of this clinical maturation process complex is that "MVP" classification schemes and numerous "prolapse" pitfalls have gradually fallen by the wayside as clinicians return to the view that the FMV is the central issue. In other words, does this individual or patient have a FMV? If so, then attention is directed to the state of FMV function, dysfunction, or complications.

Advanced perspectives of mitral valve function, which in earlier times were the purview of the morphologists, pathologists, angiographers, and surgeons dealing with the beating heart, have become basic clinical currency with the use of increasingly sophisticated imaging techniques. This renewal of coherence among clinical presentation, cardiac auscultation, FMV imaging characteristics, surgical morphology, and the natural course of the disorder contribute to greater diagnostic and nosologic precision. The FMV/MVP/MVR triad is seen in the light clinicians have traditionally used to approach and define the pathogenesis and diagnosis of the bicuspid aortic valve, mitral or aortic stenosis, aortic or tricuspid regurgitation.

Clinical investigators, morphologists, pathologists, surgeons, and imagers from around the world have defined and redefined the many facets of mitral valve structure, function, and dysfunction during the past 50 years. Upon reflection of these many advances, we reached the following conclusions that form the bases for the content of this book.

1. The FMV complex is the central issue in this category of mitral valve disorders, and it is dysfunction of the FMV that results in a broad spectrum of pathophysiological and clinical phenomena.
2. MVP associated with the FMV results from the systolic movement of portions or segments of the FMV complex into the left atrium.
3. Coaptation abnormalities or prolapse of the FMV result in unique forms of mitral valvular dysfunction and MVR.
4. These interrelated phenomena—prolapse of the FMV and MVR, associated with FMV morphology and function—constitute the FMV/MVP/MVR triad.
5. Clinical phenomena and imaging characteristics inherent in the FMV/FVP/MVR triad will be best understood when reconciled with the gross morphological, histopathological, and molecular characteristics of the FMV complex.
6. When the FMV is recognized as the basic point of reference, diagnostic and nosologic characterizations are simplified.
7. Recognition of the FMV as the hallmark of cardiac involvement in heritable cardiovascular disorders, or heritable disorders of con-

nective tissue with or without involvement of the aorta and aortic valve, involve molecular, biochemical, and genetic mechanisms.

8. Each of the consequences of FMV dysfunction—MVP, MVR, and FMV surface phenomena—are dynamic entities and contribute to the symptoms and clinical course in this patient population.

9. Although MVP may occur in the absence of a FMV in individuals with small volume, hyperdynamic, or hypercontractile left ventricles, we do not consider this phenomenon as part of the FMV/FVP/MVR triad.

10. The natural history of the FMV/FVP/MVR triad is long, and understanding the life history requires long-term follow-up with serial evaluations, i.e., both the patient and the physician must live for a long time.

11. Identification of those individuals with FMV/MVP whose symptoms are related to, or associated with, autonomic nervous system dysfunction, i.e., the *mitral valve prolapse syndrome*, is important, since this distinction has diagnostic and therapeutic implications.

Our colleagues who contributed to the present volume are responsible for many of the tenets of contemporary thought about mitral valve function and mitral valve disorders, and are widely recognized for their contributions to the FMV/FVP/MVR triad.

We are privileged to have the benefit of their wisdom.

Charles F. Wooley, MD,
Harisios Boudoulas, MD, PhD

Contents

Part I

The Floppy Mitral Valve:
The Morphologists

Introduction

The Floppy Mitral Valve:
The Morphologists

Charles F. Wooley, MD,
Harisios Boudoulas, MD, PhD

Descriptions of the valves of the heart date to antiquity. However, it remained for Leonardo da Vinci to incorporate the concepts of flow and to introduce intracardiac imaging into his anatomic sketches of the heart. The result was the application of physical laws to human anatomy.

Between 1485 and 1515, da Vinci's anatomic drawings of the heart, based primarily on careful dissections of ox hearts, presented views of the left ventricle, mitral valve, aortic valve, and aorta with three-dimensional and cross-sectional accuracy. Keele tells us how Leonardo analyzed the heart's operation in light of his earlier experiments on the mechanics of movement, projecting his views of the operating power of a machine into these anatomic images.[1] Lessons learned about the flow of water while building canals were incorporated into the analysis of blood flow through the cardiac chambers and valves.

The beginnings of cardiac imaging may be found in da Vinci's instructions for making a glass model to insert into the heart to observe the movements of water, and thus the blood, as the water passes through the aorta.

The papillary muscles, mitral valve chordae, and the mitral valve are detailed in Leonardo's drawings. The mitral chordae, arising from the papillary muscles, illustrate his thesis that the mitral valve cusps are formed by the fanning out of the thick chordae tendineae into the thin, flattened leaflets of the mitral valve. When closed, the mitral valve leaflets form the vault above, i.e., a domelike or archlike structure.

From: Boudoulas H, Wooley CF. *Mitral Valve: Floppy Mitral Valve, Mitral Valve Prolapse, Mitral Valvular Regurgitation.* Second revised edition. ©Futura Publishing Company, Armonk, NY, 2000.

The atrioventricular and arterial orifices of the heart and the mitral, aortic, pulmonary, and tricuspid valve relationships are depicted in diagrams of the ventricles of the heart (Fig. 1). Elsewhere, there are enlarged views of the H-shaped impressions on the upper surface of the mitral valve, i.e., the mitral commissures, as seen from the atrial perspective, and a sketch of the vaulted shape of the closed mitral cusps when viewed from the side.

There has been a wonderful renaissance of interest in mitral valve morphology during the cardiac surgery and cardiac imaging era.[2] Cardiovascular anatomic and morphologic studies from a number of centers have been important contributions to this morphologic renaissance. Many of these original sources are cited in the following chapter, *Anatomy of the Mitral Valve* by Annalisa Angelini and Gaetano Thiene from The Universita di Padova, Italy, working with Robert H. Anderson and Siew Ho at the National Heart and Lung Institute in London, UK.

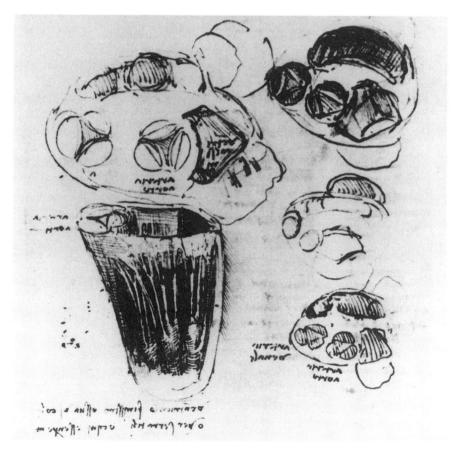

Figure 1. Used with permission of The Royal Library, Windsor Castle, London, UK.

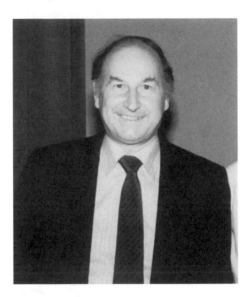

Figure 2. Dr. Robert Anderson.

The anatomic lineage at Padua dates to Andreas Vesalius (1514–1564), pre-eminent anatomist, creator of modern anatomy, and author of *De humani corporis fabrica liibri septem* in 1543. William Harvey of London trained at the Universities of Padua and Cambridge prior to establishing the scientific basis for the circulation with his publication of *Exercitatio anatomica de motu cordis et sanguinis in animalibus* in 1628. Thus, the collaboration of investigators in Padua with colleagues in London has deep historical roots.

In our opinion, Robert Anderson of London (Fig. 2) is the premier cardiac morphologist of our time; his colleagues Siew Ho, in London, and Annalisa Angelini and Gaetano Thiene from Padua, share the same high standards. The following chapter is a timeless achievement incorporating their combined wisdom.

References

1. Keele LD. Leonardo da Vinci The Anatomist. In Leonardo da Vinci Anatomical Drawings from the Royal Library Windsor Castle. New York, The Metropolitan Museum of Art, 1983, pp 10–14.
2. Wooley CF, Baker PB, Kolibash AJ, Kilman JW, Sparks EA, Boudoulas H. The floppy, myxomatous mitral valve, mitral valve prolapse, and mitral regurgitation. Progr Cardiovasc Dis 33:397–433, 1991.

1

Anatomy of the Mitral Valve

Annalisa Angelini, MD,
Siew Yen Ho, PhD,
Gaetano Thiene, MD,
Robert H. Anderson, MD

Introduction

If the mechanisms and malformations underscoring prolapse of the leaflets of the mitral valve are to be fully understood, it is axiomatic that it is first essential to have complete and secure information concerning the normal structural arrangement. Surprisingly, there is still no consensus on the number and extent of leaflets within the valve, let alone on how best to name them.[1–3] Andreas Vesalius, the preeminent anatomist who performed some of his most important works in one of our universities, is credited with having first described as mitral the valve guarding the inlet to the morphologically left ventricle. Even this precedent did not meet with universal approbation, with the eminent 19th century Viennese anatomist, Joseph Hyrtl, commenting that the adjective mitral came to the valve as the devil entering the baptismal font.[4] Be that as it may, the alternative adjective of "bicuspid" is perhaps even more questionable, since the valve in question does seem to have more resemblance to the episcopal mitre than to the surface of a bicuspid tooth, the elevations of the purported cusps being far from evident in the setting of the valve. It is against this far from settled background that we will, in this

From: Boudoulas H, Wooley CF. *Mitral Valve: Floppy Mitral Valve, Mitral Valve Prolapse, Mitral Valvular Regurgitation.* Second revised edition. ©Futura Publishing Company, Armonk, NY, 2000.

introductory chapter, give an account of our understanding of the structure of the normal valve, including the sectional anatomy as it might present to the echocardiographers.

Normal Anatomy of the Mitral Valve

The normal mitral valve is a complex anatomic structure (Fig. 1) comprising four basic components, namely the annulus, the leaflets, the tendinous chords, and the papillary muscles. Proper action of the complex depends on normal function and integration of each of the components.[5] The left atrial musculature inserting into the leaflets and the left ventricular myocardium supporting the papillary muscles are also of major significance for normal function.[6] Knowledge of the relationship of the valvar components relative to the other cardiac structures is also important in attempting to unify the terminology used by various authors and in understanding the anatomy in relation to its function as well as to its pathology.

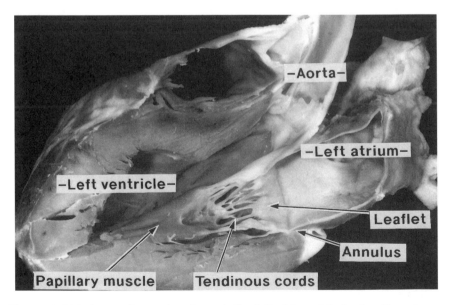

Figure 1. This long axis section through the left atrioventricular junction shows how the mitral valve is made up of an annulus, leaflets, tendinous chords, and papillary muscles.

The valvar complex is attached proximally at the left atrioventricular junction and, distally, through the papillary muscles, to the myocardial wall of the left ventricle. It bears a vital relationship to the aortic valve. This was highlighted by McAlpine,[7] who described the aorto-mitral unit. We use this relationship of the leaflets of the mitral and aortic valves, along with the relationship to the left ventricular myocardium, as the most appropriate means of naming the leaflets. The more traditional terms, such as "anterior" (or "septal") and "posterior," are less than perfect. This is because, first, the mitral valvar orifice is obliquely sited when the heart occupies its normal position within the body (Fig. 2). Second, unlike the tricuspid valve, the leaflets of the mitral valve have no chordal attachments to the ventricular septum. Indeed, an important feature of the normal morphology is the deep invagination of the left ventricular outflow tract which separates the orifice of the mitral valve from the ventricular septum (Fig. 2). It can be noted, however, that one leaflet of the valve is always in fibrous continuity with the leaflets of the aortic valve, this fibrous continuity forming one boundary of the left ventricular out-

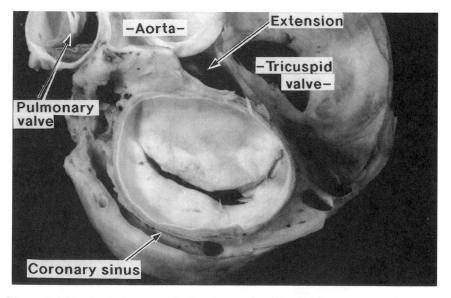

Figure 2. This dissection reveals the short axis of the heart so as to retain as far as possible the position within the body. It shows the oblique relations between the two valvar leaflets, the concave nature of the zone of apposition between them, and the deep extension beneath the aortic valve that separates the mitral valve from the septum (see also Fig. 3). The leaflets of this valve are diseased.

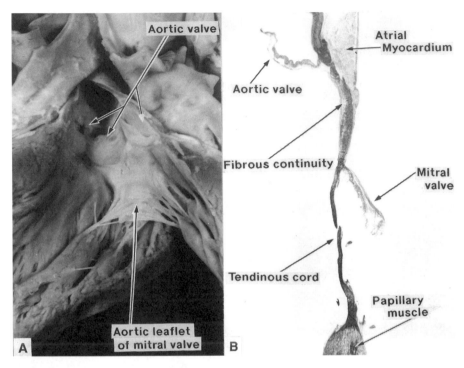

Figure 3. In this view (A), the left ventricular outflow tract is opened and photographed from the front. It is seen that one of the leaflets of the mitral valve is in extensive fibrous continuity with the leaflets of the aortic valve. We call this the *aortic* leaflet of the mitral valve. B shows a histologic section across this area, disclosing the fibrous nature of the zone of valvar continuity.

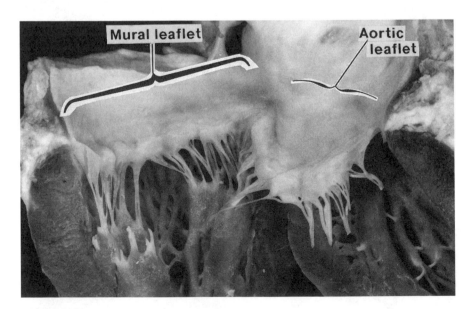

flow tract (Fig. 3). The other leaflet arises from the parietal component of the left atrioventricular junction (Fig. 4). This arrangement permits us simply and accurately to describe the leaflets as being *aortic* and *mural*, respectively. This concept of mural and aortic leaflets, which itself has a longstanding pedigree,[8] has recently been endorsed by Frater, who emphasized the functional significance of such a distinction. It is only the aortic leaflet that contracts and relaxes, while the leaflet attached to the parietal junction has the necessity of being divided so that the components can move apart from one another[10] yet fit snugly when closed.[3] The leaflets, when closed, form the floor of the left atrium. Their line of closure is markedly concave (Fig. 5). Perfect closure of the valve is ensured by the control exerted on the leaflets by the tendinous chords and

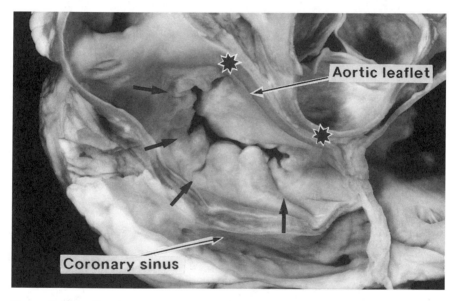

Figure 5. This dissection, photographed with the coronary sinus more horizontal than is the case in life, shows the concave zone of apposition between the aortic and mural leaflets of the mitral valve. Note the multiple slits in the mural leaflet (arrows) and the anterolateral and posteromedial locations of the ends of the zone of apposition (asterisks).

Figure 4. The left atrioventricular junction has been opened across the posteromedial end of the zone of apposition between the mitral valvar leaflets and the junction spread open. It can be seen that one leaflet of the valve has an exclusive origin from the parietal junction. We call this the *mural* leaflet. Note the markedly dissimilar dimensions of this leaflet compared to the aortic leaflet of the valve (see Fig. 3).

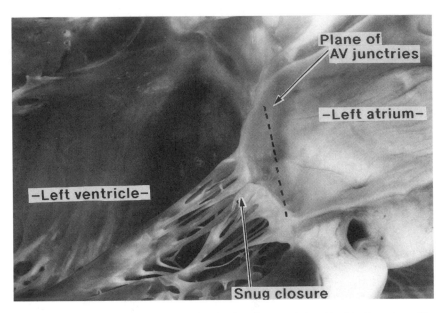

Figure 6. In this specimen, the mitral valve has been retained in its closed position by perfusion fixation. Note that the leaflets fit snugly together and that their line of closure is beneath the plane of the atrioventricular junction (dotted line).

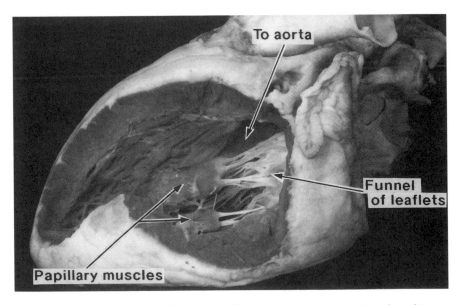

Figure 7. This mitral valve, with open leaflets, has been dissected to show its position within the left ventricle. Note that the papillary muscles are adjacent, and the overall funnel-shaped appearance of the valve.

the papillary muscles. In the normal arrangement, these sealed leaflets do not move above the plane of the atrioventricular junction (Fig. 6), a crucial point when considering the prolapsing valve. When examined intact in open position (Fig. 7), the valve has a cone-shaped appearance, with the funnel formed by the leaflets producing free continuity between the left atrium and ventricle, none of its components obstructing the orifice.

When viewed from the atrial aspect (Fig. 8), a distinct ring is seen marking the distal extent of the atrial myocardium. The relationship of this

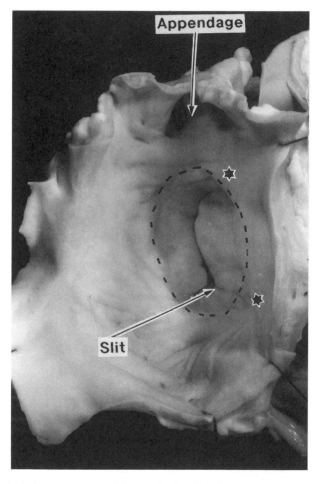

Figure 8. In this heart, prepared by perfusion fixation, the left atrium is opened widely to reveal the atrial aspect of the closed leaflets. Note the ring marking the distal extent of atrial myocardium (dotted line), and the extensively concave zone of apposition between the leaflets (the commissures are marked by asterisks).

muscular extension into the leaflets not only varies from case to case but also within the same case. The relationship is relatively constant in the area of aortic-mitral fibrous continuity. Here, the atrial myocardium overlaps the fibrous curtain seen from the ventricular aspect so that when seen from the atrial side, the level of attachment of the aortic valve is hidden behind an atrial fold. The hinge of the aortic leaflet of the valve is at the level of distal insertion of the atrial myocardium (Fig. 9). There is much more variability around the mural leaflet. The "typical" appearance is for the leaflet to hinge on the annulus (see below) with the atrial myocardium inserting at the level of the hinge. Alternatively, the myocardium can stop short of the hinge or can extend into the leaflet, both leaflet and my-

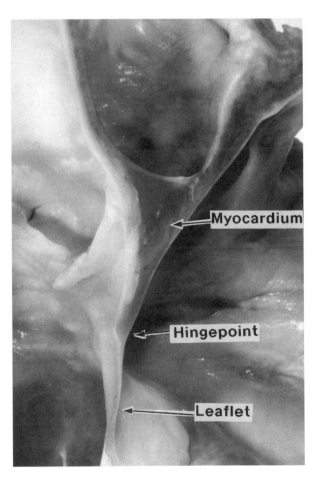

Figure 9. This closeup of a cross-section across the zone of continuity between the aortic and mitral valve leaflets shows the insertion of left atrial myocardium, which forms the hingepoint of the aortic leaflets of the mitral valve (arrows).

ocardium hinging on the fibrous annulus. The significance of these anatomic variations to valvar function is unclear. It has been suggested that the insertion of the atrial myocardium around the parietal junction can function to reduce the orificial diameter. Indeed, some have implicated such an atriogenic mechanism as part of valvar closure.[10,11] It is also suggested that enlargement of the left atrium can invoke mitral regurgitation through tension exerted by the myocardium on the mural leaflet.[12] These proposals remain as yet unproven.

The Annulus

When we use the term "annulus," we refer to the fibrous support of the leaflets of the valve. In other words, we describe part of the cardiac skeleton. Gross and Kugel, in 1931, gave an accurate description of this skeletal component of the mitral valve.[13] They distinguished, however, the concept of the *fibrous annulus* from that of the *mitral ring,* the latter representing the distal extent of the atrial myocardium (see Fig. 8). The annulus, when defined in this way, is composed of the dense connective tissue that continues into the leaflets to form their fibrous layer (the valvar "fibrosa"). Not all have followed the precedent of Gross and Kugel.[13] Subsequent authors, including ourselves, have neglected to differentiate "annulus" from "ring" but rather have used them synonymously.[6,14–18] On reflection, it seems more accurate to return to the concept of Gross and Kugel[13] (see below). With that said, the concept of a fibrous annulus must not be extended to always presume the presence of a continuous collagenous structure. Thus, McAlpine,[7] using the term "aorto-ventricular membrane," emphasized how the continuous fibrous tissue between the leaflets of the aortic and mitral valves was curtain-like rather than annular, a point endorsed from the surgical viewpoint by Loop.[19] An examination of histological sections confirms the validity of this observation. McAlpine[7] was also correct when indicating that the term "annulus" was inappropriately applied to the arterial valves, since the leaflets of these structures have semilunar rather then ring-like attachments. If we accept that the annular support of the mitral valve may in places have a curtain-like aspect, we still find the term "annulus" to be of descriptive value in this setting.

Our own studies of the annular support of the mitral leaflets have shown marked variation, not only from heart to heart but within the same heart. Thick and well-organized fibrous structures are always present at the site of the fibrous trigones. These structures, left and right, are located at the extremities of the region of fibrous continuity between the mitral and aortic valves (Fig. 3). The fibrous continuity itself is an extensive fibrous sheet joining the valvar attachments, these attachments being at markedly different levels. No dense fibrous aggregation resembling an "annulus" is seen at the hinge of the aortic leaflet, this being marked, as discussed, by the extent of atrial myocardium (Fig. 9). Prongs of fibrous tissue do extend laterally from each of the fibrous trigones and run posteriorly to embrace part of the orifice. As pointed out by Zimmerman,[20] these prongs do not always extend as solid structures throughout the circumference of the valve. It is in the extent and morphology of these prongs (the coronary files) that there is the most variation in structure from heart to heart.

The arrangement of a complete cord-like ring of connective tissue, encircling the atrioventricular junction and, on the one hand, supporting the valvar leaflets while, on the other hand, separating contiguous segments of atrial and ventricular myocardium, is very much the exception rather than the rule. Such appearances were found at limited points around the junction of all the hearts we studied (Figs. 10, 11). In most cases, however, the fibrous tissue of the annulus forms a thin curtain in many segments of

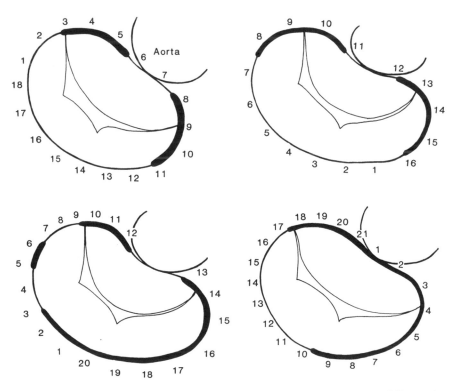

Figure 10. This diagram, shown in cross-section, illustrates the variability to be found in formation of the fibrous annulus of the mitral valve, not only from heart to heart but at different points round the junction in the same heart.

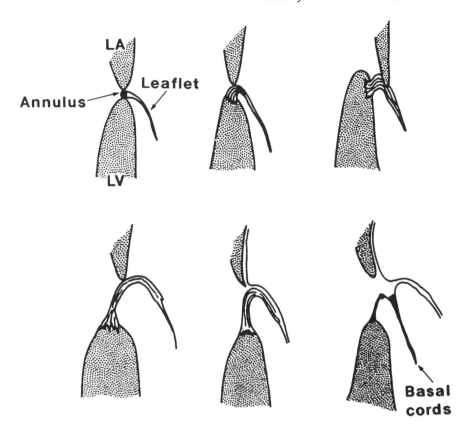

Figure 11. This diagram shows the variability found in four hearts studied by taking sections at each of the points indicated by the numbers. Only in the regions shown by a solid black line was there a true fibrous annulus.

the "ring" between the hinge of the leaflet and the crest of the ventricular myocardium. Only at selected sites is it possible to find the traditionally described relationship with an atrial myocardial wedge and a dome-shaped crest of left ventricular wall separated by a well-formed chord-like fibrous annulus giving origin to the leaflet.

Leaflets

The leaflets of the mitral valve constitute a continuous veil inserted around the entire circumference of the left atrioventricular junction.[21] Conventionally, the veil is considered to be divided into two leaflets. This is in contradistinction to the morphologically tricuspid valve, which is recognized as having three leaflets. Problems do exist, nonetheless, with making clear-cut definitions of the leaflets, since nowhere do the gaps between the components of the continuous veil extend all the way to the fi-brous annulus (Fig. 12). At best, they extend to within 2–3 mm of the an-nulus, but do so at more points around the junction than the traditional commissures. In the past, the ability to define the location of these com-missures depended on the recognition of supposed unique fan-shaped commissural chords atop a prominent papillary muscle.[16] This concept, apart from being less than perfect logically in that one variable morpho-logical feature is defined on the basis of another variable, also suffers from the fact that the supposed commissural fan-shaped chords are not unique. The chords supporting the separations between the divisions of the mural leaflet can be remarkably similar to fan-shaped chords (Fig. 13). In reality, the term "commissure" is used very loosely in the setting of the cardiac valves. When used in its literal sense, a commissure is simply the junction of two structures. If, therefore, a valve has only two leaflets, strictly it has one commissure, which itself has two ends. Conventionally, nonetheless, it is these ends of the solitary line of closure that are termed the commis-sures (Figs. 5, 8). An examination of the normal mitral valve, however, shows that the line of closure of the leaflets is not always a solitary struc-

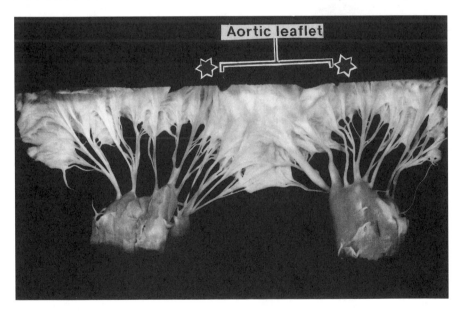

Figure 12. This preparation shows the leaflets of the mitral valve spread and viewed from the outlet (ventricular) aspect. At no point does an indentation extend to the annulus to give a clear indication of the separation of the leaflets. It is diffi-cult, therefore, to give precise definitions of "commissures" and to distinguish them from "clefts" when the valve is viewed in this fashion. The asterisks mark the tips of the traditional commissural chords, showing the dissimilar segments of the circumference guarded by the aortic versus mural leaflets.

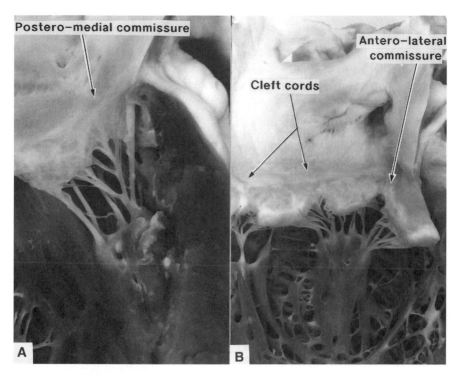

Figure 13. The panels of this illustration show **(A)** the fan-shaped chord support-ing the posteromedial end of the zone of apposition between aortic and mural leaflets, and **(B)** the equally fan-shaped chords supporting the slits in the scallops of a heart with a partially scalloped mural leaflet. It is very difficult to use the struc-ture of these chords to differentiate commissures from clefts, hence our prefer-ence to distinguish the leaflets of the valve in closed rather than open position (see Figs. 5, 8).

ture (Fig. 5). The problem is magnified when we examine a series of valves, since there is marked individual variability. It seems to us that it is best to describe this variation in terms of one major zone of apposition be-tween two primary leaflets, located in aortic and mural position, with slits formed along the mural leaflet to permit its appropriate closure. This is the morphological approach to the mitral valve also advocated by Victor and Nayak,[3] who liken the slits in the mural leaflet to the pleats of a skirt. If the line of union between the leaflets is described simply as the zone of appo-sition, it is then possible to follow the well-established convention used by both pathologists and surgeons and describe the junctions of the leaflets at their mural attachments as the commissures. These structures are found in posteromedial and anterolateral positions. As already discussed, this means that the solitary major zone of apposition between the leaflets is obliquely situated relative to the planes of the body (Figs. 1, 5, 8). In most cases, the mural leaflet is then divided into three scallops, one central and one each laterally and medially.[15,17] In some hearts, nonetheless, there may be more slits producing five or even more scallops. Taken together, the scallops of the mural leaflet make up a long, rectangular structure, whereas the aortic leaflet has the shape of an inferiorly rounded square (Figs. 4, 12). The leaflets occupy more or less the same area, but the aortic leaflet is hinged from only one-third of the overall valvar circumference.

Three zones can be defined along the mural leaflet: the rough zone, the clear zone, and the basal zone, respectively. They are delineated by the insertion of the tendinous chords. The rough zone is between the line of closure of the leaflet and its free margin. It receives the insertion of the tendinous chords on its ventricular surface. This zone represents the area of apposition of the leaflets and is marked on its atrial surface by nodular thickenings (Fig. 14). The rough zone is broadest at the lower portion of each scallop and narrower toward the slits. The clear zone does not receive any chords. It is placed between the rough and the basal zone, the latter being defined at the proximal end of the leaflets by the insertion of basal chords (Fig. 15). The bare central zone in the mural leaflets varies in width from 0.5 to 1.0 cm.[10,22] The aortic leaflet, continuous on its outflow aspect with the noncoronary and left coronary leaflets of the aortic valve, forms

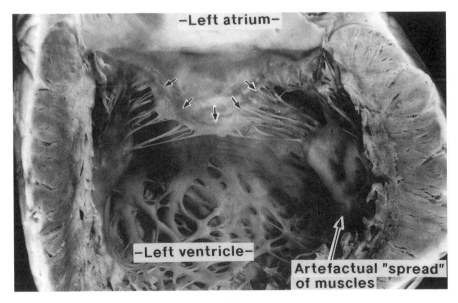

Figure 14. This valve, opened through the middle of the mural leaflet, shows the nodular thickenings (arrowed) that mark the line of closure of mural and aortic leaflets. Note that in this preparation, a false impression is given of the relationship of the papillary muscles (see Fig. 7 for correct position).

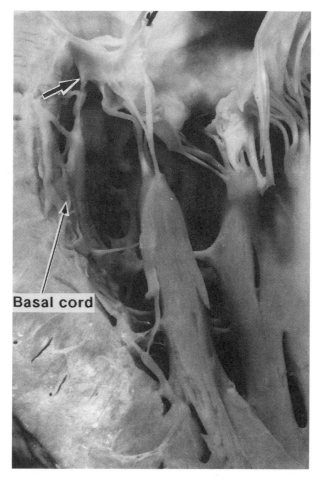

Basal cord

Figure 15. This section across the parietal atrioventricular junction shows the insertion of a basal chord into the mural leaflet (arrowed) marking the boundary between the rough and basal zones.

a boundary of the outflow tract (Fig. 3). As with the mural leaflet, it possesses rough and clear zones, but it does not have a basal zone. The clear zone is devoid of chordal insertions but may show prolongations of chordal fibers passing from their insertions in the rough zone toward the base of the leaflet.

Histologically, the leaflets have a central collagenous structure usually termed the *fibrosa*. This core is composed of fibers running parallel to the surface of the leaflet and extending down into the tendinous chords. It forms an unbroken continuation with their body and it is generally free of elastic fibrils. There is a variable amount of loose connective tissue, the spongy layer or *spongiosa*, on the atrial aspect of the fibrous core. This spongy layer is the main component of the free edge and contains sparse collagen fibrils, abundant proteoglycans, elastic fibers, and connective tissue cells.[23] The leaflets are covered for about two-thirds of their length on both surfaces by a thin, fibroelastic layer. This represents the extensions of the atrial and ventricular subendocardial layers. The atrial layer, conventionally named the *atrialis*, is usually richer in elastin. Cardiac muscle and blood vessels often extend into its proximal third. The muscle can become so prominent as to form a well-defined band and may then constitute one-fifth of the entire thickness of the leaflet.[13]

The ventricular fibroelastic layer, named the *ventricularis*, is best developed in the aortic leaflet. It shows a much denser aggregation of elastic bundles than does the atrial layer. Endothelium covers both the fibroelastic layers. The nodular thickenings at the area of apposition of the leaflets are composed of fibroelastic plaques that are independent of the fibrous layer. Marked aging changes can be seen in the leaflets. The atrial and ventricular layers both become thicker and richer in elastic and collagenous bundles with increasing age, while the spongy layer increases in thickness, probably because of destruction of part of the fibrous layer.[24,25]

The Tendinous Chords

The tendinous chords, together with the papillary muscles, constitute the tension apparatus of the valve. The chords originate from the apical portions of the papillary muscles (Figs. 12, 14), or else come directly from the posterior ventricular wall (Fig. 15). They insert either into the free edge of the leaflets or onto their ventricular surface (Fig. 12). Many attempts have been made to classify these chords. The first categorization was given by Tandler,[25] and was based on the site of insertion to the leaflets. Three different orders were recognized. The first-order chords inserted into the free edge. Second-order chords were those inserting beyond the free margin on the ventricular surface, while the third-order chords were those attached to the basal portion of the leaflet. Subsequent authors stressed the anatomy of individual chords, such as the commissural[15] and strut chords.[14] Roberts and Perloff[27] emphasized the pattern of arborization of the chords as they progressed from papillary muscle to the leaflet, while Lam and colleagues[2] classified on the basis of morphological differences, sites of insertion, and potential functional significance.

The Toronto group[2,16] emphasized the distinction between commissural chords and leaflet chords. *Commissural chords* are said to be fan-shaped structures that support each end of the primary zone of apposition between the leaflets. These chords are purported to ensure the folding and unfolding of the leaflet tissue during the cardiac cycle. They arise as a single stem from the tip of the corresponding papillary muscle and branch in a fan-like arrangement, inserting into the free margins of the adjacent leaflets (Fig. 13a). The chords of the leaflets are themselves divided into three distinct types. The first type is the *rough zone chords,* which insert into the corresponding rough zones (Fig. 12). Each of these chords usually arborizes into three branches before reaching the leaflets. One of these branches inserts to the free edge of the leaflets and the other two insert on the ventricular surface of the rough zone, reinforcing the area of apposition. If the branching pattern is deficient, this is often remedied by overlapping of contiguous chords. The *strut chords* are prominent rough zone chords, which support the aortic leaflets (Fig. 12). The second type is the *basal* chords (Fig. 15). These take origin directly from the posterior ventricular wall and insert at the base of the leaflet. The third type, distinguished by the Toronto group, is the *cleft chords.* These are remarkably similar, however, to commissural cords in having a fan-like appearance (Fig. 13b). Indeed, when seen in isolation it can be impossible to distinguish commissural and cleft chords. The latter support the contiguous free margins and the rough zone areas between the scallops (however many are present) of the mural leaflet.

The study by Becker and de Wit[28] is important in understanding the normal arrangement of chordal support. They showed a marked "spectrum of normality," with uniform support of the leaflets by the chords in normal hearts being the exception rather than the rule. The noted variation in patterns of branching usually has no deleterious effect on support because of the overlapping of neighboring chords. At times, nonetheless, minor variations in chordal architecture leave part of the leaflets less well supported than others. These arrangements favor the "hooding" deformity of the leaflets. Becker and de Wit[28] suggested that these findings may be of considerable significance in the context of prolapse of the mitral valve, introducing as they do the concept of an individual anatomical variation that could underscore functional disorder.

When studied histologically, the tendinous chords have a fibrous layer composed of collagen fibrils oriented longitudinally. This layer is surrounded by an outer layer made up of elastic fibers and proteoglycans.[29]

Papillary Muscles and Left Ventricle

The papillary muscles of the mitral valve are relatively constant in position. Although often shown as spread apart when the heart is opened by the pathologist (Fig. 14), the muscles are adjacent when dissected "in situ" (Fig. 7). As with the tendinous chords, they show marked variation in their precise architecture.[7,28,30] They are located beneath the commissures, hence occupying anterolateral and posteromedial positions. They take origin from the lower third of the left ventricular free wall and can have common or separated bases. They emerge into the left ventricular cavity and divide into a variable number of heads, each head acting as an anchor for the tendinous chords (Fig. 12). Each muscle gives attachment to chords that insert into both the aortic and the mural leaflets (Fig. 12).

The anterolateral muscle is generally the more uniform. A single head is present in 70% of cases, usually with a groove directed toward the corresponding commissure.[31] It tends to project more into the ventricular cavity than does the posteromedial muscle. The anterolateral muscle is supplied by a central artery derived either from the circumflex or the anterior descending branches of the left coronary artery. The posteromedial muscle is generally smaller than the anterolateral one and, in more than 60% of cases, consists of two or three smaller pillars.[31] It usually has several connections to the left ventricular wall in addition to the base of its major trunk. It is supplied by a branch from the right coronary artery.[32] The function of the muscles is to ensure that the tendinous chords are always under the appropriate tension.[9,22] The papillary muscles thus act as "shock absorbers" during the cardiac cycle.[33] The functional unit of the papillary muscles also includes a portion of adjacent left ventricular wall that operates as an anchoring force for the tendinous chords (Fig. 1). The geometry of the left ventricle influences markedly the position of the papillary muscles and, therefore, its directional axis.[34] It is the exertion of a vertical force by the ventricular myocardium and papillary muscles that ensures the proper apposition of the leaflets and prevents their eversion.[35]

Echocardiographic Anatomy of Mitral Valve Complex

The morphological details we have discussed above are very much the trees within the forest. It is important that the clinician recognize the overall arrangement of these various features, this being the picture revealed by cross-sectional echocardiography.

Sectional Anatomy of Mitral Valve

As anticipated, the valve can be demonstrated in each of the orthogonal planes of the left ventricle. The long-axis plane parallel to the inlet part of the septum (the so-called parasternal long-axis or two-chamber plane) is optimal for showing the mode of closure of the leaflets and their relationship to the plane of the atrioventricular junction (Figs. 1, 6). Distinction of aortic and mural leaflets is readily made in this section, and the degree of hooding, overshoot, or prolapse of each leaflet can easily be measured.

The long-axis plane at right angles to the inlet part of the septum (the so-called four-chamber plane) is not as good for distinguishing the components of the leaflets and their relations to the junction.[36,37] This is because the plane is passing more parallel relative to the different leaflets (Fig. 16). The short-axis planes reveal the arrangement of the papillary muscles and the overlapping relationship of the inlet and outlet components of the left ventricle, and confirm the disposition of the leaflets relative to the atrioventricular junction (Fig. 17). The recent introduction of transesophageal

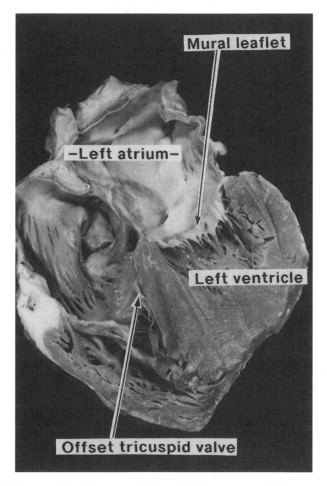

Figure 16. This so-called four-chamber echocardiographic section is more or less parallel to the zone of apposition between the aortic and mural leaflets. While showing well the offsetting of the attachment of the mitral relative to the tricuspid valve, it does not distinguish the structure of the individual leaflets.

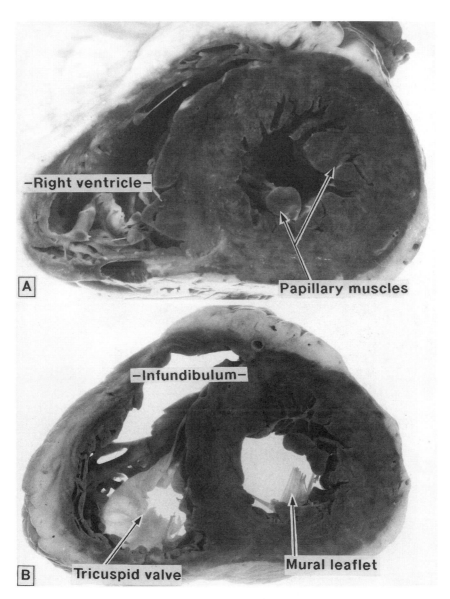

Figure 17. A, B. This series of short-axis sections of the left ventricle, viewed from the feet, show the interrelationships of the leaflets of the mitral valve and the overlapping of the inlet and outlet of the left ventricle. *Continued*

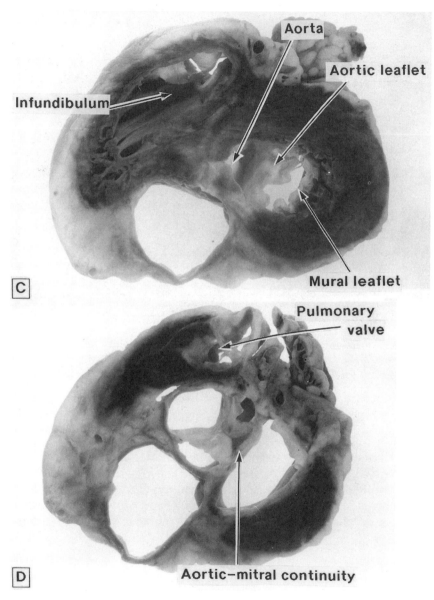

Figure 17. C, D.

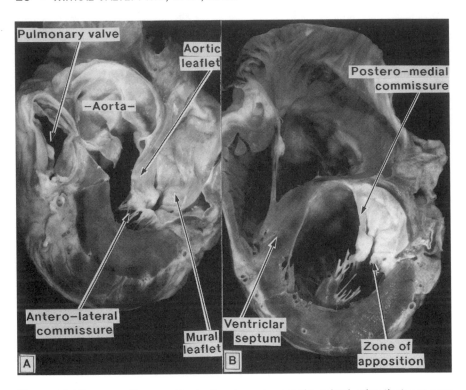

Figure 18. These sections replicate the views across the mitral valve that can now be obtained by transgastric echocardiography. They reveal the patterns of valvar closure at the anterolateral **(A)** and middle **(B)** of the zone of apposition between the aortic and mural leaflets of the valve.

echocardiography offers an important additional diagnostic tool in the noninvasive evaluation of the mitral valve. The long-axis transesophageal and transgastric planes in particular are useful in the evaluation of the entire mitral valvar complex, enabling careful study to be made of the arrangement of the tendinous chords supporting the leaflets at the commissural ends of the primary zone of apposition (Figs. 18, 19).

Conclusions

It seems unlikely that clinicians will change their practice of describing the inlet valve of the morphologically left ventricle as the mitral valve. It seems equally certain that, despite suggestions that the valve may have

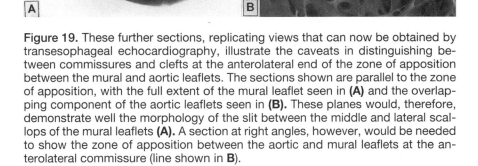

Figure 19. These further sections, replicating views that can now be obtained by transesophageal echocardiography, illustrate the caveats in distinguishing between commissures and clefts at the anterolateral end of the zone of apposition between the mural and aortic leaflets. The sections shown are parallel to the zone of apposition, with the full extent of the mural leaflet seen in **(A)** and the overlapping component of the aortic leaflets seen in **(B)**. These planes would, therefore, demonstrate well the morphology of the slit between the middle and lateral scallops of the mural leaflets **(A)**. A section at right angles, however, would be needed to show the zone of apposition between the aortic and mural leaflets at the anterolateral commissure (line shown in **B**).

four[1] or even five leaflets,[38] most will continue to recognize the two major leaflets separated by the primary zone of apposition between them. It is then advantageous for clinicians wishing to understand the function of the valve to recognize that these primary leaflets occupy aortic and mural locations within the left atrioventricular junction. They are not described to best advantage as being "anterior" and "posterior." It is these aortic and mural leaflets that are the major components of the valve, hinged from the annulus and supported and controlled by the tension apparatus. The aortic leaflet is deep, but guards only one-third of the circumference of the valve. The mural leaflet is much shallower, but guards two-thirds of the orifice. Knowledge of all these aspects, particularly together with the details of chordal support, is crucial for all those who seek to understand the prolapsed valve, as described throughout the remainder of this volume.

References

1. Yacoub M. Anatomy of the mitral valve chordae and cusps. In Kalmanson D (ed): The Mitral Valve. London, Edward Arnold, 1976, pp 15–20.
2. Lam JHC, Ranganathan N, Wigle ED, Silver MD. Morphology of the human mitral valve. I. Chordae tendineae: A new classification. Circulation 41:449–458, 1970.
3. Victor S, Nayak VM. Definitions and functions of commissures, slits and scallops of the mitral valve: Analysis of 100 hearts. Asia Pacific J Thorac Cardiovasc Surg 3:10–16, 1994.
4. Hyrtl J. Onomatologica Anatomica. Wilhelm Braumuller, Vienna, 1880, pp 328–331.
5. Silverman ME, Hurst WJ. The mitral complex. Am Heart J 76:399–418, 1968.
6. Perloff JK, Roberts WC. The mitral apparatus: Functional anatomy of mitral regurgitation. Circulation 46:227–239, 1972.
7. McAlpine WA. Heart and coronary arteries. An anatomical Atlas for Clinical Diagnosis, Radiological Investigation and Surgical Treatment. New York, Springer-Verlag, 1975, pp 39–56.
8. Walmsley T. The heart. In Sharpey Shafer G, Symington J, Byrce TH (eds): Quain's Elements of Anatomy, Volume 4, Part III. London, Longmans, Green & Co., 1929.
9. Frater RWM. The right-sided atrioventricular valve (editorial). J Heart Valve Dis 3:25–26, 1994.
10. Frater RWM, Ellis FH. The anatomy of the canine mitral valve: With notes on function and comparison with other mammalian mitral valves. J Surg Res 1:171–178, 1961.
11. Tsakiris AG. The physiology of the mitral valve. In Kalmanson D (ed): The Mitral Valve: A Pluridisciplinary Approach. Acton, Mass, Publishing Sciences Group, 1976. pp 21–26.
12. Levy MJ, Edwards JE. Anatomy of mitral insufficiency. Progr Cardiovasc Dis 5:119–144, 1962.
13. Gross L, Kugel MA: Topographic anatomy and histology of the valves in the human heart. J Pathol 7:445–473, 1931.
14. Brock RC. The surgical and pathological anatomy of the normal mitral valve. Br Heart J 14:489–513, 1952.
15. Rusted IE, Schiefley CH, Edwards JE: Studies of the mitral valve. I. Anatomic features of the normal mitral valve and associated structures. Circulation 6:825–831, 1952.
16. Ranganathan N, Lam JHC, Wigle ED, Silver MD. Morphology of the human mitral valve. II. The valve leaflets. Circulation 41:459–467, 1970.
17. Davies MJ. Pathology of Cardiac Valves. London, Butterworths, 1980.
18. Becker AE, Anderson RH. Cardiac Pathology: An Integrated Text and Colour Atlas. London, Gower Medical Publishing, 1983.
19. Loop FD: Technique for repair and replacement of the mitral valve. Surg Clin N Am 55:1193–1204, 1975.

20. Zimmerman J. The functional and surgical anatomy of the heart. Ann Royal Coll Surg Eng 39:348–366, 1966.
21. Chiechi MA, Lees WM, Thompson R. Functional anatomy of the normal mitral valve. J Thorac Surg 32:378–393, 1956.
22. Frater RWM. Mitral valve anatomy and prosthetic valve design. Proc Staff Meet Mayo Clin 36:582–592, 1961.
23. Ferrans VJ, Thiedemann K-U. Ultrastructure of the normal heart. In Silver MD (ed): Cardiovascular Pathology, vol 1. Edinburgh, Churchill Livingstone, 1983, pp 69–72.
24. Pomerance A. Ballooning deformity (mucoid degeneration) of atrioventricular valves. Br Heart J 31:343–351, 1969.
25. Sahasakul Y, Edwards W, Naessens JM, Tajik A. Age-related changes in aortic and mitral valve thickness: Implications for two-dimensional echocardiography based on an autopsy study of 200 normal human hearts. Am J Cardiol 62:424–430, 1988.
26. Tandler J. Anatomie des Herzens. Handbuch der anatomie des Menschen. Jena, Gustav Fischer, 1913, p 64.
27. Roberts WC, Perloff JK. Mitral valvular disease: A clinicopathologic survey of the conditions causing the mitral valve to function abnormally. Ann Int Med 77:939–975, 1972.
28. Becker AE, de Wit APM. The mitral valve apparatus: A spectrum of normality relevant to mitral valve prolapse. Br Heart J 42:680–689, 1980.
29. Lim KO, Boughner DR. Scanning electron microscopical study of human mitral valve chordae tendineae. Arch Pathol Lab Med 101:236–238, 1977.
30. Roberts WC, Cohen LS. Left ventricular papillary muscles: Description of the normal and a survey of conditions causing them to be abnormal. Circulation 46:138–154, 1972.
31. Rusted IE, Scheifley CH, Edwards JE, Kirklin JW. Guides to the commissures in operations upon the mitral valve. Proc Staff Meet Mayo Clin 26:297–305, 1951.
32. Reiss P, Becker AE. Dominance of the right coronary artery: What does it mean? Anat Clin 2:369–372, 1981.
33. Frater RWM. Functional anatomy of the mitral valve. In Ionescu MI, Cohn LH (eds): Mitral Valve Disease Diagnosis and Treatment. London, Butterworths, 1985, pp 127–138.
34. Burch GE, Giles TD. Angle of traction of the papillary muscles in normal and dilated hearts: A theoretical analysis of its importance in mitral valve dynamics. Am Heart J 84:141–144, 1972.
35. Shelburne JC, Rubenstein D, Gorlin R. A reappraisal of papillary muscle dysfunction: Correlative clinical and angiographic study. Am J Med 46:862–871, 1969.
36. Levine RA, Triulzi MO, Harrigan P, Weyman AE. The relationship of mitral annular shape to the diagnosis of mitral valve prolapse. Circulation 75:756–767, 1987.
37. Levine RA, Handschumacher MD, Sanfilippo AJ, Hagege AA, Harrigan P, et al. Three-dimensional echocardiographic reconstruction of the mitral valve, with implications for the diagnosis of mitral valve prolapse. Circulation 80:589–598, 1989.
38. Kumar N, Kumar M, Duran CMG. A revised terminology for recording surgical findings of the mitral valve. J Heart Valve Dis 4:70–75, 1995.

Part II

Mitral Valve Function:
Physiology

Introduction

Mitral Valve Function:
The Physiologists

Charles F. Wooley, MD,
Harisios Boudoulas, MD, PhD

Carl J. Wiggers, Dean of U.S. Cardiovascular Physiology, entitled his 1958 memoir *Reminiscences and Adventures in Circulation Research*.[1] A chronological repository of the genesis of medical thought about the circulation, the book profiles the research paths that Wiggers, his associates, and trainees explored during a golden period of investigation. Wiggers describes his experiences in terms of five research eras from 1929 to 1952; the research of each era was involved with a specific theme. His associates and trainees provide a roll call of cardiac physiology researchers and teachers who influenced the field for several generations.

Robert C. Little, MD (Fig. 1) was a member of this distinguished band in 1948–1949, and maintained a life-long interest in function of the cardiac atria and mitral[2,3] and tricuspid valve function amidst a wide spectrum of academic interests. Bob served as Chairman of the Physiology Department in the College of Medicine at the Ohio State University from 1964 to 1973 before moving to the Medical College of Georgia. William C. Little, Bob and Claire Little's son (Fig. 2), attended the College of Medicine at The Ohio State University, so that we had the opportunity of knowing Bill at the very beginnings of his career in clinical and investigative academic cardiology. Following graduation in 1975, Bill's career involved cardiology training at the University of Alabama in Birmingham, and faculty experience at the University of Texas at San Antonio, before moving to Wake Forest University School of Medicine where he is Professor of Internal Medicine and Chief of the Cardiology Section.

From: Boudoulas H, Wooley CF. *Mitral Valve: Floppy Mitral Valve, Mitral Valve Prolapse, Mitral Valvular Regurgitation.* Second revised edition. ©Futura Publishing Company, Armonk, NY, 2000.

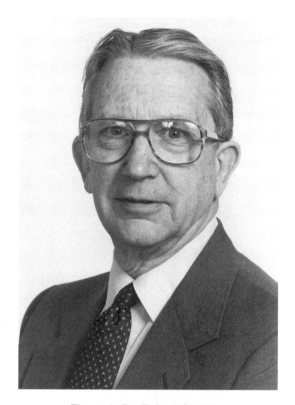

Figure 1. Dr. Robert C. Little.

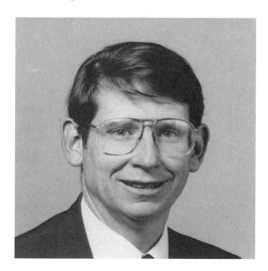

Figure 2. Dr. William C. Little.

The unique father–son collaboration has been expressed before in their physiology text.[4] Chapter 2, *Physiological Basis for Mitral Valve Function*, brings together their combined experience, wisdom, and intellectual approach to fundamental circulatory mechanisms.

The Function of the Normal Human Mitral Valve

As we have seen, mitral valve function has been a topic of great interest in cardiovascular physiology for centuries. Conjecture based on anatomic observations gradually gave way to active experimental investigation using the technology of each era. Experimental invasive methods were used initially for the observation of the beating heart and cardiac dy-

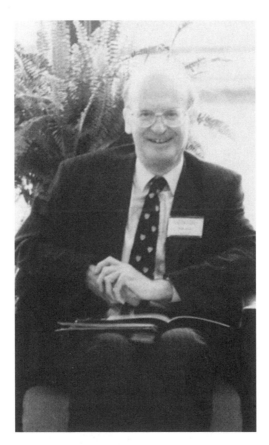

Figure 3. Dr. Derek Gibson.

namics, and later to measure left atrial, left ventricular, and aortic pressure, and to time the events of the cardiac cycle.

The study of the dynamics of individual cardiac valves was more difficult since the interventions had the inherent disadvantages of interfering with or altering the very factors and functions being studied. Certain of these limitations were overcome in the studies of mitral valve function in intact human subjects with cardiac catheterization, angiography, and surgery as each technological development added to the store of information.

However, it was the introduction of an array of noninvasive methods to the study of mitral valve function that provided the opportunity for an investigator well versed in the earlier experimental and clinical methods to develop a multidimensional approach to these dynamic processes in the intact human. Derek Gibson (Fig. 3) provides an unbridled intellectual approach to the study of mitral valve function, combining the wisdom from the past with the technology of the era. Internationally recognized as a scholar and investigator, he represents the best in British cardiac physiology.

References

1. Wiggers CJ. Reminiscences and Adventures in Circulation Research. New York and London, Grune and Stratton, 1958.
2. Little RC. Effects of atrial systole on ventricular pressure and closure of AV valves. Am J Physiol 166:178, 1951.
3. Little RC, Hilton JG, Schaeffer RD. The first heart sound in normal and ectopic ventricular contractions: Mechanism of closure of the AV valves. Circulation 2:48, 1954.
4. Little RC, Little WC. Physiology of the Heart and Circulation (4th edition). Yearbook Publishers, 1989, p 377.

2

Physiological Basis for Mitral Valve Function

Robert C. Little, MD,
William C. Little, MD

Introduction

The presence of cardiac valves has been known since antiquity. The Greek physician Philistion mentioned these structures in a manuscript written in the fourth century B.C.[1,2] A century later Erasistratos, a contemporary of Aristotle, described the atrioventricular (AV) valves with their chordae tendineae and named them the tricuspid on the right and the arterial sigmoid on the left.[1,3] Because of its resemblance to a bishop's miter,[4] the left AV valve was later renamed the mitral valve by the Flemish anatomist Andreas Vesalius (c. 1550).

Galen (c. 180 A.D.), sometimes called the first experimental physiologist, predicted on the basis of anatomical studies that the functioning mitral valve cusps would not close perfectly and thus result in some reflux back into the left atrium.[5] Thus, one may speculate that he was the first to describe mitral valve prolapse. Harvey (1628), in commenting on Galen's work, compared the cardiac valves to the "clacks" (valves) in a piston force pump and described the AV valves as the ventricular "gatekeepers" that prevented regurgitation of blood back into the atrium.[6]

While early observers recognized the one-way action of the cardiac valves, they failed to understand their full role in the pump function of the

From: Boudoulas H, Wooley CF. *Mitral Valve: Floppy Mitral Valve, Mitral Valve Prolapse, Mitral Valvular Regurgitation.* Second revised edition. ©Futura Publishing Company, Armonk, NY, 2000.

heart. Aristotle, for example, considered the heart to act like bellows with diastolic suction as its active phase. While both Galen and Leonardo da Vinci (c. 1500) understood that the left ventricle expelled blood into the aorta, the diastolic view of cardiac mechanics continued until William Harvey's classic description of the circulation in 1628.[6]

Since the time of Harvey, the function of the mitral valve has been the subject of continuous clinical and experimental study and the development of cineangiocardiographic, echocardiographic, and other sophisticated techniques has greatly expanded understanding of its dynamics. However, uncertainty remains regarding many of the details of mitral valve function.[7] It is appropriate to introduce a discussion of mitral valve prolapse with a summary of the physiology of the normal mitral valve and its role in the function of the heart. We will start with a brief discussion of the relationship of the mitral valve complex[8] to overall cardiac dynamics before considering its specific function as a gatekeeper.

The Mitral Complex and Cardiac Function

A plot of left atrial and ventricular pressure during the cardiac cycle is shown in Figure 1. From the time of aortic valve closure until mitral valve opening, the left ventricle is normally a closed chamber with a constant volume. Myocardial relaxation begins in the latter part of systole and causes a steep, exponential fall in intraventricular pressure as elastic elements of the left ventricle that compressed and twisted during ejection are allowed to recoil. Although no filling occurs during isovolumetric relaxation, the processes that determine the rate of decline of the isovolumetric pressure influence ventricular filling following opening of the mitral valve.[9,10] When left ventricular pressure falls below left atrial pressure, the mitral valve opens and left ventricular filling begins. For the first 30 to 40 ms after mitral valve opening, relaxation of left ventricle wall tension is normally rapid enough to cause left ventricular pressure to fall, despite a substantial increase in left ventricle volume.[11] This fall in left ventricular pressure produces a pressure gradient that accelerates blood from the left atrial into the left ventricle, resulting in rapid and full opening of the mitral leaflets and rapid early diastolic filling of the left ventricle. The rate of early left ventricular filling is determined by the mitral valve pressure gradient (left atrial pressure-left ventricular pressure).[9,11,12] Although peak filling occurs after the peak pressure gradient, the two are closely related. Two major factors (myocardial relaxation and left atrial pressure) determine the early diastolic mitral valve pressure gradient and the rate of left ventricular filling. Under normal circumstances more than two thirds of the stroke volume enters the left ventricle during early diastole.

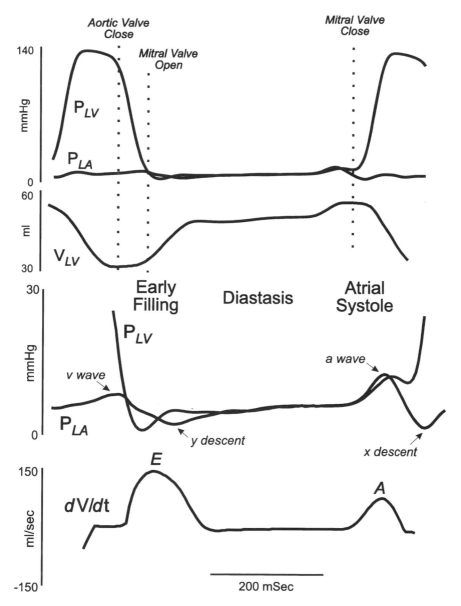

Figure 1. Recording of left ventricular pressure (P_{LV}) left atrial pressure (P_{LA}) left ventricular volume (V_{LV}), and the rate of change of left ventricular volume (dV/dT) which indicates the rate of left ventricular filling during diastolic. See text for discussion. (Used with permission from Cheng CP, et al.[11])

As filling of the left ventricle begins, the pressure gradient across the mitral valve decreases and then transiently reverses. This occurs because left ventricular relaxation is nearing completion and the flow of blood from the left atrium fills the left ventricle, raising the left ventricular pressure while lowering the left atrial pressure. This reversed mitral valve pressure gradient decelerates and then stops the rapid flow of blood into the left ventricle early in diastole.[13] The pressures in the left atrial and left ventricle equilibrate as mitral flow nearly ceases, thus little left ventricular filling occurs during the midportion of diastole. During this period of diastasis, the mitral valve leaflets drift toward the closed position.

Following activation from the sino-atrial node, a peristalsis-like contraction wave sweeps across the atrium. This causes atrial pressure to increase (the A wave) and converts the atrium from a passive conduit for pulmonary venous blood into a force pump that actively empties its contents into the left ventricle. Atrial contraction usually contributes less than 25% of the ventricular end-diastolic volume. The importance of atrial contraction to left ventricular filling is enhanced in patients with conditions that impair early diastole left ventricular filling such as left ventricular hypertrophy, ischemia, and the normal aging process.[14] This late diastolic increase in ventricular volume causes a small increase in ventricular pressure. The onset of this so-called "atrial kick" is slightly delayed from the beginning of atrial systole due to transmission through the mitral orifice. As a result, the atrial A wave has started to decline at the time ventricular pressure reaches its peak. This increase in ventricular volume determines the final end-diastolic ventricular preload (Fig. 1). Prompt closure of the mitral valve, as discussed below, then prevents this presystolic atrial contribution from regurgitating back into the left atrium during the onset of ventricular contraction. As a result, the vigor and timing of atrial contraction can serve as part of a reflex mechanism that regulates left ventricular systolic work on an essentially beat-to-beat basis.[15]

The check valve function of the mitral valve also permits the relatively continuous pulmonary vein inflow into the left atrium to be converted into an intermittent flow into the ventricle, while at the same time maintaining ventricular end-diastolic pressure at a higher level than mean left atrial pressure.[16] In this way, an adequate left ventricular preload is maintained with minimal resistance to blood flow to the left side of the heart.[16,17]

During atrial systole the left atrium maintains its roughly cylindrical shape with the decrease in its internal volume due largely to symmetrical circumferential shortening and displacement of the mitral annulus toward the atrium.[18] Following contraction, atrial pressure begins to fall as the atrial myocardium relaxes and the atrium returns to its resting configuration. This post-contraction drop in atrial pressure is abruptly stopped by closure of the mitral valve. This relationship will be discussed further below. The rapid increase in ventricular pressure due to ventricular contraction then causes the mitral leaflets to bulge into the atrium (Fig. 1). The encroachment on the left atrium may produce a small upstroke, the C wave, in left atrial pressure. Continued contraction of the ventricle and shortening of its myocardial fibers pulls the AV ring and mitral valve toward the cardiac apex. This descent of the cardiac base increases atrial volume and causes an abrupt fall in atrial pressure. The nadir of this pressure drop is the X point on the atrial pressure pulse. During the remainder of ventricular systole, atrial volume symmetrically increases as blood pools behind the closed mitral valve and atrial pressure increases to form the V wave in the pressure pulse (Fig. 1).

Ventricular pressure reaches its peak about two-thirds of the way through systole and then starts to fall as cardiac ejection begins to wane. This drop in ventricular pressure is accelerated after aortic valve closure as tension leaves the ventricular myocardium. The mitral cusps that have been bowed toward the atrium during ventricular systole now reverse direction and begin to move toward the ventricle. At the same time, the AV ring begins to move back toward its rest position. This results in a slight change in atrial volume and a small protodiastolic pressure drop in the atrial pressure pulse at the beginning of the Y descent from the peak of the V wave.[19] With opening of the mitral valve and the onset of the phase of rapid ventricular filling, blood flows into the relaxing ventricle and atrial volume decreases. The rate of this drop in atrial pressure is determined in large part by the compliance of the ventricle, the effective area of the open mitral orifice, and the elastic recoil of the atrial wall. During the remainder of atrial diastole, atrial volume gradually increases as venous inflow fills the AV cavity.

Mitral valve flow velocity patterns determined by Doppler echocardiographic studies confirm that ventricular filling occurs in two phases. The first phase follows opening of the mitral valve during the period of rapid ventricular filling and the second phase occurs during atrial contraction (Fig. 2).[20,21] Echocardiographic recordings, such as those shown for the anterior mitral valve cusp in Figure 3, permit a graphic summary of the valve movements just discussed. During isovolumic ventricular relaxation, the valve leaflets bulge into the left ventricular cavity (D). This is followed by rapid separation of the valve cusps and the beginning of the phase of rapid ventricular filling. The valve rapidly opens to its maximum position (E) and then returns to an intermediate, semiclosed, or closed position (F) during mid-diastole.[22] The valve cusps are again opened by atrial systole (A) and then begin to close as the atrium relaxes. Final closure (C) occurs with the onset of ventricular contraction.

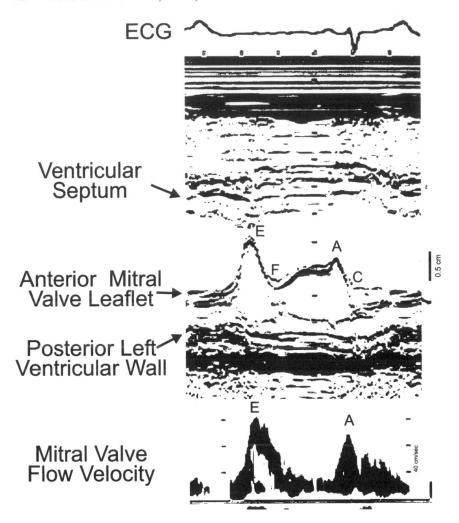

Figure 2. M-mode echocardiogram through the tips of the mitral valve and a simultaneous recording of mitral valve flow velocity obtained by Doppler echocardiography. The electrocardiogram (ECG) is also shown. See text for discussion.

The anterior mitral leaflet moves more rapidly than the smaller posterior leaflet and in its fully closed position it covers a major fraction of the mitral orifice. The slower movement of the posterior leaflet insures that coaptation of the valve cusps occurs simultaneously at or near their free margin and that they maintain a closed position throughout systole.[23,24] If there is redundant tissue or failure of the mitral support apparatus (discussed below), prolapse of part of the mitral leaflets into the left atrium may occur.

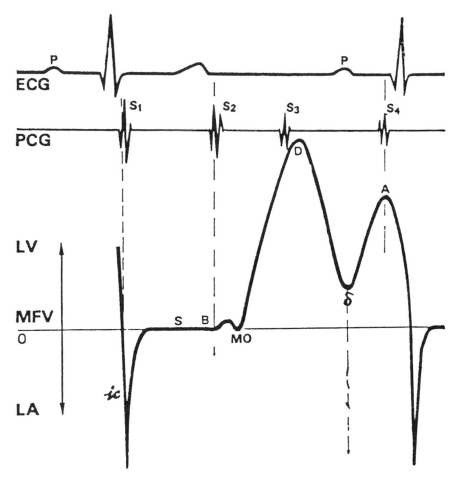

Figure 3. Drawing of mitral valve flow velocity (MFV) and simultaneous electrocardiogram (ECG) (top) and phonocardiogram (PCG) (middle). Direction of flow toward the left ventricle (LV) or the left atrium (LA) is indicated by arrows. The initial negative velocity deflection (ic) results from bulging of valve leaflets into the atrium during isovolumic contraction. The S segment shows absence of flow through closed mitral valve. The segment B-MO delineates isovolumic relaxation. The D deflection shows initial ventricular filling, and A shows the end-diastolic filling due to atrial contraction. (Modified with permission from Kalmanson A, et al.[21])

Papillary Muscle Dynamics and Mitral Valve Function

The left ventricle contains two (or rarely three) bifid papillary muscles that extend from a base in the ventricular wall and into the ventricular cavity. Each muscle connects at its free end with chordae tendineae that, in turn, insert on both mitral cusps. The papillary muscles are the only myocardial fibers that exert a direct pull between their origin and site of attachment.[25] In spite of considerable interest, the role of the papillary muscles in mitral valve function remains speculative.[23,25–46] Recent studies have, however, clarified some of the areas of uncertainty and a coherent mechanism of papillary muscle function is beginning to emerge.[28, 29]

The crossing arrangement of the chordae tendineae has been postulated to facilitate mitral valve closure when tension is applied to them by papillary muscle contraction.[26] This mechanism, however, does not appear to play a significant role in the intact heart. In vivo studies have shown, for example, that while the left papillary muscles and a segment of the ventricular free wall undergo changes in the same direction during contraction, the onset of papillary muscle systole lags behind contraction of the ventricular wall.[27,28,30] Thus, the rapid increase in ventricular pressure and final coaptation of the mitral leaflets occurs well before the development of significant papillary muscle tension.[27,30,31] The tension exerted by the papillary muscle on the mitral cusps during systole prevents prolapse of the leaflets into the left atrium and helps maintain the integrity of the valve seal.[25,26, 31–34] This mechanism is consistent with the observation that the regurgitant flow into the left atrium that accompanies surgical damage to the papillary muscle or muscle dysfunction from other causes results from a failure to maintain systolic valvular continuity and not from difficulties in valve closure.[29,35, 36, 47]

The left anterior and posterior papillary muscles contract nearly simultaneously during ventricular systole.[36] Most investigators have shown that they then elongate slowly during diastole (Fig. 4). The rate of lengthening briefly increases somewhat during atrial systole. The papillary muscles then elongate rapidly and attain their maximal length during the period of ventricular isovolumic contraction.[25,28,30,37–40] Not all studies, however, have agreed with these observations.[26,33,41] The rapid increase in length at the same time the papillary muscle begins its contraction process appears to be anomalous behavior. It may result from an overriding stretch of the papillary muscle due to alteration in ventricular dimensions during the period of isovolumic contraction as the heart changes from an ellipsoid to a more spherical systolic form.[8,37] A definitive explanation for this behavior has not been proposed. Papillary muscle lengthening at this time is apparently necessary to permit proper apposition of the valve cusps.[33,39] In any event, the maximal papillary muscular tension occurs early during ventricular ejection when the papillary muscle is at its maximal length and near the peak of its length-tension curve.[34,38]

The paradoxical shortening and the simultaneous loss of papillary muscle tension begin with closure of the aortic valve.[26,37,40,41] During isovolumic ventricular relaxation the papillary muscle shortens at an almost constant velocity and reaches its minimal length at or just after the open-

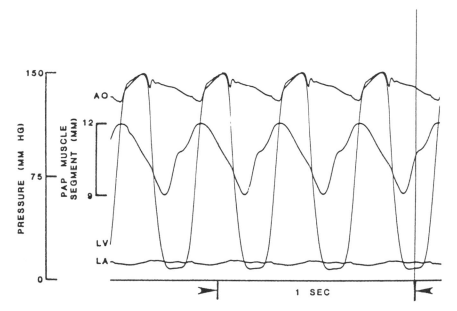

Figure 4. Record of left anterolateral papillary (PAP) muscle segment length and simultaneously recorded aortic (Ao), left ventricular (LV) and left atrial (LA) pressure. (Modified with permission from Marzilli M, et al.[38])

ing of the mitral valve.[38,42] The precise timing of mitral valve opening at the end of isovolumic relaxation is unclear.[23,43] however, recent studies suggest that the mid-portion of the valve leaflet begins to move toward the left ventricle just before the crossover of atrial and ventricular pressure.[38,44,45] This has suggested to some that during isovolumic relaxation, the shortening of the papillary muscle maintains a degree of tension on the chordae tendineae and because of the crossing arrangement of their attachment to the mitral valve leaflets that was described above, this tension leads to separation of the valve leaflets.[29,38] Others have speculated that the release of the systolic papillary muscle tension during isovolumic relaxation and the AV pressure difference are the driving force for mitral opening.[45] A resolution of this question must await further study.

Intravalvular Myocardial Fibers

The mitral valve leaflets contain a number of myocardial fibers in addition to blood vessels, nerves, collagen, elastic fibers, and endothelial cells. The muscle fibers exhibit length-tension and force-velocity characteristics[48] and electrical activity[49] that are similar to ventricular muscle. While the presence of these fibers was first described in 1839, their contractile activity was not investigated for nearly 100 years.[50] Early workers suggested that contraction of these muscle fibers might play a role in closing the mitral valve[50,51]; however, it has been only in the last 20 years that data have been available on this point.[7,52, 53]

The mitral musculature is activated nearly simultaneously with the onset of the QRS complex in the electrocardiogram.[49] Contraction causes the atrial surface of the valve leaflets to become concave in respect to the atrium.[53] This movement has been postulated to assist valve leaflet apposition at the time of ventricular contraction and to oppose bulging of the cusps into the atrium during ventricular systole.[7,54] It has also been suggested that the loss of intravalvular muscle fibers because of mitral valve fibrosis may explain the valvular insufficiency that may accompany that condition.[54]

The intravalvular muscle responds to sympathetic stimulation with an increase in its contraction force. It has been proposed[52] that the greater resistance to the systolic bulging of the mitral valve cusps into the atrium that results from this force may explain the failure of the C wave in the atrial pressure pulse to increase in amplitude during the marked increase in ventricular systolic pressure that follows sympathetic stimulation of the heart.[55]

Dynamics of the Mitral Valve Annulus

The dynamics of the mitral valve annulus and its relationship to the function of the mitral valve have been studied.[56–60] Approximately one-third of the dorsal portion of the fibrous annulus is incomplete, and both atrial and ventricular muscle fibers attach in that area directly to the base of the valve leaflets.[55] As a result, the size and configuration of the annulus can be expected to be influenced by the contraction of each muscle group.[57] Early studies in isolated, perfused hearts suggested that the area of the mitral annulus was reduced during cardiac systole.[58] Radiographic studies in man have confirmed this finding and demonstrated eccentric narrowing of the mitral ring during both atrial and ventricular contraction.[56] The mitral annular cross-sectional area reaches a maximal size in late diastole just before atrial systole (Fig. 5). Presystolic narrowing occurs with atrial contraction. This continues into early to mid-ventricular systole where it reaches its minimal size. Annular area then begins to increase throughout the remainder of the cardiac cycle.[59] The size of the valvular ring and its systolic reduction is dependent on such factors as the duration of the P-R interval and the vigor and duration of atrial and ventricular systole.[54] The normal mitral annular size corrected for body surface area varied during the cardiac cycle from $3.8 + 0.7$ cm^2/m^2 to $2.9 + 11$ cm^2/m^2. Presystolic eccentric narrowing of the mitral ring due to atrial systole acts

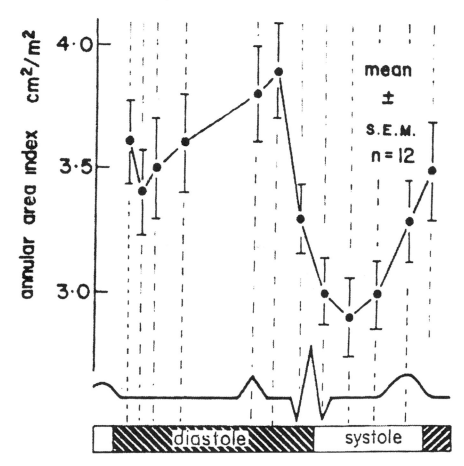

Figure 5. Mitral annular area at selected intervals during the cardiac cycle reconstructed from apical two-dimensional echocardiography in a group of normal subjects. Mitral annular area is normalized for body surface area. (Modified with permission from Shah PM, et al.[24])

to bring the mitral leaflets closer together. This finding has suggested that narrowing the mitral ring and the dynamic effects of atrial systole (see below) act together to make sure the valve is effectively closed at the onset of ventricular contraction.[55]

Closure of the Mitral Valve

The factors that lead to mitral valve closure have been the subject of debate for over a century. While most, if not all, of the forces involved with this process have been identified, a final understanding of the closing mechanism remains elusive. In fact, there may be more than one explanation; the closing mechanism may vary depending on conditions or physiological variables. This continuing controversy has been reviewed elsewhere[7] and only a summary will be presented here.

The gatekeeper function of the mitral valve requires that it be closed during ventricular contraction. Early investigators recognized the similarity between this structure and the input valve in a mechanical force pump and postulated that each was closed by the active increase in pump pressure. This ventriculogenic mechanism in its simplest form suggests that the mitral leaflets would swing closed "like barn doors in a wind storm" at the onset of ventricular contraction and that closure would be accomplished with considerable regurgitation.[61] The existence of backflow with this type of closure has, however, become a contested issue.[62] A number of studies have shown, for example, that ventriculogenic mitral closure in both animals and man is associated with significant regurgitation.[7,63–73] However, just as many careful investigators have reported that the absence of a properly timed atrial contraction results in nonregurgitant ventriculogenic mitral closure.[7,44,73–78]

A different, atriogenic, mechanism for mitral closure has been suggested.[63,64,79] This mechanism utilized the change in mitral valve flow following a normally placed atrial systole to move the valve leaflets to or toward closure before the onset of ventricular contraction. Atriogenic AV valve closure has been extensively documented.[65–67,79–83] In contrast to ventriculogenic closure, the presystolic atriogenic positioning of the AV valves prevents reflux with final closure.[84,85] Not all investigators, however, supported an atriogenic mechanism as being important for mitral closure.[76,77,86] Substantial studies have, in fact, suggested that mitral valve closure results solely from ventricular action.[44,46,58,87,88]

Other investigators have postulated that eddy currents in the area of the mitral leaflets or the formation of a ring vortex in the ventricle during late diastole will act to close the mitral valve.[61,89,90–92] Recent observations have, however, suggested that such hemodynamic factors probably do not play an important role.[93] As discussed earlier, active contraction of the intraleaflet and annular myocardial fibers probably assists in producing closure. The contribution of the papillary muscles and chordae tendineae to normal valve closure, while undoubtedly present, remains unsettled and must await further study.

The mechanism responsible for normal closure of the mitral valve must be considered to be a multifactor process in which a number of forces play a role.[7,85,93,94] It seems inappropriate to consider this process to be solely atriogenic or ventriculogenic.[93] Instead, the following analysis, as a working hypothesis, seems justified by the present state of knowledge. Movement of the mitral valve cusps results from the net effect of the mechanical and fluid forces that impinge on them. Probably the most important for mitral closure are alterations in mitral flow (Fig. 6). During atrial relaxation and before the onset of ventricular contraction, the forward flow of blood through the open mitral valve decelerates, or may even stop, in response to a reduction or even reversal of the normal AV pressure gradient. With a properly timed atrial systole, this results in movement of the valve leaflets to or toward closure. The effect of other forces on mitral valve movement, such as tension on the chordae tendineae or the whirling motion of blood as it enters the ventricle, is still undetermined but probably plays only a minor role. Reduction in the area of the mitral annulus and final apposition of the valve leaflets take place coincident with ventricular contraction and the "ventriculogenic" increase in ventricular pressure. If the interval between atrial systole (As) and ventricular systole (Vs)—the As–Vs interval—is too short, there will be insufficient time for presystolic posting of the open valve leaflets. If the interval is too long, the mitral valve will reopen in response to the reestablishment of normal AV flow. In either event, the valve will then close from its open position by the ventriculogenic action of ventricular contraction. This aspect will be discussed further below.

A. ATRIUM CONTRACTING   **B. ATRIUM RELAXING**

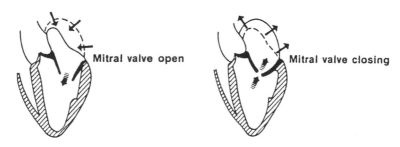

Mitral valve open

Mitral valve closing

C. VENTRICLE STARTING TO CONTRACT

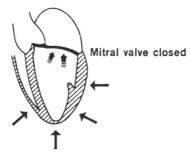

Mitral valve closed

Figure 6. Diagrammatic representation of the effect of atrial contraction (A), atrial relaxation (B), and ventricular contraction (C) on closure of the mitral valve. See text for further discussion. (Used with permission from Little RC, Ohio State Med J 65:483–486, 1969.)

Aberrant motion of the mitral valve has been reported in various disease states. Premature mitral closure may occur during mid- to late diastole in patients with severe aortic or mitral insufficiency.[95] In these individuals, left ventricular mid-diastolic pressure exceeds left atrial pressure and causes premature mitral valve closure because of near-maximal ventricular filling before the end of diastole.[96,97] Prolonged closure or locking of the mitral valve has been reported with long coupling intervals between atrial and ventricular systole.[63,84,98] The greater the ventricular volume, the longer the interval after atrial systole that is required for venous return to reestablish the AV pressure gradient and reopen the valve.[98,99] Others have reported diastolic undulations of the mitral valve apparently related to pulmonary vein flow.[100] In addition, transient mitral closure may occur following the phase of rapid ventricular filling because of an overshoot of the fluid column as it fills the ventricle.[63]

Mitral Valve Sounds

Both opening and closing of the mitral valve are temporally associated with a short series of sound vibrations. The first of these sounds, the "opening snap," is frequently absent in normal individuals or is of such low intensity that it is inaudible at the chest wall. However, in patients with uncalcified mitral stenosis or in normal subjects with markedly increased cardiac output, a characteristic short, high-pitched snapping sound occurs at the time of mitral valve opening. These sound vibrations occur coincident with a transient slowing or momentary cessation in the early opening motion of the mitral valve cusps that is perhaps due to tensing of a chorda tendinea or limitation in leaflet motion because of scar tissue.[43,100,101] The interference with the free motion of the valve cusp and the abrupt deceleration of the movement of blood into the ventricle apparently convert some of the kinetic energy of motion into vibration of the valve structures and the production of the opening snap. It has been suggested that the absence of this sound in patients with mitral stenosis and calcified valve leaflets is due to a reduced rate of valve opening. In that situation, the kinetic energy is then insufficient to produce an audible opening snap.[100]

The closure of the AV valves is associated with production of the first heart sound (S_1). The first and last components of this triad of vibrations are of low intensity and frequently are not audible. The first component probably originates in the ventricular myocardium at the beginning of ventricular contraction, and the final component is associated with opening of the pulmonary and aortic valves. The louder middle part of S_1 is temporally related to closure and tensing of the mitral and tricuspid valves at the beginning of ventricular systole. This valvular component is usually closely split into a mitral part (M_1) and a tricuspid part (T_1).[102,103]

The etiology of the M_1 component of the first sound has been controversial[104]; however, the weight of evidence now suggests that it occurs as a byproduct of mitral closure.[103,104] With a properly timed atrial contraction, presystolic positioning of the mitral valve limits the amount of regurgitation that accompanies final valve closure. However, when coaptation takes place, there is a sudden deceleration of the column of blood that is attempting to flow back into the atrium. This, plus tensing of the closed valve, liberates sufficient force to set the valve structures into vibration and produce M_1.

The intensity of M_1 is related to the position of the mitral valve cusps at the onset of ventricular contraction and the vigor of ventricular systole. A properly timed atrial contraction provides optimum time for presystolic positioning of the mitral leaflets, and they are closed or nearly closed at the onset of ventricular contraction. Under these circumstances, only minimal or no regurgitation will take place and M_1 will be soft.[94] However, if the As–Vs interval is too short, there will be insufficient time for preposition of the valve cusps. If the interval is too long, the valve leaflets will reopen and then be closed from the open position. In both situations, a loud M_1 will result.[63,79,103] This relationship between the duration of the P-R interval in the electrocardiogram and the intensity of S_1 is shown in Figure 7.

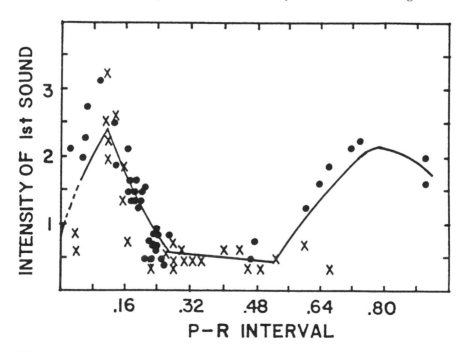

Figure 7. Plot of the relative intensity of the first heart sound taken from phonocardiograms from two patients with varying P-R intervals in the electrocardiogram. See text for further discussion. (Used with permission from Little RC; Ohio State Med J 65:483–486, 1969.)

Summary

While the major gatekeeper function of the normal mitral valve is well understood, many of the details of its dynamics are shrouded in controversy. Recent studies have clarified some of the areas of uncertainty and a coherent understanding of mitral valve dynamics is beginning to emerge.

The check valve action of the mitral valve permits the contribution of atrial systole to ventricular filling to set the left ventricular preload while maintaining a lower mean left atrial pressure. Normal closure of the mitral valve appears to be due to a combination of events. Presystolic movement of the valve cusps to or toward closure results primarily from the forces of atrial contraction with final closure due to the increase in ventricular pressure due to ventricular systole. The role of intravalvular and annular muscle fibers, the papillary muscles and chordae tendineae, the formation of intracardiac fluid vortices or jets, and other factors in mitral valve closure remains speculative. Opening of the mitral valve results largely from the developing AV pressure gradient early in diastole; however, it appears that tension from the papillary muscles and chordae tendineae probably also plays a role.

The major component of the first heart sound occurs as a byproduct of AV valve closure. With a properly timed atrial contraction and optimal presystolic positioning of the valve cusps, this valvular component is soft. If the interval between atrial and ventricular systole is too short or too long, ventriculogenic closure of the open AV valves will result in a loud sound. Opening of the normal mitral or tricuspid valve usually does not produce an audible sound; however, with mitral stenosis or increased early diastolic mitral flow even with a normal valve, a characteristic opening sound (opening snap) is produced. This sound is thought to result from sudden deceleration of the valve opening motion.

References

1. Hurlbritt FR Jr. Peri kardies: A treatis on the heart from the Hippocratic corpus. Introduction and translation. Bull History Med 1104–1113, 1939.
2. Cournard A. Air and blood. In Fishman AP, Richards DW (eds): Circulation of the Blood, Men and Ideas. New York, Oxford University Press, 1964, pp 6–7.
3. Crawford R. Our forerunners of Harvey in antiquity. The Harvein Oration. Br Med J II:551–556, 1919.
4. McKusick VA, Sharpe WD, Warner HD. An exhibition on the history of cardiovascular sound including the evolution of the stethoscope. Bull History Med 31:463–487, 1957.
5. Hall AR. Studies on the history of the cardiovascular system. Bull History Med 34:391–413, 1960.
6. Harvey W. Translated and edited by Alex Bowie. In Bowie A (ed): On the Motion of the Heart and Blood in Animals. Chicago, Henry Regnesy, 1962.

7. Little RC. The mechanism of closure of the mitral valve: A continuing controversy. Circulation 59:615–618, 1979.
8. Silverman ME, Hurst JW. The mitral complex. Am Heart J 76:399–418, 1968.
9. Yellin EL, Nikolic S, Frater RWM. Left ventricular filling dynamics and diastolic function. Prog Cardiovasc Dis 32:247–271, 1990.
10. Little WC. Enhanced load dependence of relaxation in heart failure: Clinical implications. Circulation 85:2326–2328, 1992.
11. Cheng CP, Freeman GL, Santamore WP, Constantinescu MS, Little WC. Effect of loading conditions, contractile state, and heart rate on early diastolic left ventricular filling in conscious dogs. Circ Res 66:814–823, 1990.
12. Courtois M, Mechem CJ, Barzilai B, Gutierrez F, Ludbrook PA. Delineation of determinants of left ventricular early filling: Saline versus blood infusion. Circulation 90:2041–2050, 1994.
13. Little WC, Ohno M, Kitzman DW, Thomas JD, Cheng CP. Determination of left ventricular chamber stiffness from the time for deceleration of early left ventricular filling. Circulation 92:1933–1939, 1995.
14. Little WC, Braunwald E. Assessment of Cardiac Performance. In Anonymous: Heart Disease. W. B. Saunders Company, 1996.
15. Sarnoff SJ, Gilmore JP, Brockman SK, et al. Regulation of ventricular contraction by the carotid sinus. Its effect on atrial and ventricular dynamics. Circ Res 8:1123–1136, 1960.
16. Leonard JJ, Shaver J, Thompson M. Left atrial transport function. Trans Am Clin Climatol Assoc 92:133–141, 1980.
17. Braunwald E. Symposium on cardiac arrhythmias with comments on the hemodynamics significance of atrial systole. Am J Med 37:665–669, 1964.
18. Tsakiris AG, Padiyar R, Gordon DA, et al. Left atrial size and geometry in the intact dog. Am J Physiol 232:H167-H172, 1977.
19. Payne RM, Stone HS, Engelken EJ. Atrial function during volume loading. J Appl Physiol 31:326–331, 1971.
20. Laniado S, Yellin E, Kotler M, et al. A study of the dynamic relationship between the mitral valve echocardiogram and phasic mitral valve flow. Circulation 51:104–113, 1975.
21. Kalmanson D, Veyrat C, Bouchareine F, Degroote A. Non-invasive recording of mitral valve flow velocity patterns using Doppler echocardiograph. Br Heart J 39:517–528, 1977.
22. Feigenbaum H. In Anonymous: Echocardiography. Philadelphia, Lea and Febiger, 1986.
23. Tsakiris AG, Gordon A, Mathieu Y, et al. Motion of both mitral valve leaflets: A cineroentgenographic study in intact dogs. J Appl Physiol 39:359–366, 1975.
24. Shah PM, Tei C. Functional anatomy of the mitral valve and annulus in man: Lessons from echocardiographic observations. In Duran C, Angell WW, Johnson AD (eds): Recent Progress in Mitral Valve Disease. London, Butterworth, 1984, pp 77–95.
25. Hirakawa S, Sasayama S, Tomoike H, et al. In situ measurement of papillary muscle dynamics in the dog left ventricle. Am J Physiol 233:H384-H391, 1977.
26. Rushmer RF, Finlayson BL, Nash AA. Movements of the mitral valve. Circ Res 4:337–342, 1956.
27. Cronin R, Armour JA, Randall WC. Function of the in situ papillary muscle in the canine left ventricle. Circ Res 25:67–75, 1963.
28. Hagl S, Heimisch W, Meisner H, et al. In situ function of the papillary muscle in the intact canine left ventricle. In Duran C, Angell WW, Johnson AD, Oury JH (eds): Recent Progress in Mitral Valve Disease. London, Butterworth, 1984.

29. Stein PD. Role of papillary muscle in mitral valve function. In Stein PD: A Physical and Physiological Basis for Interpretation of Cardiac Auscultation: Evaluations Based Primarily on the Second Sound and Ejection Murmurs. Mount Kisco, Futura Publishing, 1981.
30. Semafuko WEB, Bowie WC. Papillary muscle dynamics: In situ function and response of the papillary muscle. Am J Physiol 228:1800–1807, 1975.
31. Burch GE, De Pasquale NP. Time course of tension in papillary muscles of the heart. JAMA 192:701–704, 1965.
32. Armour JA, Randall WC. Electrical and mechanical activity of papillary muscle. Am J Physiol 218:1710–1717, 1970.
33. Karas S Jr., Elkins RC. Mechanism of function of the mitral valve leaflets, chordae tendineae and left ventricular papillary muscle in dogs. Circ Res 26:689–696, 1970.
34. Salisbury PF, Cross CE, Rieben PJ. Chordae tendinea tension. Am J Physiol 385–392, 1963.
35. Tsakiris AG, Rastelli GC, Des Amorin D, Titus JL, Wood E. Effect of experimental papillary muscle damage on mitral valve closure in intact anesthetized dogs. Mayo Clinic Proc 45:275–285, 1975.
36. Mittal AK, Langston M, Cohn EE, et al. Combined papillary muscle and left ventricular wall dysfunction as a cause of mitral regurgitation: An experimental study. Circulation 44:174–180, 1971.
37. Grimm AJ, Lendrum BL, Lin HL. Papillary muscle shortening in the intact dog: A cineradiographic study of tranquilized dogs in the upright position. Circ Res 36:49–59, 1975.
38. Marzilli M, Sabbah HN, Lee T, Stein PD. Role of the papillary muscle in opening and closure of the mitral valve. Am J Physiol 238:H348-H354, 1980.
39. Marzili M, Sabbah HN, Stein PP. Mitral regurgitation in ventricular premature contractions: The role of the papillary muscle. Chest 77:736–740, 1980.
40. Fisher VJ, Stuckey JH, Lee RF, Kavaler F. Length changes of papillary muscles of the canine left ventricle during the cardiac cycle. Fed Proc 24:278, 1965.
41. Bruch GJ, De Pasquale NP, Phillip JH. The syndrome of papillary muscle dysfunction. Am Heart J 75:399–415, 1968.
42. Hagl S, Heimisch, Meisner H, et al. Function of normal and ischemic papillary muscles in the canine left ventricle. Eur Surg Res 8:99–129, 1976.
43. Pohost GM, Dinsmore JJ, Rubenstein JJ, et al. The echocardiogram of the anterior leaflet of the mitral valve: Correlation with hemodynamic and cineroentgenographic studies in the day. Circulation 51:88–97, 1975.
44. Tsakiris AG, Gordon DH, Padigar R, et al. Relation of mitral valve opening and closure to left atrial and ventricular pressure in the intact dog. Am J Physiol 234:H146-H151, 1978.
45. Steffens TG, Hogan AD. Role of chordae tendineae in mitral valve opening: Two-dimensional echocardiographic evidence. Am J Cardiol 53:153–156, 1984.
46. Dent JM, Spotnitz WD, Nolan SP, Jayaweera AR, Glasheen WP, Kaul S. Mechanism of mitral leaflet excursion. Am J Physiol H2100-H2108, 1995.
47. Kaul S, Spotnitz WD, Glasheen WP, Touchstone DA. Mechanism of ischemic mitral regurgitation and experimental evaluation. Circulation 84:2167–2180, 1991.
48. Sonnenblick EH, Napolitano LM, Daggett WM, et al. An intrinsic neuromuscular basis for mitral valve motion in the dog. Circ Res 21:9–15, 1967.
49. Priola DV, Fultin RL, Napolitano LM, et al. Electrical activity of the canine mitral valve in situ. Am J Physiol 216:238–243, 1969.

50. Erlanger J. A note on the contractility of the musculature of the auriculo-ventricular valves. Am J Physiol 40:150–151, 1916.
51. Dean AL Jr. The movements of the mitral valve cusps in relation to the cardiac cycle. Am J Physiol 40:206–217, 1916.
52. Cooper T, Napolitano LM, Fitzgerald JT, et al. Structural basis for cardiac valve function. Arch Surg 93:767–771, 1966.
53. Cooper T, Doggett WM, Sonnenblick EH. Contraction of the mitral valve: An intrinsic neuromuscular basis for valve motion. J Clin Invest 45:997, 1966.
54. Priola DV, Fellows C, Moorehouse J, et al. Mechanical activity of the canine mitral valve in situ. Am J Physiol 219:1647–1651, 1970.
55. Priola DV, Randall WC. Variations in atrioventricular response to sympathetic nerve stimulation. In Randall WC (ed): Nervous Control of the Heart. Baltimore, Williams and Wilkins, 1965.
56. Smith HL, Essex HE, Baldes EJ. A study of the movement of heart valves and heart sounds. Ann Int Med 33:1357–1359, 1950.
57. Zimmerman J, Bailey CP. The surgical significance of the fibrous skeleton of the heart. J Thorac Cardiovasc Surg 44:701–712, 1962.
58. Tsakiris AG, van Bernuth G, Rastelli GC, et al. Size and motion of the mitral valve annulus in anesthetized intact dogs. J Appl Physiol 30:611–618, 1971.
59. Ormiston JA, Shah PM, Tei C, et al. Size and motion of the mitral valve annulus in man: A two-dimensional echocardiographic method and findings in normal subjects. Circulation 64:113–120, 1981.
60. Glasson JR, Komeda M, Daughters GT, Niczyporuk MA, Bolger AF, et al. Three-dimensional regional dynamics of the normal mitral anulus during left ventricular ejection. J Thorac Cardiovasc Surg 11:574–585, 1996.
61. Henderson Y, Johnson E. Two modes of closure of the heart valves. Heart 4:69–82, 1912.
62. Morgan MT, Criley JM. Mitral valve closure and first heart sound. Am J Cardiol 34:878, 1974.
63. Little RC, Hilton JJ, Schaffer RD. The first heart sound in normal and ectopic ventricular contractions. Mechanisms of closure of the A-V valves. Circ Res 2:48–52, 1954.
64. Little RC. Effect of atrial systole on ventricular pressure and closure of the A-V valves. Am J Physiol 166:289–295, 1951.
65. Sarnoff SJ, Gilmore JP, Mitchell JH. Influence of atrial contraction and relaxation on closure of mitral valve: Observations on effect of autonomic nerve activity. Circ Res 11:26–35, 1962.
66. Brockman SK. Mechanism of the movement of the atrioventricular valves. Am J Cardiol 17:682–690, 1960.
67. Skinner NS Jr, Mitchell JH, Wallace AG, et al. Hemodynamic effects of altering the timing of atrial systole. Am J Physiol 205:499–503, 1963.
68. Ankeny JL, Fishman AP, Fritts HW Jr. An analysis of normal and abnormal left atrial pressure pulses in man. Circ Res 4:95–99, 1956.
69. Ferrer MI, Harvey RM, Cathcart RT, et al. Hemodynamic studies in rheumatic heart disease. Circulation 6:688–710, 1952.
70. Daley R, McMillan IKR, Gorlin R. Mitral incompetence in experimental auricular fibrillation. Lancet 269:18–20, 1955.
71. Friedman B, Daily WM, Wilson RH. Studies on mitral valve function. Effect of acute hypervolemia, premature beats and other arrhythmias. Circ Res 4:33–37, 1956.
72. Gray IR, Joshipura CS, Macinnon J. Retrograde left ventricular cardioangiography in the diagnosis of mitral regurgitation. Br Heart J 25:145–152, 1963.

73. Nolan SP, Dixon SH, Fisher RR, et al. The influence of atrial contraction and mitral valve mechanics on ventricular filling: A study of instantaneous mitral flow. Am Heart J 77:84–91, 1969.
74. Woodward E Jr, Swan HJC, Wood EH. Evaluation of a method of detection of mitral regurgitation from indicator-dilution curves recorded from the left atrium. Mayo Clin Proc 32:525–535, 1957.
75. Braunwald E, Rockoff SD, Oldham HN Jr, et al. Effective closure of the mitral valve without atrial systole. Circulation 33:404–409, 1966.
76. Williams JCP, O'Donovan PB, Cronin L, et al. Influence of sequence of atrial and ventricular systole on closure of mitral valve. J Appl Physiol 22:786–792, 1967.
77. Williams JCP, Vandenberg RA, O'Donovan TPB, et al. Roentgen videodensitometer study of mitral valve closure during atrial fibrillation. J Appl Physiol 24:217–224, 1968.
78. Vandenberg RA, Williams JCP, Sturm RE, et al. Effect of ventricular extra systoles on closure of mitral valve. Circulation 39:197–204, 1969.
79. Zaky A, Steinmetz E, Feigenbaum H. Role of atrium in closure of mitral valve in man. Am J Physiol 17:1652–1659, 1969.
80. Shak PM, Kramer DH, Gramiak R. Influence of the timing of atrial systole on mitral closure and on the first heart sound in man. Am J Cardiol 26:231–237, 1970.
81. Burchell HB. A clinical appraisal of atrial transport function. Lancet 1:775–779, 1964.
82. Sarnoff SJ, Gilmore JP, Mitchell JH. Influence of atrial contraction and relaxation on closure of the mitral valve. Circ Res 11:26–35, 1962.
83. Meisner JS, McQueen DM, Ishida Y, et al. Effect of timing of atrial systole on LV filling and mitral valve closure: Computer and dog studies. Am J Physiol 249:H604-H619, 1985.
84. Yellin EL, Yoran C, Frater RWM. Physiology of mitral valve flow. In Duran C, Angell WW, Johnson AD, Oury JH (eds): Recent Progress in Mitral Valve Disease. London, Butterworth, 1984.
85. Perloff JK, Roberts WC. The mitral apparatus. Functional anatomy of mitral regurgitation. Circulation 46:227–239, 1972.
86. Smalcelj A, Gibson DG. Relation between mitral valve closure and early systolic function of the left ventricle. Br Heart J 53:436–442, 1985.
87. Schnittger I, Appleton CP, Hatle LK, Popp RL. Diastolic mitral and tricuspid regurgitation by Doppler echocardiography in patients with atrioventricular block: New insight into the mechanism of atrioventricular valve closure. J Am Coll Cardiol 11:83–88, 1988.
88. Reid KG. Mitral valve action and the mode of ventricular filling. Nature 223:1383–1384, 1969.
89. Bellhouse BJ. Fluid mechanics of a model mitral valve and left ventricle. Cardiovasc Res 6:199–210, 1972.
90. Taylor DEM, Wade JD. Pattern of blood flow within the heart: A stable system. Cardiovasc Res 7:14–21, 1973.
91. Lee GSF, Talbot L. A fluid-mechanical study of the closure of heart valves. J Fluid Mech 91:41–63, 1979.
92. Yellin EL, Peskin C, Yoran C, Koenigsberg M, et al. Mechanism of mitral valve motion during diastole. Am J Physiol 241:H389-H400, 1981.
93. Little RC. In Anonymous: Physiology of the Heart and Circulation. Chicago, Year Book Medical Publ, 1985, pp 399–418.

94. Mealows WR, Van Praagh J, Indreika M, et al. Premature mitral valve closure: A hemodynamic explanation for absence of the first sound in aortic insufficiency. Circulation 28:251–258, 1963.
95. Spring DA, Rowe GC. Premature closure of the mitral and tricuspid valves. Circulation 45:663–671, 1972.
96. Dianzumba SB, Montello JJ, Joyner CR. Intermittent premature mitral valve closure in combined acute severe aortic and mitral regurgitation. South Med J 77:1449–1452, 1984.
97. David D, Michelson EL, Naito M, et al. Diastolic "locking" of the mitral valve: The importance of atrial systole and intraventricular volume. Circulation 67:640–645, 1983.
98. David D, Michelson EL, Naito M, et al. Diastolic "locking" of the mitral valve: Possible importance of diastolic myocardial properties. Circulation 73:997–1005, 1986.
99. Stefadouros MA, Little RC. The cause and clinical significance of diastolic heart sounds. Arch Int Med 140:537–541, 1980.
100. Friedman NJ. Echocardiographic studies in mitral valve motion: Genesis of the opening snap in mitral stenosis. Am Heart J 80:177–187, 1970.
101. Schwartz ML, Little RC. Physiological basis for the heart sounds and their clinical significance. N Engl J Med 264:280–285, 1961.
102. Little RC. Importance of the first heart sound in cardiac diagnosis. Ohio State Med J 65:483–486, 1969.
103. Abrams J. Current concepts on the genesis of heart sounds. I: First and second sounds. JAMA 239:2787–2789, 1978.
104. Craige E. On the genesis of heart sounds: Contributions made by echocardiographic studies. Circulation 53:207–209, 1976.

3

The Function of the Normal Human Mitral Valve

Derek Gibson, MD

Introduction

The properties of the cardiac valves were already known to Galen, and William Harvey appreciated that their one-way effect on flow provided major evidence for his theory of the circulation of blood.[1] Research into mitral valve function has passed through three phases. For many centuries, ideas about mitral valve function depended on deductions from anatomy, starting with Leonardo, Vesalius, and Harvey. This was followed by a phase of animal experimentation using methods of increasing sophistication: initially pressures measured with fluid-filled manometers, and subsequently, angiography, cineradiography of radiopaque markers, catheter-tip manometry, and Doppler. Finally, it has become increasingly feasible to study mitral valve function in normal humans, using a variety of noninvasive techniques. These have included M-mode echo for mitral leaflet position, Doppler and MRI estimates of blood flow velocity and distribution, left ventricular and left atrial pressure, or surrogates for them and M-mode measurements of wall motion in the short and long axis. Three-dimensional reconstruction of valve anatomy, and of blood flow within the left ventricle are now increasingly being undertaken.

The present chapter aims to review the function of the anatomically normal mitral valve in humans, both normal subjects and patients with

From: Boudoulas H, Wooley CF. *Mitral Valve: Floppy Mitral Valve, Mitral Valve Prolapse, Mitral Valvular Regurgitation*. Second revised edition. ©Futura Publishing Company, Armonk, NY, 2000.

ventricular disease, since many of the disturbances seen in the latter seem to shed light on normal function. The experimental literature has been fully reviewed elsewhere (see also Chapter 2).[2]

Mitral Valve Function

The "function" of the normal mitral valve can be stated in terms of changes in the properties of the left atrioventricular (AV) orifice during the cardiac cycle. During systole, it remains almost completely occluded in spite of striking changes in the size and shape of the ventricular cavity. Very minor degrees of regurgitation can sometimes be detected by color flow Doppler, but these are physiologically insignificant. In contrast, during ventricular filling, a column of blood whose diameter approximates that of the ventricle itself rapidly accelerates and passes from the atrium to the ventricle without measurable resistance. The change from one state to the other is effectively a step function. It occurs over a very short time interval that is not limiting compared with the time necessary for acceleration and deceleration of the column of blood. Two further changes affect the AV orifice during the cardiac cycle: its diameter becomes smaller during systole and larger during diastole, and its position changes, moving toward the ventricular apex during systole and away during diastole. These latter two are not step functions, but change continuously throughout the cardiac cycle. Taken together, all of these changes impose directionality on the circulation, i.e., they introduce marked asymmetry in its properties with respect to direction, defining forward and retrograde flow.

The mitral valve cusps clearly play an important but not exclusive role in bringing about these changes, particularly in reducing orifice conductance during systole. Orifice diameter itself changes as the result of contraction of circumferential atrial and ventricular muscle surrounding the so-called mitral ring, itself an insubstantial fibrous structure in the normal heart. Ring motion depends on longitudinally arranged muscle in the atrium and ventricle. In the left atrium,[3] the main longitudinal component is the septoatrial bundle, which arises from the interatrial septum, passing to the anterior base of the atrium and thence to the base of the anterior cusp of the mitral valve. A second longitudinal band runs from here to the superior and posterior wall of the atrium between right and left pulmonary veins. On the ventricular side of the ring,[4] longitudinal fibers are mainly subendocardial, and to a lesser extent, subepicardial, with the papillary muscles forming as a third component of the longitudinal system within the ventricle. Circumferentially arranged fibers are largely in the mid-wall.

The properties of the valve cusps themselves are characteristic. They have high tensile strength, being virtually inextensible at physiological pressures, but are very flexible. During systole, therefore, once they are closed and locked, they effectively control flow. During the remainder of the cardiac cycle, exactly the reverse applies, since they have no motion independent of local flow and thus become markers of it. It follows, therefore, that it would be simplistic to consider motion of the mitral valve cusps in isolation. It is necessary to study interrelations between cusp motion, the other parts of the mitral valve apparatus, intraventricular blood flow, wall motion, and cavity pressures. Normal cusp motion cannot easily be dissociated from the rather specialized patterns of blood flow and wall motion seen in the normal ventricle.

The Mitral Ring

The possibility that both the cross-sectional area and shape of the orifice contained by the mitral ring might change during the cardiac cycle in humans was deduced from postmortem findings as long ago as 1909,[5] by Lian who also digitally palpated its contraction during ventricular systole in dogs. More recently, the cross-sectional area of the mitral ring has been measured echocardiographically in humans[6] and shown to be maximum just before the onset of ventricular systole, with a value of 3.8 ± 0.7 cm^2/m^2. It falls rapidly during isovolumic contraction to 2.9 ± 0.11 cm^2/m^2, and thereafter increases continuously for the remainder of the cardiac cycle. The cross-sectional area is thus at a minimum at the onset of ejection. These changes thus represent 25% of the total area of the ring. Their pathophysiological significance has not been determined in detail, although it seems possible that they may contribute to normal competence of the valve during systole.

Mitral Ring Motion

Movement of the mitral ring, also referred to as the AV plane or aortic root,[7–9] is intimately related to changes in the long axis of the ventricle. William Harvey realized that ventricular volume changes depend on the coordinate shortening of its short and long axes,[10] although changes in the long axis have received remarkably little attention in comparison with the large amount of information available about those of the minor axis and the circumferential fibers that bring them about.

Mitral ring motion can readily be studied by M-mode echocardiography with the transducer at the apex of the heart.[9] A normal trace is shown in Figure 1. The motion of the mitral ring is approximately in phase with the minor axis of the ventricle. It starts during isovolumic contraction, preceding that of the minor axis by 25 ms. Shortening continues throughout ejection and ends at the same time as that of the minor axis and of aortic valve closure. Total long-axis excursion is normally 1.5 cm and peak systolic velocity 3 cm/s^{-1}. There are minor differences in these values between the septum and the ventricular free wall. The ring remains stationary during isovolumic relaxation, but once ventricular filling begins, it moves back toward the atrium during rapid ventricular filling with a peak velocity of 8–10 cm/s, and again during atrial systole when the peak velocity is around 4 cm/s. Normally, approximately 60% of total excursion occurs during early diastole, and the remainder during atrial systole.

Motion of the mitral ring has several physiological consequences, which were predicted nearly a century ago on purely anatomical grounds by Keith[11] (Fig. 2). As the ring moves toward the apex of the left ventricle during ejection, the floor of the left atrium descends, so its capacity increases. This increase in atrial capacity may be greater than the volume of blood entering from the pulmonary veins, causing atrial pressure to fall, thus explaining the normal X' or systolic descent of the venous pulse. This unexpected combination of pressure fall and volume increase occurs because the left ventricle does external work on the left atrium; it could not occur in a chamber that was behaving passively. The pressure fall, in turn, facilitates blood flow from the pulmonary veins into the atrium during ventricular ejection.[8] Ring motion thus imposes directionality on blood flow upstream of the mitral valve itself, whose influence reaches back beyond the atrium to the pulmonary veins. On the right side of the heart, a comparable effect can be detected outside the thorax in the superior and inferior caval veins.

Patterns of blood flow in the systemic and pulmonary veins will thus depend crucially on AV ring motion. A reduction in the systolic amplitude of ring motion, as characteristically occurs when ventricular ejection fraction is reduced, will directly reduce systolic forward flow in the pulmonary veins with a corresponding increase in early diastole. This change has been documented in patients with severe ventricular disease,[12] but has been related to a high left ventricular end-diastolic pressure, which is of course frequently present when ejection fraction is low. However, the relation is likely to be an indirect one. Indeed, it is difficult to see why pulmonary venous blood flow patterns should ever be studied without reference to motion of the mitral ring.

During early diastole, blood accelerates across the mitral valve from the left atrium to the ventricle as the result of a pressure gradient directed from the atrium to the ventricle. In spite of this pressure difference, normal backward motion of the mitral ring occurs at the same time

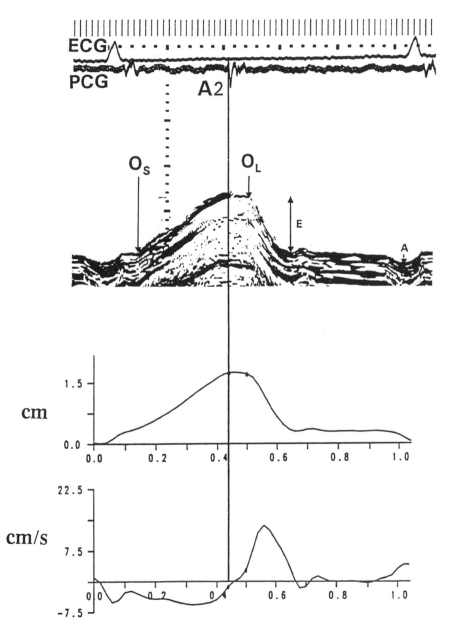

Figure 1. Normal record of the left side of the mitral valve ring, showing, from above downward, the original echogram, digitized record of its position and, bottom, velocity. A2 represents aortic valve closure on the phonocardiogram (PCG).

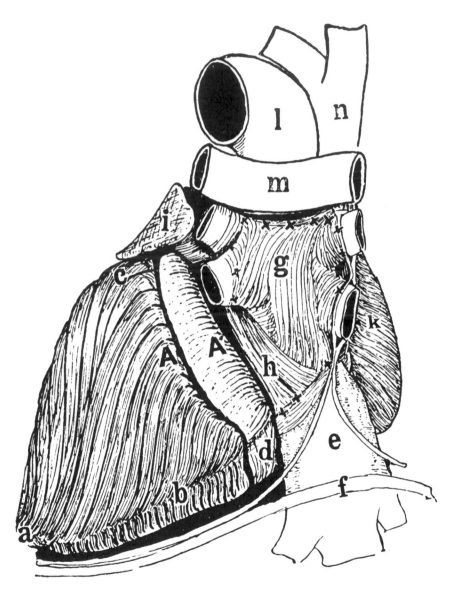

Figure 2. The heart from behind, showing the arrangements of the musculature of the left atrium and left ventricle. A' represents the mitral ring position at the time of peak atrial systole, A during ventricular systole. (Used with permission from Keith A.[11])

(Fig. 3). Ring motion must thus be brought about by a force arising in the atrium rather than by pressure in the ventricle. This atrial force is likely to be an elastic one, residing within the atrial wall and generated during the previous systole.[9,13] It tends to restore the ventricular cavity to its end-diastolic configuration, but unlike more commonly considered restoring forces, is located outside the ventricle rather than within the ventricular myocardium.

Since atrial systole itself lasts for a relatively brief period, it is tempting to consider the atria as behaving as passive chambers for the remainder of the cardiac cycle, and to describe their pressure-volume relation in

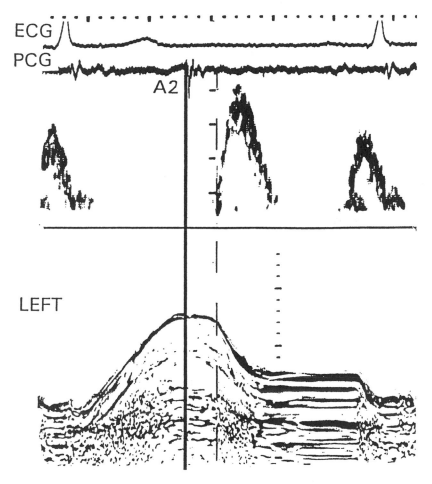

Figure 3. Records of mitral ring motion (below) and transmitral Doppler (above) synchronized with reference to A2. Note that peak early diastole filling velocity occurs at the same time as the peak rate of backward motion of the mitral valve ring.

terms of compliance. Indeed, left atrial compliance has been invoked as a major factor determining the filling pattern of the left ventricle early in diastole.[14] However, AV interactions occurring through the mitral ring must cast doubt on this interpretation. During systole, mitral ring motion indicates that external work is being done on the atrium by the ventricle, and during early diastole, stored energy is being transferred back to the circulation from its walls. The origin of this energy is deformation by the ventricle, not a pressure increase in its lumen. Only during diastasis, therefore, do the atria behave passively, and only during this period, is it permissible to speak of them as having compliance, and assume a simple analytical relation between pressure and volume.

Mitral ring motion is also a mechanism of increasing ventricular volume diastole which does not involve blood flow. Effectively, the ring mo-

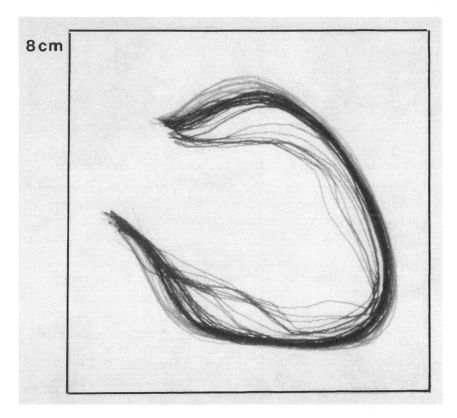

Figure 4. Superimposed left ventricular cavity outlines during diastole, derived from the cineangiogram of a normal subject, at 50 frames/s. Outlines derived from early diastole and diastasis are shown in black, and those during atrial systole in red. Note that the ventricular volume increase during atrial systole is due almost entirely to an increase in long axis. See color appendix.

tion away from the apex means that blood that was within the atrial cavity during early diastole finds itself within the ventricle during diastasis.[11,15] Exactly the same events occur during the second component of ring motion during atrial systole. Together, this volume increase accounts for 10–15% of the normal stroke volume on the left side of the heart, and more on the right. Since the blood itself does not move with respect to the chest wall, it cannot be detected by Doppler. More significant, since it does not move with respect to the center of mass of the ventricle, this volume increase is not associated with any AV pressure gradient.

Ring motion also leads to a characteristic pattern of regional left ventricular wall motion during late diastole, when the increase in ventricular volume is accounted for almost exclusively by an increase in long axis (Fig. 4). It is widely accepted that the "booster" effect of left atrial systole increases the force of left ventricular contraction by augmenting ventricular preload, an effect frequently interpreted in terms of Starling's law.[16,17] If this is indeed the case, then it would appear that Starling's law, as manifested during atrial systole, operates mainly on longitudinally rather than circumferentially directed fibers. The idea of preload, which is clearly defined with respect to an isolated muscle fiber, thus becomes complex when translated into the setting of even the intact normal heart.

Papillary Muscles

It is generally accepted that the papillary muscles support the mitral valve cusps during systole. During normal ejection, the mitral ring moves toward the apex, as the result of shortening of longitudinally directed muscle fibers within the ventricular wall.[18] At the same time, the papillary muscles also shorten, so that the position of the valve tips remain in approximately the same position with respect to the ring, although cavity volume falls. Anatomically, the papillary muscles are continuous with the subendocardial trabecula in the left ventricle, compatible with the two muscle groups functioning as a single unit.[4]

Rupture of a papillary muscle as a complication of acute myocardial infarction causes severe mitral regurgitation due to prolapse of the corresponding cusp into the left atrium. However, spontaneous papillary muscle rupture is not a satisfactory model for studying the effects of papillary muscle function in humans. Not only is it rare and usually associated with additional severe left ventricular disease due to underlying myocardial infarction, but it also causes life-threatening mitral regurgitation and pulmonary edema. Alternatively, patients can be studied after mitral valve replacement, when both papillary muscles have been sectioned in the course of operation. Although left ventricular and mitral valve function approximate to normal, clear disturbances of mitral ring motion can be seen[9]

MITRAL PROSTHESIS

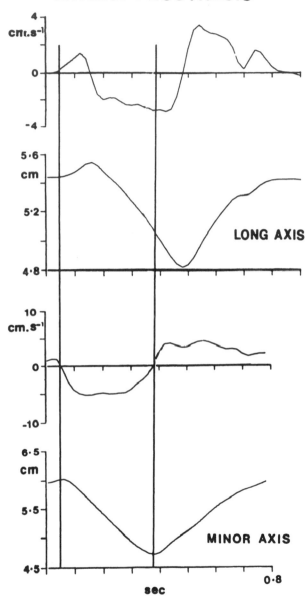

Figure 5. Left ventricular long-axis changes after mitral valve replacement (with papillary muscle section) compared with the minor axis. Note that the onset and peak of long-axis shortening are both delayed with respect both to minor axis and A2.

(Fig. 5). The onset of long-axis shortening is delayed, so that instead of preceding that of the minor axis by 25 ms, it follows it by 35 ms. Peak rate of systolic motion of the AV ring is reduced as is the overall amplitude of motion. Finally, there is striking asynchrony at end-systole, with peak shortening of the long axis following that of the minor axis by 70 ms instead of being effectively synchronous with it. These abnormalities are not seen in patients with mitral stenosis or following mitral repair, so they cannot be ascribed to the effects of mild mitral stenosis or cardiac surgery. If it is assumed that papillary muscle function represents the difference between that seen in patients in whom it is present and in those in whom it is not, its nature can be deduced. On this basis, it appears that the onset of papillary muscle contraction precedes that of the normal minor axis. The absence of its contribution during ejection impairs the force of longitudinal contraction against the normal afterload, reduces the velocity and extent of shortening, and probably increases its duration. In effect, therefore, normal papillary muscle contraction is synchronous with that of other myocardium supporting the long axis of which it forms an integral part. This conclusion is in line with recent experimental work in which care has been taken to avoid papillary muscle injury.

Mitral Cusps

In spite of the important contributions of the mitral ring and longitudinally arranged muscles, the mitral cusps play the major role in changing the conductance of the AV orifice and imparting directional asymmetry to it. The normal anterior cusp of the mitral valve has a surface area of approximately 6 cm^2. If its free margin is to move 4 cm, the normal opening amplitude, therefore, a volume of around 15 cc of blood must be displaced from its leading face, and a similar volume must move in behind its trailing edge; together these fluid shifts imply the presence of a vortex. Mitral cusp motion cannot therefore be considered in isolation. It is also necessary to show how it relates to blood flow, wall motion, and cavity pressure.

Mitral Valve Closure

The mitral valve cusps close three times in the cardiac cycle: during the deceleration phase of rapid filling, the deceleration phase following left atrial contraction, and at the onset of left ventricular systole. At all three times, there is a reverse pressure difference between the left atrium and the left ventricle. This force arises from passive diastolic properties of the left ventricle in the first two instances and from the onset of ventricular systole in the third.

Anterior cusp motion during mid-diastolic closure has been measured by M-mode echocardiography.[19] The peak closing velocity occurs at the end of the closing movement, when it has reached approximately 25 cm/s. As will be seen (Fig. 6), closing velocity increases steadily throughout mid-diastole, indicating that its acceleration is approximately constant, with a value of 0.27 ± 0.08 G. Constant acceleration implies a constant force, or in a fluid, a constant pressure gradient throughout the closure period, which, for a deceleration of 0.3 G, would correspond to a local pressure gradient of 0.22 mm Hg/cm. A constant mid-diastolic closing velocity in the presence of an unobstructed valve orifice, as implied from measurements of "diastolic closure rate" widely quoted in the early M-mode literature, would be very difficult to explain in physical terms. Closing velocity at the onset of ventricular systole is rather higher than that occurring during mid-diastole. It is approximately 30 cm/s, being the result of a higher acceleration operating over a shorter period.

In the normal subject, valve closure due to the deceleration phase of atrial systole is closely followed by that due to ventricular systole. The question thus arises as to whether atriogenic closure is essential to mitral valve function during systole. Henderson[20] likened simple ventriculogenic closure to the valves leaflets swinging closed "like barn doors in a wind storm," and suggested that it would be accompanied by significant mitral regurgitation. The conflicting experimental literature on this question remains unresolved. However, very mild mitral regurgitation can be detected in humans by color flow, which is a normal finding in about 30% otherwise healthy individuals. Neither its incidence nor is its degree significantly increased in patients with lone atrial fibrillation. The timing of mitral closure can be predicted rather precisely from its relation to peak rate of rise of pressure (as estimated from the apex cardiogram). This time is unaffected by atrial fibrillation.[21] Blood might theoretically be displaced into the left atrium as the cusps move backward to occlude the mitral orifice. Flow directly due to valve closure is not associated with blood velocities normally seen with mitral regurgitation (i.e., 5–6 m.s^{-1}), but rather with peak velocity of cusp motion (0.30 m.s^{-1}). Further, with a valve area of 6 cm^2, and a valve closure time of 20 ms, total closing volume is 3–4 mL. This small volume moving at low velocity would be difficult to detect by Doppler and is physiologically insignificant. The crucial factor limiting this regurgitant volume is thus the short duration of the closing movement, itself reflecting the sensitivity of the cusp mechanism to deceleration forces.

Atriogenic mitral valve closure becomes apparent when the normal synchrony of atrial contraction is lost, as occurs in patients with a prolonged PR interval, complete heart block, or a VVI pacemaker. As in normal sinus rhythm, closure occurs at a peak rate of 25–30 cm/s, but after 50–100 ms, the cusps drift apart again. Thus atrial systole is capable of closing the valve, but not capable of keeping it closed. Additional factors are

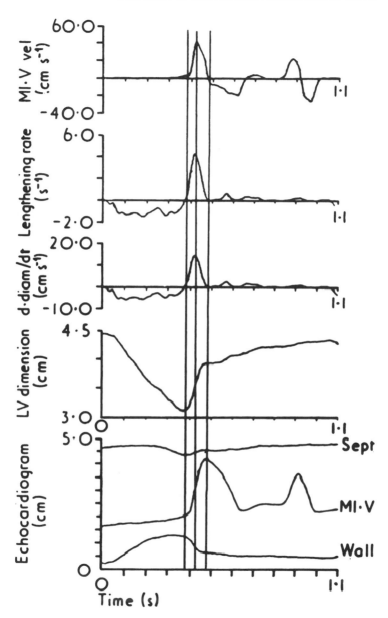

Figure 6. Normal relations between anterior mitral valve cusp motion and changes in left ventricular minor axis, showing, from below, original digitized data, changes in ventricular dimension, rate of change of dimension, normalized rate of change of dimension, and, top, rate of change of cusp position. Note the close normal time relations between dimension change and valve cusp motion (Used with permission from Upton MT, et al.[19])

necessary to lock the cusps in the closed position. The same applies to early diastolic closure; if diastasis is prolonged, the cusps drift from the closed to the half-open position. In an experimental study, David et al.,[22] by manipulating atrial coupling interval, demonstrated that the mitral cusps locked only when the pressure in the ventricle was higher than that in the atrium. This pressure difference persisted well beyond the termination of any effect of atrial relaxation. Its presence was closely related to ventricular volume and it was a function of the passive stiffness of the cavity. Evidence for prolonged pressure differences in humans can be found in patients with AV dissociation, particularly those in whom functional AV regurgitation is present during ventricular systole. An example is given in Figure 7. If the patient is in sinus rhythm, but PR interval is prolonged, then a short presystolic extension of the regurgitation is apparent, referred to as diastolic regurgitation. When atrial contraction is dissociated from that of the ventricle, the same phenomenon can be observed, but may be self-perpetuating over intervals of 100 ms or more until the onset of the next ventricular systole. Once established, therefore, the regurgitant jet appears to be very stable. Atriogenic regurgitation is probably of no

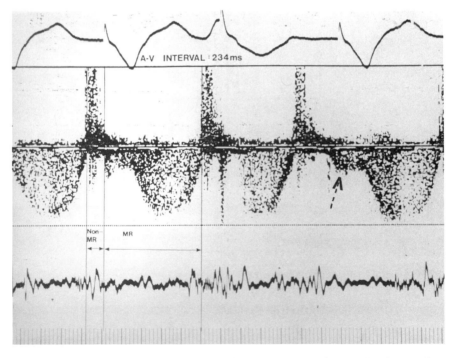

Figure 7. Presystolic mitral regurgitation (marked by arrow) occurring in a patient with a permanent pacemaker and a long AV delay. MR = total duration of mitral regurgitation; non-MR = time between pulses of mitral regurgitation during which ventricular filling can occur.

consequence as a volume load on the left ventricle, but when established, effectively prevents forward flow, and with sinus tachycardia, may even limit ventricular filling time and thus stroke volume.

A strikingly disturbed pattern of mitral valve closure occurs in patients with left ventricular disease, usually dilated cardiomyopathy, which is quantified in terms of prolongation of the PR-AC interval,[23] *A* representing the time of maximum cusp separation during atrial systole, and *C* the point of their final apposition at the onset of ventricular systole. Since these patients frequently have first degree heart block, it is necessary to correct for PR interval. The abnormality is, in fact, more complex than this, since the mitral valve cusps rapidly approximate following atrial systole; this is followed by a sudden drop in their closure rate, and they remain in a partially open position for a further 100–200 ms before finally closing (Fig. 8). This pattern characteristically occurs in patients with my-

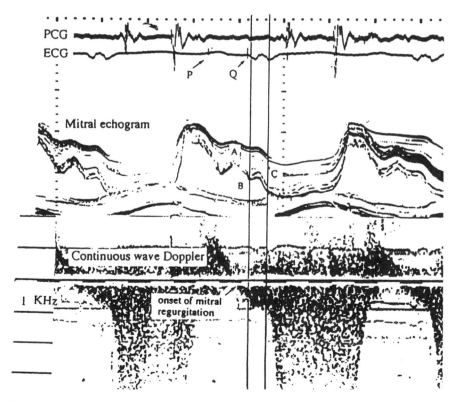

Figure 8. Simultaneous mitral echogram and functional mitral regurgitation from a patient with prolonged PR-AC interval. Note that the onset of low-velocity mitral regurgitation coincides with the B discontinuity on the mitral echogram. Final mitral cusp apposition does not occur until the onset of rapid velocity (i.e., pressure) increase. (Used with permission from Fujimoto S, et al.[23])

ocardial fibrosis and advanced activation disturbances, in whom the rate of rise of ventricular pressure is strikingly reduced as demonstrated from the continuous wave Doppler trace of functional mitral regurgitation. Final mitral closure is delayed, until peak AV pressure drop, as estimated from functional mitral regurgitation, is as high as 10–20 mm Hg. At the same time, the discontinuity in the closing motion, the so-called B wave, correlates with the onset of low-velocity regurgitation. These observations suggest that normal mitral closure requires a rapid rise of ventricular pressure. When this rate is reduced, by asynchronous ventricular contraction for example, a regurgitant jet may become established, which is suppressed only by an AV pressure difference of 10 times that normally causing valve closure.

Mitral Valve Opening

The normal mitral valve cusps separate twice during the cardiac cycle, during early diastole, and again following atrial contraction. The peak velocity of anterior cusp motion during early diastole is in the range of 40–60 cm/s, and acceleration 0.6–0.7 G.[19] Values during atrial systole are about half this value. Posterior cusp velocities are approximately half those of the anterior cusp, with peak opening velocity occurring 20 ms earlier than that of the anterior cusp. Changes in the position of the mitral ring and of the tips of the mitral valve cusps during isovolumic relaxation are both less than 1 mm, suggesting that valve geometry does not change significantly before mitral cusp separation, and eliminating the theoretical possibility that this may be a significant cause of ventricular volume change.

It is generally believed that mitral cusp separation occurs at the time of the crossover of atrial and ventricular pressures, but experimental information on this point is conflicting, with reported values ranging from 0 to 60 ms.[24] In man, for example,[25] the crossover, determined with solid state manometers, has been found to coincide with the onset of rapid cusp motion (D' point) and thus to follow initial separation. These specific difficulties, as well as the more general one of gaining access to normal subjects with catheter-tip manometers, can be approached by inverting the problem. Instead of attempting to measure pressure gradients directly, the blood itself can be used as an accelerometer.[26] Immediately following pressure crossover, an AV pressure gradient directed from atrium to ventricle will, by definition, be established. This force must cause movement of blood according to Newton's second law of motion. Using this approach, therefore, it is possible to establish not only the time of onset of a pressure gradient, but also its magnitude and direction from local blood acceleration. A pressure gradient derived in this way has the physical dimensions of mm Hg/cm, and thus differs from a simple pressure difference, e.g., that between a single atrial and a single ventricular pressure. During rapid early diastolic filling, pressure varies continuously with position along the direction of fluid movement. This constitutes a pressure field which itself changes continuously with time during the filling period. Local blood flow accelerations in the ventricular inflow tract can be estimated by pulsed Doppler mapping or MRI. Both of these techniques demonstrate that the time of onset of AV flow, and thus that of pressure crossover, varies with position along the inflow tract, being normally propagated into the ventricle with a velocity of approximately 100 cm/s[27] (Fig. 9). This implies a delay in crossover time of 10 ms for each cm from the mitral ring toward the apex of the ventricle, which may explain the variable results that have been obtained when it has been estimated from pairs of manometers in atrium and ventricle whose pressure-sensitive elements are in unspecified positions within the cardiac chambers. Direct measurement from regional blood flow ac-

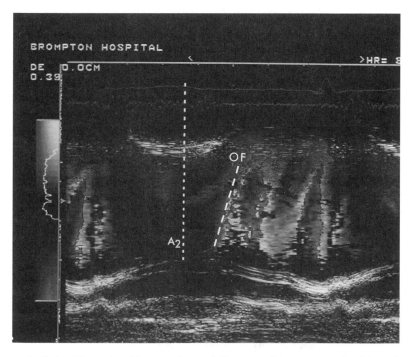

Figure 9. Color M-mode with transducer at the apex, from a normal subject showing transmitral flow velocities from the level of the mitral ring to the apex of the ventricle. A2 represents aortic valve closure. OF represents the onset of flow, which is progressively delayed with respect to A2 with distance into the cavity. See color appendix.

celeration gives a peak value of 2–3 mm Hg from atrium to ventricle during the phase of acceleration, reversing to -2–3 mm Hg during the deceleration phase.[28] If these are peak values, then the pressure gradient necessary to cause mitral cusp separation must be significantly smaller than this, demonstrating the exquisite sensitivity of the mechanisms underlying cusp motion.

In the normal subject, mitral cusp motion correlates closely with other cardiac events (Fig. 6). Cusp separation starts abruptly, 60 ± 10 ms after aortic valve closure. Cusp motion and transverse dimension are in phase with one another throughout early diastole, so that the onset of anterior cusp motion and the time of its peak velocity are both effectively synchronous with timings of the onset of dimension increase and its peak rate of increase, each to within 5 ms.[19] The E point on the mitral echogram corresponds to a sharp discontinuity on the first derivative of the transverse dimension trace at the end of rapid filling. There is similar synchrony between the mitral cusp and the long axis during early diastole. No subsequent events are recognizable on the transverse dimension trace during mid-diastolic closure or atrial systolic motion of the anterior cusp. The start of cusp separation with atrial systole, however, coincides with accelerated backward motion of the mitral ring. The onset of the E wave of the transmitral Doppler, recorded from the apex, with the sample volume at cusp level is delayed with respect to cusp separation by 25 ms, and with respect to wall motion by somewhat more.[29] The timing of peak inflow filling velocity corresponds with the end of rapid increase of the transverse dimension, and with the E point, i.e., the point of maximum cusp separation on the mitral echogram (Fig. 10a).

Normal interrelations between incoming flow, valve cusp, and ventricular wall motion seem to suggest a complex series of interlocking events. However, in disease, these apparently close relations may be lost even though mitral valve anatomy is normal. When relaxation is incoordinate, as is common in patients with coronary artery disease,[30] left ventricular wall motion and cusp separation are no longer synchronous. In Figure 10b, transverse left ventricular dimension increases strikingly before the onset of cusp separation during the period of isovolumic relaxation. Since ventricular volume is constant at this time in the cardiac cycle, cavity shape must have changed, and abnormal dimension increase in one part of the cavity must be associated with abnormal reduction elsewhere. Here, as is usually the case, the long axis continues to shorten throughout isovolumic relaxation and does not begin to lengthen again until the start of atrial systole. Though mitral cusp motion has been dissociated from changes in both axes, its opening and closing velocities are entirely normal.[30] In addition, there may be no early diastolic flow across the mitral valve detectable by pulsed Doppler, so that not only is cusp separation ab-

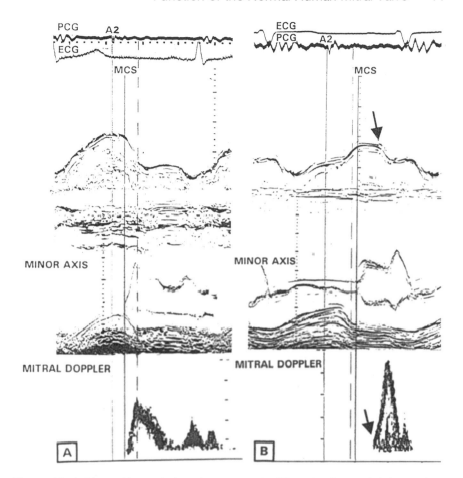

Figure 10. A. Normal interrelations between mitral Doppler (bottom), left ventricular minor axis and long axis, with individual traces synchronized on A2. Note that changes in minor and long axis occur simultaneously, and that the onset of transmitral flow is synchronous with mitral cusp separation at the onset of rapid filling. **B.** Similar data from a patient with left ventricular disease. Note that there has been a significant increase in minor dimension associated with further shortening of long axis in the period between A2 and mitral valve cusp separation. Furthermore, the onset of transmitral flow is further delayed beyond mitral cusp separation, and does not occur until atrial systole. (Used with permission from Henein M, et al.[30])

normally delayed with respect to aortic valve closure, but there is a further delay of up to 150 ms between cusp separation and the earliest detectable flow across the mitral valve.

A second group of patients showing a major disturbance of mitral cusp separation are those with dilated cardiomyopathy and functional mi-

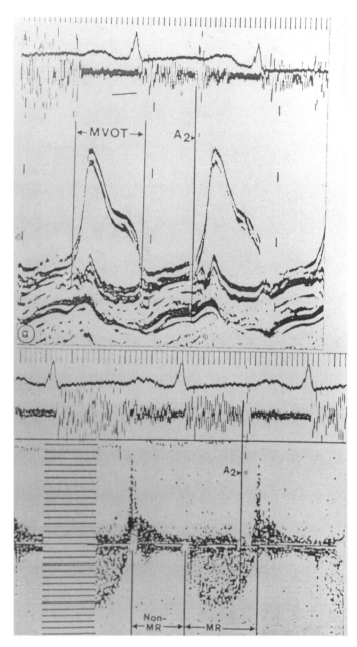

Figure 11. Interrelations between functional mitral regurgitation and mitral cusp separation in a patient with severe dilated cardiomyopathy. Note that cusp separation is effectively synchronous with A2, although mitral regurgitation persists for another 100–120 ms. (Used with permission from Ng KSK, et al.[31])

tral regurgitation, in whom filling pressures are high.[31] The interval from A2 to cusp separation is short, and indeed, the two may be synchronous when left atrial pressure is above 30 mm Hg. In spite of this, functional mitral regurgitation may continue up to 100 ms after A2 (Fig. 11). Although the mitral regurgitation itself is detected by continuous wave Doppler, color M-mode shows it to arise at the level of the line of mitral valve cusp apposition. In these patients, therefore, the mitral cusps separate when the pressure in the left ventricle is 40 mm Hg or more above that in the atrium. Interrelations between blood flow and mitral cusp motion in these two sets of circumstances, incoordinate relaxation and functional mitral regurgitation, suggest that important forces determining cusp motion act in a direction orthogonal to forward transmitral flow and are thus potentially independent of it. Their exact nature will probably be understood in detail only when methods capable of demonstrating blood flow in three dimensions are developed.

Normally, transmitral blood flow and cusp motion are also closely related during atrial systole, with valve closure starting at the peak of the A wave on the transmitral Doppler. In many patients with restrictive ventricular disease, though, active atrial contraction, as demonstrated by a pressure A wave and retrograde flow in the pulmonary veins, does not cause forward flow across the mitral valve. In spite of this, the cusps move quite normally,[32] again suggesting vortices orthogonal to the main AV axis.

The Inflow Jet

The final factor to be considered in assessing mitral valve cusp motion is the nature of the jet of blood entering the left ventricle from the atrium. Its properties are remarkable, since at peak exercise, the normal stroke volume of 70–80 mL enters the left ventricle in 100 ms or less, without appreciable elevation of left atrial pressure. The normal inflow jet is directed toward the free wall of the ventricle, probably as a result of the asymmetrical anatomy of the anterior and posterior cusps of the mitral valve[33] (Fig. 12). During ejection, the outflow jet lies alongside the interventricular septum. This organized arrangement is lost after mitral valve replacement, when the inflow jet is abnormally directed and impinges in the septum. Inflow jet diameter at valve ring level can be estimated from the ratio of stroke volume to E wave stroke distance,[34] or measured directly by color flow Doppler or MRI.[26,35,36] These approaches all agree in suggesting that it is circular in cross-section with an area of 3–5 cm² with a flow profile that is approximately rectangular. Its area thus approximates to that between the mitral valve cusps during early rapid filling. Indeed, stroke volume can be derived using the distance between the mitral valve cusps as a measure of cross-sectional area, combined with stroke distance from pulsed Doppler. Peak blood velocity is attained within 1–2 cm of the mitral ring, and then

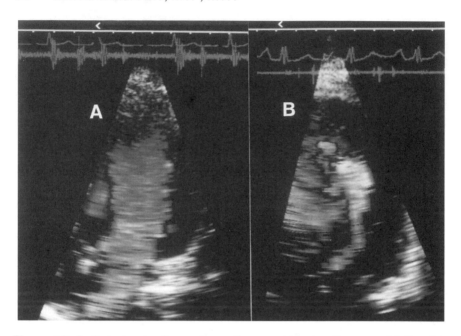

Figure 12. A. Apical color flow echocardiogram, showing the normal inflow jet, recorded at the time of peak early diastolic filling velocity. Note that the jet is directed toward the ventricular free wall, and is broad, occupying the whole mitral ring. The onset of vortex development (in blue) is also apparent. **B.** Similar recording from a patient with a restrictive filling pattern due to dilated cardiomyopathy. Note that the jet is narrow, occupying only a small part of the mitral ring. (Used with permission from Fujimoto S, et al.[37]) See color appendix.

falls off rapidly, so that by 4 cm into the cavity, it is considerably less than half the peak value. This fall in velocity is associated with momentum loss from the jet, due to lateral motion of blood in a direction perpendicular to the AV long axis.[37] The corresponding time relations show that this motion of blood out of the jet occurs within 30–40 ms of the start of flow, thus coinciding with the opening motion of the mitral valve. By 5 cm from the valve ring, there is little momentum left in the jet, but color flow demonstrates blood to move toward the outflow tract at mid-cavity level[38] during the period of mid-diastolic closure. It is this circular motion of blood from atrial to ventricular surfaces of the cusps that allows the valve to close. It can also be described in terms of a vortex, as noted in the early years of the century by Henderson.[39] More recently, in humans, they have been delineated by contrast angiography[40] and quantified from MRI images.[41] The normal filling vortex in humans has a radius of 1.6 ± 0.24 cm and an average angular velocity 30 ± 10 radians/s. Its calculated kinetic energy is thus 4.3 ± 0.7 J.10^{-4}. The properties of the inflow jet are thus those that allow the cusp movement necessary for mid-diastolic closure. In addition, its configuration greatly favors rapid filling. A large cross-sectional area, comparable to that of the ventricle at end-systole (Fig. 12), favors lower blood velocities, and thus lower accelerations and pressure gradients at any given filling rate, as expressed in mL/s. Similarly, the shorter the jet, the lower will be the pressure drop along it, as summed from the local pressure gradients. These conditions are subserved by a jet area approximately equal to the end-systolic cross-section of the ventricle, and that effectively terminates within 4 cm of the mitral ring, well short of the apex.[38]

The findings are quite different in dilated cardiomyopathy, where early diastolic inflow volumes and stroke distances are very high, although stroke volume itself is reduced.[26] This combination is due to a striking reduction in the cross-sectional area of the inflow jet often to less than 2 cm². At the same time, its length is increased to 6 cm or more, since lateral motion of blood from the jet is reduced. These abnormalities result in the total pressure drop along the jet rising to 10–15 mm Hg, suggesting that increased resistance to filling may arise purely on the basis of the hydraulic properties of the blood, quite independent of any change in the properties of the ventricle itself. In these circumstances, color flow usually shows the jet to be initially directed toward the free wall of the ventricle, forming a rotary motion around the apex and the septum. The reduced width of the jet is reflected in the smaller opening amplitude of the mitral cusps, which contributes to the increased E point septal separation characteristically seen in patients with a low ejection fraction.[42] Factors underlying this profound disturbance of the inflow jet are not understood, but may involve loss of restoring forces, which are probably responsible for the early diastolic motion of blood perpendicular to the axial jet. More puzzling is the physical basis of premature cusp separation, as it occurs both in patients with functional mitral regurgitation and also in those with incoordinate relaxation. Clearly there is an additional component of blood flow perpendicular to the AV axis whose nature and genesis is poorly understood. Techniques such as color flow Doppler, and particularly MRI, may throw further light on these problems in the near future, and in doing so, will lead to an increased understanding of flow disturbances in abnormal ventricles.

Conclusions

The function of a simple valve is to introduce an asymmetry at a single point in a circulation, making the resistance to flow in one direction much lower than that in the other. With the ideal valve, this difference should be large. If potential flow reversal should occur, and particularly with interrupted flow as occurs in a ventricle, the valve should respond rapidly and at low energy cost. These criteria are fully met by the normal mitral valve cusps whose unique anatomy and physical properties afford almost complete occlusion of the valve orifice during systole and virtually no resistance to blood flow during diastole. The change of state from one to the other is not instantaneous, but commensurate with that imposed on potential flow reversal by the inertia of blood. With the coupling between blood and valve motion imposed by the flexible cusps, the energy requirement for the change is very low, making the mechanism exquisitely sensitive to pressure differences of only 1–2 mm Hg.

A simple valve, as described above, is a bistable mechanism, alternating between very high and very low resistance to blood flow and momentum. However, the influence of the normal mitral valve is not confined to a single point in the circulation. Its asymmetrical cusps have the additional property of directing the jet of blood entering the ventricle away from the interventricular septum, thus extending its influence almost to the apex. Not only does this asymmetry appear to underlie orderly relations between ventricular filling and ejection but generates the vortices that cause mid- and late diastolic valve cusp motion, reducing the energy cost of eventual closure. This second asymmetry, by modifying jet direction, generates forces perpendicular to axial blood flow, and thus differs fundamentally from a simple change in orifice conductance.

Finally, a simple valve does not impart energy to the blood; rather it consumes a small amount to change its properties. The normal mitral apparatus, by contrast, includes longitudinally directed muscle fibers that move the ring around the blood. When it is displaced away from the cardiac apex during early diastole and atrial systole, ventricular volume increases without the necessity for an AV pressure gradient. When it moves toward the cardiac apex during ventricular systole, it does work on the left atrium, storing energy in its walls, and uses a small proportion of ventricular systolic energy to cause blood flow in the pulmonary veins. Thus, motion of the mitral ring imparts additional asymmetry to the circulation with regard to blood flow, which extends backward beyond the left atrium, by mechanisms quite independent of cusps movement. Techniques are only just becoming available by which flow in three dimensions can be studied and described. Understanding such flows within the left atrium and ventricle is a very complex field of study, but it seems likely that observations on the mitral valve in normal and abnormal hearts will play a significant part in their elucidation.

References

1. Harvey W. The movement of the heart and blood. Oxford, Blackwell, 1976, pp 124–125.
2. Little RC. Physiological basis for mitral valve function. In Boudoulas H, Woo-

ley CF (eds): Mitral Valve Prolapse and the Mitral Valve Prolapse Syndrome. Futura Publishing Co, Mount Kisco, NY, 1988, pp 67–88.

3. Wang K, Ho SY, Gibson DG, Anderson RH. Architecture of atrial musculature in humans. Br Heart J 1995;73:559–565, 1995.

4. Greenbaum RA, Ho SY, Gibson DG, Becker AE, Anderson RH. Left ventricular fibre architecture in man. Br Heart J 45:248–263, 1981.

5. Lian C. De la physiologie de l'appareil valvulaire mitral. J Anat Pathol Gen 11:597–612, 1909.

6. Ormiston JA, Shah PM, Tei C, Wong M. Size and motion of the mitral valve annulus in man: I. A two-dimensional echocardiographic method and findings in normal subjects. Circulation 64:113–120, 1981.

7. Feigenbaum H, Wolfe SB, Popp RL, Haine CL, Dodge HT. Correlation of ultrasound with angiography in measuring left ventricular volume. Am J Cardiol 23:111–120, 1969.

8. Keren G, Sonnenblick EH, LeJemtel TH. Mitral anulus motion: Relation to pulmonary venous and transmitral flows in normal subjects and patients with dilated cardiomyopathy. Circulation 78:621–629, 1988.

9. Jones CJH, Raposo L, Gibson DG. Functional importance of the long axis dynamics of the human left ventricle. Br Heart J 63:215–220, 1990.

10. Harvey W. The Movement of the Heart and Blood. Translated by G. Whitteridge. Oxford, Blackwell, 1976, pp 32–37.

11. Keith A. An account of the structures concerned in production of the jugular pulse. J Anat Physiol 42:1–25, 1907.

12. Nishimura RA, Abdel MD, Hatle LK, Tajik AJ. Relation of pulmonary vein to mitral flow velocities by transesophageal Doppler echocardiography: Effects of different loading conditions. Circulation 81:1488–1497, 1990.

13. Isaaz K, del Romeral LM, Lee E, Schiller NB. Quantification of the motion of the cardiac base in normal subjects by Doppler echocardiography. J Am Soc Echocardiogr 6:166–176, 1993.

14. Thomas JD, Weyman AE. Echocardiographic Doppler evaluation of left ventricular diastolic function. Circulation 84:977–990, 1991.

15. Jones CJH, Song GJ, Gibson DG. An echocardiographic assessment of atrial mechanical behaviour. Br Heart J 65:31–36, 1991.

16. Patterson SW, Piper H, Starling EH. The regulation of the heart beat. J Physiol 48:465–573, 1914

17. Braunwald E, Ross J Jr, Sonnenblick EH. Mechanisms of contraction in the normal and failing heart. N Engl J Med 277:1012–1010, 1967.

18. Burch GE, De Pasquale NP, Phillips JH. Clinical manifestations of papillary muscle dysfunction. Arch Intern Med 75:399–415, 1968.

19. Upton MT, Gibson DG, Brown DJ. Instantaneous mitral valve leaflet velocity and its relation to left ventricular wall movement in normal subjects. Br Heart J 38:51–58, 1976.

20. Henderson Y, Johnson E. Two modes of closure of the heart valves. Heart 14:69–82, 1912.

21. Smalcelj A, Gibson DG. Relation between mitral valve closure and early systolic function of the left ventricle. Br Heart J 53:436–442, 1985.

22. David D, Michelson EL, Naito M, Chen CC, Schaffenburg M, Dreifus L. Diastolic "locking" of the mitral valve: The importance of atrial systole and intraventricular volume. Circulation 67:640–645, 1985.

23. Fujimoto S, Parker KM, Xiao HB, Roy C, O'Sullivan C, Gibson DG. Association of reduced PR-AC interval with ventricular early potentials in dilated cardiomyopathy. Int J Cardiol 50:167–173, 1995.

24. Tsakiris AG, Gordon DA, Padiyar R, Frechette D. Relation of mitral valve opening and closure to left atrial and ventricular pressures in the intact dog. Am J Physiol (H) 234(Suppl H):146–151, 1978.
25. Shiima A. Analysis of opening and closing motion of the mitral valve by simultaneous echocardiographic and pressure tracing across the valve. J Cardiogr 6:653–662, 1976.
26. Fujimoto S, Parker KH, Xiao HB, Inge KSK, Gibson DG. Early diastolic left ventricular inflow pressures in normal subjects and patients with dilated cardiomyopathy: Reconstruction from pulsed Doppler Echocardiography. Br Heart J 74:419–425, 1995.
27. Brun P, Tribouilly C, Duval A-M, et al. Left ventricular flow propagation during early filling is related to wall relaxation: A color M-mode Doppler analysis. J Am Coll Cardiol 20:420–432, 1992.
28. Courtois M, Kovacs SJ, Ludbrook PA. Transmitral pressure-flow velocity relations: Importance of regional pressure gradients in the left ventricle during diastole. Circulation 78:661–671, 1988.
29. Park CH, Chow HW, Gibson DG. Phase differences between left ventricular wall motion and transmitral flow in man: Evidence for involvement of ventricular restoring forces in normal rapid filling. Int J Cardiol 24:347–354, 1989.
30. Henein M, Gibson DG. Suppression of left ventricular early diastolic filling by long axis asynchrony. Br Heart J 73:151–157, 1995.
31. Ng KSK, Gibson DG. Impairment of diastolic function by shortened filling period in severe left ventricular disease. Br Heart J 62:246–252, 1989.
32. Henein MY, Gibson DG. Abnormal subendocardial function in restrictive left ventricular disease. Br Heart J 72:237–242, 1994.
33. Beppu S, Izumi K, Nagata S, Park YD, Sakakibara H, Nimura Y. Abnormal blood pathways in left ventricular cavity in acute myocardial infarction. Circulation 78:157–164, 1988.
34. Singh B, Mohan JC. Atrioventricular valve orifice area in normal subjects; determination by cross-sectional and Doppler echocardiography. Int J Cardiol 44:85–91, 1994.
35. Samstad SO, Torp HG, Trinker D, et al. Cross sectional early mitral flow velocity profile from colour Doppler. Br Heart J 62:177–184, 1989.
36. Fujimoto S, Mohiaddin RH, Parker KH, Gibson DG. Magnetic resonance velocity mapping of normal human transmitral velocity profiles. Heart Vessels 10:236–240, 1995.
37. Fujimoto S, Parker KH, Xiao HB, Gibson DG. Detection and localization of early diastolic forces within the left ventricle from inflow jet dynamics: A comparison between normal subjects and patients with dilated cardiomyopathy. Heart Vessels 10:204–210, 1995.
38. Ihlen H. Assessment of diastolic function by 2-D colour flow. Heartforum 10(Suppl 1):45–48, 1996.
39. Bellhouse BJ. Mechanism of closure of the mitral valve. Clin Sci 39:13–23, 1970.
40. Reid KG. Mitral valve action and the mode of ventricular filling. Nature 223:1383–1384, 1969.
41. Kim YK, Walker PG, Pedersen EM, et al. Left ventricular blood flow patterns in normal subjects: A quantitative analysis by three-dimensional magnetic resonance velocity mapping. Circulation 26:224–238, 1995.
42. Massie BM, Schiller NB, Ratshin RA, Parmley WW. Mitral-septal separation: New echocardiographic index of left ventricular function. Am J Cardiol 39:1008–1016, 1977.

Part III

The Floppy Mitral Valve:
The Pathologists

Introduction

The Floppy Mitral Valve, Mitral Valve Prolapse, Mitral Valvular Regurgitation: *The Pathologists*

Charles F. Wooley, MD, Hariosis Boudoulas, MD, PhD

There are times when certain investigative studies open broad vistas with access to previously unexplored areas. Pathologists and morphologists pointed out the discrete characteristics of floppy mitral valves (FMVs) at autopsy in the 1940s, emphasizing that the FMVs were distinct entities when compared to chronic rheumatic valvular disease. They also recognized certain clinical correlates—the long natural history of the disorder, FMV susceptibility to infectious endocarditis, the occurrence of ruptured chordae tendinae, the progressive nature of the mitral valvular regurgitation (MVR), and the relatively late onset of congestive heart failure.

There are several clinical-pathologic studies that stand out in the development of medical thought about the FMV. In 1944, Bailey and Hickam[1] described the pathologic changes in seven patients with rupture of mitral chordae tendinae in the absence of infectious endocarditis. Six of the seven patients were men, ages ranging from 48 to 70 years. Valve cusp abnormalities not typical of chronic rheumatic valvular disease were noted in five patients. These changes included mitral valve fibrosis and thickening without stenosis, considerable ballooning of the affected posterior cusps, and dense hyaline fibrous tissue in the central portions of the valve cusps with increased connective tissue in the mitral chordae. The illustrative photographs show enlarged redundant FMVs. Clinical correlates included abrupt or insidious congestive heart failure, new or recent onset loud mitral systolic murmurs with thrills, atrial fibrillation, cardiomegaly, and systolic pulsation of the left atrium at fluoroscopy.

From: Boudoulas H, Wooley CF. *Mitral Valve: Floppy Mitral Valve, Mitral Valve Prolapse, Mitral Valvular Regurgitation.* Second revised edition. ©Futura Publishing Company, Armonk, NY, 2000.

We asked Dr. Orville T. Bailey in 1989 about his recollections of the 1944 study. His gracious reply included the following: "John Hickam and I undertook the papers at my urging to get John started writing and it was his first paper. We realized that the cases did not well fit the prevailing rheumatic fever dogma and in our own minds we left a big question mark on etiology."

"Pure" mitral regurgitation as described in England by Brigden and Leatham in 1953[2] involved 30 patients, males predominating, without a history of rheumatic fever. The authors emphasized the long natural history of the disorder, the susceptibility to bacterial endocarditis, and the late onset of congestive heart failure that was usually rapidly progressive. While the 1944 Bailey–Hickam clinical analyses were retrospective, Brigden and Leatham had been personally involved in the clinical evaluation and contemporary diagnostic studies in their patients. Eight patients had known of a murmur for more than 25 years, in one "the date being settled by an examination for military service in the First World War." The mitral orifice was dilated in eight of the nine patients who came to necropsy and the mitral valves were described as "thickened and deformed." The illustrations were those of exuberant FMVs.

Clinicians and pathologists remained preoccupied with rheumatic fever as the predominant cause of valvular heart disease and were slow to accept the etiological and pathodynamic significance of the FMVs. However, descriptions of the FMV as a discrete pathological entity accelerated during the next several decades.

Fernex and Fernex used the term "mucoid degeneration" in 1958 to describe the histologic changes in mitral valves from two older patients with mitral regurgitation; they spoke of mitral valves with multiple "domes," with "augmentation" of the valve surface without clinical evidence of the Marfan syndrome. Their study reinforced the concept of a connective tissue etiology for FMV, and may be seen as a successor of earlier papers linking the Marfan syndrome with the FMV and as the precursor to Read's 1965 clinical surgical study.

Beginning in the middle and late 1960s, multiple reports were published that described the morphology of the floppy mitral valve. In time, these studies overlapped and then complemented the numerous clinical studies dealing with the "systolic click–late systolic murmur syndrome" and mild mitral valvular regurgitation. What the FMV did, i.e., the FMV prolapsed, was linked to FMV content and composition.

Pomerance emphasized the spectrum of pathological change in the FMV in 1969 and 1972—from enlargement of only the posterior cusp of the mitral valve to involvement of both mitral cusps, and in certain cases with involvement of the tricuspid valve as well. Mitral valve cusps were thickened, opaque, and voluminous; mitral chordae became attenuated and might rupture; characteristic histologic changes involving the valve fibrosa were present; the severity of the condition was variable from localized areas of ballooning in the center of the posterior cusp to gross ectasia of the entire valve. Prolapse of the voluminous cusps into the left atrium during systole resulted in mitral regurgitation. Stretching of the affected leaflets resulted in endocardial damage; this is an important observation that requires further attention. The influence of genetic factors and the relation to heritable connective tissue disorders were also discussed as modifications of traditional concepts.

Many of the leading cardiac pathologists, among them Alfred Angrist, Jesse Edwards, and William Roberts, participated in the expansion of knowledge that occurred during the 1960s through the 1980s, as pathologists, clinicians, and cardiovascular surgeons became aware of the frequency of the FMV in the pathogenesis of mitral valvular disease. From our vantage point, the landmark FMV study by Michael Davies et al. in 1978 deserves particular attention. A prospective study of approximately 2000 consecutive autopsies in London hospitals using a standardized approach at autopsy to mitral valve morphology, function, and clinical significance was directed to evaluate the incidence and severity of FMVs. Clinically significant FMVs were found in 3.9% of the men and 5.2% of the women, severely FMVs were not apparent until age 40, and the incidence of severe FMVs increased with age. Prolapse was limited to the posterior mitral leaflet in about 67% of the hearts, affected the anterior leaflet in 10%, and involved both leaflets in 23%. Morphological grading used in this study was valuable since the more severe valvular abnormalities were associated with serious complications, while minor morphological abnormalities were not clinically significant, important natural history data.

The distinctive morphological features of the FMV, in particular, the chordal architecture, and the natural history correlations have also been studied in meticulous detail by Anton Becker and his associates. Thus, the following contribution by Anton Becker (Fig. 1) and Michael Davies (Fig. 2) in Chapter 4 represents the views of two premier cardiovascular pathologists who have been deeply involved in the genesis of thought about the FMV.[3] Their meticulous analysis of what is known about the fundamentals of FMV content, composition, organization, and expression provides the basis for understanding the clinical relevance and mechanisms of dysfunction of FMVs. Importantly, Becker and Davies also emphasize what remains unknown, providing a platform for future thought and investigation.

In Chapter 5, our colleague, Peter Baker, extends the pathomorphological approach to include the FMV structural and physical characteristics that are fundamental to our understanding of the many facets that contribute to the FMV mosaic.

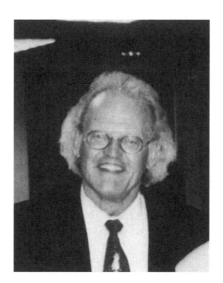

Figure 1. Dr. Anton Becker.

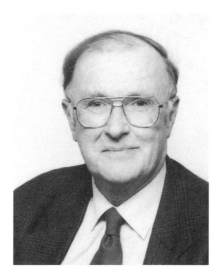

Figure 2. Dr. Michael Davies.

References

1. Bailey OT, Hickam JB. Rupture of mitral chordae tendineae. Am Heart J 28:578–600, 1944.
2. Brigden W, Leatham A. Mitral incompetence. Br Heart J 15:55–73, 1953.
3. Wooley CF, Baker PB, Kolibash AJ, Kilman JW, Sparks EA, Boudoulas H. The floppy myxomatous mitral valve, mitral valve prolapse, and mitral regurgitation. Prog Cardiovasc Dis 6:397–433, 1991.

4

Pathomorphology of Mitral Valve Polapse

Anton E. Becker, MD,
Michael J. Davies, MD

Introduction

The pathological basis of prolapse of the mitral valve remains a contentious topic despite the vast increase in clinical experiences. Indeed, the presence of prolapse may vary within a given cardiac cycle, may vary from day to day, and most significantly, may develop or disappear with aging. The pathologist is constrained having to deal with the valve as a specimen only, whether it is still within the heart or surgically excised. The clinician, however, can obtain information about the motion of the leaflets of the mitral valve in real-time and can chart variations day by day or year by year. Despite this, the morphologist can still play a major role in unraveling of the pathological background of the prolapse of the leaflets of the mitral valve. A review of the morphological evidence relevant to this event relies heavily on the understanding of the normal morphology of the mitral valve apparatus as discussed in Chapter 1. Without this information, in our opinion, it is impossible to understand the mechanics of prolapse.

Definitions

Prolapse of the leaflets of the mitral valve describes the situation in which, during ventricular systole, the leaflets extend above the plane of the

From: Boudoulas H, Wooley CF. *Mitral Valve: Floppy Mitral Valve, Mitral Valve Prolapse, Mitral Valvular Regurgitation.* Second revised edition. ©Futura Publishing Company, Armonk, NY, 2000.

atrioventricular junction so that they lie within the cavity of the left atrium (Fig. 1). In the setting of a normal mitral valve, the leaflets coapt during ventricular systole but do not extend above the level of the junction being restrained within the ventricular cavity by the tension apparatus (Fig. 2). Prolapse as thus defined can be produced by several mechanisms. For example, rupture of a papillary muscle due to myocardial infarction, or rupture of tendinous chords due to bacterial endocarditis, will certainly produce prolapse. Similarly, abnormal wall motion in the setting of myocardial ischemia can result in prolapse of a segment of valve leaflet in the dyskinetic area of the left ventricle. One may take this one step further and consider the fact that a relatively high proportion of fit young individuals may show minor upward movement of the cusps on echocardiography, often so minor that echocardiographers may disagree among themselves on its clinical significance. It is this sort of trivial "echo-prolapse" that one may consider as "physiological prolapse." A condemnable term—if one so wishes—but certainly highlighting the problems of defining precisely what is normal versus abnormal when it comes to judging mitral valve mobility, and a phenomenon with a major impact on the young if not considered in its proper perspective. Be that as it may, these, and other

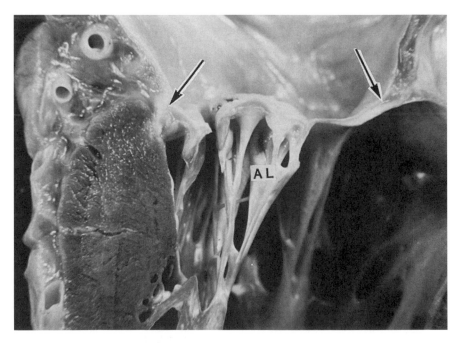

Figure 1. A long-axis section through a floppy mitral valve. The aortic leaflet (AL) extends above the plane of the atrioventricular junction (arrows) into the cavity of the left atrium. The valve has been fixed in the closed position by perfusion.

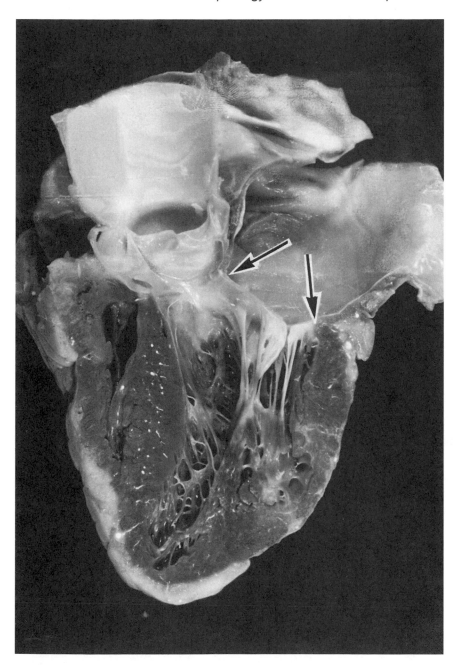

Figure 2. Long-axis section through a normal mitral valve in the closed position. The leaflets coapt but do not extend above the level of the junction, being restrained in the ventricular cavity by the tension apparatus.

manifold mechanisms, can be considered as *secondary* prolapse. We are not concerned with them in this chapter. Our topic is the lesion we describe as *primary* prolapse of the mitral valve, in which there is no identified cause other than an abnormality of the valve leaflets and their supporting chords. It is the pathology of these abnormalities that is to be described, along with discussions of their still questionable etiology and pathogenesis.

In our experience, primary prolapse is always associated with the morphological entity we will describe as the *floppy valve.* In other words, from our morphological stance, we can state that we have never seen a case of prolapse of unknown origin, at autopsy or following surgical resection, in which the valve leaflets were normal.

Our attention, therefore, will be focused on the floppy valve. Even within this setting, there are variations in the morphological appearances that require strict definition. In the normal valve, pockets between chordal insertions of the leaflets often point toward the atria without, in themselves, being abnormal. This appearance is described as *hooding* and is not indicative of prolapse. Prolapse itself can exist in two forms. In the first, the valve leaflets are noted to coapt during systole but still to extend above the level of the atrioventricular junction. We will describe this appearance as ballooning (Fig. 3). This would result hemodynamically in valve pro-

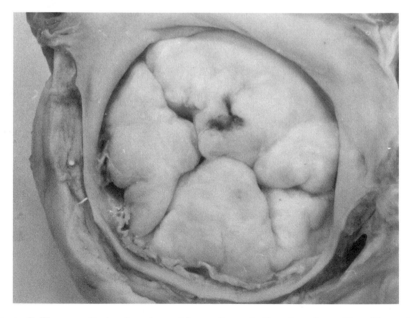

Figure 3. Floppy mitral valve viewed from above in the closed position. The valve leaflets still coapt but they bulge into the left atrium cavity giving the so-called "ballooning" appearance.

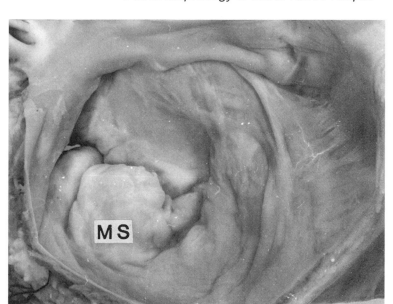

Figure 4. Floppy mitral valve. The free edge of the middle scallop (MS) of the mural leaflet overshoots above the level of the atrioventricular junction.

lapse without valvar insufficiency. The more florid form of prolapse exists when the free edge of a valve leaflet extends above the level of the atrioventricular junction (Fig. 4). Such overshoot would, in most cases, produce regurgitation through the valve.

Pathological Findings

The Atrioventricular Junction

All previous workers who have studied prolapsed valves have used the terms "ring" and "annulus" synonymously in describing dilation of the atrioventricular junction. Such dilation is regarded by some[1,2] as one of the characteristic features of the floppy valve, being said to be more marked in those patients with severe regurgitation. In these patients, the mean annular circumference was more than 65% above normal values. In contrast, in patients with floppy but competent valves, the annular circumference was found to be less than 30% above normal. Junctional dilation, however, has been found less frequently by others. In one series, studied at necropsy, the junction was found to be dilated in only 7% of the cases.[3]

When present, dilation of the junction in a minimally regurgitative valve indicates primary (or intrinsic) dilation rather than dilation due to left atrial or left ventricular enlargement.[4] In terms of the precise structure of the annulus itself, we have discovered the same range of variation as found in normal hearts. This holds both for the site of abnormalities around the junction and for the type of collagen aggregation (thread-like ring or curtain-like features). The only difference we noted between normal and floppy valves was the thickened leaflets in floppy valves. In our material, the so-called disjunction reported by Hutchins and his colleagues[5] was found as frequently in normal as in prolapsed valves.

The Leaflets

The macroscopic appearance of the floppy valve is characteristic and easily recognizable.[6] It is typified by the presence of redundant leaflets with a dome-like expansion projecting toward the left atrial cavity (Fig. 5). In some valves thus deformed, the ballooning leaflets are still able to coapt and ensure a sealed line of closure. These valves, therefore, remain com-

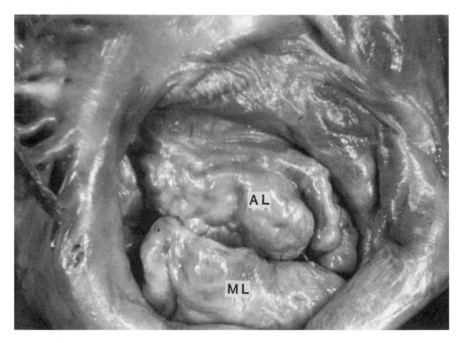

Figure 5. A floppy mitral valve viewed from above with the characteristic dome-like expansion of both aortic (AL) and mural (ML) leaflets toward the left atrial cavity.

petent. In other instances, the free edge of the affected leaflet does not appose, instead showing a distinct overshoot. Mitral regurgitation is then inevitable. In the majority of cases, the dome-shape leaflets are white and thickened. This is the result of fibrosis secondary to the impact between the leaflets (the injury lesions) or to the tension on the stretched tissue (the stress lesions).[7] The valve has a soft consistency. It does not present the rigidity felt in a valve distorted by rheumatism.[8] The opaque leaflets also lack the usual transparency of the normal valve as seen when transluminated[9] (Fig. 6). In some instances, nonetheless, the valve does appear translucent and gelatinous. The atrial aspect of the leaflets is usually smooth. When there is regurgitation, the overshooting leaflets show a rolled free edge (Fig. 7). An important gross distinction from rheumatic endocarditis is that the commissures of the floppy valve are not fused.[7]

The leaflets are not uniformly distorted and abnormal, rather presenting a spectrum of severity from partial (Fig. 8) to complete involvement (Fig. 9). The mural leaflet is most frequently involved, either in isolation or together with the aortic one. Isolated involvement of the aortic leaflet is rare (Fig. 10). When the mural leaflet is deformed, the middle

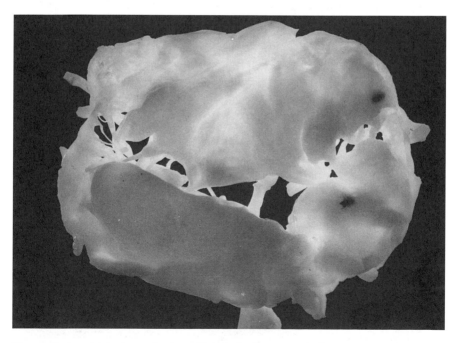

Figure 6. An atrial view of a transilluminated, resected, floppy mitral valve. The middle scallop of the mural leaflet shows a dome-like deformity with overshoot. The dome shows marked decrease in transparency because of fibrotic thickening. (Used with permission from Van der Bel-Kahn, et al.[6])

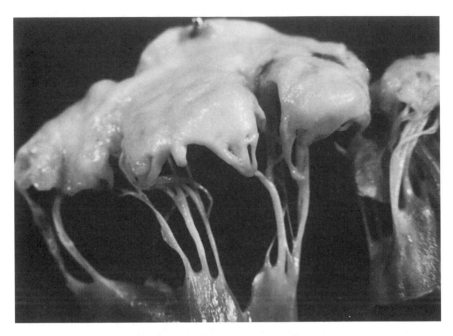

Figure 7. The mural leaflet of a resected floppy mitral valve. The overshooting leaflet shows a rolled edge.

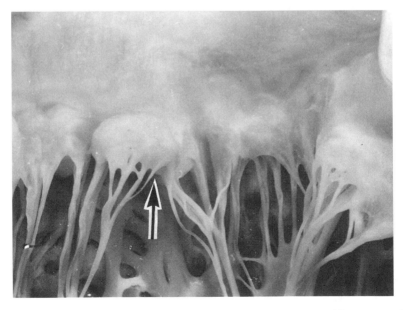

Figure 8. The mural leaflet of a floppy mitral valve in an opened heart revealing partial involvement (arrow) of the leaflet.

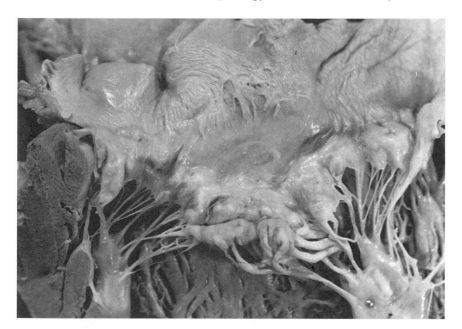

Figure 9. A floppy mitral valve in an opened heart revealing complete involvement of the leaflets.

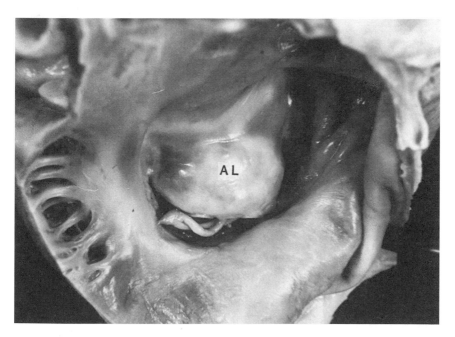

Figure 10. A floppy mitral valve viewed from above with involvement of the aortic leaflet (AL).

scallop is likely to be the portion that prolapses (Fig. 11). It is the component of the aortic leaflet closest to the posteromedial commissure that is most frequently and severely deformed. The precise configuration of leaflet involvement differs in variously reported series. According to Davies, prolapse was limited to the mural leaflet in about 67% of hearts studied, affected the aortic leaflet in 10%, and involved both leaflets in 23%.[3] In the series described by Olsen,[10] half of the patients were said to have involvement of both leaflets, but this referred to the adjacent segments of the leaflets at the posteromedial commissure.

Histologically, the leaflets show gross abnormalities of the collagen making up their central fibrous layer. Large areas show apparent loss of fibrous tissue with fragmentation, coiling, and disruption of the individual collagen bundles (Fig. 12). The fibrous layer is usually better preserved at the base of the leaflet but tapers out toward the periphery with increasing deposition of myxomatous tissue. Maximal destruction occurs around the sites of chordal insertion, although the changes may extend into the body of the leaflets. The rolled edges are made up of sponge-like tissue. The areas of destruction of collagen usually contain easily demonstrable pools of glycosaminoglycans in which lie residual strands of collagen. Some descriptions have emphasized the expansion of the spongy layer at the expense of the fibrous one.[7,11] The secondary fibrosis produces "pads" of fi-

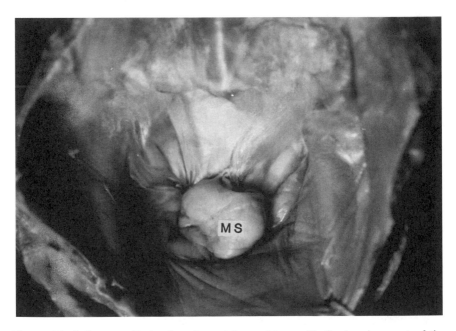

Figure 11. A floppy mitral valve viewed from above with the involvement of the middle scallop (MS) of the mural leaflet.

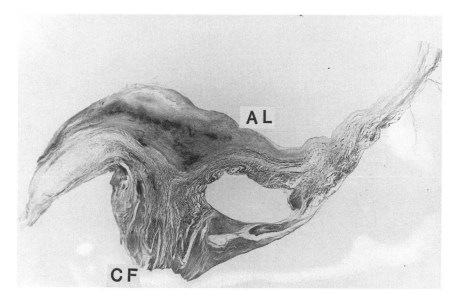

Figure 12. Histological section through a leaflet from a floppy mitral valve. There is disruption of the fibrous layer. Chordal fusion is apparent (CF). The atrial layer shows fibrotic thickening due to regurgitation (AL). Elastic tissue stain ×7.

brous tissue on the atrial and ventricular surfaces. Sometimes the fibrosis extends from the ventricular surface down to the chordal attachments.

Aggregates of fibrin and platelets (so-called platelet-rich thrombi) are commonly seen on the atrial surface near the apposition line and are also found under the mural leaflet at its junction with the ventricular wall[11] (Fig. 13). These aggregates, if embolized, are said to be responsible for the transient ischemic retinal and cerebral episodes that are suffered by some patients with floppy valves.[12,13] In the absence of a history of bacterial endocarditis, the valve leaflets are not vascularized and do not contain inflammatory cells. Calcification may occur in the leaflets of the floppy valve, even if only rarely. When present, it is mainly the basal aspect of the mural leaflet that is affected.[7] Bacterial endocarditis is another complication of the floppy valve. Signs of this inflammatory process, which begins particularly on the atrial face of the mural leaflet as a consequence of trauma, may be detected in floppy leaflets. They were seen in 18 of 300 patients (6%) with long-term follow-up in the Amsterdam series (unpublished data).

The Tendinous Chords

The tendinous chords undergo similar changes to those seen in the leaflets, becoming either elongated and attenuated or thickened and fi-

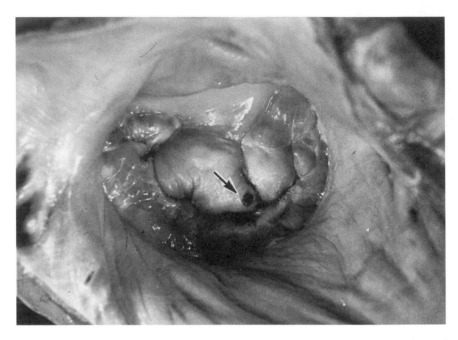

Figure 13. A floppy mitral valve viewed from above showing a thrombus (arrow) localized near the apposition line of the aortic leaflet.

brotic (Fig. 14). An inspection of the ventricular aspect of resected valves reveals major deviations in the pattern of chordal branching and anchorage[9] (Fig. 15). All type of chords are involved, although not always to the same degree and extent. The chord supporting the posteromedial commissure is the one commonly affected. The main general alteration consists of a marked decrease in chordal branching points and a wide separation of their sites of anchorage to the leaflets.[9] Whether the abnormal anchorage and branching is a primary process or secondary to the deformity of the leaflets remains controversial. The chords are often thick near the site of their insertion and are sometimes adherent, particularly at the site of doming (Fig. 16). The ventricular surface of the dome itself often shows chaotically arranged chord-like roots (Fig. 17). The chords of the mural leaflet, when elongated, constantly rub on the mural endocardium of the left ventricle. As a result, linear thickening of the mural endocardium is seen. In more advanced stages, the individual mural lesions tend to coalesce with resulting prominent white elevations of the endocardium. In extreme cases, the chords adhere to the thickened wall (Fig. 18). This process causes effective shortening of the involved chords and restraint of the motion of the mural leaflet.[14] Focal myxomatous changes or fibrosis extending from the ventricular surface of the leaflets can be noted histologi-

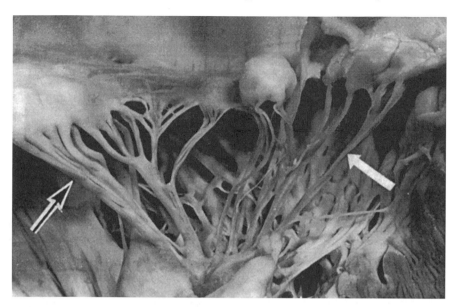

Figure 14. Tendinous chords of a floppy valve showing both elongation and attenuation (white arrow) and thickening and fibrosis (black arrow).

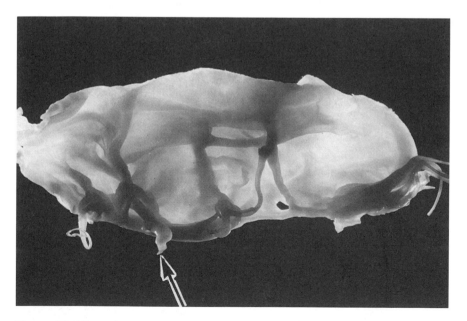

Figure 15. The ventricular view of the middle scallop of a floppy mitral valve, showing abnormal insertion and arborization of chords, together with chordal rupture (arrow).

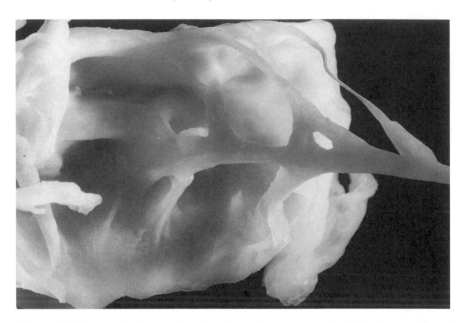

Figure 16. The ventricular surface of a dome-shaped mural leaflet with an unusual pattern of chordal insertion, associated with thickening of the chords and leaflets. (Used with permission from Van der Bel-Kahn J, et al.[9])

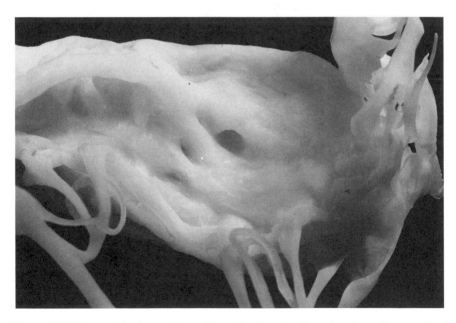

Figure 17. The ventricular surface of a prolapsing scallop showing effacement of chords, still recognizable as ridges. Part of this probably due to fusion of ruptured chords. (Used with permission from Van der Bel-Kahn J, et al.[9])

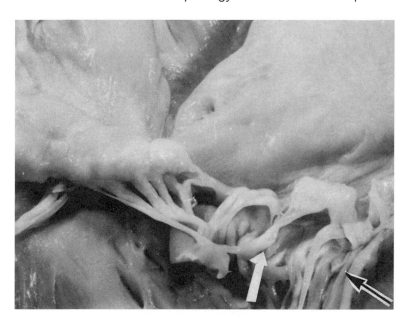

Figure 18. The mural leaflet of a floppy mitral valve showing the characteristic linear endocardial thickening (black arrow) resulting from the chords hitting the ventricle and adhesion of chords to the wall (white arrow). The head of the papillary muscle has been cut.

cally. Some chords present a thin, localized narrowing. This is held to be the point where rupture, if likely, will occur.[15] There is a different reported preponderance[2] in chordal rupture between material obtained surgically and that seen at necropsy (77% down to 30%).[16] Chords that rupture are usually related to the area with the dome-like deformity (Fig. 19). Rupture affects most frequently the mural leaflet, particulary its middle scallop (Fig. 20). Ruptured chords were observed in the mural leaflet in 54% of patients studied in one series of valves obtained at surgery. They were found in the aortic leaflet in 22.7% and were present in both leaflets in 4.5%.[3] Stumps of ruptured chords may fold back and fuse into the ventricular surface of the leaflets. The presence of fibrotic changes in the leaflets in areas that have not lost their chordal support, together with the friction lesion on the mural endocardium in correspondence to ruptured chords, gives strong support to the concept that prolapse of the leaflet was a feature present before chordal rupture.

Papillary Muscles and Ventricular Myocardium

Fibrous lesions of the left ventricular endocardium with or without chordal adhesions are well described. The lesions are regarded as friction

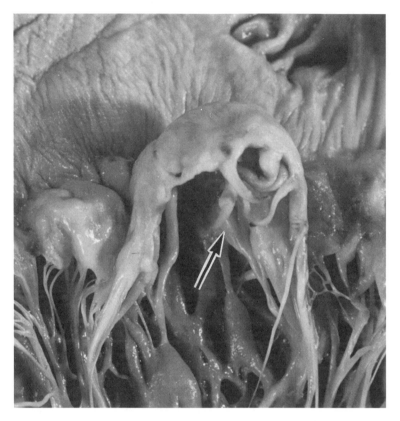

Figure 19. Chordal rupture (arrow) corresponding to the dome-like deformity in a floppy mitral valve.

lesions.[14] A few reports have described fibrosis and scarring of the papillary muscles. These are said to be the result of abnormal tension and subsequent ischemia on the papillary muscle (vasoconstriction of the artery supplying the papillary muscles).[17] Apart from these changes, there are no other myocardial abnormalities. Sudden death, even though rare, can occur in patients with floppy valve.[18] The true incidence may well have been exaggerated. From the pathologist's point of view, moreover, there is a distinct problem in "pointing the finger." For instance, in case of an individual with a clear family history of floppy mitral valve with or without ventricular arrhythmias, and normal myocardium at autopsy, the pathologist will be inclined to ascribe the floppy mitral valve as the cause of death. But, in individuals with a floppy valve associated with distinct myocardial interstitial fibrosis, often maximized in the posterolateral wall, the question arises to what extent these myocardial alterations are secondary to long-standing mitral valve prolapse and, hence, sudden death primarily of "ar-

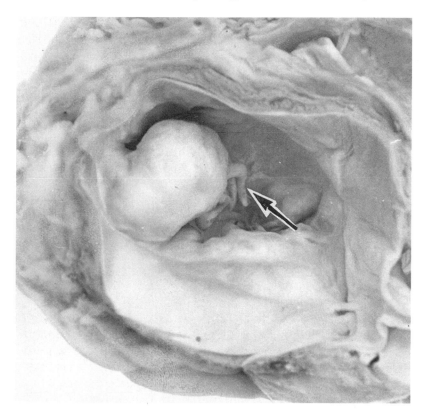

Figure 20. Chordal rupture (arrow) affecting the middle scallop of the mural leaflet.

rhythmogenic" myocardial origin. And, on top of that, the pathologist may be confronted with the individual who died suddenly and unexpectedly and in whom autopsy revealed a floppy mitral valve without a family history or prior syncopal attacks and without left ventricular myocardial abnormalities. Is this sudden death due to a floppy mitral valve? Without any further evidence to support an alternative mode of sudden death, there is the temptation to consider the floppy mitral valve as the cause of death. But, admittedly this is a calculated guess without supporting "hard facts."

Concepts of Pathogenesis

Many theories have been advanced to explain the pathogenesis of the floppy leaflets since Reid[19] proposed a mitral valvar origin for mid-systolic click and late systolic murmurs and Barlow[20] published angiographic evidence correlating the systolic click and murmurs with prolapse of the mitral valve. The prolapse was presumed due to redundancy of the leaflets and chords, these features permitting early systolic competence but late systolic overshoot. The clicks were ascribed to abrupt tension of leaflets and chords (Reid's chordal snap) in accord with the observation that these sounds coincided with maximal prolapse of the leaflets. As Jeresaty argued,[21] these theories can be considered in terms of two main viewpoints. The first stresses the abnormality of the valve, while the second postulates myocardial involvement. The so-called myocardial theory is based primarily on angiographic and hemodynamic findings. Thus, the myocardial segmental contraction anomalies designated by some authors as "segmental cardiomyopathy" could theoretically produce an abnormality in the function of the mitral valve apparatus.[22-30] While the myocardium undoubtedly plays a major role in the secondary prolapse, there are no pathological findings to support such a theory in the setting of primary prolapse. Instead, most morphological evidence lends credence to an abnormality of the valve as being responsible for prolapse.

The Valvular Hypothesis

Within the concept of the abnormality of the valve itself, there remain several schools of thought. Some ascribe the prolapse to primary deficiency of the structure of the leaflet. Myxomatous degeneration of the leaflets is said to be the underlying mechanism responsible for their prolapse.[1,3,7,10,11,31] According to this concept, the weakness of the dense collagenous fibrous layer, which is normally the supporting structure of the valve, allows stretching of the leaflets either in normal or altered hemodynamic conditions. The result is redundancy and doming of the leaflets and elongation of the tendinous chords. The fibrous friction lesions of the left posterior ventricular wall and the fibroelastic thickening of the chords are held to be secondary phenomena. Some authors[10] have suggested that the weakness of the leaflets could be due to a genetically determined increase in the thickness of the spongy layer. Support for this approach is provided by the known familial nature of the disorder[32-36] and its low incidence.[37,38] These findings can be interpreted in terms of an autosomal dominant mode of inheritance with variable expressivity.[39,40]

In this context, Read proposed, as long ago as 1965, that isolated floppy valves are a "forme fruste" of Marfan syndrome.[41] Indeed, although not a universal association, there is no question that floppy mitral valve is associated with inherited disorders of connective tissue.[42,43] Floppy valves are frequent findings in patients with Marfan syndrome,[44-47] osteogenesis imperfecta,[48,49] Ehlers-Danlos syndrome,[50,51] cutis laxa, and pseudoxanthoma elasticum.[52] These connective tissue diseases present different biochemical defects that as their final common pathway, affect the synthesis of collagen and elastin.

The most prominent in this context, is Marfan syndrome. The disease has been assigned to a "Marfan locus" on chromosome 15,[53] which harbors the gene that encodes for fibrillin, an extracellular matrix glycoprotein that serves as a precursor for elastin. However, the gene for fibrillin codes for an array of repeating structural domains and, hence, one may state that from the viewpoint of the molecular biologist, a spectrum of different genotypes exists, analogous to the spectrum of different Marfan phenotypes. Indeed, genotype-phenotype correlation becomes even more complicated, taking into account the mutated gene behind Marfan syndrome. Thus, any hint of a family history of floppy mitral valve is a marker to consider the fibrillin gene, but the size of the gene makes genetic screening a research exercise, per family, rather than a routine diagnostic test, a worthy consideration in a consultation case.

In osteogenesis imperfecta, the synthesis of type I collagen is known to be defective.[49] It is insufficient production of type III collagen that is the primary abnormality in the "type IV" variant of Ehlers-Danlos syndrome.[54] In both cutis laxa and pseudoxanthoma elasticum, there is well-recognized degeneration of elastic fibers.[55,56] Variable changes in biochemical makeup have been reported in patients with "isolated" floppy valve. The accumulation of mucopolysaccharides seems to be secondary to abnormality of collagen and elastin.[57,58] Hammer[59] found an absence of types II and V collagen. Lee,[60] in contrast, found all types of collagen to be present in the floppy valves. A defect in the synthesis of type III collagen in the skin of affected members of a family was reported.[61] Cole[62] found an increase in types III and V collagen and in glycoaminoglycans, but these were regarded as a "repair response" to repetitive injury of prolapsed leaflets. In a study of 32 floppy and 35 normal mitral valves at St. George's Hospital, it was shown that total amounts of collagen, proteoglycans, and elastin are increased approximately threefold in floppy valves. The most significant changes in floppy valves were the 59% increase in mean value of the proteoglycan content, a large increase in the ease of extractability of proteoglycans from 26.7% to 57.2% of the total, and a 62% increase in mean value of the elastin content in the anterior leaflets. The results obtained for normal and floppy valves are summarized in Table 1. As far as the type III/III + I collagen ratio is concerned, the normal human mitral valve was shown to contain a mean value of 29.3% and 26.6% type III/III + I collagen for leaflets and chords, respectively. The ratio observed in floppy valves was confirmed to be dependent on the extent of secondary fibrosis. In valves with considerable fibrosis, the percentage of type III collagen increased. In patients with negligible fibrosis, the percentage of type III collagen decreased. We still do not know whether it is diminished synthesis or increased lysis that starts the process. All the multiple steps in collagen organization could be involved. A lytic theory[63] was

Table 1
Analysis of the Leaflets and Chords from Normal and Floppy Mitral Valves

		Normal	No. of Valves	Floppy	No. of Valves
Wet weight (g)	leaflets	1.4 ± 0.4	26	*4.4 ± 2.7	24
	chords	0.2 ± 0.09	22	+0.6 ± 0.6	25
Water content	leaflets	81.8 ± 2.6	19	82.7 ± 3.8	21
(% wet weight)	chords	74.7 ± 4.7	18	80.0 ± 4.3	19
Collagen content	leaflets	57.0 ± 7.5	40	59.2 ± 15.9	32
(% dry weight)	chords	64.5 ± 12.6	32	*72.7 ± 11.1	28
Elastin content	leaflets	10.0 ± 1.7	33	12.7 ± 5.8	28
(% dry weight)	chords	9.7 ± 2.1	31	11.4 ± 4.9	28
Hexuronic acid					
content (μg/mg	leaflets	9.8 ± 0.9	20	*15.6 ± 4.2	21
dry weight)	chords	9.0 ± 1.4	19	13.2 ± 6.7	18

* Student's t test showed significant difference from the normal cusp valve $p < 0.001$, + $p < 0.005$.

proposed, although degradation by collagenase seems improbable because of the high levels of tissue inhibitor of collagenases in floppy valves.

Chordal Support

The possibility that the leaflet prolapse (particularly in older people) could be due to lack of uniform chordal support was promoted by Becker and de Wit.[64] Their hypothesis received subsequent support from the observed gross morphology of a series of floppy valves.[9] This study revealed marked deviations in both chordal branching and anchoring of the affected leaflets. The chordal concept suggests that the myxomatous degeneration of the floppy valve is a secondary result of undue stress on the connective tissue of the valve lacking uniform chordal support. Over the years, degeneration thus induced could lead to prolapse of the leaflets.

Synthesis of Theories of Pathogenesis

It is clear from our review that the pathogenesis of the floppy valve remains controversial. The gradual increase in the frequency of floppy mitral valve with age[3,31] suggests strongly that hemodynamic stresses gradually deform the weakened valves, progressively revealing the underlying defect. All of the theories postulated thus far can be interpreted in terms of the age-dependent expression of a genetically determined disorder. The body of evidence presented by different groups supporting different theories suggests the possibility of etiological heterogeneity resulting in a common morphological feature. Undue mechanical stress on leaflets with the consequent connective tissue changes could be the result of a congenitally determined chordal pattern that fails to support the leaflets adequately. Alternatively, it may represent a biochemical disorder of collagen that may have no apparent effect in childhood but, instead expresses itself later in life. Furthermore, the biochemically determined weakness could be present in the same anatomically weakened valve. Indeed, both may be necessary for manifestation of the prolapse. The observed biochemical and pathological findings suggest the existence of a repair process with an increased production of glycoaminoglycans and collagen. At the present time our opinion is that these are a secondary response to a primary defect not yet defined with precision, but with genetic influences and a well-recognized spectrum of insufficient chordal support being important factors.

References

1. King BD, Clark MA, Baba N, Kilman JW, Wooley CF. "Myxomatous" mitral valves: Collagen dissolution as the primary defect. Circulation 66:288–296, 1982.
2. Bulkley BH, Roberts WC: Dilatation of the mitral annulus: A rare cause of mitral regurgitation. Am J Med 59:457–463, 1975.
3. Davies MJ, Moore BP, Braimbridge MV. The floppy mitral valve. Study of incidence, pathology, and complications in surgical, necropsy, and forensic material. Br Heart J 40:468–481, 1978.
4. Ormiston JA, Shah PM, Tei C, Wong M. Size and motion of the mitral valve annulus in man. II. Abnormalities in mitral valve prolapse. Circulation 65:713–719, 1982.
5. Hutchins GM, Moore GW, Skoog DK. The association of floppy mitral valve with disjunction of the mitral annulus fibrosus. N Engl J Med 314:535–540, 1986.
6. Van der Bel-Kahn J, Becker AE. The surgical pathology of rheumatic and floppy mitral valves: Distinctive morphologic features upon gross examination. Am J Surg Pathol 10:282–292, 1986.
7. Shrivastava S, Guthrie RB, Edwards JE. Prolapse of the mitral valve. Mod Concepts Cardiovasc Dis 46:57–61, 1977.
8. Davies MJ. Aetiology and pathology of the diseased mitral valve. In Ionescu MI, Cohn LH (ed.): Mitral Valve Disease Diagnosis and Treatment. London, Butterworths, 1985, pp 27–42.
9. Van der Bel-Kahn J, Duren DR, Becker AE. Isolated mitral valve prolapse: Chordal architecture as an anatomic basis in older patients. J Am Coll Cardiol 5:1335–1340, 1985.
10. Olsen EGJ, Al-Rufaie HK. The floppy mitral valve: Study on pathogenesis. Br Heart J 44:674–683, 1980.
11. Guthrie RB, Edwards JE. Pathology of the myxomatous mitral valve: Nature, secondary changes and complication. Minn Med 59:637–647, 1976.
12. Kostuk WJ, Bougher DR, Barnett HJM, Silver MD. Strokes: A complication of mitral-leaflet prolapse. Lancet 1:313–316, 1977.

13. Wilson LA, Keeling PWN, Malcolm AD, Russell RWR, Webb-Peploe MM. Visual complications of mitral leaflet prolapse. Br Med J 2:86–88, 1977.
14. Salazar AE, Edwards JE. Friction lesions of ventricular endocardium. Relation to chordae tendineae of mitral valve. Arch Pathol 90:364–376, 1970.
15. Davies MJ: Pathology of Cardiac Valves. London, Butterworths, 1980.
16. Grenadier E, Alpan G, Keider S, Palant A. The prevalence of ruptured chordae tendineae in the mitral valve prolapse syndrome. Am Heart J 105:603–610, 1983.
17. Trent JK, Adelman AG, Wigle ED, Silver MD. Morphology of a prolapsed posterior mitral valve leaflet: A case report. Am Heart J 79:539–543, 1970.
18. Marshall CE, Shappell SD. Sudden death and the ballooning posterior leaflet syndrome: Detailed anatomic and histochemical investigation. Arch Pathol 98:134–138, 1974.
19. Reid JVO: Mid-systolic clicks. S Afr Med J 35:353–355, 1961.
20. Barlow JB, Pocock WA, Marchand P, Denny M. The significance of late systolic murmurs. Am Heart J 66:443–452, 1963.
21. Jeresaty RM. Etiology of the mitral valve prolapse-click syndrome. Am J Cardiol 36:110–113, 1975.
22. Grossman H, Fleming RJ, Engle MA, Levin AH, Ahlers KH. Angiocardiography in the apical systolic click syndrome: Left ventricular abnormality, mitral insufficiency, late systolic murmur, and inversion of T waves. Radiology 91:898–904, 1968.
23. Liedtke AJ, Gault JH, Leaman DM, Blumenthal MS. Geometry of left ventricular contraction in the systolic click syndrome: Characterization of a segmental myocardial abnormality. Circulation 47:27–35, 1973.
24. Gooch AS, Vicencio F, Maranhao V, Goldberg H. Arrhythmias and left ventricular asynergy in the prolapsing mitral leaflet syndrome. Am J Cardiol 29:611–620, 1972.
25. Scampardonis G, Yang SS, Maranhao V, Goldberg H, Gooch AS. Left ventricular abnormalities in prolapsed mitral leaflet syndrome: Review of eighty-seven cases. Circulation 48:287–297, 1973.
26. Jeresaty RM. The syndrome associated with mid-systolic click and/or late systolic murmur: Analysis of 32 cases. Chest 59:643–647, 1971.
27. Gulotta SJ, Gulco L, Padmanabhan V, Miller S. The syndrome of systolic click, murmur, and mitral valve prolapse: A cardiomyopathy? Circulation 49:717–728, 1974.
28. Mathey DG, Decoodt PR, Allen HN, Swan HJC. Abnormal left ventricular contraction pattern in the systolic click-late systolic murmur syndrome. Circulation 56:311–315, 1977.
29. Steelman RB, White RS, Hill JC, Nagle JP, Cheitlin MD. Midsystolic clicks in atherosclerotic heart disease: A new facet in the clinical syndrome of papillary muscle dysfunction. Circulation 44:503–515, 1971.
30. Cheng TO. Late systolic murmur in coronary artery disease. Chest 61:346–356, 1972.
31. Pomerance A. Ballooning deformity (mucoid degeneration) of atrioventricular valves. Br Heart J 31:343–351, 1969.
32. Hancock EW, Cohn K. The syndrome associated with midsystolic click and late systolic murmur. Am J Med 41:193–196, 1966.
33. Barlow JB, Bosman CK. Aneurysmal protrusion of the posterior leaflet of the mitral valve: An auscultatory-electrocardiographic syndrome. Am Heart J 71:166–178, 1966.

34. Pocock WA, Barlow JB. Etiology and electrocardiographic features of the billowing posterior mitral leaflet syndrome. Am J Med 57:731–739, 1971.
35. Rizzon P, Biasco G, Brindicci G, Mauro F. Familial syndrome of midsystolic click and late systolic murmur. Br Heart J 35:245–259, 1973.
36. Weiss AN, Mimbs JW, Ludbrooke PA, Sobel BE. Echocardiographic detection of mitral valve prolapse: Exclusion of false positive diagnosis and determination of inheritance. Circulation 52:1091–1096, 1975.
37. Scheele W, Allen HN, Krans R, Rubin PJ. Familial prevalence and genetic transmission of mitral valve prolapse [abstract]. Circulation 54(III):111, 1976.
38. Devereux RB, Brown WT, Kramer R, Sachs I. Inheritance of mitral valve prolapse: Autosomal dominant with reduced expression in children and adult males [abstract]. Clin Res 29:512A, 1981.
39. Schutte JE, Gaffney FA, Blend L, Blomquist CG. Distinctive anthropometric characteristics of women with mitral valve prolapse. Am J Med 71:533–538, 1981.
40. Devereux RB, Brown WT, Kramer-Fox R, Sachs I. Inheritance of mitral valve prolapse: Effect of age and sex on gene expression. Ann Int Med 97:826–832, 1982.
41. Read RC, Than AP, Wendt VE. Symptomatic valvular myxomatous transformation (the floppy valve syndrome): A possible forme fruste of the Marfan syndrome. Circulation 32:897–910, 1965.
42. Pyeritz RE. In Steinberg AG, Bearn AG, et al. (eds): Medical Genetics New Series, vol. V. Genetics of Cardiovascular Diseases. Philadelphia, W.B. Saunders, 1983, pp 191–302.
43. Prockop DJ, Kivirikko KI. Heritable diseases of collagen. N Engl J Med 311:376–386, 1984.
44. McKusick VA. The cardiovascular aspects of Marfan's syndrome: A heritable disorder of connective tissue. Circulation 11:321–342, 1955.
45. Shankar KR, Hultgren MK, Lauer RM, Diehl AM. Lethal tricuspid and mitral regurgitation in Marfan's syndrome. Am J Cardiol 20:122–128, 1967.
46. Bowers D. Pathogenesis of primary abnormalities of the mitral valve in Marfan's syndrome. Br Heart J 31:679–683, 1969.
47. Murdoch JL, Walker BA, Halpern BL, Kuzman JW, McKusick VA. Life expectancy and causes of death in Marfan's syndrome. N Engl J Med 286:804–808, 1982.
48. Criscitiello MG, Ronan JA, Besterman EMM, Schoenwetter W. Cardiovascular abnormalities in osteogenesis imperfecta. Circulation 31:255–262, 1965.
49. Wood SJ, Thomas J, Braimbridge MV. Mitral valve disease and open heart surgery in osteogenesis imperfecta tarda. Br Heart J 35:103–106, 1973.
50. McKusick VA. Heritable Diseases of Connective Tissue. 3rd ed. St Louis, Mosby, 1966.
51. Brandt KD, Sumner RD, Ryan TJ, Cohen AS. Herniation of mitral leaflets in Ehlers-Danlos syndrome. Am J Cardiol 36:524–528, 1975.
52. Huang S, Kumar G, Steele HD, Parker JO. Cardiac involvement in pseudoxanthoma elasticum. Am Heart J 74:680–686, 1967.
53. Kainulainen K, Pulkkinen L, Savolainen A, Kaitila I, Peltonen L. Location on chromosome 15 of the gene defect causing Marfan syndrome. N Engl J Med 323:935–939, 1990.
54. Jaffe AS, Geltman EM, Rodey GE, Uitto J. Mitral valve prolapse: A consistent manifestation of type IV Ehlers-Danlos syndrome. The pathogenetic role of the abnormal production of type III collagen. Circulation 64:121–125, 1981.

55. Brown FR III, Holbrook KA, Byers PH, Stewart D, Dean J, Pyeritz RE. Cutis laxa. Johns Hopkins Med J 150:148–153, 1982.
56. Hashimoto K, Kanzani T. Cutis laxa. Ultrastructural and biochemical studies. Arch Dermatol 111:861–873, 1975.
57. Shappell SD, Marshall CE, Brown RE, Bruce TA. Sudden death and the familial occurrence of mid-systolic click, late systolic murmur. Circulation 48:1128–1134, 1973.
58. Sherman EB, Char F, Dungan WT, Campbell GS. Myxomatous transformation of the mitral valve producing mitral insufficiency. Am J Dis Child 119:171–175, 1970.
59. Hammer D, Leier CV, Baba N, Vasco JS, Wooley CF, Pinnell SR. Altered collagen composition in a prolapsing mitral valve with ruptured chordae tendineae. Am J Med 67:863–866, 1979.
60. Lee YS, Lee FY, Lu AH, Chang CH, Chen HC, Liang KF, Chang CS. Biochemical analysis and electron microscopy of human mitral valve collagen in patients with various etiologies of mitral valve diseases. Jpn Heart J 24:529–538, 1983.
61. Aumailley R. MD thesis. University of Bordeaux, 1982.
62. Cole WG, Chan D, Hickey AJ, Wilcken DEL. Collagen composition of normal and myxomatous human mitral heart valves. Biochem J 219:451–460, 1984.
63. Caulfield JB, Page DL, Kastor JA, Saunders S. Connective tissue abnormalities in spontaneous rupture of chordae tendineae. Arch Pathol 91:537–541, 1971.
64. Becker AE, de Wit APM. The mitral valve apparatus: A spectrum of normality relevant to mitral valve prolapse. Br Heart J 42:680–689, 1980.

5

The Floppy Mitral Valve:

Structural and Physical Characteristics

Peter B. Baker, MD,
Harisios Boudoulas, MD, PhD,
Charles F. Wooley, MD

Introduction

The floppy mitral valve (FMV) morphological, histopathological, and tissue content characteristics are the fundamental determinants of the degrees of mitral valvular redundancy, mitral valve prolapse, and mitral valvular dysfunction. A broad spectrum of FMV pathological changes may alter each of the components of the FMV complex, thus precise FMV morphological definition of each of the components of the FMV complex provides the basis for understanding of mechanisms of FMV complex dysfunction, as well as for surgical reconstructive procedures.

Structural and Physical Characteristics

Floppy Mitral Valve: Dimensions

Precise definition of the dimensions of the myxomatous FMV became increasingly important as imaging techniques matured and the surgical

From: Boudoulas H, Wooley CF. *Mitral Valve: Floppy Mitral Valve, Mitral Valve Prolapse, Mitral Valvular Regurgitation.* Second revised edition. ©Futura Publishing Company, Armonk, NY, 2000.

approach to FMV repair, reconstruction, or replacement became feasible. A broad spectrum of quantitative changes has been described.

Dimensional changes in FMV include significant increases in commissural length, commissural diameter, longest and shortest diameter, length of the line of coaptation, surface area, and chordae tendineae length (Fig. 1). In circumstances when the FMV surface area of both leaflets is increased, the usual 2:1 ratio of anterior leaflet to posterior leaflet surface area (anterior greater than posterior) is altered by virtue of enlargement of all or portions of the posterior leaflet.[1] In addition, the weight of myxomatous FMV is significantly greater than control valves.

Floppy Mitral Valve: Valve Thickness

Varying degrees of thickness occur in the FMV (Table 1). FMV leaflet thickness, a basic morphological consideration, has clinical relevance in establishing imaging diagnostic criteria.

Morphological measurements were made on autopsy-procured normal mitral valves (normal mitral valves, n=17, 8 men, 9 women) and surgically excised FMVs (n=13, 7 men, 6 women). The data includes anterior

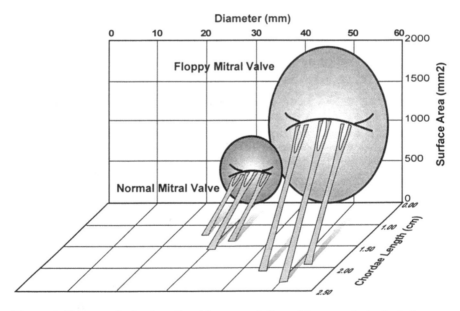

Figure 1. Floppy mitral valve. Graphic presentation of the morphological characteristics of normal mitral valve and floppy mitral valve associated with severe mitral valvular regurgitation. Valve diameter (mm), valve surface area (mm²), and chordal length (cm) are presented. AL = anterior leaflet.

Table 1
Cusp Thickness (mm) in Floppy Mitral Valves (FMV) and Normal Mitral Valves (NMV)

	Anterior Cusp			Posterior Cusp		
	Free Edge	*Mid-Point*	*Base at the Annulus*	*Free Edge*	*Mid-Point*	*Base at the Annulus*
NMV	1.6 ± .4	0.6 ± 0.2	1.1 ± .3	0.6 ± .3	0.8 ± 0.2	0.9 ± .2
FMV	2.0 ± .8	2.3 ± 1.0	1.3 ± .8	2.2 ± .8	2.2 ± 1.1	2.1 ± .6
P	N/S	<0.001	N/S	<.001	<.001	<.001

and posterior cusp thickness at three points: free edge, base at the annulus, and midpoint between base and free edge (Table 1).

Maximum thickness in normal mitral valves, defined as two standard deviations above the mean, was 2.4 mm and was found at the anterior cusp free edge. The entire posterior cusp and the anterior cusp were thicker in FMVs compared with normal mitral valves. Different thicknesses at different points should be considered for cusp thickness evaluation, since these anatomic measurements provide the basis for imaging data interpretation.

Floppy Mitral Valve: Histopathology

Histologically, mitral valve cusps consist of four connective tissue layers, which are oriented parallel to the inflow and outflow surfaces of the cusps. Proceeding from the atrial to the ventricular side of the valve cusps, the layers are the atrialis, spongiosa, fibrosa, and ventricularis.

FMV leaflets have a large central zone of loose myxomatous connective tissue (Figs. 2 , 3). This zone focally extends into the fibrosa, producing disruption of the collagen. In the myxomatous areas, the collagen bundles are short, fragmented, disoriented, and separated by acid mucopolysaccharides. Myxomatous tissue is found in the free edge and line of closure of many normal mitral valves, but is more prominent in FMV (Fig. 4). It has been suggested that the myxomatous tissue in FMV represents expansion of the valve cusp spongiosa. Myxomatous areas with associated collagen dissolution are present in the fibrosa and chordae tendineae of FMV, but not in the corresponding areas of normal mitral valves. Alterations in the collagenous supporting structures of FMV, particularly the valve cusp fibrosa and chordae tendineae, are involved in the pathological process. Additional histopathological changes in the cusps of

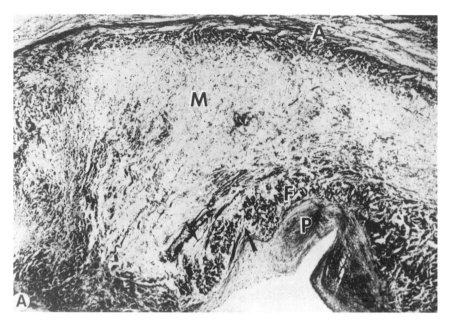

Figure 2. Floppy mitral valve leaflet oriented with the inflow (atrial) surface at the top and ventricular (outflow) surface at the bottom. The histological layers shown from top to bottom are atrialis with fibrosis (A), large zone of loose myxomatous tissue (M), fibrosa (F), which is attenuated and focally disrupted by myxomatous tissue (arrows), and fibrous pads (P) on the ventricular endocardium. Jones's methenamine silver stain; original magnification x16.

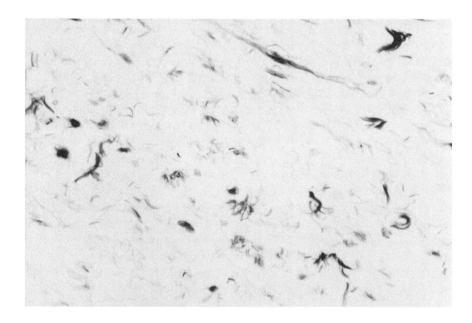

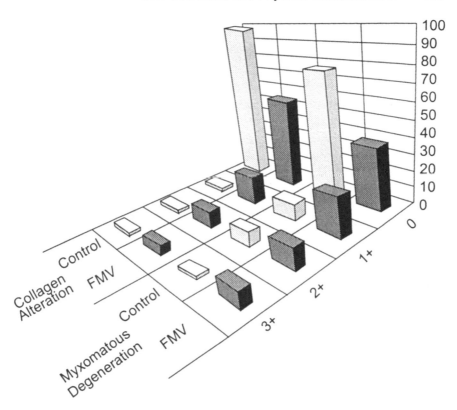

Figure 4. Floppy mitral valve (FMV). Graphic presentation of collagen alteration and myxomatous degeneration. Control mitral valve (control) compared with FMV. Severity and percentage of patients with collagen degeneration or myxomatous degeneration are shown. 0 = no change; 1+ = mild change; 2+ = moderate change; 3+ = severe change.

FMV include thickening of the atrialis and deposition of fibrous connective tissue "pads" on the ventricular surface.[1-21]

Floppy Mitral Valve: Surface Characteristics

Vascular endothelial surface activities have been studied extensively; however, whether normal valvular endothelial cell properties are similar

---

Figure 3. Floppy mitral valve cusp. A high magnification view of the myxomatous area seen in Figure 2 shows short, disoriented, separated collagen bundles. A Mowry's colloidal iron stain demonstrated abundant accumulation of acid mucopolysaccharides in this area (Jones's methenamine silver stain, original magnification x80).

is unclear. Abnormal valve endothelial cells from FMV have not been studied in detail.

A variety of molecules interact to form the extracellular matrix and then adhere to the matrix. The resultant nonthrombogenicity of the vascular endothelial cell surface represents the normal state in health, whereas thrombogenicity occurs when these complex processes at the endothelial cell surface are disturbed. Composition of the vascular endothelial cell and the extracellular matrix involves several types of collagen, von Willebrand factor, fibronectin, thrombospondin, vitronectin, laminin, elastin, and proteoglycans. Fibrinolytic constituents on the endothelial cell surface involve the known coagulant factors and pathways, a family of adhesive proteins such as vitronectin and thrombospondin, which interact with endothelial cell surface adhesive receptors, in addition to platelet adhesive interactions and receptors. Laminar or disturbed blood flow and shear rates appear to be additional important modifiers.

The interactions, signals, and genetics that modulate assembly and otherwise regulate, stimulate, and inhibit these processes are currently subjects of intense investigation using a variety of in vitro and in vivo vascular endothelial cell systems. To date, little has been done to identify the characteristics of FMV endothelial cell systems. FMV surface phenomena and reactions most likely result from the interactions between specialized endothelial cell composition further modified by chronic mechanical forces acting on the valve structure in a disturbed hemodynamic environment.

Normal mitral valves have tightly packed, organized collagen fibers with a linear orientation and a relatively smooth, continuous endothelial surface (Fig. 5A,B). FMV surfaces display folding and surface irregularities as a result of the underlying collagen disruption, dissolution, and separation (Figs. 6A,B, 7A,B), the elastin fragmentation, and the mucopolysaccharide deposition in the FMV substrate; the net result is an internal "swiss cheese" effect.[1] Pomerance suggested that the endocardial surface changes were secondary to these underling fibrosal disruptions and that with cusp stretching the endothelial layer was subjected to abrupt changes in tension with resultant loss in endothelial continuity, rupture of subendothelial connective tissue fibers, and fibrin deposition.[11]

Alterations in surface endothelial cell morphology, chemistry, or integrity factors have been postulated to precede platelet adherence to fibrin and the development of nonbacterial thrombotic endocardial (NBTE) lesions with embolic and infectious potential. Binding of circulating microorganisms from bacteremia to the NBTE lesions has been presumed to be a pathogenetic mechanism for certain forms of infective endocarditis, and such model systems have been developed and studied in animals. Endothelial cell surface or bacterial binding characteristics influence adhesion to surface receptor protein complexes.

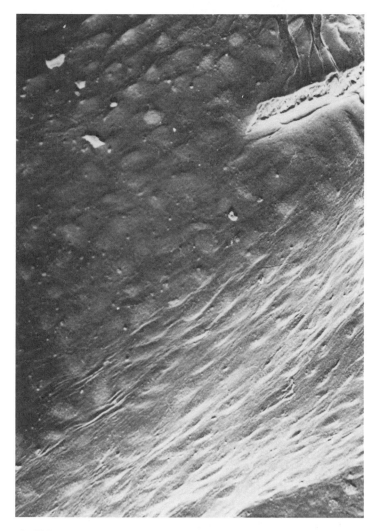

Figure 5A. This normal mitral valve leaflet inflow surface is smooth with a gently rolling appearance. Scanning electron micrograph; original magnification x130.

The extent to which FMV surface molecular characteristics differ from normal mitral valves has not been analyzed critically. Thrombus formation with thromboembolic complications and infective endocarditis are recognized complications of FMV and are related in part to the hemodynamics of turbulence contributing further to valve surface irregularities. The unusual susceptibility of patients with FMV to these complications is probably related to alterations in the extracellular matrix molecules and valve surface receptors but this is as yet unstudied in FMV.[22–28]

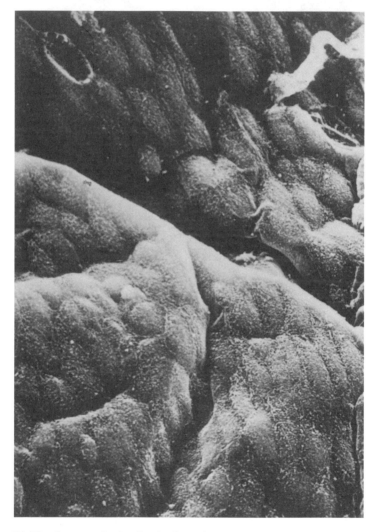

Figure 5B. The floppy mitral valve leaflet inflow surface is characterized by irregular folding forming narrow indentations. Scanning electron micrograph; original magnification x280.

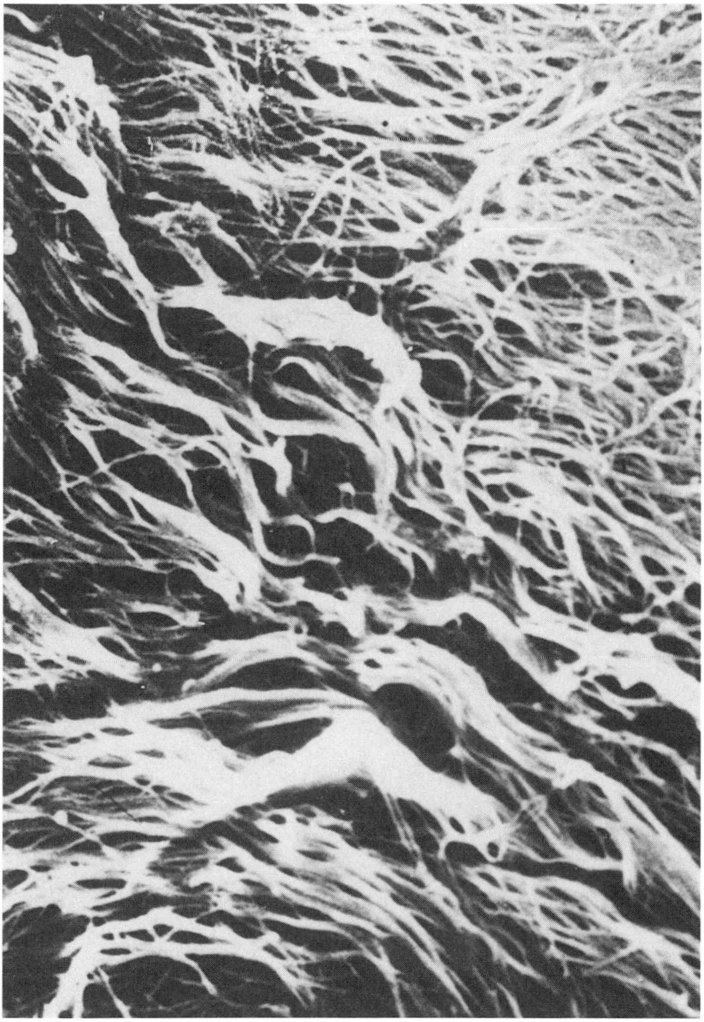

Figure 6A. A normal mitral valve was snap frozen in liquid nitrogen and the cusps were cracked. A leaflet fragment with the cracked surface oriented perpendicular to the inflow surface was digested with hyaluronidase. Collagen fibers are observed to be tightly packed and arranged in parallel. Scanning electron micrograph; original magnification x2300.

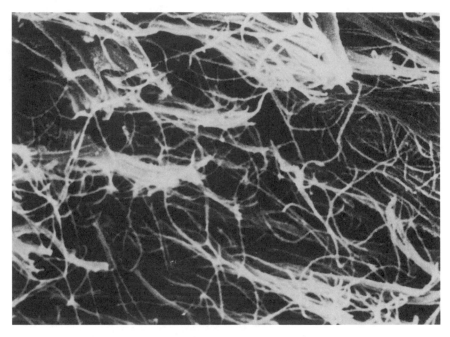

Figure 6B. Using the same preparation described for normal mitral valve, the floppy mitral valve demonstrates loosely arranged collagen fibers with disruption of the parallel orientation. Scanning electron micrograph; original magnification x2500.

Floppy Mitral Valve: Mitral Annulus

A spectrum of annular involvement has been described in patients with FMV.[11,14,15,18] The mean annular circumference in patients with FMV and severe mitral valvular regurgitation is greater than 65% above normal valves, and approximately 30% above normal in patients with competent floppy mitral valves.[29] Annular dilatation was present in 7% in Davies large necropsy series.[14] Annular dilatation is a consistent finding in patients with Marfan syndrome and FMV.

Mitral annular calcification may occur in patients with FMV (Fig. 8). Mitral annular calcific deposits are actually located between the undersurface of the posterior mitral leaflet and the left ventricular wall endocardium. The association of the FMV with mitral annular calcification usually occurs in older individuals, but may be seen in younger patients with Marfan syndrome. Mitral annular calcification also poses problems for surgical repair of the FMV.

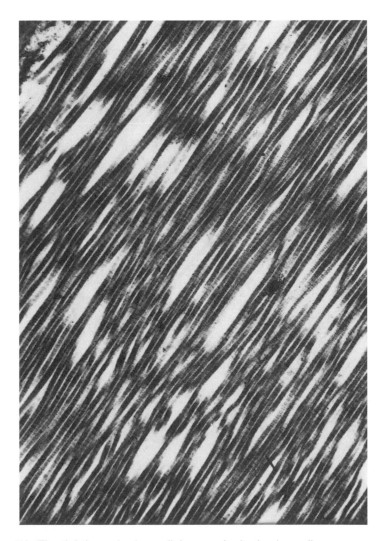

Figure 7A. The tightly packed, parallel, normal mitral valve collagen corresponds with the cracked valve leaflet surface in Figure 6. Transmission electron micrograph; original magnification x12,000.

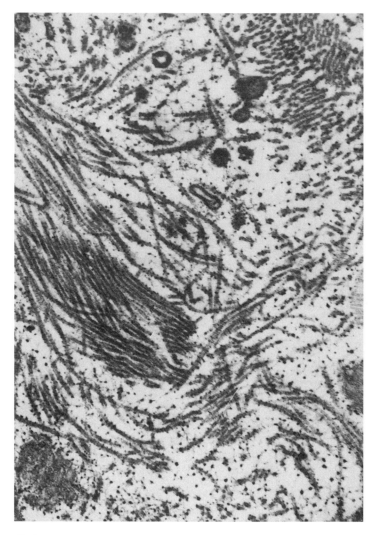

Figure 7B. Separated disorganized collagen fibers characterize myxomatous areas of the floppy mitral valve; this appearance corresponds with the cracked floppy valve leaflet surface in Figure 6. Transmission electron micrograph; original magnification x12,000.

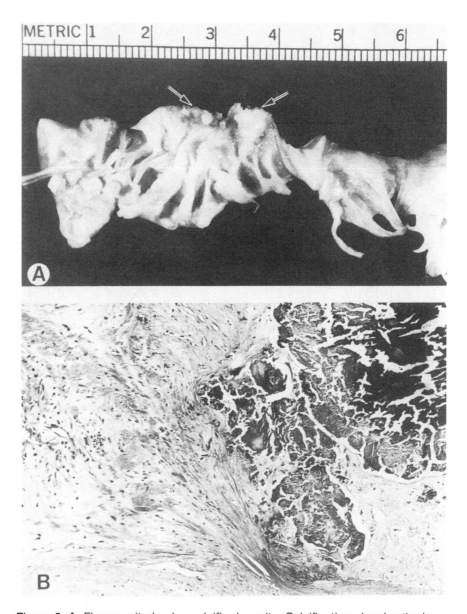

Figure 8. A. Floppy mitral valve calcific deposits. Calcifications involve the base of this posterior leaflet, forming irregular nodules on the ventricular aspect (arrows). **B.** Floppy mitral valve calcific deposits. This tissue section shows the irregular calcifications that involve the leaflet tissue (on the right); the loose myxomatous connective tissue is noted on the left. Hematoxylin and eosin; original magnification x107.

Floppy Mitral Valve: Chordae Tendineae

Gross pathological changes have been consistently observed in FMV chordae tendineae; however, the results of histopathological studies have been variable. Our studies of the histopathology and mechanical properties of FMV chordae tendineae and previous studies by other investigators form the basis for the following discussion.

Floppy Mitral Valve: Chordal Rupture

Before the FMV was recognized as a distinct pathological entity, several reports of spontaneous chordal rupture appeared in the literature. As early as 1934, Frothingham described spontaneous rupture of chordae tendineae in a mitral valve in the absence of any known predisposing cardiac pathology; description of the valve indicates that it was probably a FMV. In subsequent reports of spontaneous chordal rupture, the mitral valves also had characteristic FMV pathological features.[30–32]

A strong association exists between chordal rupture and the FMV. Although this association has been questioned by some investigators, recent studies of consecutive patients with ruptured chordae tendineae demonstrated that approximately 90% had FMV. In addition, most ruptured chordae have not been attributed to bacterial endocarditis.[33–36]

Ruptured chordae tendineae have been documented in 22–80% of FMVs that were surgically excised or observed at autopsy.[14,18,37–40] Echocardiographic studies of consecutive patients with mitral valve prolapse revealed evidence of chordal rupture in 7% and 11%.[41,42] Thus, clinical and pathological studies have documented that ruptured chordae tendineae are frequently present in patients with floppy or myxomatous mitral valves.

Floppy Mitral Valve: Chordal Elongation

Other gross pathological alterations observed in FMV chordae tendineae include elongation, thickening, and thinning.[14,34–39,43–46] Previous studies have not quantitatively documented elongation of FMV chordae tendineae. We measured the lengths of normal and FMV chordae tendineae, dividing the chordae into three anatomic categories according to the location of attachment to the valve cusps. The categories included chordae attached to the anterior or posterior cusp and commissural chordae with branches that insert on both cusps near the commissural areas. The chordal measurements are shown in Table 2. FMV chordae tendineae were significantly longer compared with the corresponding normal mitral valve chordae.

Table 2
Average Lengths of Chordae Tendineae (cm) Shown as Mean ± Standard Deviation

Chordal Attachment Site	Normal Mitral Valve (n = 10)	Floppy Mitral Valve (n = 8)
Anterior cusp	1.54 ± 0.33 (n = 59)	2.30 ± 0.35 (n = 48) p < 0.01
Posterior cusp	1.32 ± 0.30 (n = 73)	2.31 ± 0.34 (n = 66) p < 0.001
Commissure	1.34 ± 0.35 (n = 20)	2.17 ± 0.45 (n = 14) p < 0.001

Floppy Mitral Valve Chordae: Microscopic Findings

Histological studies of FMV chordae tendineae have produced conflicting results. Alterations have been observed by some investigators, while others have found no histological abnormalities in nonruptured FMV chordae tendineae.

Marchand described collagen fragmentation in ruptured chordae tendineae but found that adjacent nonruptured chordae, which were thin and elongated, had no histopathological change.[45] Similar observations were made by Scott-Jupp who studied ruptured and nonruptured chordae by light and electron microscopy and found that collagen "degeneration" was confined to ruptured chordae with only one exception.[32] Lucas and Edwards were "unable to find a consistent explanation based on gross anatomy or histologic study" for chordal abnormalities in FMV.[15] Guthrie mentioned that "mucinous" alteration might contribute to chordal elongation;[43] however, Marchand, Scott-Jupp, and Guthrie independently suggested that FMV chordal abnormalities were probably due to abnormal chordal tension.

In contrast to the above studies, other authors have described generalized collagen alterations in FMV chordae tendineae. Caulfield, observing connective tissue dissolution in ruptured and nonruptured FMV chordae while additional nonruptured chordae showed normal histology, concluded that chordal rupture was due to collagen dissolution.[31] McKay found "disorganization" of collagen in FMV chordae from "all parts of the valve."[18] King observed that collagen dissolution, present in FMV chordae, was absent in normal mitral valve chordae.[13]

A systematic histological study of chordae tendineae was performed on nonruptured chordae tendineae from eight surgically excised FMVs, and compared with chordae tendineae from 10 normal mitral valves obtained at autopsy. The accumulation of acid mucopolysaccharides and al-

Table 3

Histopathological Grading of Normal and Floppy Mitral Valve Chordae
Tendineae Shown as Percent of Chordae

	Grade	FMV (n = 128)	NMV (n = 152)
Acid	0	27	80
Mucopolysaccharide	1	34	18
Accumulation (%)	2	20	1
	3	19	<1
Collagen	0	62	98
Alterations (%)	1	16	<1
	2	10	<1
	3	12	<1

FMV = floppy mitral valve; NMV = normal mitral valve.

terations in collagen were semiquantitatively graded from 0 to 3, with 3 indicating severe changes.[47]

The results are summarized in Table 3 and Figure 9. Normal mitral valve chordae tendineae uniformly had a dense central collagenous core surrounded by a thin layer of compact elastic fibers with or without small deposits of acid mucopolysaccharides (Fig. 10). Collagen alterations and moderate to severe acid mucopolysaccharide accumulation, rarely found in normal mitral valve chordae tendineae, were frequently present in FMV chordae tendineae (p<0.001). The collagen alterations in FMV chordae tendineae are illustrated in Figure 11).

The histopathology of FMV chordae was nonuniform, however, ranging from a normal histological appearance to severe collagen fragmentation, attenuation, and separation, with associated severe acid mucopolysaccharide accumulation. Histopathological alterations were found in FMV chordae tendineae from all valve cusp attachment sites without predilection for any particular site.

Ultrastructural studies have supported and expanded on the light microscopic observations. Chordae from normal mitral valves had a central core of closely packed collagen fibers surrounded by a thin zone of elastic fibers. FMV chordae had increased proteoglycans, degraded collagen and elastic fibers in the central core and degeneration of the surrounding elastic layer.[48] Using immunologic cytochemistry, nonspecific electron dense material was found to label by alpha elastin antibody. Other electron dense aggregates labeled by collagen types I and III as well as fibronectin antibodies.[49] These observations further document the presence of collagen and elastic fiber degradation in FMV chordae.

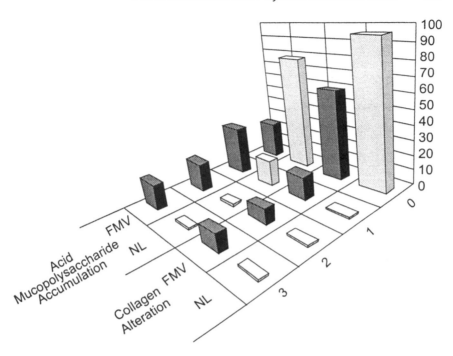

Figure 9. Floppy mitral valve (FMV) chordae tendineae. Graphic presentation of histopathological characteristics. Normal control (NL) mitral valve compared with FMV. Severity and percentage of patients with collagen alteration and acid mucopolysaccharide accumulation are presented. 0 = no change; 1+ = mild change; 2+ = moderate change; 3+ = severe change.

Floppy Mitral Valve Chordae: Mechanical Properties

The histopathological alterations identified in FMV chordae tendineae might be expected to result in altered mechanical properties when compared with normal mitral valve chordae tendineae. We tested this hypothesis using 15 chordae from five FMV, and 20 chordae from six normal mitral valves. The chordae were tested in a uniaxial tension mode. Load versus elongation curves were obtained for each chorda by increasing the load until the chorda fractured. Fracture stress (fracture load/original chordal cross-sectional area) and fracture strain (total chordal elongation/original chordal length) are given in Table 4 and Fig. 12). The fracture stress in FMV chordae tendineae was significantly lower (p<0.01) compared with that in normal mitral valve chordae tendineae.

These results indicate a loss of tissue strength that accompany the histopathological changes and may contribute further to chordal elonga-

Table 4
Mechanical Properties of Normal and Floppy Mitral Valve Chordae
Tendineae Shown as Mean ± Standard Deviation

	Fracture Stress (dyne/cm²) ×10⁸	Fracture Strain %
FMV Chordae (n = 15)	2.96 ± 1.96	27.3 ± 6.5
NMV Chordae (n = 20)	5.62 ± 1.60	27.6 ± 11.9
	p < 0.01	NS

FMV = floppy mitral valve; NMV = normal mitral valve; NS = not significant.

tion and rupture. Alterations in collagen represent structural changes that account for reduced fracture stress in FMV chordae tendineae. The similar fracture strain in normal and FMV chordae tendineae may indicate that collagen, representing the major structural component, is not qualitatively altered in FMV chordae tendineae.

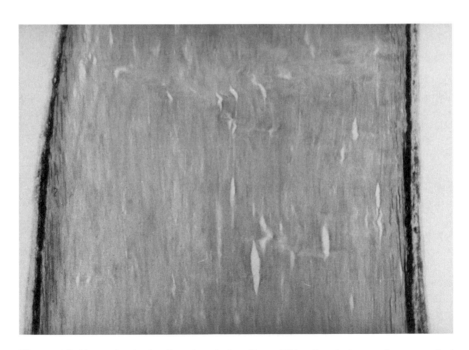

Figure 10. Normal mitral valve chorda tendinea. This chorda has a dense central collagenous core surrounded by a thin zone of compact, dark-staining elastic fibers. This histological appearance was uniformly seen in normal mitral valve chordae (Weigert's elastic stain, original magnification x40).

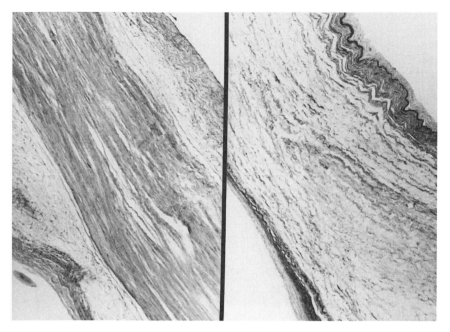

Figure 11. Floppy mitral valve chordae tendineae. These chordae show two patterns of histopathological alterations. The chorda on the left shows myxomatous expansion of the peripheral connective tissue with loss of the distinct elastic layer. The chorda on the right has severe separation and attenuation of collagen in the central core while the peripheral elastic layer remains intact. Mowry's colloidal iron stain demonstrated abundant acid mucopolysaccharide accumulation in both chordae (Weigert's elastic stain, original magnification x25).

Floppy Mitral Valve Chordae: Clinical Implications

Identification of the histopathological and mechanical property abnormalities in the FMV complex and FMV chordae tendineae may lead to a better understanding of the natural history of FMV. Salisbury demonstrated in experimental studies in dogs that severing some of the mitral valve chordae tendineae resulted in increased tension on the remaining intact chordae.[50] Chordal elongation, rupture, or severe alterations in the collagen content of individual chordae would also be expected to produce increased tension on adjacent chordae. Increased chordal tension with gradual elongation and occasional chordal rupture may contribute to the progressive increase in valvular prolapse and regurgitation observed in some patients with FMV.[50,51] Other mechanical and hemodynamic factors may further increase chordal tension in FMV.

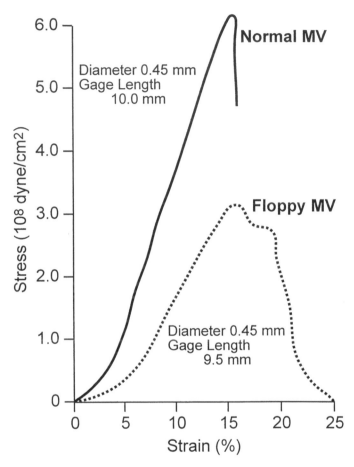

Figure 12. Stress-strain relationship of a chordae tendineae of a normal mitral valve (MV) and a floppy mitral valve.

Chordal rupture may produce a sudden increase in valvular regurgitation;[18,51,52] however, many patients with chordal rupture do not experience an episode of sudden cardiac decompensation.[53,54] A ruptured FMV chorda is likely to be adjacent to chordae tendineae with mild or no histopathological alterations. Since these chordae probably remain intact despite increased tension, the chordal rupture may not result in a sudden increase in valvular regurgitation. Rupture of an FMV chorda in a location critical for valve cusp support or rupture of several adjacent chordae would account for a sudden worsening of valvular regurgitation.

The histopathological alterations and changes in mechanical properties in FMV chordae tendineae predispose to chordal elongation and rupture, which may contribute to progressive FMV prolapse and mitral valvular regurgitation.

Floppy Mitral Valve: Structural and Physical Characteristics: Perspective

The sum total of the broad spectrum of FMV complex morphological, histopathological, pathogenetic, and tissue content changes account for the variable FMV clinical characteristics and expressions. However, although a great deal has been learned about the FMV structure and physical characteristics, much remains to be done if we are to understand the basis for progressive FMV dysfunction.

References

1. Wooley CF, Baker PB, Kolibash AJ, Kilman JW, Sparks EA, Boudoulas H. The floppy myxomatous mitral valve, mitral valve prolapse, and mitral regurgitation. Progr Cardiovasc Dis 32:397–433, 1991.
2. Boudoulas H, Wooley CF (eds). Mitral Valve Prolapse and the Mitral Valve Prolapse Syndrome. Mount Kisco, NY, Futura Publishing Co, 1988.
3. Boudoulas H, Kolibash AJ, Baker P, King BD, Wooley CF. Mitral valve prolapse and the mitral valve prolapse syndrome: A diagnostic classification and pathogenesis of symptoms. Am Heart J 118:796–818, 1989.
4. Read RC, Thal AP, Wendt VE. Symptomatic valvular myxomatous transformation (the floppy valve syndrome): A possible forme fruste of the Marfan syndrome. Circulation 32:897–910, 1965.
5. Aslam PA, Eastridge CE, Bernhardt H, et al. Myxomatous degeneration of cardiac valves. Chest 57:535–539, 1970.
6. McCarthy LJ, Wolf PL. Mucoid degeneration of heart valves: Blue valve syndrome. Am J Clin Pathol 54;852–856, 1970.
7. Sherman EB, Char F, Dungan WT, et al. Myxomatous transformation of the mitral valve producing mitral insufficiency. Am J Dis Child 119:171–175, 1970.
8. Edwards JE. Mitral insufficiency resulting from "overshooting" of leaflets. Circulation 43:606–612, 1971.
9. Cooley DA, Gerami S, Hallman GL, et al. Mitral insufficiency due to myxomatous transformation: Floppy valve syndrome. J Cardiovasc Surg 13:346–349, 1972.
10. Rippe J. Fishbein MC, Carabello B, et al. Primary myxomatous degeneration of cardiac valves. Clinical, pathological, hemodynamic and echocardiographic profile. Br Heart J 44:621–629, 1980.
11. Pomerance A. Ballooning deformity (mucoid degeneration) of atrioventricular valves. Br Heart J 31:343–351, 1969.
12. Kern WH, Tucker BL. Myxoid changes in cardiac valves: Pathologic, clinical and ultrastructural studies. Am Heart J 84:294–301, 1972.
13. King BD, Clark MA, Baba N, et al. Myxomatous mitral valves: Collagen dissolution as the primary defect. Circulation 66:288–296, 1982.
14. Davies MJ, Moore BP, Braimbridge MV. The floppy mitral valve: Study of incidence, pathology, and complications in surgical, necropsy and forensic material. Br Heart J 40:468–481, 1978.

15. Lucas RV, Edwards JE. The floppy mitral valve. Curr Probl Cardiol 7:1–48, 1982.
16. Becker AE, DeWit APM. Mitral valve apparatus: A spectrum of normality relevant to mitral valve prolapse. Br Heart J 42:680–689, 1979.
17. Carpentier A, Guerinon J, Deloche A, et al. Pathology of the mitral valve. In Kalmanson D (ed): The Mitral Valve: A Pluridisciplinary Approach. Action, MA, Mass Publishing Sciences Group, 1976, pp 65–77.
18. McKay R, Yacoub MH. Clinical and pathological finding in patients with "floppy" valves treated surgically. Circulation 47(Suppl):63–73, 1973.
19. Barlow JB, Pocock WA. Mitral leaflet billowing and prolapse. In Barlow JB (ed). Perspective on the Mitral Valve. Philadelphia, PA, Davis 1987, pp 45–111.
20. Roberts WC. Morphologic features on the normal and abnormal mitral valve. Am J Cardiol 51:1005–1028, 1983.
21. Boudoulas H, Wooley CF. Mitral valve prolapse and the mitral valve prolapse syndrome. In Yu PN, Goodwin JF (eds). Progress in Cardiology 14:275–309, 1986.
22. Campbell KM, Johnson CM. Identification of *Staphylococcus aureus* binding proteins on isolated porcine cardiac valve cells. J Lab Clin Med 115:217–223, 1990.
23. Courtney HS, Stanislawski L, Ofek I, et al. Localization of a lipoteichoic acid binding site to a 24-kilodalton NH2 terminal fragment of fibronectin. Rev Infect Dis 10(Suppl 2):S360-S362, 1988.
24. Schauer R. Sialic acids and their role as biological masks. Trends Biochem Sci 10:357–360, 1985.
25. Baddour LM, Bisno AL. Infective endocarditis complicating mitral valve prolapse: Epidemiological, clinical, and microbiological aspects. Rev Infect Dis 8:117–137, 1986.
26. Cole WG, Chan D, Hickey AJ, et al. Collagen composition of normal and myxomatous human mitral heart valves. Biochem J 219:451–460, 1984.
27. Henney AM, Tsipouras P, Schwartz RC, et al. Genetic evidence that mutations in the COL1A1, COL1A2, COL3A1, or COL5A2 collagen genes are not responsible for mitral valve prolapse. Br Heart J 61:292–299, 1989.
28. Wordsworth P, Ogilvie D, Akhras F, et al. Genetic segregation analysis of familial mitral valve prolapse shows no linkage to fibrillar collagen genes. Br Heart J 61:300–306, 1989.
29. Ormiston JA, Shah PM, Tei C, et al. Size and motion of the mitral valve annulus in man. Circulation 1982;65:713–719, 1982.
30. Singh R, Schrank JP, Nolan SP, McGuire LB. Spontaneous rupture of mitral chordae tendineae. JAMA 219:189–193, 1972.
31. Caulfield JB, Page DL, Kastor JA, Sanders CA. Connective tissue abnormalities in spontaneous rupture of chordae tendineae. Arch Pathol 91:537–541, 1971.
32. Scott-Jupp W, Barnett NL, Gallagher PJ, Monro JL, Ross JK. Ultrastructural changes in spontaneous rupture of mitral chordae tendineae. J Pathol 133:185–201, 1980.
33. Selzer A. Nonrheumatic mitral regurgitation. Mod Concepts Cardiovasc Dis 48:25–30, 1974.
34. Oliveira DBG, Dawkins KD, Kay PH, Paneth M. Chordal rupture I: Etiology and natural history. Br Heart J 50:312–317, 1983.
35. Hickey AJ, Wilcken DEL, Wright JS, Warren BA. Primary (spontaneous) chordal rupture: Relation to myxomatous valve disease and mitral valve prolapse. J Am Coll Cardiol 5:1341–1346, 1985.
36. Jeresaty RM, Edwards JE, Chawla SK. Mitral valve prolapse and ruptured chordae tendineae. Am J Cardiol 55:138–142, 1985.

37. Olsen EGJ, Al-Rufaie HK. The floppy mitral valve: Study on pathogenesis. Br Heart J 44:674–683, 1980.

38. Yacoub M, Halim M, Radley-Smith R, McKay R, Nijveld A, Towers M. Surgical treatment of mitral regurgitation caused by floppy valves: Repair versus replacement. Circulation 64(Suppl 2):210–216, 1981.

39. Waller BF, Morrow AG, Maron BJ, Del Negro AA, Kent KM, McGrath FJ, et al. Etiology of clinically isolated, severe, chronic, pure mitral regurgitation: Analysis of 97 patients over 30 years of age having mitral valve replacement. Am Heart J 104:276–288, 1982.

40. Hanson TP, Edwards BS, Edwards JE. Pathology of surgically excised mitral valves. One-hundred consecutive cases. Arch Pathol Lab Med 109:823–828, 1985.

41. Chandraratna PAN, Aronow WS. Incidence of ruptured chordae tendineae in the mitral valvular prolapse syndrome: An echocardiographic study. Chest 75:334–339, 1979.

42. Grenadier E, Alpan G, Keidar S, Palant A. The prevalence of ruptured chordae tendineae in the mitral valve prolapse syndrome. Am Heart J 105:603–610, 1976.

43. Guthrie RB, Edwards JE. Pathology of the myxomatous mitral valve: Nature, secondary changes and complications. Minn Med 59:637–647, 1976.

44. Roberts WC. Congenital cardiovascular abnormalities usually "silent" until adulthood: Morphologic features of the floppy mitral valve, valvular aortic stenosis, discrete subvalvular aortic stenosis, hypertrophic cardiopmyopathy, sinus of valsalva aneurysm and the Marfan syndrome. Cardiovasc Clin 10:407–453, 1979.

45. Marchand P, Barlow JB, DuPlessis LA, Webster I. Mitral regurgitation with rupture of normal chordae tendineae. Br Heart J 28:746–758, 1966.

46. Van der Bel-Kahn J, Becker AE. The surgical pathology of rheumatic and floppy mitral valves. Am J Surg Pathol 10:282–292, 1986.

47. Baker PB, Bansal G, Boudoulas H, Kolibash AJ, Kilman J, Wooley CF. Floppy mitral valve chordae tendineae: Histopathological alterations. Human Pathol 19:507–512, 1988.

48. Akhtar S, Meek KM, James V. Ultrastructure abnormalities in proteoglycans, collagen fibrils and elastic fibers in normal and myxomatous mitral valve chordae tendineae. Cardiovasc Pathol 8:191–201, 1999.

49. Akhtar S, Meek KM, James V. Immunolocalization of elastin, collagen type I and III, fibronectin and vitronectin in extracellular matrix components of normal and myxomatous mitral heart valve chordae tendineae. Cardiovasc Pathol 8:203–211, 1999.

50. Salisbury PF, Cross CE, Rieben PA. Chordae tendinea tension. Am J Physiol 205:385–392, 1963.

51. Kolibash AJ, Kilman JW, Bush CA, Ryan JM, Fontana ME, Wooley CF. Evidence for progression from mild to severe mitral regurgitation in mitral valve prolapse. Am J Cardiol 58:762–767, 1986.

52. Nishimura RA, McGoon MD, Shub C, Miller FA, Ilstrup DM, Tajik AJ. Echocardiographically documented mitral valve prolapse: Long-term follow-up of 237 patients. N Engl J Med 313:1305–1309, 1985.

53. Goodman D, Kimbiris D, Linhart JW. Chordae tendineae rupture complicating the systolic click-late systolic murmur syndrome. Am J Cardiol 33:681–684, 1974.

54. Child JS, Cabeen WR, Roberts NK. Mitral valve prolapse complicated by ruptured chordae tendineae. West J Med 129:160–163, 1978.

Part IV

The Floppy Mitral Valve, Mitral Valve Prolapse, Mitral Valvular Regurgitation:
The Triad

Introduction

The Floppy Mitral Valve, Mitral Valve Prolapse, Mitral Valvular Regurgitation:

Keys To Understanding

Charles F. Wooley, MD,
Harisios Boudoulas, MD, PhD

There are relatively few instances in cardiovascular medicine where controversy and wrong-headedness delayed the recognition of discrete clinical entities and their interrelationships as in the case of the floppy mitral valve (FMV), mitral valve prolapse (MVP), and mitral valvular regurgitation (MVR).

If the delayed recognition was due solely to a series of historical detours, then the topic *Keys To Understanding* could be omitted and emphasis directed to the here and now. However, the way that clinicians learn is an integral and continuing part of the FMV-MVP-MVR narrative. Years, or decades, pass between the time of the initial clinical or pathological descriptions before clinical comprehension occurs. The process may be further delayed by controversies fueled by dogma without critical and supportive data.

The discriminating reader should be aware that a number of our 19th century predecessors had a fine sense of appreciation for the variety of systolic murmurs associated with MVR, the clinical recognition of MVR, and the long-term consequences of MVR. In the 1850s, Austin Flint was well aware that MVR could be "long borne" without serious inconvenience, i.e., the natural history of the patient with MVR was different from that of patients with other forms of valvular heart disease. This concept was lost and rediscovered several times since.

From: Boudoulas H, Wooley CF. *Mitral Valve: Floppy Mitral Valve, Mitral Valve Prolapse, Mitral Valvular Regurgitation.* Second revised edition. ©Futura Publishing Company, Armonk, NY, 2000.

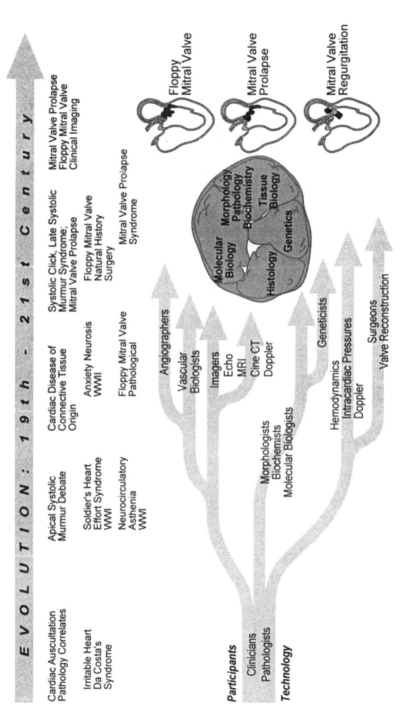

Figure 1.

The paths to our current recognition and comprehension of the FMV-MVP-MVR triad have been multiple and tortuous, extending over two centuries. However, the narrative is inhabited by many of our illustrious predecessors and contemporaries and is enriched with the sense of discovery that makes clinical cardiology so exciting. The ways our predecessors and contemporaries approached and solved many of the dilemmas along the way are presented in Chapter 6. Beyond providing pertinent background information, these observations reveal the breadth and depth of their accomplishments, leaving us with multiple basic and clinical challenges as we move into the 3rd century of inquiry (Fig. 1).

6

The Floppy Mitral Valve, Mitral Valve Prolapse, Mitral Valvular Regurgitation:

Keys to Understanding

Charles F. Wooley, MD,
Harisios Boudoulas, MD, PhD

Introduction

The path to understanding the etiology and pathogenesis of mitral valvular regurgitation (MVR) has been the most tortuous of all the individual valvular lesions. This is related primarily to the complexity and interrelationships of the function of the mitral valve complex within the left atrium and left ventricle. Ignoring or forgetting astute clinical observations by our predecessors has also contributed to the process.

Nineteenth century pathologists and clinicians based their insights about MVR on clinical assessments correlated with autopsy findings (Fig. 1). These physical diagnosis correlations with autopsy findings came into existence and reached new levels in 19th century France when Corvisart refined percussion of the thorax and its contents in 1808, and Laennec introduced cardiopulmonary auscultation in 1819. Cardiovascular physical diagnosis developed through the stages of observation, inspection, and

---

From: Boudoulas H, Wooley CF. *Mitral Valve: Floppy Mitral Valve, Mitral Valve Prolapse, Mitral Valvular Regurgitation.* Second revised edition. ©Futura Publishing Company, Armonk, NY, 2000.

Mitral Valvular Regurgitation

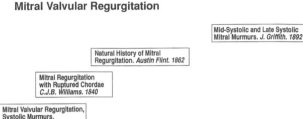

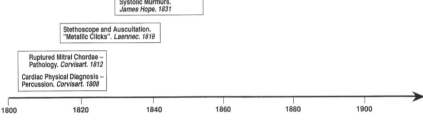

19th Century Cardiac Pathology and Auscultation

Figure 1. Mitral valvular regurgitation. Nineteenth century concepts based primarily on cardiac pathology, cardiac auscultation, and early natural history observations.

palpation to the application and interpretation of the acoustic information inherent in percussion and auscultation. Thus, the presence and interpretation of cardiac murmurs and the detection of cardiac enlargement lead to the more precise diagnosis of valvular heart disease. Physical diagnosis became a subject of intense interest to clinicians.[1]

Before clinicians could accurately time cardiac murmurs, it was necessary to understand the timing and origin of the first and second heart sounds. Laennec's belief that the first sound resulted from ventricular contraction and that contraction of the auricles caused the second heart sound led to a period of confusion. Studies during the 1830s by Rouanet, Bouillaud, Magendie, Hope and CJB Williams led to clarification of the heart sound sequence, i.e., that the first heart sound was related to ventricular contraction with closure of the mitral and tricuspid valves, and the second heart sound was related to aortic and pulmonic valve closure. Once clinicians could separate systole from diastole, the timing of murmurs and their interpretation became useful clinical currency.

In England, James Hope established the relationship of apical systolic thrills and systolic murmurs to the diagnosis of mitral regurgitation as a distinct valvular lesion in the 1830s. Hope incorporated Newtonian principles into the heart's action when he introduced his modern perspectives in 1839.[2] In particular, he displayed an extraordinary grasp of the hemodynamics of mitral regurgitation.

When the mitral orifice is permanently patescent [wide open] so that, at each ventricular contraction, blood regurgitates into the auricle, this cavity suffers in a remarkable degree, for it is not only gorged with the blood which it cannot transmit, but, in addition, sustains the pressure of the ventricular contraction. Permanent patescence of the mitral orifice, therefore, constitutes an obstruction on the left side of the heart, and the effect of this, as of contraction of the orifice, may be propagated backwards to the right side. The regurgitation is always considerable when it renders the pulse small and weak.

When the impediment to the circulation is primitively seated in the lungs, the right ventricle, situated immediately behind them, is the first to experience its influence, and when the cavity is so far overpowered by the distending pressure of the blood as to be incapable of adequately expelling its contents, the obstruction extends to the auricle—the process being exactly the same as that which I have already described, in reference to the left ventricle and auricle.[3]

Hope's contemporary, CJB Williams, provided the pathological correlation for a loud apical systolic murmur heard during life in a patient when the autopsy demonstrated ruptured mitral chordae associated with abnormalities of the mitral valve leaflets.

In the United States in the 1850s, Austin Flint recognized and taught that mitral regurgitation could be long borne without serious inconvenience, with a natural history quite distinct from other forms of valvular disease. This important concept was lost and then resurfaced again later in the 20th century. JP Crozer Griffith, Professor of Clinical Medicine at the University of Pennsylvania, discussed apical mid- and late systolic murmurs of mitral origin as instances of mitral regurgitation at the Association of American Physicians meeting in 1892. JN Hall, in Colorado, encountered late systolic murmurs of mitral insufficiency frequently and considered sudden yielding of the valve unable to withstand left ventricular systolic pressure as the probable mechanism.[4]

Thus, by the beginning of the 20th century, the auscultatory diagnosis of MVR was clearly described, mid- and late systolic murmurs were recognized as variant forms of MVR murmurs, ruptured mitral chordae as a cause of MVR was recognized, and the long natural history of patients with MVR had been defined. So where did clinicians go wrong for the next 100 years?

As is usually the case, the answer involved dogma without data. Information from the cardiovascular physiologists about mitral valve function was just beginning to have an impact in the clinical area. Authoritative French auscultators regarded apical systolic clicks and apical mid-

and late systolic murmurs as nonorganic or extracardiac in origin. A coherent approach to the pathophysiology and etiology of mitral regurgitation had not yet surfaced.

British cardiologists—initially Graham Steell and James Mackenzie, and later Thomas Lewis and John Parkinson—downplayed the diagnostic significance of apical systolic murmurs (Fig. 2). Mackenzie's original intent was to overcome the "tyranny of the stethoscope" and to spare a host of individuals from invalidism and cardiac neurosis. However, during World War I, the concept was expanded on a grand scale so that medical officers could deal specifically with the large numbers of young men with apical systolic murmurs, soldier's heart, and the effort syndrome that presented extraordinary diagnostic, disposition, and pension problems during the war. The doctrine that the apical systolic murmur should be disregarded when not accompanied by other signs of heart disease was developed and implemented under the wartime manpower pressures. The approach became military policy first in Great Britain and then in the United States as the war progressed. Intended to provide medical officers with guidelines about fitness for military service, the net result of setting

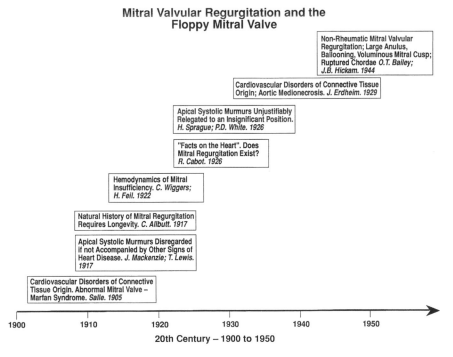

Figure 2. Mitral valvular regurgitation and the floppy mitral valve. Progression of concepts and controversies in the first one-half of the 20th century.

dogma about individuals with apical systolic murmurs without data was the inhibition of inquiry for several decades.[4]

Thus, as the result of the physical examination of millions of young men in the United States during World War I, several controversial issues regarding physical fitness for military service surfaced. The unexpected frequency of apical systolic murmurs and the interpretation and significance of these murmurs were the primary cardiovascular dilemmas. Following the war, in 1926 in the United States, Richard Cabot attacked the basic concept of mitral regurgitation as a clinical entity in his text, *Facts on the Heart*,[5] when he stated that mitral regurgitation was a lesion almost never verified at post mortem. He thought physicians were in error when they diagnosed mitral regurgitation on the basis of the loud apical systolic murmurs, and made the outrageous statement that these murmurs were extraordinarily common in all sorts of noncardiac disease as in health. He dated this pernicious habit to the World War I wartime experience noted above. "Fortunately the mistake was discovered and the rule put into effect that no man should be rejected from military service on account of a sytolic murmur no matter how loud it might be." Cabot expressed doubts that mitral regurgitation could be diagnosed in life, but did grant that it might exist as a great rarity. It is not a "clinical entity, for it cannot, so far as I can see, be recognized in life. Mackenzie has told us how he gradually came to recognize that no one ever died of mitral regurgitation."

Cabot was widely recognized in the United States for his emphasis on clinical and autopsy correlations and his contributions to medical progress with the case history method of teaching. The Case Records of the Massachusetts General Hospital published in *The New England Journal of Medicine* had their origins in the Clinicopathological Exercises founded by Cabot. Thus, the Mackenzie and Cabot dogma without data came from authoritative sounces and had a significant and negative impact on the mitral regurgitation debate that lasted for several decades.

Sir Thomas Lewis continued to teach that "the diagnosis of mitral regurgitation has a very limited importance" in the 1930s. However, clinical cardiologists such as Paul Dudley White and Samuel Levine in Boston realized that these positions were incorrect and developed a more reasonable approach to the apical systolic murmur-mitral regurgitation association in the early 1930s.[4]

As Paul Wood realized in 1956, the pendulum had swung much too far. The mid-20th century introduction of mitral valve surgery forced the pace, the whole subject received "the concentrated attention of investigators all over the world," and mitral regurgitation was seen in the "proper perspective."[6]

There were some data developing from experimental studies. When Wiggers and Feil described the cardiodynamics of mitral insufficiency in

1922, they incorporated and analyzed the earlier German experimental experience.[7] Their state-of-the-art studies involved recording optical pressure curves from the left atrium, left ventricle, and aorta, left atrial and left ventricular volumes, and arterial resistance. The timing of mitral regurgitation was related to the temporal events of the cardiac cycle described earlier by Wiggers. Determining the time of onset and duration of valvular regurgitation, quantitating the increased left atrial and left ventricular volumes, and documenting the marked increase in valvular regurgitation associated with increasing arterial resistance were among the results in this classic study.

The Floppy Mitral Valve and Mitral Valvular Regurgitation

The clinical emphasis on inflammatory diseases with scar formation as residual of previous inflammation causing chronic cardiac valvular disorders was appropriate at a time when life span was short, infections were prevalent, and rheumatic fever and syphilis were rampant. There were exceptions to these categorical classifications based on pathological observations. As early as 1912, Salle described mitral leaflet and chordal abnormalities in a postmortem examination of a patient with Marfan syndrome (Fig. 2). Bailey and Hickam (1944) made the association of severe mitral regurgitation with rupture of elongated, thin mitral chordae not related to infectious endocarditis.[8] Mitral cusps were voluminous and showed "fibrosis without stenosis" and ballooned or bulged upward into the left atrium. Dilatation of the mitral annulus was a consistent finding. Valvular connective tissue changes were present without inflammation, a gross anatomic and histologic profile that led the investigators to exclude a rheumatic etiology. The illustrations in the article establish the paper as a fundamental floppy mitral valve (FMV) study.

When Brigden and Leatham (1953) described "pure" mitral incompetence in males without a rheumatic history, the clinical features included a long natural history, susceptibility to bacterial endocarditis, and the late onset of rapidly progressive congestive heart failure, forerunners to the FMV natural history studies later in the century.[9]

A new group of cardiac morphological pathologists described valvular stretch as opposed to valvular scar and contraction as a cause of chronic valvular heart disease (Fig. 3). They introduced terms such as mucoid degeneration (Fernex and Fernex, 1958),[10] billowing sail deformity (Oka and Angrist, 1961),[11] or floppy, myxomatous, mucinous, hooded, or balloon mitral valves. The Fernex article, describing cardiomegaly in two patients who had mitral valves with multiple domes, augmentation of the mitral valve surface, and MVR without clinical evi-

Mitral Valvular Regurgitation, the Floppy Mitral Valve and Mitral Valve Prolapse

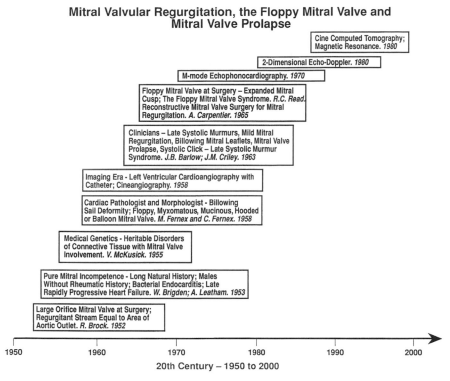

Figure 3. Mitral valvular regurgitation, the floppy mitral valve, and mitral valve prolapse. Progression of concepts and observations during the second half of the 20th century in parallel with the evolution of the technology of the era.

dence of Marfan syndrome, was a key article emphasizing a connective tissue etiology for FMVs.

At about the same time, an important symposium on MVR in 1958 presented a historical background, clinical and hemodynamic characteristics of MVR, and the important distinctions between mitral valve stenosis and MVR.[1] However, there was no clear-cut consideration of the FMV as an etiologic factor in patients with MVR.

The state-of-the-art in the recognition of MVR in 1961 was succinctly stated by an eminent cardiologist who was also an astute medical historian:

Physical diagnosis came into being shortly after the turn of the 19th century. Before that time mitral insufficiency was not diagnosable during life. After the introduction of the stethoscope, some 15 years elapsed before murmurs were distinguishable as systolic or diastolic. Very quickly thereafter, mitral insufficiency became recognizable and there followed a period of diagnostic overemphasis until Graham Steell and Mackenzie pushed the pendulum too far in the opposite direction. The disease is now recognized as one that has several etiologies (not rheumatic fever alone) and that may have fatal issue. Some types of it are coming to be correctable surgically and the most significant recent contributions are in the field of angiocardiography and hemodynamics. The lesion is still the least well understood of all valve lesions, however, and a great deal remains to be done.—CB Chapman, 1961[12]

For a variety of reasons, medical thought about MVR matured in a more controversial fashion than it did about other forms of valvular disease. More of nature's secrets were involved, there was diagnostic uncertainty about the significance of apical systolic murmurs, and a peculiar emotional bias toward symptomatic young people with apical systolic murmurs contributed to the controversy.

During the 1960s the association of nonejection clicks and apical mid- and late systolic murmurs with billowing mitral leaflets, mitral valve prolapse, and MVR was defined, initially by auscultation with phonocardiographic and cineangiographic correlates, and later by various imaging techniques.[13] An extensive reorganization of medical thought about the pathogenesis and classification of MVR followed (Fig. 3).

The rediscovery of nonrheumatic forms of MVR accompanied mid-20th-century cardiovascular diagnosis and surgery. One of the basic questions reviewing the floppy, "myxomatous" mitral valve lineage has been: Where were these valves in earlier days, and what were they called?

Pomerance, whose appreciation of these valves dates back to the 1960s, answered this in part: "Pathologists unfamiliar with the condition tend to attribute the appearances to previous rheumatism. . ."[14] The development of a small subspecialty group of cardiac morphologists and pathologists, whose new observations and clinical correlations about mitral valve anatomy and pathology influenced the way that clinicians presently think about mitral valve function and the pathogenesis of MVR, contributed significantly to progress in this area.

The Natural History of Mitral Regurgitation

The prolonged natural history of most forms of mitral regurgitation required that the patient live a long life before developing symptoms and disability, and also that the clinician be long-lived in order to follow such patients and understand the process. One such clinician was Clifford Allbutt, who lived 89 years, and was engaged in a consulting practice in Leeds, England, for 28 years (from 1861 to 1889) and learned these lessons.

Allbutt straddled the 19th and 20th centuries, and participated in both the "old" and the "new" cardiology.[15] Many years later, at age 81, he reviewed the World War I British Military Heart Hospital experience in 1917, and differed with Mackenzie and Lewis regarding the long-term significance and prognosis of apical systolic murmurs in young soldiers. Allbutt filed a minority dissenting opinion and presented a clear-cut picture of progressive mitral regurgitation:

> In looking back upon many years of practice I recall very vividly . . .the subsequent lives of many a patient in whom a mitral regurgitant murmur was for years the precursor of subsequent cardiac incapacity and ultimate failure. . .For many a year perhaps a young or comparatively young heart, out of its abundant stores, can meet excessive demands, and build itself up at threatened points; but if the interval is often a long one the event is none the less manifest. The murmur in crucial cases has been discovered accidentally; as for example in an examination for some temporary disorder, or for life insurance; though cardiac incapacity may not have ensued for years afterwards. After an uncertain period, however, the heart begins to enlarge, and the patient to feel a little transient dyspnea on unusual effort; this symptom increases, and the heart begins to make itself felt; yet even thus the patient may live still a few more years, and under due precautions do not a little work of a sedentary kind. It is then that effort tests may betray myocardial default, but the patient has then entered not upon his disease but upon the last stage of it. Then nocturnal dyspnea will appear, the ankles puff up, and other symptoms of the final phase of the malady accumulate. . .Scores of such cases arise in my mind as I turn my eyes to the past. . .

Although mitral regurgitation was treated in early medical and cardiological textbooks, etiological and pathophysiological classifications were late developments and for the most part are products of mid-late 20th century diagnostic, surgical, and pathological correlations. With these developments has come the rather belated recognition that, in contrast to mitral stenosis, for example, MVR is a phenomenon or manifestation with its own differential diagnosis that must be corrected for age, genetic setting, and region of the world. Diagnostic considerations must address mitral valve complex function, the integration of the entire mitral valve apparatus within the left atrium, left ventricle, and the circulation, as well as the total body economy.

The transition from the clinical, pathological, necropsy experience to the cardiovascular diagnostic and surgical era was reflected in the work of

Read et al. (1965), "symptomatic valvular myxomatous transformation (the floppy valve syndrome)"[16]; Carpentier and associates (1969), with reconstructive surgery for mitral regurgitation[17]; and McKay and Yacoub (1973), "clinical and pathological findings in patients with floppy valves treated surgically,"[18] when floppy or myxomatous mitral valves became a frequent reason for mitral valve reconstruction or replacement in the Western world.

The Floppy Mitral Valve: Mortality and Morbidity–A Family of Curves

The cumulative FMV data that provide a contemporary definition of natural history come from various sources—necropsy studies, cardiac surgical pathology, cardiac epidemiology, and diagnostic cardiac imaging studies—each with its own built-in bias and selectivity. However, certain profiles have emerged, and a collective analysis of carefully performed studies permits a definition of subgroups of patients. Data from major studies of patients with FMVs provide a family of curves providing greater insight into the natural history of individuals with FMVs and illustrating the varying modes of clinical presentation (Fig. 4).[19,20]

Nosology

King has noted that we take the classification of disease for granted, expect our medical textbooks to have detailed tables of contents, and tend to forget this orderly arrangement did not arise spontaneously but represents a slow and painful development that reaches back to the 18th century.[21] As clinicians we find it difficult to appreciate that the classification of disease is a continuous, dynamic process. Nowhere has this been more apparent than in reviewing the past 150-year history of MVR, and even more so in the accelerated pace of the past three decades.

We must continue to integrate basic and clinical studies in order to develop a new and improved nosology as we proceed with the definition of MVR. We address this question in Chapter 7, dealing with the floppy mitral valve in heritable cardiovascular disorders.

Cardiovascular Disorders of Connective Tissue Origin, Heritable Disorders of Connective Tissue, and the Floppy Mitral Valve

The history of the FMV is set against this background of medical thought about the natural history of MVR and the late-developing etiological and pathophysiological classifications.

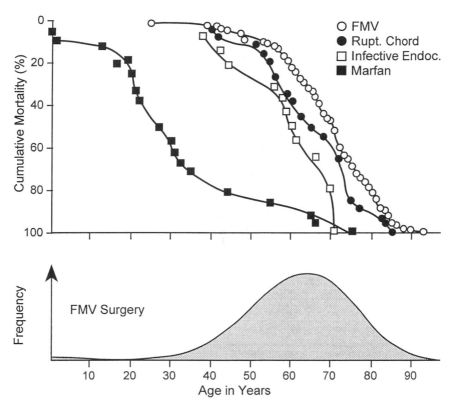

Figure 4. There are a series of natural history curves in patients with floppy mitral valves, with a prolonged natural history influenced or modified by the presence of a recognizable heritable disorder of connective tissue (Marfan syndrome), progressive mitral valvular regurgitation resulting in cardiovascular surgery, or specific complications such as infective endocarditis or ruptured chordae tendineae. Cumulative mortality from complications and associated conditions of the floppy mitral valve. The cumulative mortality of 102 patients with floppy mitral valves from a community hospital autopsy population of 1,376 (incidence 7.4%; 62 men, 40 women) is presented in the open circles (FMV). The other curves represent the cumulative mortality from the specific complication or associated conditions in a combined series, the community hospital cases noted above, and registry cases referred from elsewhere. Solid circles represent 26 patients with ruptured chordae; open triangles represent 14 patients with infective endocarditis; closed triangles represent 21 patients with Marfan syndrome. The lower curve represents the number and age of patients with floppy mitral valves who had valve replacement surgery for severe mitral valvular regurgitation reported in the 21-year surgical pathology of the mitral valve study at the Mayo Clinic during 1965, 1970, 1975, 1980, and 1985.[20] (Modified from Lucas RV and Edwards JE, reproduced with permission of Year Book Medical Publishers.)

That connective tissue abnormalities, expressed either as recognizable heritable disorders of connective tissue (syndromes), or as inherited isolated cardiovascular defects, are important causes of symptomatic cardiovascular disease is a relatively recent concept in the development of medical thought; it led to the realization that there is a broad spectrum of inherited or spontaneous cardiovascular disorders of connective tissue origin.[22] As a result, molecular biology and medical genetics have come to occupy an increasingly important place in establishing cardiovascular etiological diagnoses. We are gradually learning to identify and separate genetic factors from the influences of aging itself, a process that is particularly relevant in understanding the expression of clinical entities with a long natural history such as MVR associated with FMVs.

Recognition of aortic involvement appeared to take precedence in the definition of cardiovascular disorders or connective tissue origin. Erdheim described aortic medionecrosis in association with spontaneous rupture of the aorta in 1929.[23] This type of change was noted in the unruptured aorta by Rottino in 1940[24]; a similar histopathology was associated with aneurysmal dilatation of the aorta and arachnodactyly, and aortic dissection with Marfan syndrome in 1943.[25,26] These developmental steps brought the connective tissue concept into focus at the time of the mid-20th century revolution in cardiovascular diagnosis and surgery.

Mitral valve abnormalities occurring as isolated inherited connective tissue phenomena or within the spectrum of syndromes of heritable disorders of connective tissue, were actually recognized earlier than aortic involvement, and this has continued with increasing frequency during the past 75 years.[27] FMV may be inherited as an isolated defect, or as *the* or *a* cardiac manifestation of Marfan syndrome, Ehlers-Danlos syndrome[28], and polycystic kidney disease.[29] This realization placed the matter in an entirely new perspective for contemporary and future physicians.[30]

Perspective

Why did the medical giants of yesteryear have so much difficulty with the apical systolic murmur–mitral valvular regurgitation–floppy mitral valve connection? Why did the MVR odyssey turn into a trip on the merry-go-round or the swings of childhood rather than traverse a well-plotted path of discovery? And why did the evolution of medical thought reach such a crescendo in the mid-to-late 20th century?

The lack of technology and, after it was introduced, the distrust of technology by late-19th century and early-20th century clinicians were factors. The arduous transition from the "old" cardiology to the "new" cardiology, which has been expressed and analyzed by Lawrence, is a repetitive theme for each generation of clinicians.[31]

The antigenicity of new ideas, the arrogance without data expressed by key figures who failed to ask the right questions or do the experiments, the physicians' traditional stranglehold on medical thought about cardiovascular diseases until the relatively late appearance of the surgeons and cardiac pathologists were all contributory factors.

The prolonged natural clinical history of MVR, the subordination of careful medical epidemiology and analyses of natural history to World War I wartime military manpower needs, the lack of understanding about heritable cardiovascular disorders of connective tissue origin, and the prolonged, forceful use of the rheumatic fever etiology for many forms of heart disease were all influences that are difficult to weigh individually.[4]

Early 20th century concepts about the incidence, etiology, and pathogenesis of MVR were revised during the second half of the century by cardiac morphologists and pathologists, clinical cardiologists, cardiac imagers, and cardiovascular surgeons. The culmination of these basic and clinical developments are best exemplified in the current approaches to the diagnosis of FMV, mitral valve prolapse, and the documentation of the natural history of MVR .[4] The sophisticated imaging and surgical approaches to FMV recognition and reconstruction utilize principles developed by multiple basic and clinical investigators.

While it must be acknowledged that we stand on the shoulders of the giants who preceded us, it is also important for us to realize that while they stood amid rich archeological ruins, they frequently mistook the Rosetta stone for a platform, and because their gaze rested upon residual statuary and edifices, they overlooked the keys to understanding.

References

1. Vander Veer JB. Mitral insufficiency: Historical and clinical aspects. Am J Cardiol 2:1–6, 1958.
2. Keele KD. The application of the physics of sound to 19th century cardiology: With particular reference to the part played by CJB Williams and James Hope. Clio Medica 8:191–221, 1973.
3. Hope J. A Treatise on Diseases of the Heart and Great Vessels. Wm. Kidd, London, 1832.
4. Wooley CF, Baker PB, Kolibash AJ, Kilman JW, Sparks EA, Boudoulas H. The floppy, myxomatous mitral valve, mitral valve prolapse, and mitral regurgitation. Prog Cardiovasc Dis 33:397–433, 1991.
5. Cabot RC. Facts on the Heart. Philadephia and London, WB Saunders, 1926, pp 290–295.
6. Wood P. Diseases of the Heart and Circulation. London, Eyre and Spottiswoode, 1956, p 503.
7. Wiggers CJ, Feil H. The cardiodynamics of mitral insufficiency. Heart 9:149–174, 1922.
8. Bailey OT, Hickam JB. Rupture of mitral chordae tendineae. Am Heart J 28:578–600, 1944.
9. Brigden W, Leadham A. Mitral incompetence. Br Heart J 15:55–73, 1953.

10. Fernex PM, Fernex C. La degenerescence mucoide des valvules mitrales. Ses repercussions fonctionnelles. Helv Medica Acta 25:694–705, 1958.
11. Oka M, Angrist A. Fibrous thickening with billowing sails distortion of the aging heart valve. Proc NYS Assoc Publ Hlth Lab 46:21–23, 1961.
12. Mitral insufficiency: An annotated bibliography, 1803–1961. Private printing, Carleton B. Chapman, 1961.
13. Barlow JB, Bosman CK. Aneurysmal protrusion of the posterior leaflet of the mitral valve: An auscultatory-electrocardiographic syndrome. Am Heart J 71: 166–178, 1966.
14. Pomerance A, Davies M, eds. The Pathology of the Heart. London, Blackwell Scientific Publishing, 1975, p 68.
15. Wooley CF. From irritable heart to mitral valve prolapse: World War I, the British experience and Clifford Allbutt. Am J Cardiol 59:353–357, 1987.
16. Read RC, Thal AP, Wendt VE. Symptomatic valvular myxomatous transformation (the floppy valve syndrome). Circulation 32:897–910, 1965.
17. Carpentier A, Guerinon J, Deloche A, Fabiani JN, Relland J. Pathology of the mitral vlave. The Mitral Valve: A Pluridisciplinary Approach. Kalmanson D (ed): Acton, Mass, Publishing Sciences Group, 1976, pp 65–77.
18. McKay R, Yacoub MH. Clinical and pathological findings in patients with "floppy" valves treated surgically. Circulation 47 (Suppl 3):63–73, 1973.
19. Lucas RV, Edwards JE. The floppy mitral valve. Curr Prob Cardiol 7:1–48, 1982.
20. Olson LJ, Subramanian R, Ackermann DM, Orszulak TA, Edwards WD. Surgical pathology of the mitral valve: A study of 712 cases spanning 21 years. Mayo Clin Proc 62:22–34, 1987.
21. King LS. The Medical World of the Eighteenth Century. Chicago, The University of Chicago Press, 1958, pp 193–226.
22. McKusick VA. The cardiovascular aspects of Marfan's syndrome: A heritable disorder of connective tissue. Circulation 11:321–341;1955.
23. Erdheim J. Medionecrosis aortae idiopathica. Virchows Arch (Pathol Anat) 273: 454–479, 1929.
24. Rottino A. Medial degeneration, cystic variety, in unruptured aortas. Am Heart J 19:330–337, 1940.
25. Baer RW, Taussig HB, Oppenheimer EN. Congenital aneurysmal dilatation of the aorta associated with arachnodactyly. Bull Hopkins Hosp 72:309–331, 1943.
26. Etter LE, Glover LP. Arachnodactyly complicated by dislocated lens and death from rupture of dissecting aneurysm of aorta. JAMA 123:88–89, 1943.
27. Pyeritz RE. Mitral valve dysfunction in the Marfan syndrome. Am J Med 74; 797–707, 1983.
28. Leier CV, Call TD, Fulkerson PK, Wooley CF. The spectrum of cardiac defects in the Ehlers-Danlos syndrome, types I and III. Ann Int Med 921:171–178, 1980.
29. Leier CV, Baker PB, Kilman JW, Wooley CF. Cardiovascular abnormalities associated with adult polycystic kidney disease. Ann Int Med 100:683–688, 1984.
30. Bowen J, Boudoulas HB, Wooley CF. Cardiovascular disease of connective tissue origin. Am J Med 82:481–488, 1987.
31. Lawrence C. Moderns and ancients: The "new cardiology" in Britain 1880–1930. Med History (Suppl 5):1–33, 1985.

Part V

The Floppy Mitral Valve, Mitral Valve Prolapse, Mitral Valvular Regurgitation:

Heritable Aspects

Introduction

The Floppy Mitral Valve, Mitral Valve Prolapse, Mitral Valvular Regurgitation:
Heritable Aspects

Charles F. Wooley, MD,
Harisios Boudoulas, MD, PhD

When should a clinical phenomenon be considered as an isolated phenotype, or a phenotype within the continuum of a heritable disorder or syndrome?

This is a question that faces all clinicians, and in particular those involved in the detection, diagnosis, and care of individuals, patients, and families with heritable disorders. It is also a question that our predecessors did not envision when they developed categories and classifications of disorders and disease that became standard dogma for successive generations. For once established, medical nosology tends to become rigid and slow to change. In turn, the rigidity inhibits critical thinking and assimilation of new data into clinical classification schemes.

The ferment in clinical and molecular genetics, and the associated or underlying science, is changing our comprehension of inherited biological traits and challenging our comprehension and classification of disorders and disease. The impact of these changes and their clinical application has been phenomenal in certain areas, changing medical concepts and practice, with the promise of continuing progress. The clinician, however, working in the here and now, must, in order to reach a diagnosis, rely on identifying the clinical phenomena that are isolated phenotypes, or phenotypes within the spectrum or continuum of heritable disorders or syndromes.

From: Boudoulas H, Wooley CF. *Mitral Valve: Floppy Mitral Valve, Mitral Valve Prolapse, Mitral Valvular Regurgitation.* Second revised edition. ©Futura Publishing Company, Armonk, NY, 2000.

This brings us to the interface between genealogy and genetics, clinical identification and genetic testing, and the role of inheritance in the floppy mitral valve (FMV), mitral valve prolapse (MVP), mitral valvular regurgitation (MVR) triad.

That the FMV is a heritable disorder was a revolutionary concept at a time when rheumatic fever and syphilis were the main causes of valvular heart disease. When it was further postulated that the FMV was either an isolated phenotype or a phenotype in individuals with heritable disorders of connective tissue, this was equally confounding. As we will see in Chapter 7, both the concept and the postulate required decades for clarification and acceptance.

The FMV as a heritable disorder, and as a phenotype within recognized heritable syndromes, demonstrating genetic heterogeneity, with variable expression, are underlying themes in Chapter 7. Advances in molecular biology and contemporary genetics provide keys to understanding the mechanisms involved in this wide spectrum of heritable disorders, and to identify individuals as affected, at risk, or uninvolved.

The emphasis placed on individual patient analysis in the detection of individuals with heritable disorders is extremely important for the clinician and is highly dependent on the development of carefully constructed clinical pedigrees. In order to clarify the full expression of FMV mutations, long-term follow-up of individuals and family members is necessary, placing new obligations on clinicians interested in full participation in the new order of clinical cardiology.

Chapter 8, from our French colleagues, presents the provocative message that myxomatous mitral valvular disease might be inherited in an X-linked fashion. The spectrum of clinical involvement, the modes of inheritance, the genetic analyses, and the distinctions in severity of disease in men compared to women, expand the etiopathogenetic horizons in heritable valvular heart disease.

Taken together, Chapters 7 and 8 present an approach to the clinical assessment of individuals with the FMV/MVP/MVR triad, emphasizing a more global evaluation than is generally performed.

Enhanced awareness of the clinical environment, in which the FMV occurs, i.e., the clinical syndromes described in Chapter 7, is a prerequisite for new diagnostic matrices.

Utilization of the clinical history, the family history, pedigree development, phenotype analysis, and genetic technology will permit clinicians to identify individuals or families with an isolated form of the FMV/MVP/MVR triad, or patients with the FMV/MVP/MVR phenotype within the continuum of a systemic heritable disorder, with greater precision (Figure 1).

Individual Patient Analysis

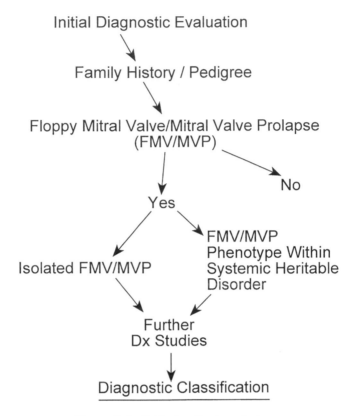

Figure 1. Individual patient analysis.

Close associations between clinicians with genetic interests and geneticists with clinical interests will improve diagnostic precision while creating new cross-specialty disciplines. As these improvements occur, emphasis will shift from FMV recognition and diagnosis to informed long-term management and preventative therapy.

The Floppy Mitral Valve/Mitral Valve Prolapse/Mitral Valvular Regurgitation:

Heritable Disorders

Elizabeth H. Sparks, MS, RN,
Harisios Boudoulas, MD, PhD,
Charles F. Wooley, MD

Mitral valve prolapse appears to be the most common Mendelian cardiovascular abnormality in humans.[1]

Introduction

This is a time of transition for clinicians concerned with the diagnosis and care of patients and families with heritable disorders, since the ferment in medical and molecular genetics has both elevated and complicated clinical comprehension. While it is obvious that medicine is at a threshold rich with promise and expectations, the clinician, working with both feet in the present, is frequently dealing with clinical phenomena that in reality are phenotypes in a continuum within incompletely understood heritable disorders. Yet the reality of the moment is that the diagnosis of most heritable cardiovascular disorders is still based on clinical recognition of phenotypes, the development of informed family his-

From: Boudoulas H, Wooley CF. *Mitral Valve: Floppy Mitral Valve, Mitral Valve Prolapse, Mitral Valvular Regurgitation.* Second revised edition. ©Futura Publishing Company, Armonk, NY, 2000.

tories and pedigrees correlated with evolving laboratory and imaging techniques.

Our entire comprehension of disease or disorders is under challenge in the molecular genetic era as investigative and diagnostic methods proliferate. While our understanding of genotype-phenotype relations expands diagnostic and classification concepts, at the same time the clinical implications of genetic defects that have already been identified are incompletely understood.

With these concerns in mind, let us consider the role of inheritance in the floppy mitral valve (FMV), mitral valve prolapse (MVP), mitral valvular regurgitation (MVR), and the FMV/MVP/MVR triad.

Genealogy Meets Genetics

The interface between genealogy and genetics is an important facet in the recognition of those heritable disorders with a broad spectrum of clinical expression, variable penetrance, and a long natural history.

An example may be found in a report in 1981 describing an Israeli kindred of North African Sephardic descent.[2] Following the diagnosis of MVP in an 8-year-old boy, an extensive family investigation yielded information about age-related progressive autosomal dominant mitral valve disease involving 15 members in four generations of the kindred (Fig. 1). Four of the 15 affected members were young children. The spectrum of involvement in the 15 affected members ranged from asymptomatic family members with auscultatory evidence of a systolic click and late systolic murmur, to those with pansystolic murmurs, ectopic ventricular activity, severe MVR, and congestive heart failure. A cluster of family members with sudden death at about age 40 was also identified. Skeletal abnormalities included pectus excavatum, kyphoscoliosis, and narrow anterior-posterior thoracic diameter. These phenotypic observations demonstrate the full spectrum of the FMV/MVP/MVR triad.

The authors of this chapter had a similar experience in 1971, with the additional benefit of a 25-year follow-up. The proband is a 66-year-old female who presented at age 41 with history of a heart murmur, intermittent palpitations, and episodes of chest heaviness. She was slender, with long fingers and a mild pectus excavatum. An apical nonejection systolic click was followed by a late systolic murmur. Electrocardiographic findings included sinus rhythm and frequent premature atrial contractions with aberrant conduction. Left ventricular cineangiography demonstrated FMV, posterior mitral valve leaflet prolapse, no mitral regurgitation, and normal coronary anatomy. Low-dose propranolol therapy minimized the frequency of premature atrial contractions. Antibiotic prophylaxis for dental, gastrointestinal, or genitourinary procedures was recommended.

Generation

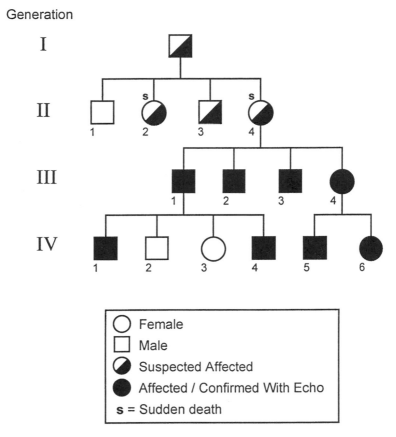

Figure 1. Pedigree demonstrates four generations of a family with mitral valve prolapse. Circles denote females; squares denote males. Fully shaded symbols represent members with MVP confirmed by echocardiography; partially shaded symbols represent members suspected of MVP by clinical examination. Members in generations I and II were not studied by echocardiography. Members in generations III and IV had thoracic skeletal abnormalities. Small case "s" identifies members with sudden death. See text for details. (Used with permission from Cooper MJ, et al.[2])

Over a 25-year-period her symptoms of chest discomfort were more noticeable during physical exertion and emotional stress, and the palpitations were especially noticeable at night while in the left lateral decubitus position. Overall, however, her symptoms were well controlled. The most recent physical examination showed slender body habitus, nonejection systolic click, and a late systolic murmur, grade I/VI increasing to grade II/VI with prompt squatting and standing post squatting.

Both maternal grandparents had long fingers and lived long lives.

The grandfather was tall and slender with long arms. The patient's mother was examined at age 75, had long fingers, cardiomegaly, an apical systolic thrill with a grade V/VI mitral regurgitation murmur; death at age 85 was due to congestive heart failure. The proband's three older sisters are alive and well (Fig. 2).

The proband's daughter presented at age 14 with a 4-year history of fatigue, dull chest pain, and lightheadedness. Physical examination showed slender habitus, long fingers, long thorax, hyperextensible joints, pectus excavatum, apical mid-systolic click, and grade II/VI late systolic murmur in the recumbent position which became holosystolic in the upright posture. She returned with proximal muscle weakness at age 17. Electromyogram and nerve conduction studies were negative for neuropathic and myopathic processes; homocystinuria screen was negative.

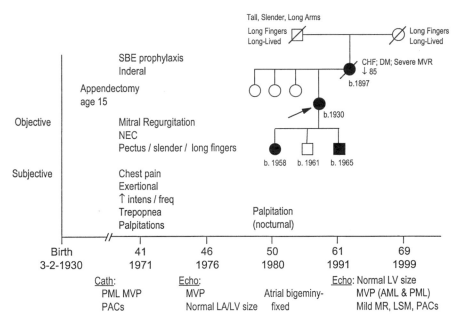

Figure 2. Four-generation pedigree of family members with heritable FMV. Proband is illustrated by arrow. Circles represent females; squares represent males. Shaded symbols denote family members with floppy mitral valve, mitral valve prolapse or mitral valvular regurgitation. Diagonal slashes through symbols denote deceased members. b. = year born; NEC = nonejection click; SBE = subacute bacterial endocarditis; CHF = congestive heart failure; DM = diabetes mellitus; PAC's = premature atrial contractions; MVP = mitral valve prolapse; LV = left ventricular; LA = left atrial; AML = anterior mitral leaflet; PML = posterior mitral leaflet; MR = mitral regurgitation; LSM = late systolic murmur. See text for details.

Echocardiogram showed MVP; left ventricular cineangiography showed an FMV with posterior mitral leaflet prolapse.

The proband's 7-year-old son, asymptomatic at the initial evaluation, had a late systolic murmur in the recumbent posture that became holosystolic in the upright posture. At age 11 auscultation was unchanged; an echocardiogram showed FMV, MVP, normal left atrial and left ventricular size and systolic function. He developed mild exertional chest discomfort in his mid-teen years. He became active in track and field activities and bicycling and the episodic chest discomfort resolved spontaneously. He returned at age 17, was quite active, however, considered himself "undermuscled." Physical examination showed slender build and pectus excavatum. He was 25 years old at his most recent evaluation, asymptomatic, auscultation was unchanged, and his echocardiogram showed anterior leaflet MVP.

These two family studies emphasize the need to obtain an extended family history, perform thorough clinical evaluations of individual family members, and arrange follow-up evaluations. Long-term, multigenerational family data are invaluable in the assessment of risk for progression of disease, and are fundamental to clinical comprehension, classification, and evaluation of the mode of FMV clinical expression and the natural history in families.

The Classification of Cardiovascular Disease

Discussions of heritable cardiovascular diseases and disorders are restricted by traditional classifications of cardiovascular disease that were constructed without genetic data. This situation persists despite the increasing awareness that heritable cardiovascular disorders occupy the high ground in the etiology of cardiac disease.

Classification of cardiovascular diseases is rooted in the 19th century anatomic and pathologic constructs when the medical history, physical diagnosis, the clinical course, and the autopsy were the bases for clinical diagnosis. The resulting classification placed emphasis on the "structural" or "anatomic" aspects of cardiovascular disease (Fig. 3).

Richard Cabot's classification scheme emphasized pathophysiology and an understanding of the specific cause of cardiovascular disorders in 1914: rheumatic fever, syphilis, hypertension, and atherosclerosis; "etiology" became a cornerstone augmenting the anatomic approach.[3] The introduction of exercise testing as a screening device in the assessment of physical fitness of soldiers during World War I, or as a therapeutic modality in symptomatic young men with soldier's heart, added another dimension to the cardiac classification process based on physical capability-the "functional classification."

Classification of Cardiovascular Disease

		Nomenclature and Criteria
		(NYHA - 1928)
		Etiology
		Anatomic
		Physiologic
	Cause	Functional
	(Cabot - 1914)	
	Rheumatic	
	Syphilitic	
	Atherosclerotic	
Functional State	Hypertensive	
Exercise Testing		
Early 20th Century		
Structural		
Anatomic Pathology		
19th Century		

Traditional Classification of Cardiovascular Disease

Figure 3. Traditional classifications of cardiovascular disease beginning in the 19th century when anatomic pathology defined structural abnormalities. Early in the 20th century when pathophysiology and exercise testing were used to define functional state the functional classification followed. Etiologic considerations including rheumatic, syphilitic, atherosclerotic, or hypertensive causes of cardiovascular disease were introduced. The New York Heart Association Classification identified nomenclature and criteria for cardiovascular disease based on etiology, anatomy, physiology, and function.

The New York Heart Association incorporated all of these elements into a multiple axial classification system in 1928.[4] Although modified with time, this basic classification continues to be widely used at present, with nomenclature and criteria arranged into categories for etiology, anatomy, physiology, and functional class (Fig. 3).

Awareness of the origins of cardiac classification schemes assumes increasing significance in view of the impact of molecular genetics in the clinical environment. The traditional classifications of cardiac disease came into existence long before heritable cardiovascular disorders, heritable disorders of connective tissue with cardiac involvement, and contemporary genetic concepts intruded upon modern cardiology. New, expanded, and flexible cardiovascular classification schemes are required in order to integrate the evolving concepts in medical genetics and vascular biology into traditional classifications.[5,6] Examples of recent revisions of diagnostic criteria that extend and affect traditional classification schemes will be presented in the Marfan syndrome and Ehlers-Danlos syndrome sections that follow.

Heritable Cardiovascular Disorders

The lineage of heritable cardiovascular disorders reflects the prolonged interval between the initial description of specific clinical phenomena and the clinician's awareness that the phenomena are in actuality phenotypes within the spectrum of a heritable disorder (Fig. 4). The next level of comprehension occurs when clinicians realize that two or more phenotypes linked together form a syndrome, and that familial patterns of inheritance exist. In the past, the time interval from description to com-

Heritable Cardiovascular Disorders

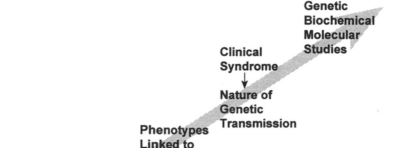

Figure 4. Evolution of a classification of heritable cardiovascular disorders over time (X axis) and through a series of developmental stages (Y axis). Classification begins with a description of the clinical phenomena, followed by the recognition of clinical phenomena as phenotypes. When phenotypes are linked, clinical syndromes are defined. These steps are fundamental to the recognition of genetic transmission of clinical syndromes. Genetic, biochemical, and molecular studies in individuals and families within clinical syndromes provide the bases for classification of heritable cardiovascular disorders, and putative pathogenetic mechanisms.

prehension has been measured in decades. Once the clinical syndrome has been described and the nature of genetic transmission is established, these steps must withstand critical scrutiny and sensitivity-specificity characteristics must be developed.

Eventually the clinical syndromes must be understood in terms of the basic structural, biochemical, and molecular mechanisms (Fig. 4). Frequently these mechanisms are interrelated in ways that are beyond comprehension or the available technology when the search is initiated. The time intervals for each of these steps is extremely variable, often prolonged beyond our recollection. Solutions to diagnostic dilemmas are dependent on the appropriate technology, which in turn may be beyond the horizon. Intensity of the search and the fund of knowledge available to the investigators and clinicians in pursuit of diagnostic coherence are other important factors.

A recurrent theme in these transitions has been the relatively late recognition of cardiovascular involvement in heritable disorders of connective tissue, and of cardiovascular disease as heritable entities per se (Fig. 4). Thus the chronology of heritable cardiovascular disorders is not a straight shot from point to point, rather a profile of various works in progress over prolonged intervals.

Terminology

Terms such as etiology, variability, pleiotropy, penetrance, genetic heterogeneity, and pathogenesis are basic to the language of the geneticists. However, not all clinicians are comfortable with this language and the terms are not always used precisely in the clinical environment. Since the concepts have diagnostic overtones, a brief review of the terms may be appropriate (Table 1).

A Three-Dimensional Approach

As Burn et al.[7] noted, clinical understanding of the genotype-phenotype relations is complex and requires a three-dimensional approach. *First* is the clinical picture, or the phenotype, i.e., the structural changes, the nature and severity of the clinical disease. There are important roles for clinicians and clinician-investigators in these areas. *Second* are the gene, its DNA sequence, and the protein it encodes. Although frequently presented as a straightforward quest, these steps may be quite complex. *Third*, in order to complete the cycle, how does the abnormal protein product produce the phenotype?

The three-dimensional approach forms a substrate for clarification of

Table 1
Glossary

Allele – one of the variant forms of a gene at a particular locus, or location, on a chromosome. Different alleles produce variation in inherited characteristics such as hair color or blood type. In an individual, one form of the allele (the dominant one) may be expressed more than another form (the recessive one).

Etiology – involves the study of cause.

Genetic heterogeneity – refers to an identical phenotype that may be inherited in different ways, or from more than a single gene.

Genotype – the genetic identity of an individual that does not show as outward characteristics.

Inherited – transmitted through genes from parents to offspring.

Pathogenesis – refers to the process by which the causative factors operate.

Penetrance – is an all or none expression of the genotype: the percentage of people carrying the gene who express the phenotype.

Phenotype – the observable traits or characteristics of an organism. For example, hair color, weight, or the presence or absence of a disease. Phenotypic traits are not necessarily genetic.

Pleiotropy – relates to multiple phenotypic expressions arising from the same genetic mutation.

Polymorphism – a gene that exists in more than one version (allele), and where the rare allele can be found in more than 1% of the population.

Variable expression – the gene can be associated with clinical manifestations exhibiting varying degrees of severity in different individuals; refers to the varying intensity of the symptoms.

diagnostic criteria, i.e., a fourth dimension, refinements that extend beyond individual patient analysis and extensive pedigree analysis, establishing new diagnostic criteria with sensitivity and specificity analyses (Fig. 5). Evaluating FMV genotype-phenotype relations provides the basis for current understanding and a platform for future developments.

Inheritance Patterns in Families with the Floppy Mitral Valve

The changes in FMV nosology and the introduction of specific FMV diagnostic criteria during the past five decades influence the interpretation of earlier publications about FMV inheritance patterns, as does the growing awareness of a broad spectrum of FMV clinical expression and the long natural history. Familial occurrence of MVP or FMV was described during the clinical recognition phase based on auscultation, angiography, and early echocardiography during the 1960s and 1970s.[8-15]

When Strahan[16] et al. reported the families of 12 probands with auscultatory and echocardiographic criteria for MVP in 1983, 70 parents, sibs,

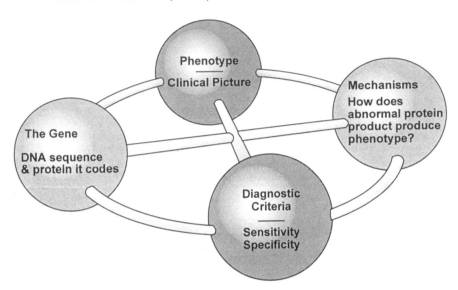

Figure 5. Clinical appraisal provides the basis for defining the phenotype. DNA sequences and the proteins they encode contribute information about the gene itself. How an abnormal protein product produces specific phenotypes is the next step, and requires confirmation via established diagnostic criteria. When diagnostic criteria are subjected to critical analysis, sensitivity and specificity criteria are established.

and progeny were included in the analysis. Forty-seven percent of progeny were affected compared with 30% of parents; 38% of sibs were affected. The authors proposed a three-compartmental penetrance model to account for the variation in expression with age. This included a latent stage, the time before onset of signs; an affected stage; and a stage in which the subjects are withdrawn because of treatment, regression, or death.

A detailed review of the inheritance and phenotypic features of MVP was presented by Devereux and Kramer-Fox in 1988.[17] Based on their own experience and that of others, Devereux and Kramer-Fox found that the family studies were consistent with autosomal dominant inheritance, although reduced expression in children, adult males, and older women kept the proportion of affected first degree relatives below the expected 50% for a fully expressed dominant condition. Prevalence figures far exceeded MVP prevalence among unselected subjects. In addition, expression of the MVP gene was affected by sex, and an age-dependent expression of MVP was noted. The phenotype of inherited MVP included thoracic bony abnormalities, low body weight and blood pressure, and palpitations; however, the authors did not confirm further associations between MVP and other symptoms. Devereux and his associates have continued to emphasize the importance of family studies in the definition of subtypes within the inherited condition using demographic, clinical, and echocardiographic findings in relatives of MVP index cases.[18]

Clinicians have described a number of skeletal and anthropometric phenotypes in patients with FMV/MVP from the earliest studies to the present, wrestling with connective tissue etiologic concerns, i.e., the Marfan versus non-Marfan categorization. These concerns were similar to those expressed even earlier by clinicians and cardiac pathologists dealing with patients with aneurysmal aortic disease, aortic dissection, and annuloaortic ectasia.

The Floppy Mitral Valve: Marfan and "Overlap" Connective Tissue Disorders

Clinical and biological pathways to understanding the etiology of the FMV have evolved from the recognition and increasingly precise definition of Marfan syndrome during the past century. Mitral valve leaflet and chordae abnormalities in Marfan syndrome were described as early as 1912.[19] After a long period of relative inactivity, attention then shifted to the aorta when the occurrence and severity of cardiovascular complications due to aortopathy with aortic root dilatation and aortic dissection were described in the 1940s. The clinical and pathological expression of the FMV within Marfan syndrome was recognized and accelerated with more precise definition of Marfan syndrome per se[20] and FMV angiographic and echocardiographic diagnostic criteria.[21]

FMV dysfunction in a study of 166 patients with Marfan syndrome was described by Pyeritz and Wappel in 1983.[19] The relative concordance of auscultatory and echocardiographic findings of MVP was noted, and progressive FMV dysfunction presenting as MVP/MVR was extremely common in young patients with Marfan syndrome. Serious MVR developed in one of every eight patients by the third decade, much earlier than FMV expression in patients without Marfan syndrome. By the time of this report a certain degree of clinical and pathologic coherence had developed about the ubiquitous nature of the FMV. Although the pathologic changes and natural history were accelerated and exaggerated in Marfan syndrome patients, similarities of FMV expression-heritable nature, basic histopathology, and mechanisms of dysfunction were consistent with FMV clinical expression in general.[21]

Throughout the evolving medical literature about patients with the systolic click, late systolic murmur, and MVP inheritance patterns during the 1960s and 1970s, the frequent references to body habitus, anthropometrics, and skeletal abnormalities provoked discussion. Similar to the Marfan non-Marfan distinctions in the literature about thoracic aortic aneurysms, annuloaortic ectasia, and aortic dissection, recurrent diagnostic or classification concerns involved the presence of the cardiovascular lesions without overt skeletal or ocular lesions, i.e., the "complete" Marfan syndrome.

Glesby and Pyeritz addressed these concerns about the association of MVP and systemic abnormalities of connective tissue in an important paper in 1989.[22] Their study involved patients or individuals who, although they could not be precisely classified within a recognized heritable syndrome using contemporary nosology, had clinical evidence of a systemic defect of the extracellular matrix. This differential diagnosis was a clinical conundrum facing physicians concerned with precise diagnosis in patients and families who presented with connective tissue abnormalities, the FMV/MVP/MVR triad, or combinations therein. These were patients who shared certain manifestations of Marfan syndrome, including long limbs, thoracic cage deformities, striae atrophicae, FMV with MVP, and mild dilatation of the aortic root. The authors concluded that the clinical phenotype of patients with MVP constitutes a continuum, from the "complete" Marfan syndrome at one extreme to isolated MVP due to FMV at the other end. These observations resonated with clinicians concerned with these clinical distinctions. Thus the expanding concept of an "overlap" heritable connective tissue disorder was introduced to describe familial FMV/MVP. The MASS phenotype was suggested as an acronym to emphasize involvement of the mitral valve, aorta, skeleton, and skin, pending greater precision in genetic investigations.

The Marfan Syndrome as Prototype

Marfan syndrome, a systemic disorder of connective tissue with autosomal dominant inheritance results in ocular, skeletal, and cardiovascular abnormalities. Although penetrance is complete, variability in the time of onset, tissue distribution, and severity of clinical manifestations occur between and within families. The molecular mechanisms involved in Marfan syndrome are multiple, and tracing the pathways involves a variety of disciplines.

Revised Diagnostic Criteria

Reliance solely on clinical criteria has resulted in either diagnostic dilemmas or overdiagnosis of Marfan syndrome. Revised diagnostic criteria for Marfan syndrome were presented in 1996 along with a chronology; clinical criteria and molecular analysis were incorporated.[20] The revised diagnostic criteria continue to be based on a combination of major and minor clinical expressions, however, the revisions include "more stringent diagnostic requirements in relatives of an unequivocally affected individual; skeletal involvement as a major criterion if at least four of eight typical skeletal manifestations are present; potential contribution of molecular analysis to the diagnosis of Marfan syndrome; and delineation of initial criteria for diagnosis of other heritable conditions with partially overlapping phenotypes." The authors emphasize that the presence of a major criterion in a system carries higher diagnostic specificity than a system "being involved." An outline of the revised Marfan syndrome diagnostic criteria is presented in Table 2.

Requirements of the diagnosis of Marfan syndrome in the index case include: in the noncontributory family or genetic history, major manifestations in at least two different organ systems with involvement of a third organ system; or if the mutation known to cause Marfan syndrome in other family members is detected, one major criterion and a second organ system involvement.

The importance of the revised diagnostic criteria for Marfan syndrome extends beyond the syndrome. Enhanced diagnostic precision and coherence, with the introduction of biochemical, molecular, and genetic factors provide the bases and an evolving template for the classification of heritable cardiovascular disorders in general.

Basic Abnormalities

Understanding the basic abnormalities in the heritable connective tissue disorders has evolved during the past several decades. Developments in medical genetics, protein chemistry, and analysis of the extracellular matrix, introduced fibrillin, microfibrillar proteins, calcium binding proteins, contractile proteins, and extracellular matrix proteins into the clinical literature dealing with heritable connective tissue disorders.

Fibrillin-1, a modular glycoprotein and major component of 10–12 nm microfibrils of the extracellular matrix, and the fibrillin-1 gene, FBN1, became clinical concerns as attention was directed toward defects in elastin and the microfibrillar fibers, integral components of elastic components. Located on chromosome 15 q21.1, the FBN1 gene encodes fibrillin-1, and mutations in this gene cause Marfan syndrome.[23] This is a very large gene, and genetic changes or mutations may be responsible for the disorder in one family, while an entirely different mutation may be found in another affected family. The large number of mutations responsible for Marfan syndrome means that at present the diagnosis of Marfan syndrome remains primarily a clinical diagnosis.

Table 2
Marfan Syndrome: Diagnostic Criteria

Index Case

If noncontributory family history or genetic history:

Must have major criteria in two or more different organ systems + involvement of a 3rd organ system; or

Mutation in the family that is known to cause Marfan syndrome + one major criterion in an organ system and involvement in a 2nd organ system

Relative of the Index Case

Family history + 1 major criterion in an organ system + involvement of a 2nd organ system

Skeletal System

Major Criteria	Minor Criteria	Involvement
• 4 of 8 required: • Pectus carinatum • Pectus excavatum requiring surgery • Upper to lower segment ratio <0.85 and arm span to height ratio >1.05 • Wrist + thumb signs • Scoliosis >20° or spondylolisthesis • Reduced elbow extension (<170°) • Medial malleolus displacement medially causing pes planus • Protrusio acetabulae (radiographically)	• Pectus excavatum of moderate severity • Joint hypermobility • Highly arched palate with crowding of the teeth • Facial appearance: dolichocephaly, malar hypoplasia, enophthalmos, retrognathia, downslanting palpebral fissures	two major; or one major and two minor criteria

Ocular System

Major Criteria	Minor Criteria	Involvement
Ectopia lentis	Abnormally flattened corneas (by keratometry) Increased axial globe length (by ultrasound) Hypoplastic iris or hypoplastic ciliary muscle causing miosis	two minor criteria

Cardiovascular System

Major Criteria	Minor Criteria	Involvement
Ascending aortic dilatation involving the sinuses of Valsalva Ascending aortic dissection	Mitral valve prolapse Pulmonary artery dilatation without valvular or peripheral pulmonary stenosis and age <40 years	one major and one minor criteria

Table 2
Continued

| | Mitral annular calcification and age <40 years | |
| | Descending thoracic or abdominal aortic dilatation or dissection and age <50 years | |

Pulmonary System

Major Criteria	**Minor Criteria**	**Involvement**
None	Spontaneous pneumothorax	one minor criterion
	Apical blebs	

Skin and Integument

Major Criteria	**Minor Criteria**	**Involvement**
None	Striae atrophicae not associated with marked weight changes, pregnancy or repetitive stress	one minor criterion
	Recurrent or incisional herniae	

Dura

Major Criteria	**Minor Criteria**	
Dural ectasia on MRI or CT	None	

Family/Genetic

Major Criteria	**Minor Criteria**	**Involvement**
Child, sib, or parent who meets criteria independently	None	one major criterion
• FBN1 mutation known to cause Marfan syndrome is detected		
• Affected haplotype around FBN1 gene is inherited by descent and is known to be associated with Marfan syndrome		

The immunohistochemistry of connective tissue matrix proteinases and the role of these enzymes in Marfan syndrome are involved in the pathogenesis of the cardiovascular tissue lesions. When Segura et al.[24] analyzed the changes in matrix metalloproteinases and their tissue inhibitors as potential factors in damage to connective tissue in Marfan syndrome, their findings led them to propose the following sequential hypotheses. Defects in fibrillin-1 in Marfan syndrome lead to formation of elastin that is abnormally aggregated and more easily degraded by matrix metalloproteinases than normal elastin. Upregulation of matrix metalloproteinase synthesis occurs, leading to progressive destruction of connective tissue by these enzymes with the development of the cardiovascular tissue abnormalities expressed in the aorta and cardiac valves.

FBN1 gene mutations have been associated with a spectrum of milder overlap phenotypes, from the MASS phenotype described above at the mild end, to the classic Marfan syndrome at the other end. The FBN1 genotype and phenotype relationships were examined in families with mild phenotypes, and also in those with striking clinical variability among apparently affected family members.[25] Multiple molecular mechanisms were identified underlying the subdiagnostic variants of Marfan syndrome. One family was shown to cosegregate the MVP syndrome with a mutation in FBN1 that could be distinguished from those associated with the classic Marfan phenotype.

Fibrillin-1 has a modular organization that includes 43 calcium binding epidermal growth factor-like domains and seven transforming growth factor beta binding protein-like domains. The calcium binding epidermal growth factor-like domain is the predominant structure motif of the protein and it is estimated that over 70% of the mutations leading to Marfan syndrome disrupt this domain.[26,27] The structural and functional consequences of defective calcium binding to fibrillin-1 and the effects on assembly and properties of the microfibrils are subjects of active investigation.

These basic observations provide insights into clinical concerns that extend back for a century,[28] while offering the potential for increased precision in diagnosis and counseling.

Uniform diagnostic criteria for Marfan syndrome and other heritable connective tissue disorders are important since the phenotypic continuum among heritable disorders of connective tissue involves a broad spectrum of clinical expression. Considering the vast array of diagnostic dilemmas frequently associated with cardiovascular involvement, in heritable disorders with FMV/MVP/MVR triad, aortopathy and its consequences, or combinations of FMV and aortopathy,[29,30] one can begin to appreciate the enormity of the task at hand as well as the potential for future interventions and therapy (Fig. 6).

Ehlers-Danlos Syndrome

The Ehlers-Danlos syndrome (EDS) is a heterogeneous connective tissue disorder characterized by abnormalities of the skin and joints. Fragile

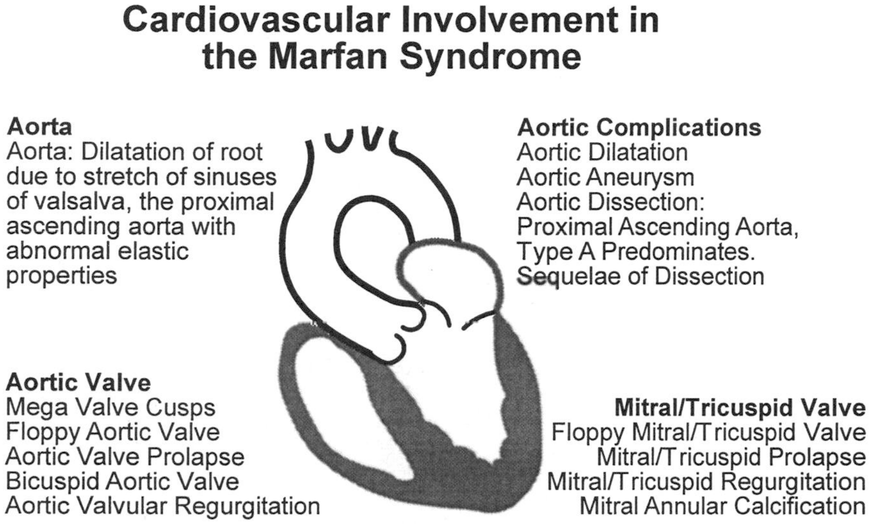

Cardiovascular Involvement in the Marfan Syndrome

Aorta
Aorta: Dilatation of root due to stretch of sinuses of valsalva, the proximal ascending aorta with abnormal elastic properties

Aortic Complications
Aortic Dilatation
Aortic Aneurysm
Aortic Dissection:
Proximal Ascending Aorta,
Type A Predominates.
Sequelae of Dissection

Aortic Valve
Mega Valve Cusps
Floppy Aortic Valve
Aortic Valve Prolapse
Bicuspid Aortic Valve
Aortic Valvular Regurgitation

Mitral/Tricuspid Valve
Floppy Mitral/Tricuspid Valve
Mitral/Tricuspid Prolapse
Mitral/Tricuspid Regurgitation
Mitral Annular Calcification

Figure 6. The spectrum of cardiovascular involvement in Marfan syndrome.

skin that is hypertextensible, bruises easily, and forms abnormal scars, as well as joint hypermobility with loose-jointedness and joint dislocation are characteristics of the disorder. Major fibrillar collagen abnormalities have been identified in EDS subgroups,[23] however, at present, as with Marfan syndrome, the EDS diagnosis remains primarily a clinical diagnosis.

The EDS classification was initially based on clinical signs and the mode of inheritance; as biochemical and molecular information became available, the classification was further modified. With increases in the number of subtypes, and the biochemical and molecular data, the classification lost coherence.

Thus, the revised nosology proposed by Beighton et al. in 1998[31] is helpful to clinicians concerned with greater precision in diagnosis and communication. Six major types based on major and minor diagnostic criteria have been proposed. The major criteria are intended to provide higher diagnostic specificity, important considerations when dealing with distinctions between other heritable conditions and the general population. The mode of inheritance, major and minor diagnostic criteria, cause and laboratory diagnosis, and special comments provide greater degrees of nosologic coherence. More specific methods of assessing skin hyperextensibility and joint hypermobility also assist the clinical appraisal (Table 3).

Within this proposed classification, the classical, hypermobility, and arterial types are more common, while the kyphoscoliosis, arthrochalasis, and dermatosparaxis types are considerably less common.

Table 3
Ehlers-Danlos Diagnostic Criteria

Classic Type
Autosomal Dominant

Major Criteria	Minor Criteria	Laboratory
Skin hyperextensibility	Smooth velvety skin	Proα1(V) or
Widened atrophic scars	Molluscoid pseudotumors	Proα2(V) collagen type V chains
Joint hypermobility	Subcutaneous spheroids	Abnormal collagen fibril structure
	Sprains, dislocations, subluxations, pes planus	"Cauliflower deformity"
	Muscle hypotonia, delayed gross motor development	
	Easy bruising	
	Tissue extensibility and fragility (i.e., hiatus hernia, anal prolapse in childhood, cervical insufficiency)	
	Postoperative hernias	
	Positive family history	

Hypermobility Type
Autosomal dominant

Major	Minor
Hyperextensible and/or smooth velvety skin	Recurring joint dislocations
	Chronic joint/limb pain
Generalized joint hypermobility	Positive family history

Vascular Type
Autosomal dominant

Major Criteria	Minor Criteria	Laboratory
Thin, translucent skin	Acrogeria	Abnormal collagen type III;
Arterial/intestinal/ uterine fragility or rupture	Tendon and muscle rupture	Mutation in COL3A1 gene
	Talipes equinovarus	
Would dehiscence	Early-onset varicose veins	
Hypermobility of small joints	Arteriovenous, carotid cavernous sinus fistula	
Extensive bruising	Pneumothorax/ pneumohemothorax	
Facial appearance: thin delicate pinched nose; thin lips, tight skin; hollow cheeks; prominent staring eyes; tight firm lobeless ears	Gingival recession	
	Family history, sudden death in a close relative	

Table 3
Continued

Kyphoscoliosis Type
Autosomal recessive

Major Criteria	Minor Criteria
Generalized joint laxity	Tissue fragility, atrophic scars
Severe muscle hypotonia at birth	Easy bruising
	Arterial rupture
	Marfanoid habitus
Scoliosis at birth, progressive	Microcornea
scleral fragility, and rupture of the ocular globe	Radiologically considerable osteopenia
	Family history

Arthrochalasia Type
Autosomal dominant

Major Criteria	Minor Criteria	Laboratory
Severe generalized joint hypermobility with recurrent subluxations	Skin hyperextensibility	pNα1(I) or pNα2(I) dermal collagen or cultural skin fibroblast chains
	Tissue fragility, atrophic scars	
	Easy bruising	
	Muscle hypotonia	
Congenital bilateral hip dislocation	Kyphoscoliosis	Exon 6 (complete or partial) dipping in cDNA of COL1A or COL1A2
	Radiologically mild osteopenia	

Dermatosparaxis Type
Autosomal recessive

Major Criteria	Minor Criteria	Laboratory
Severe skin fragility	Soft, doughy skin	pNα1(I) or pNα2(I) collagen type I dermis chains in the presence of protease inhibitors; or from fibroblasts
Sagging, redundant skin	Easy bruising	
	Premature rupture of fetal membranes	
	Large umbilical inguinal hernias	

Our experience with cardiac defects in the EDS would fit within the classic type in the proposed classification described above. Leier described the spectrum of cardiovascular involvement in 19 EDS patients in 1980.[32] The cardiovascular abnormalities fell into two categories: connective tissue defects and congenital lesions. Fifteen of the patients had floppy mitral valves with MVP. Congenital lesions included bicuspid aortic valve, atrial septal defects, and ventricular septal defects. Aortic root or sinus of Valsalva dilatation was present in 6 of 19; aortic dissection complicated chronic aortic regurgitation in 1 patient.

A more recent report from Guys Hospital in London of EDS patients, 30 types I-III or classic, 3 type IV or arterial, was based on clinical evaluation and two-dimensional echo.[33] Although MVP was found in 6% of EDS patients, 7% of the control group had MVP. Contrary to earlier published observations the authors found no increase in the incidence of cardiac abnormalities in the EDS patients studied, leading to the conclusion that the syndrome may be relatively more benign from the cardiac point of view than was previously thought. Conversely, a report of five cases of aortic root dilatation in five families with individuals affected with EDS types I, II, and III parallels Leier's observations, supporting the wisdom of cardiac evaluation in EDS patients.[34]

The Stickler Syndrome

The Stickler syndrome, described in 1965, is an autosomal dominant osteochondrodysplasia with ocular, orofacial and skeletal abnormalities that result in myopia, retinal detachment, facial changes, and precocious osteoarthritis.[35] Other manifestations include deafness and Marfanoid habitus, with interfamilial variability. A variety of mutations in the COL2A1 gene, Stickler syndrome type 1; the COL11A2 gene, Stickler type 2; and the COL11A1 gene, Stickler type 3 have been identified. When 57 patients with the Stickler syndrome were evaluated with auscultation and two-dimensional echocardiography, 26 were diagnosed with MVP, however only 9 of the 26 had the auscultatory systolic click-systolic murmur syndrome.[36] Conversely, there was no evidence of MVP in a recent study of children with Stickler syndrome.[37] The incidence of cardiac abnormalities or the extent of cardiac involvement in the Stickler syndrome awaits further clarification.

X-Linked Myxomatous Valvular Disease

A detailed consideration of this clinical entity is presented by our French colleagues in Chapter 8. Inherited in an X-linked fashion, the disorder is characterized by multivalvular myxomatous degeneration, histopathologic changes that are described as not differing significantly from FMV, an association with mild hemophilia A in males, more severe expression in males, with no male to male transmission.[38] Heterozygous women were mildly affected. All of the nine men had MVR; MVP of the myxomatous mitral valve was present in eight of the nine, and MVR was moderate to severe in all. Six of the nine men also had aortic valvular regurgitation. The gene maps to chromosome Xq28.

The clinical phenotypic distinctions are of significance in the overall interpretation of the mode of FMV inheritance, given the spectrum of clinical involvement, the severity of the disease in men, and the mildly affected heterozygous women.

Autosomal Dominant Polycystic Kidney Disease

Expanding awareness of the relationship between adult polycystic kidney disease (APKD) chromosome locus, and cardiovascular abnormalities is relatively recent. The association of APKD characterized by autosomal dominant transmission with heritable and congenital cardiovascular abnormalities was presented by Leier et al.[39] Eleven of 62 patients with APKD seen at the Ohio State University Hospitals had one or more cardiovascular lesions. Seven had marked dilatation of the aortic root and annulus with aortic valvular regurgitation, three had mitral regurgitation and/or aortic regurgitation related to a bicuspid aortic valve, and one had coarctation of the aorta. Aortic and mitral valve tissue was characterized by myxomatous degeneration with loss and disruption of collagen, suggesting that these cardiovascular abnormalities associated with APKD were related to heritable developmental metabolic abnormalities of connective tissue.

Annuloaortic ectasia, abdominal aortic aneurysms, and mitral valve and tricuspid valve prolapse with valvular insufficiency have been the subject of studies from other laboratories. An extensive echo Doppler study of 163 patients with autosomal dominant polycystic kidney disease (ADPKD) demonstrated MVP (26%), mitral regurgitation (31%), aortic regurgitation (18%), tricuspid regurgitation (15%), and tricuspid valve prolapse (6%). These findings were considered to be a reflection of the systemic nature of polycystic kidney disease, and supported the hypothesis that the disorder involves a defect in the extracellular matrix and that the cardiac abnormalities are an expression of that defect.[40]

Echocardiography was used in a study of 154 children of 66 families in which one parent has ADPKD; 86 affected children and 68 unaffected children were defined on the basis of those with any cysts on a concurrent renal ultrasound or those predicted to be gene carriers by gene linkage analysis. There was a 12% incidence of MVP in the affected children compared to 3% in the unaffected children. ADPKD children, but not their unaffected siblings, demonstrated a significant correlation between left ventricular mass index and systolic blood pressure.[41] Systemic manifestations of ADPKD, particularly cardiovascular abnormalities, are present in childhood and warrant the clinician's attention.

Intracranial aneurysms occur in patients with ADPKD, probably with greater frequency than the general population; however, gathering control data has been a confounding issue. Intracranial aneurysms are an important cause of the mortality and morbidity in patients with ADPKD associated with subarachnoid hemorrhage from rupture. The association of ADPKD with extrarenal manifestations affecting the cardiovascular and gastrointestinal systems led to the classification of ADPKD as a systemic disorder. In particular, the cardiovascular involvement is quite similar to that noted in heritable connective tissue disorders.

A kindred in which ADPKD and a connective tissue disorder appeared to cosegregate has been described.[42] The connective tissue phenotype included aortic root dilatation, aortic and vertebral artery aneurysms with dissection, and aortic valve incompetence, as well as musculoskeletal phenotypes. Cosegregation of ADPKD and the connective tissue phenotype was observed and markers for PKD 1 were tightly linked to both. The ADPKD and connective tissue mutations were genetically linked. The presence of the connective tissue disorder in this family with ADPKD identified patients at significantly greater risk for sudden death from aortic root and vascular aneurysmal dissection and rupture.

The Floppy Mitral Valve and Other Heritable Disorders

MVP has been described in other heritable disorders: osteogenesis imperfecta, pseudoxanthoma elasticum, fragile-X syndrome, Down syndrome, cutis laxa, Fabry's disease, and epidermolysis bullosa. However, to date, the FMV has not been firmly established in these disorders as a distinct phenotype as described above in Marfan syndrome, EDS, or ADPKD. We look forward to additional, clinical, pathological, molecular, genetic, and natural history correlates in these heritable disorders.

The association of FMV with disorders that have heritable overtones has been the subject of numerous reports. Malcolm addressed the question, "Causal coincidence, common link, or fundamental genetic disturbance?", in an excellent review, and provides a balanced response.[43] Some of the best answers to these questions may be found in careful pathological studies with precise definition of the FMV[44,45] while the earlier echocardiographic studies that placed emphasis on MVP must be viewed with discernment. The association of FMV with other heritable disorders are outlined in a categorical fashion in Table 4.

The overlap between cardiac defects or disorders classified as congenital heart disease or as heritable cardiovascular disorders is a subject of renewed analysis. Two statements in the late 1980s point the way toward 21st century approaches to the genetic-molecular study and analysis of maternal, paternal, and fetal congenital cardiac defects.

Clark moved beyond the traditional anatomic classification and approached congenital cardiac malformations from a point of disordered mechanisms, placing emphasis on the developmental mechanisms of car-

---

Table 4
Heritable Cardiovascular Disease

Heritable Disorders of Connective Tissue
  Recognized syndromes
    Marfan syndrome
    Homocystinuria
    Ehlers-Danlos syndrome
    Combined Ehlers-Danlos and Marfan syndromes
    Stickler syndrome
  Cardiac Abnormalities
    Floppy mitral valve
    Combined floppy valves
    Annuloaortic ectasia
    Pulmonary artery aneurysm
  Heritable Matrix Disorders
    Autosomal dominant polycystic kidney disease
Heritable Vascular Defects
  Aortopathy
  Familial aortic dissecting aneurysm
  Cerebral cavernous disorders
  Hereditary hemorrhagic telangiectasia
Heritable Disorders of Vascular Biology
  Endothelial disorders
Heritable Cardiac Conduction System Disorders
  Familial conduction defects
  Familial preexcitation
Heritable Cardiac Conduction and Myocardial Disorders
Hypertrophic Disease of the Ventricles
  Hypertrophic cardiomyopathy

---

diac morphogenesis in the fetus.[46] He analyzed the stages of fetal maturation, the temporal effects of perturbations in embryogenesis, and related the resulting cardiac defect to this temporal-pathogenetic framework. The major developmental mechanisms under consideration included: (1) mesenchymal tissue migration; (2) cardiac hemodynamics; (3) cellular death; and (4) extracellular matrix abnormalities, considered either singularly or in combination. Disruptions in mesenchymal tissue migration were held responsible for: conotruncal cardiac malformations, and for cardiac malformations in the branchial arch syndromes; altered cardiac hemodynamics for coarctation of the aorta, left heart syndromes, valvular aortic stenosis, and atrial septal defects; alterations in cellular death patterns, normally responsible for molding and removal of cardiac tissue, for muscular ventricular defects and Ebstein's anomaly; and abnormalities of the extracellular matrix for cushion defects and outflow tract lesions.

The second statement came from Pyeritz and Murphy.[47] They addressed what was known about embryogenesis and analyzed the limitations of our current understanding of normal and abnormal embryogenesis. "The major task of determining how a one-dimensional code specifies a three-dimensional structure demands an understanding of biologic systems considerably beyond the current level." Emphasis was placed on the basic limitations of contemporary genetic counseling, while the impact of the new biology in the "fundamental investigations of highly complex, interactive systems" was anticipated.

The overlap between heritable cardiovascular disease and certain congenital cardiac defects has been further clarified by laboratory and clinical investigations providing evidence that human congenital heart disease has genetic origins. A review of causative mechanisms in the molecular era by Payne et al.[48] reflects these conceptual and nosologic

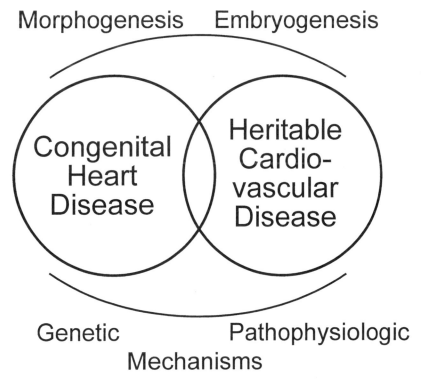

Figure 7. Classification of congenital cardiac defects, heritable cardiovascular disease, with emphasis on the overlap between the two. Clarifying morphogenesis, embryogenesis, molecular, genetic, and pathophysiological mechanisms will result in new classifications of congenital and heritable cardiovascular disease.

changes. Several of their conclusions are appropriate to this discussion. First, human congenital heart disease (CHD) is frequently due to single gene defects. Second, clinically useful classifications of CHD must not interfere with critical thinking concerning similar genetic and pathophysiological causative mechanisms. Third, elucidation of the genetic basis of CHD will provide additional insights into normal cardiovascular developmental biology. Fourth, mutations at a single locus cause multiple, different cardiac phenotypes (pleiotropy). Fifth, the same cardiac malformation is caused by specific gene defects at different loci, indicating that several different, but single gene defects may cause the same apparent phenotype (genetic heterogeneity).

Efforts directed toward developing a pathogenetic classification for congenital cardiac defects and for heritable cardiovascular disorders will continue to evolve as more is learned of embryogenesis, cardiac development, and genetic control mechanisms[49,50] (Fig. 7).

The Floppy Mitral Valve as a Heritable Disorder: Futuristic Changes

The FMV has emerged as a major cardiac valvular disorder during the past century and has been subsequently identified as a heritable cardiovascular disorder. To date, the well-defined heritable aspects include the FMV occurring as an isolated valvular abnormality; the FMV associated with the floppy tricuspid valve, floppy aortic valve, or both; the FMV associated with aortopathy, aortic root dilatation, or both. Recognition of the FMV as *a* or *the* cardiovascular manifestation of heritable disorders of connective tissue as described above has been an important milestone, since the advances in understanding the metabolic, biochemical, molecular, and genetic components of these systemic disorders form the bases for assembling the various components that constitute the FMV mosaic (Fig. 8).

Our anticipation of future developments involving the FMV as a heritable disorder is based in part on the following:

1. Emphasis on the FMV as the central, primary component of the FMV/MVP/MVR triad is the fundamental issue in the identification and classification of FMV as a heritable cardiac disorder.
2. Enhanced awareness of the clinical environment, e.g., clinical syndromes described above, in which the FMV occurs is a prerequisite for new diagnostic matrices.
3. Utilization of the clinical history, family history, pedigree development, phenotype analysis, genetic, and imaging technology in appropriate combinations will permit clinicians to identify indi-

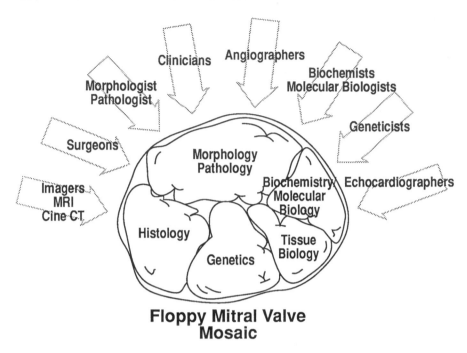

Floppy Mitral Valve Mosaic

Figure 8. Floppy mitral valve mosaic. Emphasis on contributions of various disciplines to date.

viduals or families with heritable forms of the FMV/MVP/MVR triad.

4. Close associations and joint participation between clinical cardiologists with genetic interests but without expertise in genetics, and geneticists interested in cardiovascular diseases but without broad clinical experience, are requisites to continued progress. In fact, we anticipate that the distinctions among the next generation of specialists will be blurred with the creation of new cross-specialty disciplines.

5. Efforts directed toward developing more precise pathogenetic classifications for congenital cardiac defects and for heritable cardiovascular disorders will continue to evolve as more is learned of embryogenesis, cardiac development, and genetic control mechanisms.

6. A shift in focus, once the diagnosis of FMV is established or individuals or families at risk are identified, from FMV recognition and diagnosis to informed long-term management and preventative therapy.

References

1. McKusick VA. Mitral valve prolapse, familial; MVP. In Online Mendelian Inheritance in Man, OMIM™. Baltimore, MD, Johns Hopkins University. MIM Number {157700}:{6–2-97}. http://www3.ncbi.nlm.nih.gov/omim/

2. Cooper MJ, Abinader EG. Family history in assessing the risk for progression of mitral valve prolapse: Report of a kindred. Am J Dis Child 135:647–649, 1981.

3. Cabot RC. The four common types of heart disease: An analysis of six hundred cases. JAMA 63:1461–1463, 1914.

4. Criteria Committee, New York Heart Association, Nomenclature and Criteria for Diagnosis of Diseases of the Heart and Great Vessels, Ninth Edition. New York, NY, Little Brown, 1994.

5. Pyeritz RE. Heritable disorders of connective tissue. In Boudoulas H, Wooley CF (eds). Mitral Valve Prolapse and the Mitral Valve Prolapse Syndrome. Mount Kisco, NY, Futura Publishing Co., Inc., 1988, pp 129–146.

6. Bowen JM, Boudoulas H, Wooley CF. Cardiovascular disease of connective tissue origin. Am J Med 82:481–488, 1987.

7. Burn J, Camm J, Davies MJ, Peltonen L, Schwartz PJ, Watkins H. The phenotype-genotype relation and the current status of genetic screening in hypertrophic cardiomyopathy, Marfan syndrome, and the long QT syndrome. Heart 78:110–116, 1997.

8. Barlow JB, Bosman CK. Aneurysmal protrusion of the posterior leaflet of the mitral valve. Am Heart J 71:166–178, 1966.

9. Stannard M, Sloman JG, Hare WSC, Goble AJ. Prolapse of the posterior leaflet of the mitral valve: A clinical, familial, and cineangiographic study. Br Med J 3:71–74, 1967.

10. Leachman RD, DeFrancheschi A, Zamalloa O. Late systolic murmurs and clicks associated with abnormal mitral valve ring. Am J Cardiol 23:679–683, 1969.

11. Shell WE, Walton JA, Clifford ME, Willis PW III. The familial occurrence of the syndrome of mid-late systolic click and late systolic murmur. Circulation 39:327–337, 1969.

12. Fontana ME, Pence HL, Leighton RF, Wooley CF. The varying clinical spectrum of the systolic click-late systolic murmur syndrome. Circulation 41:807–816, 1970.

13. Rizzon P, Biasco G, Brindicci G, Mauro F. Familial syndrome of midsystolic click and late systolic murmur. Br Heart J 35:245–258, 1973.

14. Hunt D, Sloman G. Prolapse of the posterior leaflet of the mitral valve occurring in eleven members of a family. Am Heart J 78:149–153, 1969.

15. Weiss AN, Mimbs JW, Ludbrook PA, Sobel BE. Echocardiographic detection of MVP. Circulation 52:1091–1096, 1975.

16. Strahan NV, Murphy EA, Fortuin NJ, Come PC, Humphries JO. Inheritance of the mitral valve prolapse syndrome: Discussion of a three-dimensional penetrance model. Am J Med 74:967–972, 1983.

17. Devereux RB, Kramer-Fox R. Inheritance and phenotypic features of mitral valve prolapse. In Boudoulas H, Wooley CF (eds). Mitral Valve Prolapse and the Mitral Valve Prolapse Syndrome. Mount Kisco NY, Futura Publishing Co., 1988, pp 109–127.

18. Zuppiroli A, Roman MJ, O'Grady M, Devereux RB. A family study of anterior mitral leaflet thickness and mitral valve prolapse. Am J Cardiol 82:823–826, 1998.

19. Pyeritz RE, Wappel MA. Mitral valve dysfunction in Marfan syndrome: Clini-

cal and echocardiographic study of prevalence and natural history. Am J Med 74:797–807, 1983.

20. DePaepe A, Devereux RB, Dietz HC, Hennekam RCM, Pyeritz RE. Revised diagnostic criteria for the Marfan syndrome. Am J Med Genet 62:417–426, 1996.

21. Wooley CF, Baker PB, Kolibash AJ, Kilman JW, Sparks EA, Boudoulas H. The floppy, myxomatous mitral valve, mitral valve prolapse, and mitral regurgitation. Prog Cardiovasc Dis 33:397–433, 1991.

22. Glesby MJ, Pyeritz RE. Association of mitral valve prolapse and systemic abnormalities of connective tissue: A phenotypic continuum. JAMA 262:523–528, 1989.

23. Milewicz DM. Molecular genetics of Marfan syndrome and Ehlers-Danlos type IV. Curr Opin Cardiol 13:198–204, 1998.

24. Segura AM, Luna RE, Horiba K, Stetler-Stevenson WG, McAllister HA Jr, Willerson JT, Ferrans VJ. Immunohistochemistry of matrix metalloproteinases and their inhibitors in thoracic aortic aneurysms and aortic valves of patients with Marfan's syndrome. Circulation 98(19 Suppl):II331–337, 1998.

25. Montgomery RA, Geraghyt MT, Bull E, Gelb BD, Johnson M, McIntosh I, Francomano CA, et al. Multiple molecular mechanisms underlying subdiagnostic variants of Marfan syndrome. Am J Hum Genet 63:1703–1711, 1998.

26. Kettle S, Yuan X, Grundy G, Knott V, Downing, Handford PA. Defective calcium binding to fibrillin-1: Consequence of an N2144S change for fibrillin-1 structure and function. J Mol Biol 285:1277–1287, 1999.

27. Cardy CM, Handford PA. Metal ion dependency of microfibrils supports a rodlike conformation for fibrillin-1 calcium-binding epidermal growth factor-like domains. J Mol Biol 276:855–860, 1998.

28. Periera L, Andrikopoulos K, Tian J, Lee SY, Keene DR, Ono R, Reinhardt DP, et al. Targeting of the gene encoding fibrillin-1 recapitulates the vascular aspect of Marfan syndrome. Nat Genet 17:218–222, 1997.

29. Wooley CF Sparks EH, Hirata K, Boudoulas H. The aortopathy of heritable cardiovascular disease. In Boudoulas H, Toutouzas PK, Wooley CF (eds): Functional Abnormalities of the Aorta. Armonk NY, Futura Publishing Co. 1996, pp 295–320.

30. Hirata K, Triposkiadis F, Sparks E, Bowen J, Wooley CF, Boudoulas H. The Marfan syndrome: Abnormal aortic elastic properties. J Am Coll Cardiol 18:57–63, 1991.

31. Beighton P, DePaepe A, Steinmann B, Tsipouras P, Wenstrup RJ. Ehlers-Danlos syndromes: Revised nosology, Villefranche, 1997. Ehlers-Danlos National Foundation (USA) and Ehlers-Danlos Support Group (UK). Am J Med Genet 77:31–37, 1998.

32. Leier C, Call T, Fulkerson P. The spectrum of cardiac defects in Ehlers-Danlos syndrome, types I and III. Ann Intern Med 92:171–178, 1980.

33. Dolan AL, Mishra MB, Chambers JB, Grahame R. Clinical and echocardiographic survey of the Ehlers-Danlos syndrome. Br J Rheumatol 36:459–462, 1997.

34. Tiller GE, Cassidy SB, Wensel C, Wenstrup RJ. Aortic root dilatation in Ehlers-Danlos syndrome types I, II and III: A report of five cases. Clin Genet 53:460–465, 1998.

35. Stickler GB, Belau PG, Farrell FJ, Jones JD, Pugh DG, Steinberg AG, Ward LE. Hereditary progressive arthro-ophthalmopathy. Mayo Clin Proc 40:433–455, 1965.

36. Liberfarb RM, Goldblatt A. Prevalence of mitral valve prolapse in the Stickler syndrome. Am J Med Genet 24:387–392, 1986.

37. Snead MP, Yates JR. Clinical and molecular genetics of Stickler syndrome. J Med Genet 36:353–359, 1999.
38. Kyndt F, Schot JJ, Trochu JN, Baranger F, Herbert O, Scott V, Fressinaud E, et al. Mapping of X-linked myxomatous valvular dystrophy to chromosome Xq28. Am J Hum Genet 62:627–632, 1998.
39. Leier CV, Baker PB, Kilman JW, Wooley CF. Cardiovascular abnormalities associated with adult polycystic kidney disease. Ann Intern Med 100:683–688, 1984.
40. Hossack KF, Leddy CL, Johnson AM, Schrier RW, Gabow PA. Echocardiographic findings in autosomal dominant polycystic kidney disease. N Engl J Med 319:907–912, 1988.
41. Ivy DD, Shaffer EM, Johnson AM, Kimberling WJ, Dobin A, Gabow PA. Cardiovascular abnormalities in children with autosomal dominant polycystic kidney disease. J Am Soc Nephrol 5:2032–2036, 1995.
42. Somlo S, Rutecki G, Giuffra LA. A kindred exhibiting cosegregation of an overlap connective tissue disorder and the chromosome 16 linked form of autosomal dominant polycystic kidney disease. J Am Soc Nephrol 4:1371–1378, 1993.
43. Malcolm AD. Mitral valve prolapse associated with other disorders: Casual coincidence, common link, or fundamental genetic disturbance? Br Heart J 53:353–362, 1985.
44. Lucas RV Jr, Edwards JE. Floppy mitral valve and ventricular septal defect: An anatomic study. J Am Coll Cardiol 1:1337–1347, 1983.
45. Roberts WC, Honig HS. The spectrum of cardiovascular disease in the Marfan syndrome: A clinicomorphologic study of 18 necropsy patients and comparison to 151 previously reported necropsy patients. Am Heart J 104:115–135, 1982.
46. Clark EB. Mechanisms in the pathogenesis of congenital cardiac malformations. In Pierpont ME, Moller JH (eds). Genetics of Cardiovascular Disease. Boston, MA, Martinus Nijhoff, 1986.
47. Pyeritz RE, Murphy EA. Genetics and congenital heart disease: Perspectives and prospects. J Am Coll Cardiol 13:1458–1468, 1989.
48. Payne RM, Johnson MC, Grant JW, Strauss AW. Toward a molecular understanding of congenital heart disease. Circulation 91:494–504, 1995.
49. Wooley CF, Sparks EH. Congenital heart disease, heritable cardiovascular disease, and pregnancy. Prog Cardiovasc Dis 35:41–60, 1992.
50. Mikawa T. Cardiac Lineages. In Harvey RP, Rosenthal N (eds): Heart Development. Boston, MA, Academic Press, 1999, pp 19–33.

8

Mapping of a Gene for an X-Linked Myxomatous Valvular Disease

Hervé Le Marec, MD, PhD,
Jean-Noël Trochu, MD,
Jean-Jacques Schott, PhD,
Florence Kyndt, PhD,
Bernard Bénichou, MD, PhD

Introduction

Nonsyndromic valvular dystrophies with myxomatous degeneration are among the most frequent inherited cardiac diseases; two forms have been described. Idiopathic mitral valve prolapse is by far the most common defect, occurring in 2–4% of the population[1] and displaying a broad clinical spectrum from mild valve defects without clinical repercussions to severe valvular disease.[2] Although the exact prevalence of familial cases is still uncertain, most familial forms appear to be inherited in an autosomal dominant manner with incomplete penetrance.[3] There is also clinical evidence of genetic heterogeneity.[4] A second type of inherited nonsyndromic valvular dystrophy was identified three decades ago by Monteleone and Fagan.[5] This rare disease, known as sex-linked valvular dysplasia, is supposedly transmitted as an X-linked recessive trait and may involve one or

From: Boudoulas H, Wooley CF. *Mitral Valve: Floppy Mitral Valve, Mitral Valve Prolapse, Mitral Valvular Regurgitation.* Second revised edition. ©Futura Publishing Company, Armonk, NY, 2000.

191

several valves in affected males. Both forms display classic histological abnormalities of myxomatous valve degeneration, with fragmentation of collagenous bundles within the valve fibrosa and accumulation of proteoglycan.

Valvular diseases with myxomatous degeneration form a complex group of disorders. Common histological features and a clinical continuum from isolated nonsyndromic valvular diseases (e.g., idiopathic mitral valve prolapse) to multivalvular diseases and syndromic disorders (e.g., Marfan and Elhers-Danlos syndromes) make it difficult to subclassify these heterogeneous and complex pathologies. In this instance, the identification of the genetic defects would be the ultimate tool for classification. Because of common histological features in type IV Elhers-Danlos syndrome and Marfan syndrome, it has been suggested that gene coding for these diseases, in particular collagen isoforms, could be implicated in nonsyndromic valvular diseases. However, genetic studies have failed to find a link between these genes and familial mitral valve prolapse.[6,7] Even though there is a high incidence of mitral valve prolapse, none of the nonsyndromic valvular dysplasias have been mapped, despite significant developments in molecular biology leading to the identification of a growing number of genes implicated in human pathology.

The purpose of this study was to describe the genetics and the clinical characteristics of inherited X-linked valvular dystrophy (XLVD). Its cosegregation with mild hemophilia A in a large French family enabled us to map the disease gene on Xq28 and characterize the genetic status of each patient. These studies showed that heterozygous women, in addition to obviously affected monozygous men, can be mildly affected by the disease. The fact that penetrance is complete in men and incomplete in heterozygous women (for whom it increases with age) provides new insight into the clinical characteristics of myxomatous valvular diseases and should improve genetic analysis of inherited valvular diseases in general. Determination of the localization of the gene for nonsyndromic valvular dystrophy is the first step in identifying it and defining the subclassifications of these diseases.

Methods

In our familial study, the probant was a 16-year-old boy with severe aortic regurgitation as a result of valvular dystrophy. During his hospitalization for clinical evaluation before valvular surgery, mild asymptomatic hemophilia A was detected. Subsequent inquiry revealed that a cousin had mitral valve regurgitation due to valvular dystrophy and the same hematologic defect. This led to the identification of a very large five-generation family.

The study was conducted according to French guidelines for genetic research. After informed written consent was received from each family member, the following evaluation was conducted: a review of medical history, a physical examination with particular attention to the cardiovascular system and any connective tissues diseases, a 12-lead electrocardiogram, and two-dimensional echocardiography with color-coded Doppler analysis. Blood samples were collected for genetic studies and quantification of antihemophilic factor VIII.

Physical Examination

Age, height, and weight were determined for each participant in the study, and conventional cardiac auscultation was performed. Clinical signs of valvular disease, such as dyspnea and/or palpitations, were investigated in each patient.

Echocardiography

The phenotypic assignment of family members was based on echocardiographic examination.

Transthoracic M-mode and two-dimensional echocardiograms were recorded according to the criteria of the American Society of Echocardiography[8] using a Hewlett-Packard Sonos 2000™ (Hewlett-Packard Inc., Andover, MA) with a 3.5-MHz probe, or an Acuson Sequoia™ C256 (Acuson Inc., Mountain View, CA) equipped with a multifrequency probe (3.5-2 MHz). Examinations were recorded on SVHS videotapes for further analysis. All data were analyzed in a blinded manner by two experienced physicians. Measurements of mitral valves were performed on parasternal long-axis two-dimensional images.[9] The length of each leaflet was determined just before valve closure, from its hinge point to the free edge, excluding the chordae. The thickness of the free edge of the mitral leaflets was measured on a selected diastolic frame that clearly separated the mitral leaflets and chordae. Mitral annular diameter was calculated by measuring the length of the line between the anterior and the posterior leaflet hinge points at end-diastole, just before the onset of the QRS complex, and at end-systole, before valve opening. Mitral valve prolapse was considered to exist when two-dimensional recordings in the parasternal long-axis view showed protrusion of mitral leaflets into the left atrium, crossing the line between the annular hinge points, and when the coaptation point of the leaflets remained at or above the mitral annular plane during systole.[10] Mitral regurgitation was estimated quantitatively by transthoracic color Doppler flow mapping in three spatial planes. Doppler color gain was optimized by first turning down the setting completely and then increasing the scale gradually until static background noise appeared.[11] The severity of mitral regurgitation was assessed by calculating the maximum regurgitating jet area (RJA) expressed as a percentage of left atrial area (RJA/LAA). Regurgitant flow signals localized in the vicinity of valve closure were considered as physiological regurgitation, and these patients were classified as unaffected.[12] Mitral regurgitation was rated as mild when RJA/LAA was ≤20%, moderate when >20% to ≤40%, and severe when >40%.[13]

Measurements of left ventricular outflow tract diameter (LVOTD) were obtained for the aortic device from parasternal long-axis two-dimensional images at the level of aortic cusp insertion, and aortic root dimensions were calculated from M-mode tracings. Aortic regurgitation was considered to exist if an abnormal diastolic flow originating from aortic cusps was identified in the left ventricular outflow tract. Color flow gain was adjusted as described above. The diameter of the regurgitated jet (AJD) was measured at its origin in the left outflow tract. The AJD/LVOTD ratio was calculated for quantification of aortic regurgitation[14] which was rated as mild when ≤25%, moderate when AJD/LVOTD >25% to ≤40% and severe when >40%. Tricuspid valve images were recorded in four-chamber apical views, and the pulmonary valve was analyzed in high left parasternal short-axis view.

Biological Analysis

Antihemophilic factor VIII activity was estimated by a one-stage clotting assay based on activated partial thromboplastin time, using factor VIII-deficient plasma (Diagnostica Stago, France) on an STA analyzer (Diagnostica Stago). The Second International Reference Preparation for factor VIII-related activity (National Institute for Biological Standards and Control, London, UK) was used as a standard.

Genetic Study

Phenotypes were defined as affected, unaffected, or undetermined. Patients were considered clinically affected when echocardiographic analysis identified at least mild regurgitation of one of the left cardiac valves and/or obvious dystrophy of the mitral valve was present, associated or not with billowing, and unaffected when the echocardiogram was normal or regurgitation was physiological. Finally, status was considered to be undetermined when only the right cardiac valves were abnormal or another disease such as hypertension could have caused the valve defect.

DNA was extracted from whole blood by means of standard protocols. Since the F8 gene lies in Xq28 and XLVD cosegregate with hemophilia A, a series of microsatellite markers spanning the entire Xq28 region were analyzed.

PCR reactions were carried out in 20 μl volumes, containing 2 μl diluted genomic DNA (approximately 200 ng), 1 × Taq buffer (50 mM KCl, 1.5 mM MgCl2, 10 mM Tris-HCl pH 9), 0.2 mM each dNTP, 1 μM each of both oligonucleotide primers and 1 unit Taq polymerase (Pharmacia); the mix was then subjected to 30 cycles of PCR amplification under annealing conditions adapted for each primer with a Peltier Thermal Cycler 200 (MJ Research); 2 μl of each PCR product were then diluted with 1 μl of loading buffer, denatured for 2 min at 94°C, and kept on ice until separation on a 6% denaturing polyacrylamide gel; the DNA was then transferred onto a nitrocellulose membrane (Hybond, Amersham), hybridized to a labeled 18-mer CA repeat oligonucleotide probe, revealed as recommended by the company (ECL direct nucleic acid labeling and detection system, Amersham) and visualized by autoradiography.

Linkage Analyses

The linkage analyses were carried out on a personal computer using the MLINK features of the LINKAGE program 5.2.[15] The XLVD diseaseallele frequency was assumed to be .00001, based on the rareness of reported cases. A value of .02 and .04 was used to account for possible phenocopies for males and females, respectively, which correspond to idopathic mitral valve prolapse frequency in the general population.[1] Allele frequencies were arbitrarily assigned a value of 1/n, where n refers to the number of alleles observed. Since incorrect parameters for linkage analysis may give false results, positive LOD scores were tested for robustness using either published frequencies or the frequencies observed in this family. The results were almost identical in every case, suggesting that the number of members in this family was sufficient to obtain very consistent results.

Statistical Methods

Statistical analysis was performed using Student's *t*-test and the Mann-Whitney test. A p value of less than 0.05 was considered significant. Results are expressed as the mean ±SD.

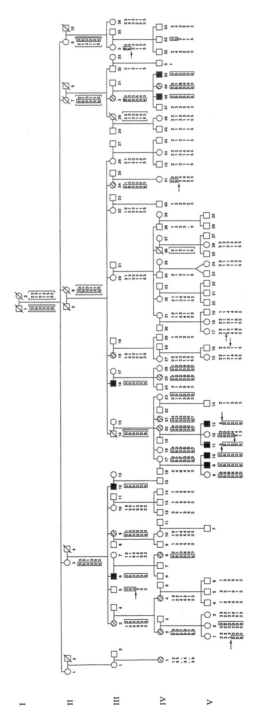

Figure 1. Pedigree of the family. Black symbols denote males simultaneously affected by severe X-linked myxoid valvular dysplasia and hemophilia A, and grey symbols indicate women showing abnormalities in echocardiography. Black bars represent the markers inherited from the ancestor who transmitted the disease. Marker order was as follows (top to bottom): DXS998, DXS8091, DXS8011, DXS8061, INT-13, and DXS1108. Blackened arrows indicate recombinations of parental alleles. A recombination event in male III-5 with a normal phenotype allowed us to delineate the linked area between markers DXS8011 and Xqter.

Results

The probant, a 16-year-old boy (patient V-11), had class II dyspnea according to the NYHA classification. He was of normal size and morphology, and a physical examination found no connective tissue or joint abnormalities. Cardiac auscultation revealed aortic regurgitant murmur, and echocardiography showed severe aortic regurgitation. Aortic root dimensions were normal as confirmed by a nuclear magnetic resonance study of the thoracic aorta. The left ventricle was enlarged, with normal systolic function. Mild hemophilia A was diagnosed at the time of aortic valve replacement.

Histological examination of the excised valves showed typical features of myxomatous valvular disease, with marked thickening of the free edge of the valve and extensive accumulation of proteoglycan that fragmented the collagenous bundle of the pars fibrosa. Aortic root analysis was strictly normal.

Among the 318 members of the pedigree, 302 are still alive and 97 participated in the study (Fig. 1): 43 women (36 ± 17 years), 46 men (22 ± 15 years) and 8 spouses (4 men and 4 women, mean age 48 ± 12 years). A valve defect was found in 22 (9 men and 13 women) of these nonconsanguineous subjects. No family members showed clinical evidence of syndromic disorders such as Marfan syndrome or Elhers-Danlos disease. Because of the far greater severity of myxomatous valvular disease in males, the absence of male-to-male transmission and a constant association with mild hemophilia A, it soon became apparent that the disorder was X-linked. Moreover, analysis of obligate carriers, the daughters or mothers of affected men (Fig. 1), showed that penetrance was incomplete in heterozygotes. Consequently, it was decided to analyze males and females separately.

Clinical Characteristics of Males

Among the 46 males (Table 1), nine had obvious aortic and/or mitral valve defect and were classified as affected, including four who underwent valvular surgery. Subsequent to surgery, one patient was asymptomatic and three had dyspnea (two class II; one class I). Seven of the nine affected males had mitral regurgitant murmur. No differences were found between affected and unaffected patients concerning age and body surface area.

Mitral Valve Defect

All affected males had mitral valvular dystrophy, and one had undergone mitral valvuloplasty when he was 18 (patient V-9). Mitral valves

Table 1
Echocardiographic Characteristics of Male Subjects

	Affected Males (n = 9)	P Value	Unaffected Males (n = 37)
Age (years)	31 ± 17	Ns	20 ± 14
Body surface area (m²)	1.70 ± 0.25	Ns	1.43 ± 0.51
Thickness of AML (mm)	4.7 ± 0.7	<0.0001	2.0 ± 0.4
Thickness of PML (mm)	3.8 ± 0.6	<0.0001	1.8 ± 0.4
Length of AML (mm)	28.1 ± 2.4	0.0004	22.1 ± 4.4
Length of PML (mm)	13.6 ± 1.7	0.0002	10.1 ± 1.8
DMAD (mm)	31.3 ± 3.0	0.0002	23.8 ± 5.1
SMAD (mm)	35.2 ± 3.3	0.0004	27.5 ± 5.3
ARD (mm)	30.6 ± 2.2	Ns	27.1 ± 1.1
LVDD (mm)	53.7 ± 6.8	0.0014	43.5 ± 7.8
LAD (mm)	36.7 ± 10.0	Ns	29.8 ± 6.0
Ejection fraction (%)	69 ± 8	Ns	68 ± 7

AML = anterior mitral leaflet; PML= posterior mitral leaflet; DMAD = diastolic mitral annulus diameter; SMAD = systolic mitral annulus diameter; LVOTD = left ventricular outflow tract diameter; LVDD = left ventricular diastolic diameter; LAD = left atrial diameter.

were characterized by thicker anterior (AML) and posterior (PML) leaflets, longer AML and PML, and larger mitral annular diameters at end-diastole and end-systole (Fig. 2). Mitral valve dystrophy was associated with moderate billowing in all but one (V-10) of the affected males (mean anterior leaflet prolapse: 3.1 ± 1.5 mm). Mitral regurgitation was moderate in four patients (IV-48, V-10, V-11, V-13; RJA/LAA = 0.37 ± 0.02) and severe in five (III-12, III-6, III-16, IV-50, V-9; RJA/LAA = 0.46 ± 0.07).

Aortic Valve Defect

As aortic valve dystrophy is difficult to assess by transthoracic echocardiography, we chose to quantify aortic regurgitation, which was associated with mitral valve dystrophy in six affected men. In three of these patients (III-6, III-16, and V-11), the severity of aortic regurgitation led to valve replacement, respectively, at 42, 24, and 16 years of age. Histological examination of the aortic valves found abnormalities similar to those described in the probant. In the other three men (III-12, IV-50, and V-10), aortic regurgitation was quantified as mild or moderate, with an AJD/LVOTD of 0.1, 0.24, and 0.26, respectively. Aortic root diameters and the left ventricular outflow tract were normal and did not differ significantly in affected and unaffected men. The three remaining affected men had no detectable aortic valve defect.

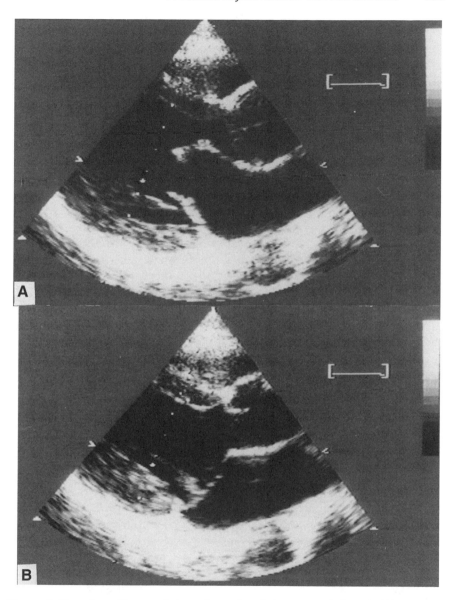

Figure 2. Parasternal long-axis two-dimensional view, at end diastole (**A**) and end systole (**B**), performed in an affected male (patient IV 49) showing the structural abnormalities of the mitral valve. Thickening of mitral valve leaflets (**A**) and a mild prolapse (**B**) were present in all affected males.

Affected males had larger left ventricular diastolic diameters, whereas left atrial diameters did not differ significantly. Ejection fractions were similar in the two groups.

Finally, the phenotypic status of men could easily be characterized since affected patients had obvious valvular dystrophy clearly differentiating them from the normal phenotype.

Hematologic Defect

Because of low factor VIII biological activity in the probant and his cousin (respectively, 0.31 and 0.29), hemophilia A was suspected in cosegregation with the valve defect. Von Willebrand disease was excluded, and mild hemophilia A was detected in all males affected by valvular disease, whereas all unaffected males had normal factor VIII activity (0.32 ± 0.05 vs. 0.91 ± 0.29, $p<0.0001$). These findings suggested that the X-linked valvular dysplasia gene and the factor VIII gene are closely related.

Linkage Analysis

Only male phenotypes were used to calculate the LOD score since the number of affected males was sufficient to produce a highly significant score. Moreover, penetrance in obligate female carriers (Fig. 1), unlike that in males, was not complete and could have been misleading.

Patient DNAs were typed with 6 CA repeat polymorphic markers, one of them being intronic to the F8 gene, spanning a total of 19 cM, and haplotypes were reconstructed for important absent or deceased family members (Fig. 1).

Since the occurrence of this disease has been reported only twice, and for very small pedigrees, the definition of the parameters for LOD score calculations was not obvious. Only male phenotypes were first used to calculate the LOD scores, thus avoiding the use of an arbitrary penetrance value for females.

The result of the two-point linkage analysis is given in Table 1. An identical maximum LOD score of 5.91 at $\theta = 0$ was obtained for INT-13 and DXS1108. Recombination events occurring in patients III-34, IV-41, IV-53, V-1, V-11, V-12, and V-13 allowed delineation of the candidate region (Fig. 3) to an 8cM interval between marker DXS8011 and Xqter.[16]

Clinical Characteristics of Females

This first linkage study was the key factor for detailed clinical analysis of X-linked valvular dystrophy, allowing identification of female carri-

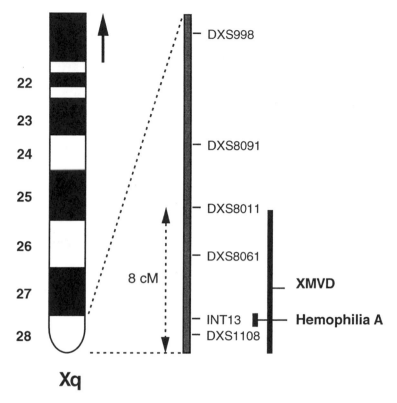

Figure 3. Chromosome Xq28 backbone. Polymorphic markers used for linkage analysis have been represented. The XLVD gene has been mapped between DXS8011 and Xqter. Factor VIII gene, that is mutated in hemophilia A, has been represented as well.

ers on the basis of their haplotypes and analysis of the expression of the diseased gene in heterozygotes (Fig. 1).

Among the 43 females in the pedigree, 17 who inherited the entire diseases-associated haplotype were heterozygous to the disease-associated gene. Four other females (III-34 IV-41, V-1, and V-12) had inherited part of the haplotype, with recombination events within the candidate region, so that their genetic status is unknown.

Characteristics of the 17 Heterozygous Females

All females were asymptomatic, but physical examination detected holosystolic murmur in four, and echocardiography identified 10 (mean age 40 ± 15 years) with mitral and/or aortic valve abnormalities. Eight (III-3, III-8, III-24, III-30, IV-18, IV-25, and IV-49) had moderate mitral regurgitation (mean RJA/LAA = 0.31 ± 0.04), with mitral valve prolapse in one and mild aortic regurgitation in three. Two women had isolated mild aortic regurgitation.

None of the affected women had obvious valvular dystrophy, and echocardiographic parameters such as leaflet thickness and mitral annulus, aortic root, left ventricular outflow tract, and the left ventricle diastolic diameters did not differ in heterozygous and unaffected women (Table 2).

According to the criteria used to characterize the phenotype, the valvular status of two heterozygous women was considered as undetermined. Patient II-3, the 83-year-old mother of two affected males, had isolated moderate mitral regurgitation without valvular dystrophy or mitral valve prolapse and a history of systemic hypertension that could have accounted for the valvular disorder. Patient IV-26, the 19-year-old daughter of an affected male, had an atypical valve defect with moderate pulmonary regurgitation without left valve defect.

The penetrance of the disease in heterozygotes was estimated as between 0.59 and 0.71, depending on the status of the two undetermined cases. The penetrance of the disease-associated gene in heterozygous women was age-dependent, with valve defect in five out of seven females over 40 years of age and in only five out of 10 under 40 (none under 20).

Table 2
Echocardiographic Characteristics of Women

	Heterozygous Females (n = 17)	P Value	Normal Females (n = 24)
Age (years)	38 ± 18	Ns	37 ± 17
Body surface area (m²)	1.59 ± 0.13	Ns	1.61 ± 0.31
Thickness of AML (mm)	2.5 ± 0.5	Ns	2.3 ± 0.5
Thickness of PML (mm)	2.1 ± 0.3	Ns	2.0 ± 0.3
Length of AML (mm)	24.0 ± 2.9	Ns	22.7 ± 2.9
Length of PML (mm)	11.2 ± 1.5	Ns	10.6 ± 1.6
DMAD (mm)	25.5 ± 3.4	ns	26.2 ± 3.2
SMAD (mm)	29.8 ± 3.5	ns	28.8 ± 4.1
ARD (mm)	28.4 ± 4.4	ns	28.1 ± 3.8
LVDD (mm)	47.7 ± 2.7	ns	44.7 ± 2.7
LAD (mm)	31.1 ± 4.4	ns	29.7 ± 3.8
Ejection fraction (%)	72 ± 6	ns	68 ± 6

AML = anterior mitral leaflet; PML= posterior mitral leaflet; DMAD = diastolic mitral annulus diameter; SMAD = systolic mitral annulus diameter; LVOTD = left ventricular outflow tract diameter; LVDD = left ventricular diastolic diameter; LAD = left atrial diameter.

Characteristics of Females with Undetermined Genetic Status

Echocardiographic examinations were normal for the four females (III-34, IV-41, V-1, and V-12) with recombination events in the candidate area. As the son of patient III-34 inherited the same haplotype and was unaffected, her genetic status was considered as normal.

Characteristics of Females with Normal Genetic Status

If it is assumed that patient III-34 did not inherit the "diseased" haplotype, 23 females can be considered to have normal genetic status, including three with a valve defect and 20 with normal echocardiography.

Patient III-20, a 64-year-old woman with isolated mild mitral regurgitation (RJA/LAA = 0.12) without valvular dystrophy or mitral valve prolapse, had received thoracic radiotherapy for breast cancer 10 years earlier. Patient IV-1 with severe mitral regurgitation (RJA/LAA = 0.49) had experienced an episode of prolonged fever shortly after delivery 10 years earlier which had been treated with antibiotics. A diagnosis of endocarditis was considered but never confirmed, despite the occurrence of mitral regurgitation. In these two cases, the valve defect could have been secondary to radiotherapy or endocarditis. Patient IV-4, a 33-year-old woman with mild mitral regurgitation (RJA/LAA = 0.20) associated with moderate aortic regurgitation (AJD/LVOTD = 0.27), had no clinical history indicative of acquired valvular disease. When these cases were taken into consideration, a risk of phenocopy of 0.12 was found for heterozygotes.

Finally, the eight spouses studied were all asymptomatic, although two had echocardiographic abnormalities. Patient III-7, a 60-year-old woman with moderate mitral regurgitation (RJA/LAA = 0.27) without valvular dystrophy or mitral valve prolapse, had a history of hypertension and breast cancer treated by radiotherapy. Patient III-15, a 47-year-old woman with mild aortic regurgitation (AJD/LVOTD = 0.17), had no clinical history of acquired valvular disease.

Discussion

Valvular dystrophy with myxomatous degeneration is a frequent cause of valve defects. It has been well-described in mitral valve prolapse[17] and also occurs in aortic regurgitation.[18,19] Although most affected patients are asymptomatic, they risk complications such as endocarditis, spontaneous chordal rupture, and sudden death. Moreover, progressive worsening of valvular regurgitation can lead to heart failure. Within the last decade, this disease has become an increasing cause of valvular surgery [representing almost 20% of such patients in our institution (unpublished data)].

The clinical spectrum of myxomatous valvular disorders, ranging from isolated mild defects to severe multivalvular lesions, is in favor of a heterogeneous disease that is in fact difficult to subclassify because of the absence of specific features, even at the histological level. To date, only genes for syndromic diseases have been mapped or cloned,[20–22] but the identification of genetic defects would appear to be the key factor for determining subclassifications, as demonstrated with some cardiac genetic diseases (e.g., long QT syndrome). In the long QT syndrome, despite the description of several electrocardiographic features,[23] the genetic heterogeneity of this syndrome was only confirmed when several loci were mapped, which has led to the cloning of the genes and a more precise clinical analysis of patients, facilitating the identification of specific phenotypes for each genetic defect.[24]

Isolated mitral dystrophy associated with billowing is the most common form of myxomatous valvular disease. It is easy to diagnose an obviously affected patient on echocardiographic data, but the continuum from normal to severely affected valves, and from isolated to multivalvular defects, can complicate the identification of affected patients.[2] In the family studied here, it was not difficult to identify the phenotype of affected men since they were either clearly normal or affected. The latter all had an obvious mitral valve dystrophy with thicker and longer leaflets and a mild prolapse associated with aortic regurgitation in two-thirds of cases. Valvular degeneration was not associated with other detectable cardiovascular or morphological defects. Clinical examination of affected patients indicated a nonsyndromic disease since no features of a connective tissue disease such as Marfan or Elher-Danlos syndrome were detected, and no signs of osteogenesis imperfecta were detected. Moreover, the thoracic aorta, particularly the aortic root, was echocardiographically and histologically normal, and skin histology performed in one affected patient was normal.

Several factors indicated that the inherited valvular disease was X-linked. There was no male-to-male transmission, and all affected men had mild hemophilia, whereas those with normal valves showed normal factor VIII activity. This suggested that both valvular dysplasia and hemophilia A were cosegregated in the family and that the gene responsible for valvular dysplasia was closely related to the factor VIII gene.

One of the most striking features of this disease is a tendency toward earlier severity from generation to generation. Reconstruction of the haplotype of ancestors indicated that the male in generation I was probably genetically affected and responsible for the transmission of the disease. Although no clinical cardiac analysis exists for this man, it is unlikely that he had severe valvular disease since he died at age 65 from peritonitis without any indication of cardiovascular symptoms. In generation III, three males were affected. The disease was identified when they were in their forties, and two of them underwent valvular surgery at age 51 and 49. In generation IV, two men are affected. The diagnosis of valvular disease was made during their twenties, and at age 30 and 24 they are still asymptomatic with moderate mitral regurgitation. Finally, four males of generation V are affected by the disease. Two underwent valvular surgery at the age of 17 because of severe mitral (V-11) or aortic (V-9) valvular regurgitation and two others (16 and 12 years old) are severely affected. This apparent tendency toward earlier severity could actually be due to improvement of echocardiographic techniques. However, similar tendencies were noted in two previous descriptions of this disease. In the family reported by Monteleone and Fagan,[5] a fourth-generation patient died of cardiac failure due to valvular disease when he was 8 months old, whereas several men from the previous generation were still alive, although clinically affected. In the family described by Newbury-Ecob et al.,[25] a fourth-generation baby died from valve defect and cardiac failure 24 hours after birth, whereas his grandfather in the second generation was asymptomatic until the age of 25 and underwent valve replacement at age 41. This tendency toward earlier severity, called anticipation, needs to be confirmed in other families.

On the basis of these clinical data, and because of uncertainty concerning the female phenotype, linkage analysis was performed only on males, starting on Xq28, the region in which the factor VIII gene is located. The gene for X-linked valvular disease was clearly localized on Xq28 between marker DXS8011 and Xqter. Given the size of the family and the ability to identify heterozygous women, this first genetic localization allowed us to provide new information on the characteristics of this apparently nonsyndromic valvular disease.

Our clinical observations differ from those previously described for X-linked valvular dysplasia, even though the same genetic disease is probably involved. An important result not previously described is the identification of an intermediate phenotype in heterozygous females.

With the mapping of the gene in monozygous males, it has become possible to identify female carriers on the basis of their haplotypes and to analyze the expression of the diseased gene. As has been demonstrated for idiopathic mitral valve prolapse,[2] there was no clear delineation between normal and abnormal valves. There is a continuum from normal to abnormal valves since some heterozygous women in the family studied here had normal echocardiography, whereas others had mitral or aortic regurgitation, giving a penetrance value of 60–70% which increased with age. Furthermore, valve defects were less severe than in men, as shown by the absence of differences in mitral valve thickness, length and diameter between affected heterozygous and normal women, and by a better outcome (no valvular surgery). Furthermore, dystrophic valves could not be identified (contrary to the situation for males). This could have been due to the low accuracy of transthoracic echocardiography in identifying small valve defects. Heterozygous women can be affected in X-linked diseases, though with less severity and/or a later age of onset. All of the echocardiographic results as well as the significantly lower factor VIII activity in carriers than noncarriers (Fig. 3) are indicative of an X-linked disease.

It is quite likely that nonsyndromic myxomatous valvular diseases are heterogeneous and that myxoid degeneration is the final pathway for several protein defects. Although few studies have been conducted, at least two nonsyndromic inherited forms of myxomatous valvular disease have already been identified. Idiopathic mitral valve prolapse is by far the most frequent syndrome, whereas X-linked valvular dystrophy seems to be a rare disease described only twice. In idiopathic mitral valve prolapse, one study has identified at least two different phenotypes with a strong family pattern,[4] but both forms appear to be inherited in an autosomal dominant manner.[3] However, several studies have reported striking cases that can hardly be explained by this mode of inheritance. Several epidemiological studies have shown that the disease is twice as frequent in females as in males[26] and that no clear delineation exists between normal and affected patients. Furthermore, the disease is more severe in males than in females,[27] as confirmed by several surgical series of mitral valve prolapse as well as myxoid aortic valve regurgitation in which the patients were largely male.[18,19] Although these results could have been due to hormonal as well as environmental factors, they are still surprising for an autosomal dominant disease.

X-linked valvular dystrophy has rarely been reported although idiopathic mitral valve prolapse is a frequent disease. This could have been due to the rarity of the disease or to misinterpretation of the mode of inheritance of the valvular defect. Due to the heterogeneity of the disease and the nonspecificity of echocardiographic criteria, as well as the presence of mildly affected heterozygous women and a tendency toward earlier severity in X-linked valvular disease that could have been clinically misleading, it is hardly possible that some patients with myxomatous valve defects may have been affected by an unidentified X-linked valvular disease. In analysis of the inheritance mode, only male-to-male transmission could rule out the possibility of an X-linked disease. In this respect, the identification of genetic defects will be the ultimate tools allowing subclassification of this complex group of diseases.

Pathophysiology

Although myxomatous valve degeneration is common in various diseases, particularly syndromic connective tissue disorders such as Elhers-Danlos and Marfan syndromes, its pathogenesis in nonsyndromic valvular dysplasia is unknown. The valve anomaly is the main defect but some studies are in favor of a more diffuse disease affecting other cardiac structures.[28] It has been suggested that genes coding for collagen isoforms are implicated in mitral valve prolapse. However, despite several studies, no forms of nonsyndromic valvular dysplasia have been found to be associated with collagen defects. Concerning the mild hemophilia A affecting all men with myxomatous valve dystrophy, we do not know yet if they inherited two different genetic defects or if the genetic defect implicated in the myxomatous valve dystrophy is by itself responsible for the alteration factor VIII gene expression.

Conclusion

This first localization of a gene for nonsyndromic myxomatous valvular diseases should facilitate the subclassification of this complex group of diseases. Ultimately, the cloning of the gene will give new insight into the pathophysiology of these diseases.

Author's Note: Since the submission of this chapter, a second locus for mitral vale prolapse, transmitted in an autosomal dominant manner, has been mapped to chromosome 16 (16p11.2-p12.1), confirming the genetic heterogeneity of myxomatous valvular dystrophy.

Disse S, Abergel E, Houot AM, LeHeuzey JF, Diebold B, Carpentier A, Corvol P, Jeunemaitre X. Mapping of a first locus for autosomal dominant myxomatous mitral valve prolapse to chromosome 16p11.2-p12.1 Am J Hum Genet 65:1242–1251, 1999.

References

1. Savage D, Garrison RJ, Devereux RB, Castelli WP, Anderson SJ, Levy D, McNamara PM, et al. Mitral valve prolapse in the general population. I. Epidemiologic features: The Framingham study. Am Heart J 106:571–576, 1983.
2. Wooley CF, Baker PB, Kolibash AJ, Kilman JW, Sparks EA, Boudoulas H. The floppy, myxomatous mitral valve, mitral valve prolapse, and mitral regurgitation. Prog Cardiovasc Dis 33:397–433, 1991.
3. Devereux RB, Brown TW, Kramer-Fox R, Sachs I. Inheritance of mitral valve prolapse: Effects of age and sex on gene expression. Ann Intern Med 97:826–832, 1982.
4. Pini R, Greppi B, Kramer-Fox R, Roman MJ, Devereux RB. Mitral valve dimen-

sions and motion and familial transmission of mitral valve prolapse with and without leaflet billowing. J Am Coll Cardiol 12:1423–1431, 1988.

5. Monteleone OL, Fagan LF. Possible X-linked congenital heart disease. Circulation 39:611–614, 1969.

6. Wordsworth P, Ogilvie D, Akhras F, Jackson G, Sykes B. Genetic segregation analysis of familial mitral valve prolapse shows no linkage of fibrillar collagen genes. Br Heart J 61:300–306, 1989.

7. Henney AM, Tsipouras P, Schwartz RC, Child AH, Devereux RB, Leech GJ. Genetic evidence that mutations in the COL1A1, COL1A2, COL3A1 or COL5A2 collagen genes are not responsible for mitral valve prolapse. Br Heart J 61:292–299, 1989.

8. Henry WL, DeMaria A, Gramiak R, King DL, Kisslo JA, Popp RL, Sahn DJ, et al. Report of the American Society of Echocardiography committee in nomenclature and standards in two-dimensional echocardiography. Circulation 62;212–217, 1980.

9. Weissman NJ, Pini R, Roman MJ, Kramer-Fox R, Andersen HS, Devereux RB, Spitzer MC. In vivo mitral valve morphology and motion in mitral valve prolapse. Am J Cardiol 73:1080–1088, 1994.

10. Devereux RB, Kramer-Fox R, Shear MK, Kligfield P, Pini R, Savage DD. Diagnosis and classification of severity of mitral valve prolapse: Methodologic, biologic and prognostic considerations. Am Heart J 113:1265–1280, 1987.

11. Miyatake K, Izumi S, Okamoto M, Kinoshita N, Asonuma H, Nakagawa H, Yamamoto K, et al. Semiquantitative grading of severity of mitral regurgitation by real-time two dimensional Doppler flow image technique. J Am Coll Cardiol 7:82–88, 1986.

12. Yoshida K, Yoshikawa J, Shakudo M, Akasak T, Takao S, Shiratori K, Koisumi K, et al. Color Doppler evaluation of valvular regurgitation in normal subjects. Circulation 78:840–847, 1988.

13. Helmcke F, Nanda NC, Hsiung MC, Soto B, Adey CK, Goyal RG, Gatewood RP. Color Doppler assessment of mitral regurgitation with orthogonal planes. Circulation 7:175–183, 1987.

14. Dolan MS, Castello R, St Vrain JA, Aguirre F, Labovitz AJ. Quantitation of aortic regurgitation by Doppler echocardiography: A practical approach. Am Heart J 129:1014–1020, 1995.

15. Lathrop GM, Lalouel JM. Easy calculations of LOD scores and genetic risks on small computers. Am J Hum Genet 36:460–465, 1984.

16. Kyndt F, Schott JJ, Trochu JN, Baranger F, Herbert O, Scott V, Fressinaud E, et al. Mapping of X-linked myxomatous valvular dystrophy to chromosome Xq28. Am J Hum Genet (in press).

17. Malkowski MJ, Boudoulas H, Wooley CF, Guo R, Pearson AC, Gray PG. Spectrum of structural abnormalities in floppy mitral valve echocardiographic evaluation. Am Heart J 132(1 Pt 1):145–151, 1996.

18. Allen WM, Matloff JM, Fishbein MC. Myxomatous degeneration of the aortic valve and isolated severe aortic regurgitation. Am J Cardiol 55:439–444, 1985.

19. Tonnemacher D, Reid C, Kawanishi D, Cummings T, Chandrasoma P, McKay CR, Rahimtoola SH, et al. Frequency of myxomatous degeneration of the aortic valve as a cause of isolated aortic regurgitation severe enough to warrant aortic valve replacement. Am J Cardiol 60:1194–1196, 1987.

20. Dietz HC, Cutting GR, Pyeritz RE, Maslen CL, Sakai LY, Corson GM, Puffenberger EG, et al. Marfan syndrome caused by a recurrent de novo missense mutation in the fibrillin gene. Nature 352:337–339, 1991.

21. Putnam EA, Zhang H, Ramirez F, Milewicz DM. Fibrillin-2 (FBN2) mutations

result in the Marfan-like disorder congenital contractural arachnodactyly. Nature Genet 11:456–458, 1995.

22. Superti-Furga A, Gugler E, Gitzelmann R, Steinmann B. Ehlers-Danlos syndrome type IV: A multi-exon deletion in one of the two COL3A1 alleles affecting structure, stability, and processing of type III procollagen. J Biol Chem 263:6226–6232, 1988.

23. Moss AJ, Robinson J. Clinical features of the idiopathic long QT syndrome. Circulation. 85(1 Suppl):I140-I144, 1992.

24. Moss AJ, Zareba W, Benhorin J, Locati EH, Hall WJ, Robinson JL, Schwartz PJ, et al. ECG T-wave patterns in genetically distinct forms of the hereditary long QT syndrome. Circulation 92:2929–2934, 1995.

25. Newbury-Ecob RA, Zucollo JM, Rutter N, Young ID. Sex linked valvular dysplasia. J Med Genet 30:873–874, 1993

26. Levy D, Savage D. Prevalence and clinical features of mitral valve prolapse. Am Heart J 113:1281–1290, 1987.

27. Devereux RB, Hawkins I, Kramer-Fox R, Lutas EM, Hammond IW, Spitzer MC, Hochreiter C, et al. Complications of mitral valve prolapse: Disproportionate occurrence in men and older patients. Am J Med 81:751–758, 1986.

28. Morales AR, Romanelli R, Boucek RJ, Tate LG, Alvarez RT, Davis JT. Myxomatous heart disease: An assessment of extravalvular cardiac pathology in severe mitral valve prolapse. Hum Pathol 23:129–137, 1992.

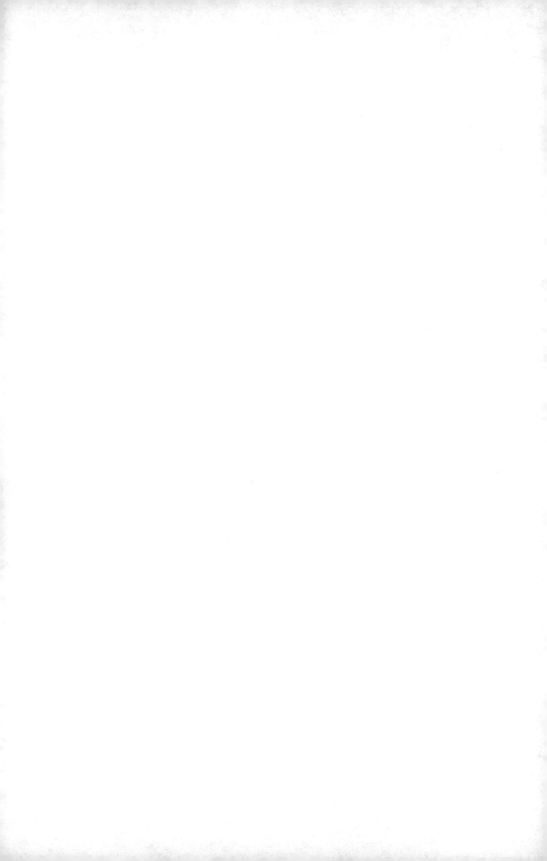

Part VI

The Floppy Mitral Valve, Mitral Valve Prolapse, Mitral Valvular Regurgitation:
The Imagers

Introduction

The Floppy Mitral Valve, Mitral Valve Prolapse, Mitral Valvular Regurgitation:
The Imagers

Charles F. Wooley, MD,
Harisios Boudoulas, MD, PhD

We are visual creatures. The reduction of dynamic events to fixed or moving images involves complex integrative functions in regions of our brains where reconstruction occurs and comprehension resides. The resulting mental or pictorial images constitute our true universal language.

Images and imagery have been vital components of cardiovascular morphology, physiology, and pathodynamics for centuries; however, the advances from the angiographic studies of the 1950s and 1960s to the evolving imagery of the present time would hold our predecessors spellbound.

Imaging the floppy mitral valve has been a central issue in the development of clinical wisdom about the floppy mitral valve/mitral valve prolapse/mitral valvular regurgitation (FMV/MVP/MVR) triad. The FMV morphologic characteristics should be viewed as part of a continuum from the cardiac surgeons' views of the FMV in the beating heart, the cardiac pathologists' approach to the FMV, and the sophisticated angiographic, echo Doppler, and evolving MRI images. As each of these techniques have been integrated with the clinical phenomena, the more certainty clinicians bring to comprehensive clinical profiles.

The 1950s and early 1960s were times of great activity in cardiac catheterization, hemodynamics, and surgery. It is difficult to believe just how remote the territory of the left heart was prior to the introduction of cardiac catheter techniques to enter the left heart via retrograde arterial or

From: Boudoulas H, Wooley CF. *Mitral Valve: Floppy Mitral Valve, Mitral Valve Prolapse, Mitral Valvular Regurgitation.* Second revised edition. ©Futura Publishing Company, Armonk, NY, 2000.

transseptal approaches. The excitement that accompanied left heart visualization with contrast media, initially as seen with cut-film techniques and then with cineangiographic studies, was palpable. The precise identification of left heart structures, in particular the mitral valve complex, required various projections in order to enhance anatomic certainty. These steps would be repeated with the introduction of each subsequent imaging technique.

The anatomic, functional, and cross-sectional characteristics of the normal mitral valve complex—the mitral valve leaflets, annulus, and support structures operating within the left ventricle and left atrium gradually became apparent, as did the selective and global changes that accompanied disease states. A series of cut-film angiographic studies from Sweden in the 1950s with emphasis on mitral stenosis and the size and volume of left heart chambers were landmarks at the time.

In the United States a series of cineangiographic studies by John Michael Criley, Richard Ross, and associates, published in 1961 and 1962 provided detailed identification of mitral valve leaflet structure and analysis of mitral valve complex movement, with emphasis on use of right and left anterior oblique projections. Cineangiographic demonstration of "prolapse" of the mural leaflet of the FMV into the left atrium, with mitral valvular regurgitation occurring in late systole in a 39-year-old man with an apical mid- and late systolic murmur was a defining moment in the 1962 publication. By 1966 Criley and co-investigators extended the prolapse concept and terminology, using cineangiography with simultaneous phonocardiography to time the FMV auscultatory phenomena and relate the systolic clicks and late systolic murmurs to the angiographic events. Thus the cineangiographic characteristics of the FMV were described in detail, and most importantly, integrated with the clinical auscultatory phenomena. With time as the angiographic criteria for normal mitral valve morphology, motion, and function were established, a reasonable degree of consensus was reached about specific FMV/MVP/MVR angiographic criteria as well.

The advent of ultrasonography provided advantages for patient and clinician alike. Multiple views and projections with prolonged sampling times provided a tremendous impetus to the study of valvular heart disease. However, problems in diagnostic specificity and sensitivity multiplied as the number of participants in the diagnostic process increased, and with the use of these testing devices without strict clinical correlates. When "prolapse" was the M-mode echo criterion for diagnosis, the entire FMV/MVP/MVR triad came under siege. Although the previous cineangiographic observations had been based on FMV morphology in carefully selected patients, some of the early echocardiographic imagers lost sight of the clinical auscultatory and FMV angiographic diagnostic imaging criteria.

The subsequent rediscovery of the fundamental FMV morphologic characteristics by the echocardiographers, correlated with the clinical auscultatory criteria and morphologic observations by the cardiac surgeons, placed the diagnosis of the FMV/MVP/MVR triad on solid grounds. Thus, the current FMV imaging literature deals with specific FMV phenomena. FMV leaflet morphology, FMV complex dynamics, which leaflet or segment is prolapsing, chordal and papillary muscle morphology and function, the location, complex geometry, and volumes of MVR jets, and the quantitative assessment of the MVR, all have applicability to patients with the FMV/MVP/MVR triad.

However, while the transition from the early M-mode echocardiographic studies to two-dimensional, color flow Doppler, transesophageal, and three-dimensional techniques during the past several decades had a major impact on cardiovascular investigation and diagnosis, several caveats should be mentioned.

Patients frequently have symptoms while upright, active, and during the activities of daily living, while many of our cardiac examinations and tests are still performed with the patient recumbent. The recumbent posi-

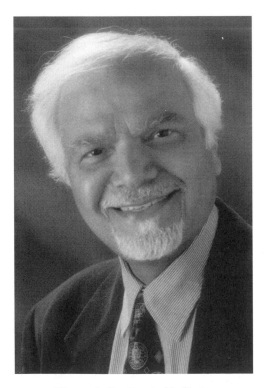

Figure 1. Dr. Pravin M. Shah.

tion is part of the legacy of many diagnostic tests in cardiology. The use of recumbent, passive imaging studies in patients with the FMV/MVP/MVR triad translates to an incomplete evaluation of patients with the dynamics of FMV function and dysfunction. We learned these lessons during the past decades using dynamic, postural auscultation, phonocardiography, cineangiography, and nuclear stress testing in patients with the FMV/MVP/MVR triad. Unless the diagnostic testing is tailored to the dynamics and mechanisms operative in patients with the FMV/MVP/MVR triad, the assessment remains incomplete.

Throughout the past four decades, the editors of this book have had the benefit of the wisdom of many of our colleagues involved in these imaging developments. We alluded to the importance of Criley's observations in the 1960s. Some of our earliest experiences with the echocardio-

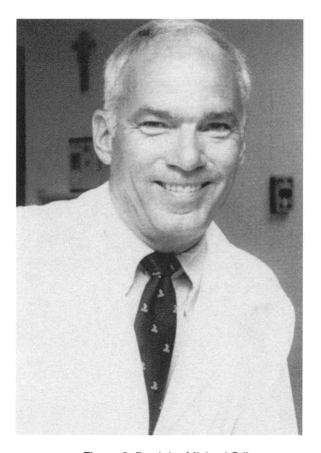

Figure 2. Dr. John Michael Criley.

graphic approach to the FMV came in 1970 when we exchanged visits with Pravin M. Shah (Fig.1). His early work with Gramiak was important in many ways; however, his consistent insistence that the evolving imaging techniques should be correlated with the characteristic physical findings was an equally important message.

The list of important contributors to the imaging of the FMV/MVP/MVR triad includes many respected colleagues, and their many contributions have been incremental with time. Most of the original contributors are referenced in the text or bibliographies of the next three chapters. To attempt to list them all here would risk omitting individual contributions and would require an additional chapter.

In the next three chapters we have the benefit of clinical investigators sharing their approaches to the FMV imaging phenomena, always with an eye toward the basic FMV morphology.

John Michael Criley (Fig. 2) and his son, David G. Criley, provide an elegant introduction to the functional anatomy of the normal mitral appa-

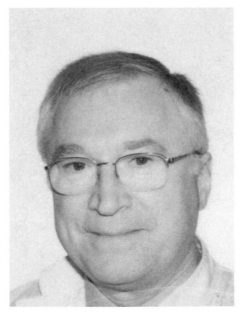

Figure 3. Dr. Jos R.T.C. Roelandt.

ratus, the functional anatomy of the FMV/MVP, and the correlation of these observations and concepts with the clinical manifestations.

Our colleagues in Cardiology at The Ohio State University, Michael Malkowski and Anthony Pearson, refer to many of the hallmark imaging studies in their chapter, while reconciling the echocardiographic assessment of the FMV with basic FMV morphology, function, and dysfunction.

In the third chapter in this section, Jos R.T.C. Roelandt (Fig. 3), Director of the Heart Centre at Rotterdam, and internationally known for his innovative work in cardiac imaging, explores the three-dimensional echocardiographic reconstruction approach to the FMV, presenting images that will resonate with the morphologists, pathologists, and surgeons.

9

Functional Anatomic, Angiographic, and Clinical Correlates in Mitral Valve Prolapse

John Michael Criley, MD,
David G. Criley

Introduction

The constellation of signs and symptoms that frequently accompany mitral prolapse were reported long before the underlying valvular abnormalities were first delineated. Using cineangiography synchronized with heart sound recording, plausible explanations of the previously enigmatic auscultatory findings were proposed.[1-3] The click was found to be temporally related to the full inflation of the billowing leaflet(s), shown angiographically in Figure 1 and the resultant loss of leaflet apposition in late systole caused late systolic regurgitation and its accompanying murmur. Abnormal mitral leaflet configuration and excursions were later detected by echocardiography.[4]

The relationship between the movements of the valve leaflets and the systolic auscultatory events, as shown in Figure 2, are consistent with the angiographic-phonocardiographic temporal correlations. We believe that the origin of the unique early diastolic sound[5,6] that we have termed the

From: Boudoulas H, Wooley CF. *Mitral Valve: Floppy Mitral Valve, Mitral Valve Prolapse, Mitral Valvular Regurgitation.* Second revised edition. ©Futura Publishing Company, Armonk, NY, 2000.

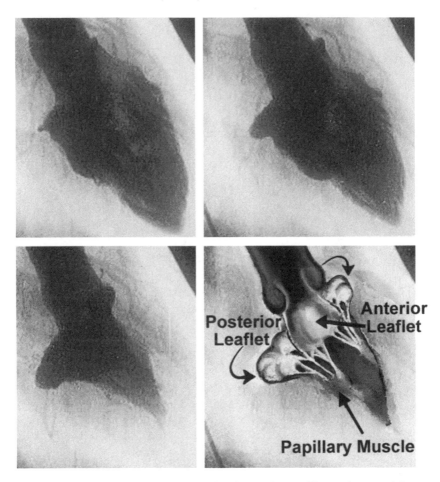

Figure 1. Left ventriculography in mitral valve prolapse. Three phases of the cardiac cycle are shown in frames from a right anterior oblique (RAO) left ventriculogram. The upper left panel represents end diastole, the upper right panel isovolumic systole, and the lower panels mid-systole, at the time of maximal inflation of the mitral leaflets. The "spare tire" at the base of the left ventricle inflates as the ventricular chamber decreases in size, and represents aneurysmal protrusion of the posterior mitral leaflet as shown in the overlay drawing in the lower right panel. The anterior leaflet does not form a border of RAO silhouette since it is engulfed within the croissant-shaped posterior leaflet. An indentation in the inferior aspect of the ventricular silhouette represents the posteromedial papillary muscle, which is being pulled inward by the inflated valve leaflets.

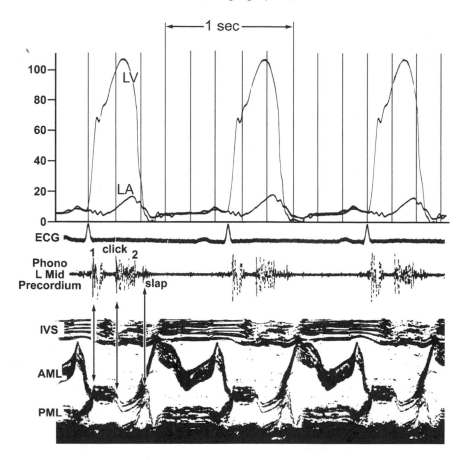

Figure 2. The temporal relationships between the auscultatory events, mitral valve excursions, and pressure events in the left heart chambers. The anterior mitral leaflet (AML) and posterior mitral leaflet (PML) come into apposition coincident with the first heart sound (1, first arrow) during the electrocardiographic (ECG) R wave and the systolic rise in left ventricular (LV) pressure. An abrupt dorsal (downward) excursion of both leaflets in mid-systole coincides with a mid-systolic click (second arrow). A late systolic murmur occupies the space between the click and the second sound (2). These events are in turn followed by an early diastolic sound (third arrow). We have termed this early diastolic sound a "slap shot" sound because of its relationship to the impact of the posterior leaflet against the anterior leaflet. The slap sound coincides with an abrupt reapposition of the leaflets; the posterior leaflet pivots on the annulus, moving in an arc from its dorsal position within the atrium to strike the anterior leaflet and then moves dorsally into the inferior wall of the ventricle. With dynamic imaging by two-dimensional echocardiography (not shown), the blood-laden PML can be seen to strike the AML and impel it across the subaortic vestibule toward the interventricular septum (IVS) coincident with this sound. The pressures in the left heart in this patient with 2+ mitral regurgitation exhibit enlarged v waves, whereas most patients with mitral prolapse have normal pressures in the left heart.

"slap shot" sound is caused by the sharp impact of the posterior leaflet against the anterior leaflet. The blood-laden posterior leaflet pivots on its annular attachment from its systolic position within the atrium and slaps the anterior leaflet in the act of opening.

Since angiography and echocardiography depict the heart differently, it is our intention, in this chapter, to create a three-dimensional concept of the left ventricle and mitral valve in an effort to enhance appreciation of the spatial relationships and unique functional anatomy that characterize mitral prolapse.

Functional Anatomy of the Normal Mitral Apparatus

Figure 3 contrasts normal and prolapsing mitral valves in cartoons that can be viewed either as radiographic left anterior oblique (LAO) projections, or by turning the page 90° clockwise, into a parasternal long-axis echocardiographic format. The orifice of the mitral valve is depicted widely open in diastole, with the anterior leaflet adjacent to the ventricular septum and the annular attachment of the posterior leaflet forming a semicircle at the interface with the left atrium. The leaflets of the valve close competently to initiate isovolumic systole, but the elongated leaflets of mitral valve prolapse (MVP) overinflate in mid-systole. The increased leaflet surface exposed to the pressure in the ventricle exerts excessive lift on the valve apparatus so that the papillary muscles are unable to hold the valve in a competent subannular position within the cavity of the left ventricle. The leaflets are then shown to lose apposition, and a fine jet of mitral regurgitation is indicated in the right lower panel.

Since the left heart chambers appear to be hollow (echo free) by echocardiography and solid (opaque) by angiocardiography, it is appropriate to relate the two as a "mold" and a "cast," respectively. If the left heart chambers, as shown in Figure 4, were used to make a plaster cast, it would contain the mitral and aortic valves, since they are both within the hollow portion of the mold. The mold has been cut open to reveal the mitral apparatus and depicted in two standard radiographic projections. The mitral sleeve is invaginated into the conical cavity of the left ventricle and normally held in a subannular position by chordal attachments to the papillary muscles. Both papillary muscles receive chordae from the anterior and posterior leaflets, and share nomenclature with the commissures with which they are aligned.[7–9] The posteromedial papillary muscle, shown arising from the inferior left ventricular (LV) wall in the right anterior oblique (RAO) view, is in line with the posteromedial commissural scallop (PMCS), while the anterolateral papillary muscle, cephalad in the RAO view, is aligned with the anterolateral commissural scallop (ALCS). The

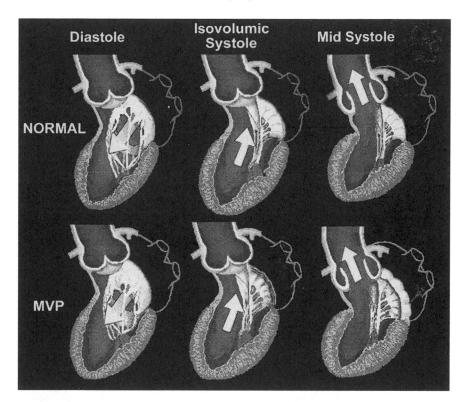

Figure 3. Normal and prolapsing mitral valve function. Three phases of the cardiac cycle are depicted, contrasting normal (above) and mitral valve prolapse (MVP) in a left anterior oblique projection. The position of the valve leaflets is comparable in diastole and at the time of initial mitral closure (isovolumic systole), but the inflated, elongated leaflets in MVP herniate into the left atrium in mid-systole. A fine spray of mitral regurgitation is indicated in the lower right figure. This figure represents a left anterior oblique (LAO) radiographic projection; by turning it 90°, it resembles a left parasternal long-axis echocardiographic view.

posterior mitral leaflet is divided into three sections, with the middle scallop bracketed by the commissural scallops.[9]

At the onset of systole (Fig. 3) both the normal and prolapsing mitral valves inflate because of the rising pressure in the left ventricle. The inflated posterior mitral leaflet (PML) engulfs and supports the anterior mitral leaflet (AML) within its concave aspect. Contraction of the papillary muscles counters the parachute-like pull of the inflating leaflets to maintain the normal leaflets in a competent subannular position. The plane of the closed PML is bent along the point of apposition. The basal attachments of the closed PML form a plane nearly at right angles to the long axis of the ventricle while the AML's plane and the plane of apposition are

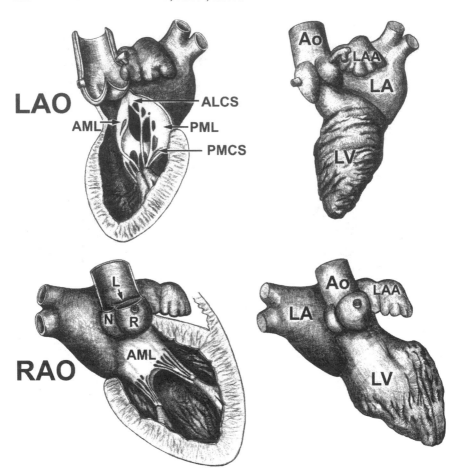

Figure 4. Molds and casts of the left heart. Normal left heart chambers in diastole are shown in left anterior oblique (LAO) and right anterior oblique (RAO) projections, representing the concept of "mold" and "cast" as described in the text. The mold has been cut open to reveal the mitral apparatus invaginated into the cavity of the left ventricle. In the RAO view, only the anterior mitral leaflet (AML) is seen, immediately adjacent to the buttocks-like aortic sinuses. The left (L) and non-coronary (N) aortic sinuses of Valsalva are in direct continuity with AML, while the right (R) sinus is in front of the plane of the mitral valve. The origins of the coronary arteries are indicated as they emerge from the aortic sinuses. The posterior mitral leaflet (PML) comprises three scallops. The posteromedial papillary muscle, arising from the inferior LV wall in RAO view, is in line with the posteromedial commissural scallop (PMCS), while the anterolateral papillary muscle is aligned with the anterolateral commissural scallop (ALCS). These commissural scallops bracket the middle scallop, which is indicated by the arrow labeled PML.

more nearly parallel to the long axis. In changing from the systolic to the diastolic configuration, the PML deflates and drops down in tailgate fashion into the left ventricular inflow tract. Meanwhile, the AML makes a larger excursion as it changes its systolic position as the posterolateral boundary of the cylindrical LV outflow tract to its diastolic position as the anteromedial boundary of the inflow tract. This excursion of the anterior leaflet into the subaortic vestibule in diastole is accompanied by a change from systolic concavity to diastolic convexity relative to the left ventricle.

Other actions not readily depicted in still pictures are contraction of the mitral annulus and descent of the base. Contraction of the annulus begins at the onset of atrial systole and progressively constricts in drawstring fashion throughout ventricular systole, and is thought to be an important component of competent closure. A progressive descent (movement toward the apex) of the base, represented by the mitral and aortic valves, occurs throughout systole. This descent can be seen in Figures 1 and 3 by noting that more of the aortic root is seen in the mid-systolic frame, and the inflated mitral valve has moved downward, or away from the top of the frame despite being herniated upward into the left atrium.

Functional Anatomy of Mitral Prolapse

It is our thesis that mitral prolapse results from a valvoventricular disproportion[10] in which the mitral valve apparatus is anatomically or functionally too big for the left ventricle in systole. This disproportion can result from a valve that is structurally or functionally too big, a ventricle that is functionally or structurally too small, or combinations of both. Two disease entities that represent two ends of this spectrum are Marfan syndrome, in which the mitral valve apparatus is overtly voluminous, and hypertrophic cardiomyopathy, in which the left ventricular systolic cavity size is miniscule. Both lead to functional prolapse as defined by failure to maintain the mitral valve in a competent subannular position throughout systole. Both of these entities also share common auscultatory features with "primary" mitral valve prolapse.

Since it was through left ventricular cineangiography that the functional anatomy of mitral prolapse was first defined,[1-3] the bases for the abnormal ventriculographic silhouettes will be described. The "spare tire" appearance of the base of the ventricle in Figure 1 inflates after competent valve closure, and disappears in diastole. In the RAO projection the posterior mitral leaflet and the atrioventricular annulus to which it is attached are projected on edge; the aneurysmally dilated PML forms the basal ventricular border. The exaggerated concavity of the inferior wall of the ventricular silhouette is the result of traction on the posteromedial papillary muscle engendered by inflating leaflets.

LAO   RAO   RPO

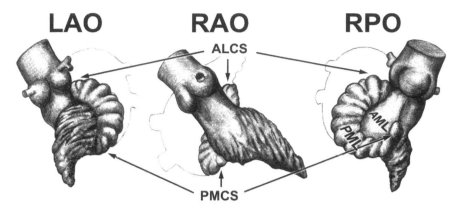

Figure 5. Three-dimensional angiographic depictions of mitral valve prolapse. Three views of a cast of the left ventricle and aortic root, with the left atrium removed to reveal the prolapsed valve leaflets, are shown as though it is rotated on a turntable in 90° increments. Rotation from LAO through RAO to the right posterior oblique (RPO) projection permits identification of the leaflets and the scallops involved in the prolapse. The exaggerated "croissant" appearance seen from the atrial aspect in the RPO view represents the hyperinflation of all three scallops of PML and bulging of their interchordal hoods. A "potbelly" appearance of prolapse of AML, above the line of coaptation, results from lack of support from the encircling posterior leaflet. These projections were developed from biplane angiography of the patient shown in Figure 1.

Figure 5 depicts renderings of a three-dimensional model of the left ventriculogram shown in Figure 1 demonstrating extensive mitral valve prolapse as it is rotated into three projections each separated by 90°. In many instances of MVP, a localized prolapse may involve only one or two scallops of PML, and since AML is well supported, there may be little or no abnormal motion or systolic billowing of that leaflet.

The variable nature of these functional anatomic and associated bedside physical findings can be conveniently explained by the concept of a functionally variable valvoventricular disproportion.[10] Perturbations that increase ventricular volume or retard the emptying of the ventricle (e.g., squatting, and vasopressors) diminish the disproportion, while standing (or amyl nitrite inhalation) augments the disproportion. It is useful to consider that there is a "prolapse threshold" LV volume at which leaflets can no longer be maintained in a competent subannular position as shown in Figure 6. When this volume is achieved during LV ejection, leaflet slippage occurs. When this slippage is abruptly checked by chordal restraints, the click is generated. If the slippage causes leaflet separation, the murmur ensues. In those instances where multiple clicks occur, they can be attributed to the asynchronous prolapse of inter-

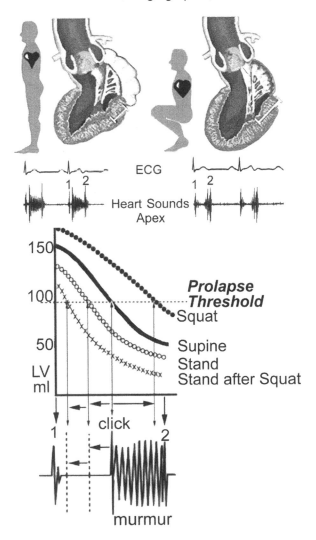

Figure 6. Postural effects on the click and murmur of mitral valve prolapse: the prolapse threshold. The valvo-ventricular disproportion concept is illustrated by cartoons related to a hypothetical plot of systolic ventricular volume curves under different loading conditions. A prolapse threshold that indicates the volume at which the ventricle is unable to hold the mitral apparatus in a competent subannular position intercepts each curve at different times following the onset of systole. The timing of these intercepts determine the time at which the prolapse, click, and murmur occur following the first heart sound (1). Squatting increases ventricular volume and retards ejection, moving the click and murmur later in systole, while standing moves the intercept earlier. Calipers superimposed on the images of the left ventricle denote the distance between the annular and papillary muscle points of attachment of the posterior leaflet. There is a shorter separation resulting in more inflation when the ventricular volume is reduced, permitting earlier prolapse and earlier occurrence of the associated auscultatory events.

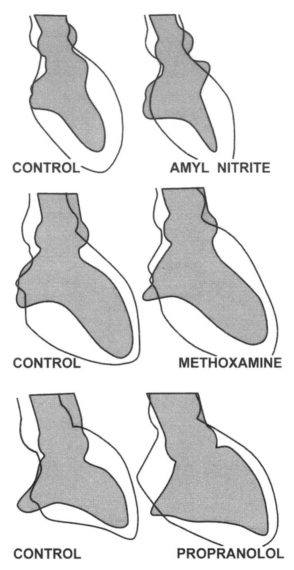

Figure 7. Response to pharmacological interventions. Drugs that affect the rate and degree of left ventricular emptying were administered to three patients prior to obtaining a left ventriculogram following a control recording. The resulting RAO ventriculographic silhouettes in diastole (dashed line) and systole (shading) demonstrate lesser degrees of prolapse after administration of a negative inotrope, propranolol, and a pressor agent, methoxamine. Conversely, inhalation of amyl nitrite reduced filling and enhanced emptying of the ventricle, causing a greater degree of prolapse. These responses to pharmacological stimuli mimic the volumetric and auscultatory effects of the postural maneuvers shown in Figure 6.

chordal hoods of the valve as might be imagined from viewing the valve morphology in Figure 5.

Silhouettes derived from left ventriculograms taken before and after vasoactive drug administration, shown in Figure 7, emulate the postural effects on the ventricular volume and the magnitude of prolapse. Amyl nitrite inhalation decreases ventricular volume in a manner similar to sudden standing after squatting, increasing the magnitude of the disproportion between the ventricle and mitral valve. Methoxamine administration decreases that disproportional relationship similar to squatting. Propranolol reduces the ejection fraction and minimizes the magnitude of the aneurysmal billowing of the leaflets. These pharmacological agents have been shown to affect the timing of the click and murmur in a manner similar to the postural maneuvers[10] that achieve comparable volumetric changes in the left ventricle.

Conclusions

We believe that a spatial concept of the relationship of the unique actions of the mitral valve to the variable auscultatory findings enhances understanding of the clinical manifestations of mitral valve prolapse. Since left heart catheterization is no longer required as a diagnostic procedure in patients with suspected MVP, having been superceded by echo Doppler ultrasonography, we have attempted to create a three-dimensional concept that can be applied to invasive as well as noninvasive imaging. It is hoped that the depictions in this chapter will enhance the understanding of the often-confusing manifestations of mitral valve prolapse.

Acknowledgments: The graphics used in Figures 1, 3, and 6 were adapted with permission from Criley JM, Criley DG, and Zalace C: The Physiological Origins of Heart Sounds and Murmurs: The Unique Interactive Guide to Cardiac Diagnosis. Lippincott, Williams & Wilkins, 1998.

References

1. Ross RS, Criley JM. Contrast radiography in mitral regurgitation. Prog Cardiovasc Dis 5:195–217, 1962.
2. Barlow JB. Conjoint clinic on the clinical significance of late systolic murmurs and nonejection systolic clicks. J Chron Dis 18:665, 1965.
3. Criley JM, Lewis KB, Humphries JO, Ross RS. Prolapse of the mitral valve: Clinical and cineangiocardiographic findings. Br Heart J 28:488–496, 1966.
4. Kerber RE, Isaeff DM, Hancock EW. Echocardiographic patterns in patients with the syndrome of systolic click and late systolic murmur. N Engl J Med 284: 691–693, 1971.
5. Bonner AJ, Noble RJ, Feigenbaum H. Early diastolic sound associated with mitral valve prolapse. Arch Intern Med 136:347–349, 1976.

6. Wei JY, Fortuin NJ. Diastolic sounds and murmurs associated with mitral valve prolapse. Circulation 63:559–564, 1981.
7. Walmsley R, Watson H. The outflow tract of the left ventricle. Br Heart J 28: 435–447, 1966.
8. du Plessis LA, Marchand P. The anatomy of the mitral valve and its associated structures. Thorax 19: 221–227, 1964.
9. Ranganathan N, Silver MD, Robinson TI, Wilson JK. Idiopathic prolapsed mitral leaflet syndrome: Angiographic-clinical correlation. Circulation 54:707–716, 1976.
10. Fontana ME, Kissel GL, Criley JM. Functional anatomy of mitral valve prolapse. In Leon DF, Shaver JA (eds): Physiologic Principles of Heart Sounds and Murmurs. New York, American Heart Association, 1975, p 126.

10

The Echocardiographic Assessment of the Floppy Mitral Valve:

An Integrated Approach

Michael J. Malkowski, MD,
Anthony C. Pearson, MD

Introduction

In the past two decades, with the evolution and widespread use of M-mode and two-dimensional echocardiography, considerable attention has been paid to prolapse of the mitral leaflets.[1,2] The ubiquity of the term "mitral valve prolapse" for the condition characterized by floppy mitral valves is testimony to the overwhelming attention paid to this echocardiographic phenomenon. Prolapse was first described angiographically as a buckling motion of the mitral leaflets into the left atrium.[3] It has also been described as having a billowing appearance.[4] Echocardiographically it is usually described as part or all of the mitral leaflet "breaking the plane of the mitral annulus" during systole with displacement into the left atrium (Fig. 1).

Most pathologic studies indicate that a spectrum of mitral valve pathology exists with the greatest morbidity occurring in patients with the

From: Boudoulas H, Wooley CF. *Mitral Valve: Floppy Mitral Valve, Mitral Valve Prolapse, Mitral Valvular Regurgitation.* Second revised edition. ©Futura Publishing Company, Armonk, NY, 2000.

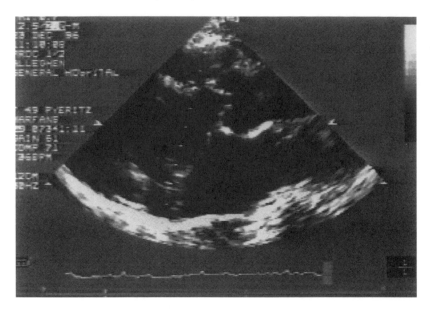

Figure 1. Example of prolapse of the anterior and posterior mitral leaflets across the mitral annulus into the left atrium from the transthoracic parasternal long-axis view.

most severe valvular deformities.[5–7] Fortunately, echocardiography provides excellent characterization of the underlying valvular anatomy and pathology of the floppy mitral valve.[8,9] In addition, echocardiography provides an assessment of associated functional abnormalities and secondary structural deformities.[10–13]

In this chapter the evaluation of valvular morphology in patients with floppy mitral valves and the relationship of the echocardiographic observations to surgical and pathologic findings as well as clinical phenomena will be reviewed. Finally, the utility of transesophageal echocardiography in patients with floppy mitral valves and severe mitral regurgitation in predicting the feasibility of mitral valve repair and timing of surgical intervention[14] will be discussed.

The Echocardiographic Diagnosis of Mitral Valve Prolapse

Webster defines prolapse as an object being out of place. With respect to the mitral valve, prolapse refers to protrusion of the mitral leaflets beyond their normal coaptation point at the plane of the mitral annulus, into the left atrium. Despite the apparent simplicity of this definition, the echocardiographic diagnosis of prolapse has been the subject of much controversy. Initially, prolapse was diagnosed from M-mode echocardiography.[15] However, this technique resulted in the diagnosis being made in a number of patients with normal mitral valves.[16] Due to its low sensitivity and low specificity, M-mode echocardiography has been supplanted by two-dimensional echocardiography in the assessment of the mitral valve.

The two-dimensional criteria initially proposed for mitral valve prolapse required the detection of either mitral leaflet protruding beyond the leaflet hinge points of the mitral annulus into the left atrium in any imaging plane. However, many normal hearts display the mid-portion of the anterior leaflet protruding across the plane of the mitral annulus when imaged from the apical four-chamber view. Because this criterion was nonspecific, many normal patients were diagnosed with prolapse and the significance of this disease was debated.[17] Levine et al.[1] postulated that the mitral annulus was saddle-shaped, thus, portions of the leaflet would normally appear to prolapse in the apical four-chamber view.[2] When the echocardiographic diagnosis of mitral valve prolapse is made from the parasternal long-axis view, specificity is raised and the association of mitral valve prolapse and abnormalities such as left atrial enlargement and mitral regurgitation is improved.[2]

The current two-dimensional diagnositic criterion for mitral valve prolapse is the displacement of one or both mitral leaflets across the mitral annulus in the parasternal long-axis view.[1] By limiting the diagnosis to strict criteria again provides meaning to the diagnosis. The most common pathologic process that results in prolapse of the mitral valve is the presence of a floppy mitral valve. When a patient population is defined by the floppy mitral valve that results in prolapse, clear separation between normal subjects and patients becomes evident. Abnormal physical findings and complications related to the mitral valve are frequently present in the group with floppy mitral valves.[18] Currently, the floppy mitral valve is the most common etiology of pure mitral regurgitation and the most common underlying abnormality in patients requiring mitral valve replacement.[19] The echocardigraphic presentation of the floppy mitral valve, which is central to this disease state, is the subject of the rest of this chapter.

The Structural Assessment of Floppy Mitral Valve Disease

Mitral Leaflet Thickness

The preferred method for measuring mitral leaflet thickness utilizes the parasternal long-axis two-dimensional images from the diastolic still

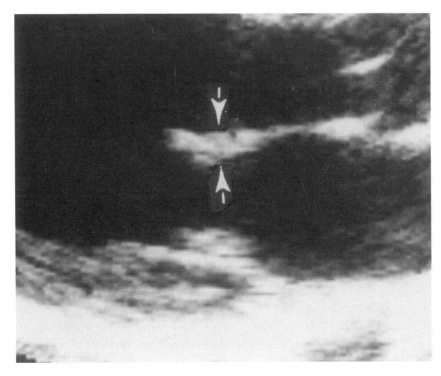

Figure 2. Transthoracic two-dimensional echocardiographic image from the parasternal long-axis view demonstrating the site used for the measurement of anterior leaflet margin thickness.

frame with the mitral leaflet maximally opened (Fig. 2). Previous reports have utilized measurements of mitral leaflet thickness from M-mode echocardiography, but this method may significantly overestimate leaflet thickness if the ultrasound beam is directed tangential to the leaflet and should not be considered a reliable method of determining leaflet thickness.

When measuring leaflet thickness, the normal leaflet morphology should be considered. The thickest site of the normal mitral leaflets corresponds with the line of closure, resulting from a more expansive spongiosum and the insertion of multiple chordae tendineae.[20,21] This region has been referred to as the rough zone or margin of the leaflet. The mid-region or clear zone is the area between the annulus and the margin and is generally thin, translucent, and devoid of chordal insertions. These differences in leaflet thickness need to be considered when assessing leaflet pathology. Consistent with the previously reported anatomic findings, two-dimensional echocardiography easily differentiates the mid- from

Table 1
Differences by Transthoracic Echocardiography in Anterior and Posterior
Leaflet Thickness in Floppy Mitral Valve Patients and Normal Subjects
(All Mean Values in mm ± SD)

	NI Anterior	FMV Anterior	NI Posterior	FMV Posterior
Chandraratna[22]	3.5 ± 0.8	3.6 ± 0.6	NR	NR
Weissman[8]	2.2 ± 0.57	3.94 ± 0.98	2.25 ± 0.46	3.50 ± 0.92
Malkowski[9]	4.1 ± 0.4	5.3 ± 0.7	3.2 ± 0.4	4.7 ± 0.9

FMV = floppy mitral valve group; NI = normal subjects; NR = not reported.

margin regions and consistently finds the margin the thickest portion of the leaflet.[8,9]

Thickness of both the anterior and the posterior mitral leaflets are greater in patients with floppy mitral valves than in normal subjects (Table 1). Malkowski et al.[9] found anterior leaflet thickness was increased in 48% and posterior leaflet thickness was increased in 66% of floppy mitral valve patients without significant regurgitation. In the same study, patients with moderate to severe regurgitation had a greater percentage of increased anterior and posterior leaflet thickness, 91% and 88%, respectively.[9] Weissman et al.[8] similarly found that over 50% of floppy mitral valve patients displayed increased leaflet thickness and over 60% of patients with significant regurgitation were identified as having increased thickness. The increased thickness in both studies was associated with mitral regurgitation as assessed by color Doppler echocardiography (Table 2).

Table 2
Differences by Transthoracic Echocardiography in Leaflet Thickness in
Floppy Mitral Valve Patients with and without Mitral Regurgitation
(All Mean Values in mm ± SD)

	FMV without MR		FMV with MR	
	Anterior	Posterior	Anterior	Posterior
Chandraratna[22]	3.6 ± 0.6	NR	8.8 ± 1.2	NR
Weissman[8]	3.84 ± 0.95	3.36 ± 0.92	4.53 ± 0.99	4.20 ± 0.78
Malkowski[9]	5.2 ± 0.7	4.5 ± 0.9	5.8 ± 0.8	5.3 ± 0.7

FMV = floppy mitral valve; MR = mitral regurgitation; NR = not reported.

Clinical Significance of Leaflet Thickness by Transthoracic Echocardiography in Floppy Mitral Valves

Patients with floppy mitral valves are at higher risk for complications related to their valvular pathology. In one of the first studies to examine the association of mitral leaflet thickness with clinical phenomena, Chandraratna et al.[22] found that patients with abnormal mitral valve thickness or an increased mitral valve thickness to aortic wall thickness ratio had a greater incidence of cardiovascular abnormalities noted on echocardiography including significant mitral regurgitation, tricuspid valve prolapse, and ascending aorta dilatation. Nishimura et al.[23] followed 237 mitral valve prolapse patients who were asymptomatic or minimally symptomatic for an average of 6.2 years. The subgroup of patients with the presence of increased thickness by M-mode echocardiography had a higher incidence of sudden death, infectious endocardititis, and stroke during the follow-up period. Marks et al.[24] compared the clinical course of mitral valve prolapse patients with and without leaflet thickening by two-dimensional echocardiography. In this retrospective study, patients with leaflet thickness greater than 5 mm had a higher rate of endocarditis, mitral regurgitation, and mitral valve replacement. Grayburn et al.[10] found mitral regurgitation was present in a greater number of mitral valve prolapse patients with mitral leaflet thickness greater than 5 mm compared to patients without increased leaflet thickness (Table 2).

Although the mechanism is not completely clear, patients with increased leaflet thickness have greater morbidity related to the floppy mitral valve that results in mitral valve prolapse. These findings are consistent with pathologic observations that a spectrum of valve morphology is present in floppy mitral valve disease. Patients with multiple and more severe structural abnormalities are more likely to suffer serious complications while mitral valve prolapse with minor morphologic abnormalities is rarely clinically significant.[5] Although posterior displacement of the mitral valve has been the major echocardiographic criterion used for the diagnosis of mitral valve prolapse, the degree of billowing is influenced by ventricular volume[25] and has not been shown to have prognostic importance or predict symptoms.[26] Increased mitral thickness appears to be much more important in the definition and risk stratification of the floppy mitral valve than leaflet displacement.

Measurement of Leaflet Length

Pathologic studies of floppy mitral valves indicate that in addition to increased thickness, the surface area and length of the valves are also increased.[6,7,27] Leaflet length can be measured off the two-dimensional transthoracic echocardiogram (Fig. 3). The best view for the assessment of leaflet length is the parasternal long-axis view with the leaflets maximally open. The anterior leaflet is measured from the mitral annulus at the hinge point of the anterior leaflet to the tip of the leaflet, being careful not to include chordae tendineae. Similarly, the posterior leaflet can be measured from the mitral annulus to the tip of the leaflet.

Malkowski et al.[9] found that anterior and posterior leaflet length are greater in patients with floppy mitral valves than in normal subjects when assessed by echocardiography (Table 3). Forty-eight percent of patients with floppy mitral valves displayed abnormal posterior leaflet length and 21% had abnormal anterior length. In patients with floppy mitral valves and significant mitral regurgitation, 55% had abnormal leaflet length. Weissman et al.[8] also demonstrated increased anterior length in patients with floppy mitral valves but not increased posterior length (Table 3). Although the anterior leaflet length in the two studies was similar, the posterior length in the study by Malkowski et al. is more consistent with pathologic findings. In fact, Dollar and Roberts have used a posterior leaflet length of greater than 15 mm as an anatomic criterion for floppy mitral

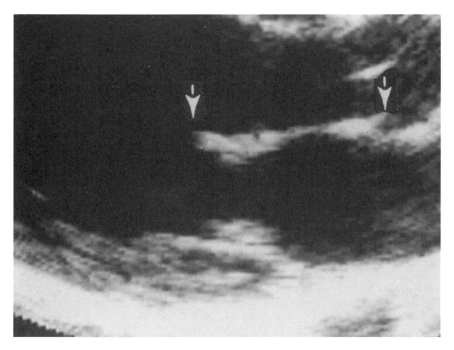

Figure 3. Transthoracic two-dimensional echocardiographic image from the parasternal long-axis view demonstrating the sites used for the measurement of anterior leaflet length.

Table 3

Leaflet Length by Transthoracic Echocardiography in Normal Subjects, Patients with Floopy Mitral Valves without Mitral Regurgitation, and Patients with Floppy Mitral Valves with Mitral Regurgitation (Mean Values Reported in mm ± SD)

	Weissman[8]	Malkowski[9]
Normals:		
Anterior	21.8 ± 2.8	22.8 ± 2.0
Posterior	12.6 ± 1.9	12.8 ± 1.0
Floppy Mitral Valves without Mitral Regurgitation:		
Anterior	23.4 ± 2.7	25.6 ± 1.7
Posterior	12.8 ± 2.4	15.1 ± 1.6
Floppy Mitral Valves with Mitral Regurgitation:		
Anterior	25.8 ± 4.0	26.2 ± 1.6
Posterior	14.7 ± 2.1	17.9 ± 4.2

mm = millimeters; SD = standard deviation.

valves and emphasized that frequently in severe cases the posterior annulus to margin length may approach the length of a normal anterior leaflet.[28]

Measurement of Annular Diameter

The annulus of the mitral valve is structurally and functionally abnormal in the floppy mitral valve and may significantly contribute to mitral regurgitation in patients with floppy mitral valves.[29] Annular diameter can be measured from either the parasternal long-axis view, the apical four-chamber view, or the apical two-chamber view (Fig. 4). In addition to recognizing an increase in the annular diameter in patients with floppy mitral valves, Ormiston et al.[30] also noted that the change in circumference that normally occurs with each cardiac cycle is attenuated in floppy mitral valve patients. These abnormalities in annular function may contribute to regurgitation by diminishing the sphincter effect the annulus has in preventing regurgitation against the high pressure of the left ventricle.

Malkowski et al.[9] found that the annular diameter was greater in patients with floppy mitral valves and was frequently abnormal in patients with significant valvular regurgitation (Table 4). Weissman et al.[8] also found a significant percentage of patients with increased annular diameter with mitral valve prolapse, especially in patients with significant mitral regurgitation (Table 4). These studies confirmed the work by Pini et

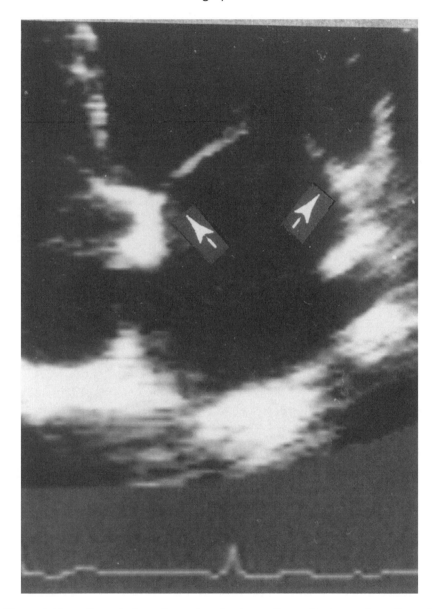

Figure 4. Transthoracic two-dimensional echocardiographic image from the apical four-chamber view demonstrating the sites used to measure annular diameter.

Table 4

Table Summarizing the Studies That Examined the Mitral Annulus in Patients with Floppy Mitral Valves

	Normal	FMV without Regurgitation	FMV with Regurgitation
Ormiston[30] (circumference, cm)	9.3 ± 1.0	9.8 ± 0.6	14.2 ± 1.2
Pini[31] (diameter, mm)	26.8 ± 3.9	27.1 ± 3.6	42.2 ± 9.0
Weissman[8] (diameter, mm)	26.4 ± 3.1	29.4 ± 3.3	34.3 ± 4.5
Malkowski[9] (diameter, mm)	28.9 ± 1.5	30.6 ± 2.0	33.3 ± 2.1

FMV = floppy mitral valve group.

al.[31] who demonstrated that patients with floppy mitral valves and severe mitral regurgitation had markedly increased annular diameters compared to normal subjects and patients with uncomplicated mitral valve prolapse. In addition to finding abnormal annular contraction with each cardiac cycle, Ormiston et al.[30] also found that the overall annular circumference was greater in patients with floppy mitral valves and greatest in those patients with regurgitation (Table 4). Most laboratories, however, report annular diameter. With abnormal defined as two standard deviations above the mean, an annular diameter measured by echocardiography of greater than 32 mm is abnormal from the parasternal long-axis view.

These echocardiographic observations regarding the mitral annulus in the floppy mitral valve coincide with pathologic studies. Roberts et al.[29] reported that significant annulus dilatation was frequently present in patients with floppy mitral valves requiring mitral valve surgery for severe regurgitation.

Integrated Approach to Assessing the Floppy Mitral Valve

As noted above, the floppy mitral valve may have structural abnormalities in one or several components of the valve apparatus. Gross and histologic–pathologic reports indicate a spectrum of mitral valve pathology exists in this patient population.[5] The spectrum described at surgery, pathology, and autopsy is mirrored by the spectrum now observed in these patients with two-dimensional echocardiography. Malkowski et al.[9]

found that 80% of the patients with floppy mitral valves and mitral valve prolapse had at least one structural abnormality and over 50% had two or more abnormalities (Fig. 5A). Patients with floppy mitral valves and significant mitral regurgitation were more likely to demonstrate multiple abnormalities than patients without significant regurgitation (Fig. 5B). These observations are consistent with a necropsy study that demonstrated that minor degrees of abnormalities are rarely clinically significant whereas severe thickening and elongation of the leaflets or elongation of the chordae tendineae are potentially more serious.[5]

Although the focus of the clinical and echocadiographic evaluation of these patients has been on the presence or absence of mechanical prolapse across the mitral annulus, the fundamental abnormalities in the valve structure appear to be the critical factor in the risk stratification of these patients. The spectrum of abnormalities seen in this disease process needs to be considered in the diagnosis and management of these patients and their complications (Table 5).

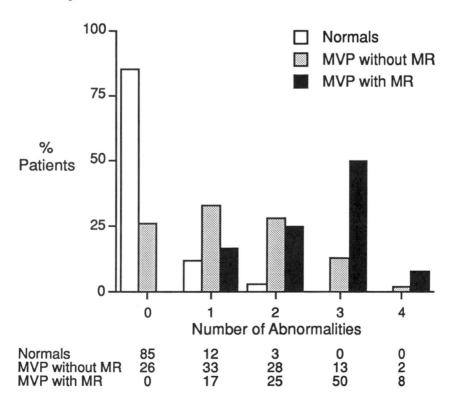

	0	1	2	3	4
Normals	85	12	3	0	0
MVP without MR	26	33	28	13	2
MVP with MR	0	17	25	50	8

Figure 5A. Bar graph indicating the percentage of normal subjects and floppy mitral valve patients with zero through four structural abnormalities. (Used with permission.[9])

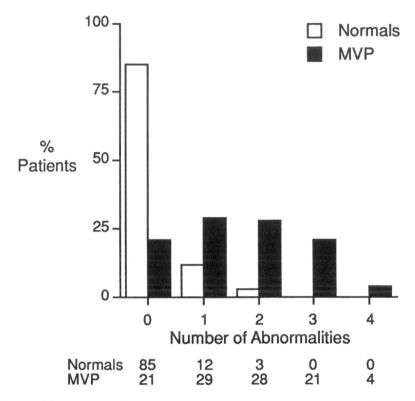

Number of Abnormalities	0	1	2	3	4
Normals	85	12	3	0	0
MVP	21	29	28	21	4

Figure 5B. Bar graph indicating the percentage of normal subjects and floppy mitral valve patients with and without mitral regurgitation with zero through four structural abnormalities. (Used with permission.[9])

Assessment of Mitral Regurgitation

Mitral regurgitation in the floppy mitral valve appears to be related to several potential mechanisms (Table 6). The most dramatic and frequently devastating mechanism of severe mitral regurgitation is the flail mitral leaflet.[32,33] Pathologic studies have demonstrated that the chordae tendineae of floppy mitral valves are grossly and histologically abnormal.[34] The structural abnormalities predispose these patients to rupture of the chordae tendineae and flail mitral leaflets. Echocardiography is an excellent method for the diagnosis of flail leaflet. The diagnosis of flail leaflet can be made by two-dimensional echocardiography from the transthoracic or the transesophageal approach.[35] Flail leaflet is defined echocardiographically by visualizing the free leaflet tip directed toward the left atrium with the body of the leaflet concave toward the left ventricle. The

Table 5
Important Structural Abnormalities of the Floppy Mitral Valve by Echocardiography

Leaflet thickness;	Abnormal leaflet thickness is present when the thickness of either the anterior or the posterior leaflet is greater than 5 mm. Measurements are usually made in the parasternal long-axis view. It is more common to find an increased thickness of anterior leaflet. Increased leaflet thickness has been related to mitral regurgitation, risk of endocarditis, sudden death, stroke, and need for valve replacement.
Leaflet length:	Anterior leaflet length is abnormal when it is greater than 27 mm. Posterior leaflet length is abnormal when it is greater than 15 mm. Leaflet length is best measured in the parasternal long-axis view from the hinge point at the mitral annulus to the leaflet tip. Increased leaflet length has been related to mitral regurgitation and in a transesophageal echocardiography study was an independent predictor of flail leaflet.
Mitral annulus:	Annular diameter is abnormal when it exceeds 32 mm. The annulus can be measured from the parasternal long-axis or apical views. Increased annular diameter has been related to mitral regurgitation in two recent echocardiographic studies. In addition, the change in annular diameter with the cardiac cycle has also been shown to be abnormal.
Chordae Tendineae:	There are no specific guidelines for abnormal chordal length by two-dimensional echocardiography. The distance from the papillary muscle to the anterior leaflet can be measured and should be considered abnormal if the distance is greater than 32 mm. Occasionally systolic anterior motion of the chordae can be seen but the significance of this finding is not well defined. Mobile chordae can be seen in patients with flail leaflets and indicates torn or ruptured chordae tendineae.

diagnosis is supported by visualizing unattached chordae tendineae within the left atrium. Recent studies suggest the identification of a flail mitral valve is associated with a poor prognosis and that early surgical intervention improves patient outcome.[36,37]

Color Doppler is very useful in assessing mitral regurgitation due to flail leaflets.[12] Frequently these patients have highly eccentric and turbulent jets that are dictated by the involved mitral leaflet (Fig. 6). Posterior flail leaflets generally create anteriorly directed color Doppler jets, which are directed along the posterior surface of the anterior leaflet and behind the posterior surface of the aorta while anterior flail leaflets direct the color

Table 6
Summary of the Mechanisms of Mitral Regurgitation Associated with Floppy Mitral Valves

Flail mitral leaflet:	The chordae tendineae of the floppy mitral valve are abnormally long and have abnormal physical properties. The histopathologic alterations result in weakening of the chordae which predisposes these patients to ruptured chordae tendineae and flail leaflets. Flail leaflet is diagnosed on echocardiography by recognizing the leaflet tip pointing into the left atrium and occasionally the visualization of unattached chordae. Color Doppler frequently reveals severe mitral regurgitation with an eccentric jet of regurgitation.
Annular dilatation:	The annulus may become dilated and display abnormal sphincter function resulting in the incomplete coaptation of the mitral leaflets. The leaflets become displaced outward from the center of the mitral orifice resulting in regurgitation. This is recognized on echocardiography by identifying an abnormal annular diameter or circumference.
Chordal lengthening:	Due to chordal lengthening one or both mitral leaflets may protrude into the left atrium and incompletely coapt. This mechanism may lead to severe mitral regurgitation but is usually mild or moderate in severity. The regurgitation associated with chordal lengthening may increase during periods when the left ventricular volume is decreased and the relationship of the papillary, chordal apparatus, and the mitral annulus changes.
Leaflet size:	The increased surface area of the mitral leaflets leads to a mismatch of the annular circumference and the leaflet surface area which is usually equal in the normal valve. This mismatch can lead to abnormal apposition of the leaflets and cause regurgitation. This mechanism usually results in mild or moderate regurgitation but may result in severe regurgitation in cases of extreme leaflet to annular mismatch.

Doppler jet posteriorly.[12] Unfortunately, these eccentric jets usually are adjacent to the atrial septum or atrial free wall, which contributes to the significant underestimation of the severity of regurgitation when utilizing color Doppler alone.[38] A study by Chen et al.[38] demonstrated that compared to centrally directed jets, wall-hugging eccentric jets frequently lead to an underestimation of the degree of regurgitation as compared to regurgitatant fraction. Since floppy mitral valves with prolapse and flail leaflets frequently produce eccentric jets of regurgitation, underestimation

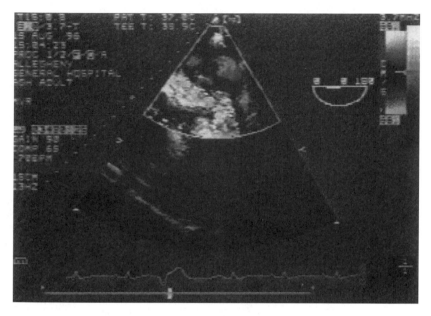

Figure 6. Transesophageal two-dimensional color Doppler image demonstrating eccentric and anteriorly directed jet of mitral regurgitation caused by a floppy mitral valve with flail posterior leaflet. See color appendix.

of the severity of regurgitation must be avoided. Although eccentric jets add to the difficulty of estimating the severity of mitral regurgitation by color Doppler, the recognition of the eccentric jet should alert the sonographer and/or physician to search for the mechanism of regurgitation, which is usually a flail or severely prolapsed mitral leaflet.

A more common mechanism of mitral regurgitation in floppy mitral valves is mismatch between valve leaflet area and annular circumference. Redundant and elongated chordae and leaflet tissue allow the leaflets to protrude into the left atrium. Roberts has observed that the increased leaflet area that is greater than the annular circumference results in an undulating surface with multiple folds and poor leaflet coaptation.[7] In addition, abnormal annular function and increased annular diameter may also prevent normal leaflet coaptation. One or all of these factors may contribute to the presence of mitral regurgitation (Table 6).

In addition to color Doppler estimates of mitral regurgitation, pulsed Doppler, which measures flow velocities, may be used to evaluate the degree of regurgitation. By using the time velocity integral of the pulsed Doppler flow at the mitral and aortic orifices and an estimate of the mitral and aortic orifice area from two-dimensional echocardiography, the flow through the mitral and aortic annulus may be calculated.[39] In the absence of aortic insufficiency, the difference in flow across the two valves divided by the transmitral flow will estimate a regurgitant fraction. The regurgitatant fraction as estimated by pulsed Doppler correlates very well with in vivo measurements of regurgitation using electroflowmeters and appears to be an accurate method of determining the severity of regurgitation regardless of the etiology. A regurgitant fraction of greater than 40% is considered to be severe.

Pulsed Doppler of pulmonary venous flow may also help to estimate the severity of mitral regurgitation. In a study utilizing transesophageal echocardiography, Castello et al.[40] found that peak systolic flow and systolic flow velocity integral were significantly lower in patients with moderate or severe mitral regurgitation when compared to patients with mild or no regurgitation. In addition, Castello et al.[40] reported that systolic flow reversal in the pulmonary veins was a sensitive and specific marker for severe mitral regurgitation. Klein et al.[41] also identified reversal of pulmonary venous systolic flow to be a very sensitive and specific marker for severe mitral regurgitation. This group also reported that discordant flow between right and left pulmonary veins may occur when eccentric jets are present, which underscores the necessity of evaluating all pulmonary viens during the echocardiographic evaluation of mitral regurgitation in patients with floppy mitral valves.[41]

Transesophageal Echocardiography and the Preoperative Evaluation of Floppy Mitral Valves

Floppy mitral valve disease resulting in mitral valve prolapse is a common valvular abnormality in the United States[42] and is the most common cause of pure severe mitral valve regurgitation requiring mitral valve surgery.[43] Recent improvements in surgical techniques have resulted in a marked increase in the number of valves that are surgically repaired rather than replaced.[14] Compared to mitral valve replacement, mitral valve repair has been reported to have lower morbidity and mortality, improved hemodynamic profile, fewer thromboembolic complications, and less bleeding complications.[44] A major complication of chronic mitral regurgitation is the development of severe left ventricular dilatation and systolic dysfunction which can result from chronic left ventricular volume overload. Abnormal left ventricular contractile function may be difficult to assess due to the reduced afterload on the left ventricle present with mitral regurgitation.[45] The risk of permanent left ventricular dysfunction and heart failure postoperatively makes the timing of surgery critical.[46,47] A lower risk procedure with less postoperative morbidity such as mitral valve repair affords the clinician and patient the option to proceed earlier to surgery avoiding the prospect of pre- and postoperative heart failure, left ventricular dilatation and systolic dysfunction, atrial dilatation and dysfunction, and atrial dysrrhythmias. In addition, the preservation of left ventricular geometry with mitral valve repair helps preserve left ventricular systolic function postoperatively.[14] The likelihood of a successful and safe repair is critically important information in timing mitral valve surgery.

The feasibility of repairing floppy valves is greatest when there is posterior chordal rupture or prolapse, elongated and redundant chordae, or annular dilatation, and least when there is chordal rupture to the anterior leaflet or both leaflets.[14] Transesophageal echocardiography has provided excellent information regarding the valvular anatomy in addition to the severity of mitral regurgitation, presence of prolapse or flail leaflets, and the presence or absence of ruptured chordae[48–50] (Fig. 7). Additional information including the jet direction by Doppler color flow mapping is helpful in evaluating these patients. Stewart et al.[11] demonstrated that two-dimensional and Doppler accurately diagnosed the mechanism of regurgitation compared to surgical findings in 93% of their surgical series. Since the feasibility of mitral repair is largely dependent on the mechanism of dysfunction, echocardiography is vital in the evaluation of these patients.

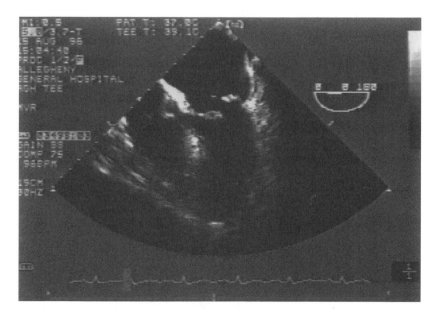

Figure 7. Transesophageal two-dimensional echocardiographic image demonstrating a floppy mitral valve with flail posterior leaflet due to torn chordae tendineae.

Although the severity of mitral regurgitation by color Doppler echocardiography has limitations,[38] in most cases the semiquantitative estimates are accurate and useful clinically.[13] Frequently, patients with mitral valve prolapse or flail mitral leaflets have very eccentric jets of mitral regurgitation.[12] With such eccentric, "wall-hugging" jets, especially those directed toward the atrial septum, the severity of mitral regurgitation may be underestimated. Transesophageal echocardigraphy may be superior to transthoracic echocardiography in the evaluation of severity of mitral regurgitation when the regurgitant jet is eccentric.[48] Findings such as color flow extending into the pulmonary veins, pulmonary venous systolic flow reversal by pulsed Doppler,[40,41] and atrial septal bowing are all evaluated superbly by transesophageal echocardigraphy and indicate severe regurgitation.[48]

In a recent transesophageal study of 72 patients, Malkowski et al.[51] assessed mitral valvular morphology in three groups (24 normal, 26 mitral valve prolapse without significant mitral regurgitation, and 22 with flail mitral leaflets with severe mitral regurgitation) to evaluate the relationship between morphologic characteristics of floppy mitral valves and clinical phenomena. In the flail leaflet group, two-thirds had posterior leaflet flail. Compared with the normal subjects, patients with mitral valve prolapse had greater anterior and posterior thickness and anterior length. The flail mitral leaflet group when compared to the mitral valve prolapse group were older and had significantly greater posterior leaflet thickness, anterior leaflet length, and posterior leaflet length. In addition, posterior leaflet length was the only predictor of flail mitral leaflet. These results indicated that older patients with increased leaflet length and thickness are predisposed to flail leaflets.

Since the valvular anatomy dictates the surgical approach in mitral regurgitation, accurate identification of valvular pathology is imperative. When chordal rupture to the posterior leaflet results in severe regurgitation, a quadrilateral resection frequently results in satisfactory leaflet coaptation and integrity.[14] Because the anterior leaflet is longer, quadrilateral resection for ruptured chordae to the anterior leaflet may result in residual regurgitation. Alternatively, chordal transfer may repair the mechanism of regurgitation when the anterior leaflet is flail but this approach is less frequently used.

Transesophageal echocardiography is superior to transthoracic echocardiography in the assessment of valvular pathology and is helpful preoperatively in the planning and timing of surgery for severe mitral regurgitation from floppy mitral valve disease. Finally, intraoperative transesophageal echocardiography has become invaluable in patients undergoing mitral valve repair.[52] The postoperative assessment helps identify the effectiveness of the repair as well as assessing for systolic anterior motion of the mitral valve, an infrequent but important complication of the procedure.[52]

Summary

The integrated approach to the echocardiographic evaluation of the floppy mitral valve, which incorporates the structural and functional information, correlates well with clinical phenomena. The improved imaging technology allows us to progress beyond the simple evaluation of leaflet prolapse and adds significantly to the clinical characteristics used to risk-stratify patients.[53] Our approach establishes coherence between imaging and pathologic findings in patients with floppy mitral valves. The quantitative assessment of valvular structures and function by echocardiography provides the framework to accurately define and risk stratify patients with floppy mitral valves.

References

1. Levine RA, Triulzi MO, Harrigan EW, Weyman AE. The relationship of mitral annular shape to the diagnosis of mitral valve prolapse. Circulation 75:756–767, 1987.
2. Levine RA, Stathogiannis E, Newell JB, Harrigan P, Weyman AE. Reconsideration of echocardiographic standards for mitral valve prolapse: Lack of association between leaflet displacement isolated to the apical four-chamber view and independent echocardiographic evidence of abnormality. J Am Coll Cardiol 11:1010–1019, 1988.
3. Criley JM, Lewis KB, Humphries JO, Ross RS. Prolapse of the mitral valve: clinical and cine-angiographic findings. Br Heart J 28:588–596, 1966.
4. Barlow JB, Pocock WA. Mitral leaflet billowing and prolapse. In Barlow JB (ed): Perspective on the Mitral Valve. Philadelphia, PA, Davis, 1987, pp 45–111.
5. Davies MJ, Moore BP, Bainbridge MV. The floppy mitral valve: Study of incidence, pathology, and complications in surgical, necropsy and forensic material. Br Heart J 40:468–481, 1978.
6. Van der Bel-Kahn J, Becker AE. The surgical pathology of rheumatic and floppy mitral valves: Distinctive morphologic features upon gross examination. Am J Surg Pathol 10:282–292, 1986.
7. Roberts WC. Morphologic aspects of cardiac valve dysfunction. Am Heart J 123:1610–1632, 1992.
8. Weissman NJ, Pini R, Roman MJ, Kramer-fox R, Andersen HS, Devereux RB. In vivo mitral valve morphology and motion in mitral valve prolapse. Am J Cardiol 73:1080–1088, 1994.
9. Malkowski MJ, Boudoulas H, Wooley CF, Guo R, Pearson AC. The spectrum of structural abnormalities in the floppy mitral valve echocardiographic evaluation. Am Heart J 132:145–151, 1996.
10. Grayburn PA, Berk MR, Spain MG, Harrison MR, Smith MD, DeMaria AN. Relation of echocardiographic morphology of mitral valve apparatus to mitral re-

gurgitation in mitral valve prolapse: Assessment by Doppler color flow imaging. Am Heart J 119:1095–1102, 1990.
11. Stewart WJ, Currie PJ, Salcedo EE, Klein AL, Marwick T, Agler DA, Homa D, et al. Evaluation of mitral leaflet motion by echocardiography and jet direction by Doppler color flow mapping to determine the mechanism of mitral regurgitation. J Am Coll Cardiol 20:1353–1361, 1992.
12. Pearson AC, St. Vrain J, Mrosek D, Labovitz AJ. Color Doppler echocardiographic evaluation of patients with a flail mitral leaflet. J Am Coll Cardiol 16:232–239, 1960.
13. Helmke F, Nanda NC, Hsuing MC, Soto B, Adey CK, Goyal RG, Gatewood RP. Color Doppler assessment of mitral regurgitation with orthogonal planes. Circulation 75:175–183, 1987.
14. Cosgrove DM, Stewart WJ. Mitral valvuloplasty. Curr Probl Cardiol 14:359–415, 1989.
15. Kerber RE, Isaeff DM, Hancock EW. Echocardiographic patterns in patients with the syndrome of click and late systolic murmur. N Engl J Med 284:691–693, 1971.
16. Savage DD, Garrison RJ, Devereux RB, Castelli WP, Anderson SJ, Levy D, McNamara PM, et al. Mitral valve prolapse in the general population. 1. Epidemiologic features: The Framingham Study. Am Heart J 106:571–576, 1983.
17. Warth DC, King ME, Cohen JM, Tesoriero VL, Marcus E, Weyman AE. Prevalence of mitral valve prolapse in normal children. J Am Coll Cardiol 5:1173–1177, 1985.
18. Wooley CF, Sparks EH, Boudoulas H. The floppy mitral valve–mitral valve prolapse–mitral valvular regurgitation triad. ACC Current J Rev 3 (4):23–26, 1994.
19. Hickey AJ, Wilcken DEL, Wright JS, Warren BA. Primary (spontaneous) chordal rupture: Relation to myxomatous valve disease and mitral valve prolapse. J Am Coll Cardiol 5:1341–1346, 1985.
20. Sahasakul Y, Edwards WD, Naessens JM, Tajik AJ. Age-related changes in aortic and mitral thickness: Implications for two-dimensional echocardiography based on an autopsy study of 200 normal human hearts. Am J Cardiol 62:424–430, 1988.
21. Ranganathan N, Lam JHC, Wigle ED, Silver MD. Morphology of the human mitral valve. II. The valve leaflet. Circulation 41:459–467, 1970.
22. Chandraratna PAN, Nimalasuriya A, Kawanishi D, Duncan P, Rosen B, Rahimtoola SH. Identification of the increased frequency of cardiovascular abnormalities associated with mitral valve prolapse by two-dimensional echocardiography. Am J Cardiol 54:1283–1285, 1984.
23. Nishimura RA, McGoon MD, Shub C, Miller FA, Ilstrup DM, Tajik AJ. Echocardiographically documented mitral valve prolapse: Long-term follow-up of 237 patients. N Engl J Med 313:1305–1309, 1985.
24. Marks AR, Choong CY, Sanfilippo AJ, Ferre M, Weyman AE. Identification of high-risk and low-risk subgroups of patients with mitral valve prolapse. N Engl J Med 320:1031–1036, 1989.
25. Fontana ME, Wooley CF, Leighton RF, Lewis RP. Postural changes in left ventricular and valvular dynamics in the systolic click–late murmur syndrome. Circulation 51:165–173, 1975.
26. Labovitz AJ, Williams GA, Pearson AC. Clinical significance of echocardiographic degree of mitral valve prolapse. Am Heart J 115:1305–1309, 1988.

27. King BD, Clark MA, Baba N, Kilman JW, Wooley CF. Myxomatous mitral valve disease: Collegen dissolution as the primary defect. Circulation 66:288–296, 1982.
28. Dollar AL, Roberts WC. Morphologic comparison of patients with mitral valve prolapse who died suddenly with patients who died from severe valvular dysfunction or other conditions. J Am Coll Cardiol 17:921–931, 1991.
29. Roberts WC, McIntosh CL, Wallace RB. Mechanisms of severe mitral regurgitation in mitral valve prolapse determined from analysis of operatively excised valves. Am Heart J 113:1316–1323, 1987.
30. Ormiston JA, Shah PM, Tei C, Wong M. Size and motion of the mitral valve annulus in man. Circulation 65:713–719, 1982.
31. Pini R, Devereux RB, Greppi B, Roman MJ, Hochreiter C, Kramer-Fox R, Niles NW, et al. Comparison of mitral valve dimensions and motion in mitral valve prolapse with severe mitral regurgitation to uncomplicated mitral valve prolapse and to mitral regurgitation without mitral valve prolapse. Am J Cardiol 62:257–263, 1988.
32. Kolibash AJ, Kilman JW, Bush CA, Fontana ME, Wooley CF. Evidence for progression from mild to severe mitral regurgitation in mitral valve prolapse. Am J Cardiol 58:762–767, 1986.
33. Wooley CF, Baker PB, Kolibash AJ, Kilman JW, Sparks EA, Boudoulas H. The floppy, myxomatous mitral valve, mitral valve prolapse and mitral regurgitation. Prog Cardiovasc Dis 33:397–433, 1991.
34. Baker PB, Bansal G, Boudoulas H, Kolibash AJ, Wooley CF. Floppy mitral chordae tendineae: Histopathologic alterations. Hum Pathol 19:507–512, 1988.
35. Mintz GS, Kotler MN, Parry WR, Segal BL. Statistical comparison of M-mode and two-dimensional echocardiographic diagnosis of flail mitral leaflets. Am J Cardiol 45:253–259, 1980.
36. Ling LH, Enriquez-Sarano M, Seward JB, et al. Clinical outcome of mitral regurgitation due to flail leaflet. N Engl J Med 335:1417–1423, 1996.
37. Ling LH, Enriquez-Sarano M, Seward JB, Orszulak TA, Schaff HV, Bailey KR, Tajik AJ, et al. Early surgery in patients with mitral regurgitation due to flail leaflets: A long-term outcome study. Circulation 96:1819–1825, 1997.
38. Chen C, Thomas J, Anconina J, Harrigan P, Mueller L, Picard MH, Levine RA, et al. Impact of impinging wall jet on color Doppler quantification of mitral regurgitation. Circulation 84:712–720, 1991.
39. Rokey R, Sterling LL, Zoghbi WA, Sartori MP, Limacher MC, Kuo LC, Quinones MA. Determination of regurgitant fraction in isolated mitral or aortic regurgitation by pulsed Doppler two-dimensional echocardiography. J Am Coll Cardiol 7:1273–1278, 1986.
40. Castello R, Pearson AC, Lenzen P, Labovitz AJ. Effect of mitral regurgitation on pulmonary venous velocities derived from transesophageal ecocardiography color-guided pulsed Doppler imaging. J Am Coll Cardiol 17:1499–1506, 1991.
41. Klein AL, Obarski TP, Stewart WJ, Casale PN, Pearce GL, Husbands K, Cosgrove DM, et al. Transesophageal Doppler echocardiography of pulmonary venous flow: A new marker of mitral regurgitation severity. J Am Coll Cardiol 18:518–526, 1991.
42. Devereux RB, Kramer-Fox R, Kligfield P. Mitral valve prolapse: etiology, clinical manifestations and management. Ann Intern Med 111:305–317, 1989.
43. Agozzino L, Falco A, de Vivo F, de Vincentiis C, de Luca L, Esposito S, Cotrufo M. Surgical pathology of the mitral valve: Gross and histological study of 1288 surgically excised valves. Int J Cardiol 37:79–89, 1992.

44. Enriquez-Sarano M, Schaff HV, Orszulak TA, Tajik AJ, Bailey KR, Frye RL. Valve repair improves the outcome of surgery for mitral regurgitation: A multivariate analysis. Circulation 91:1022–1028, 1995.
45. Enriquez-Sarano M, Tajik J, Schaff HV, Orszulak TA, McGoon MD, Bailey KR, Frye RL. Echocardiographic prediction of left ventricular function after correction of mitral regurgitation: Results and clinical implications. J Am Coll Cardiol 24:1536–1543, 1994.
46. Stewart WJ. Choosing the "golden" moment for mitral valve repair. J Am Coll Cardiol 24:1544–1546, 1994.
47. Starling MR, Kirsh MM, Montgomery DG, Gross MD. Impaired left ventricular contractile function in patients with long-term mitral regurgitation and normal ejection fraction. J Am Coll Cardiol 22:239–250, 1993.
48. Schiller NB, Foster E, Redberg RF. Transesophageal echocardiography in the evaluation of mitral regurgitation: The twenty-four signs of severe mitral regurgitation. Cardiol Clin 11:399–408, 1993.
49. Grewal K, Malkowski MJ, Kramer CM, Dianzumba S, Reichek N. Multiplane transesophageal echocardiography predicts the involved scallop in patients with posterior flail mitral leaflet and severe mitral regurgitation: An intraoperative correlation. J Am Coll Cardiol 29:340A, 1997.
50. Stewart WJ, Griffin B, Thomas JD. Multiplane transesophageal echocardiographic evaluation of mitral valve disease. Am J Cardiac Imaging 9:121–128, 1995.
51. Malkowski MJ, Guo R, Orsinelli DA, Wooley CF, Tice FD, Pearson AC, Boudoulas H. The morphologic characteristics of mitral valve prolapse with flail mitral leaflets by transesophageal echocardiography. J Heart Valve Dis 6:54–59, 1997.
52. Freeman WK, Schaff HV, Khandheria BK, Oh JK, Orszulak TA, Abel MD, Seward JB, et al. Intraoperative evaluation of mitral valve regurgitation and repair by transesophageal echocardiography: Incidence and significance of systolic anterior motion. J Am Coll Cardiol 20:599–609, 1992.
53. Zuppiroli A, Rinaldi M, Kramer-Fox R, Favilli S, Roman MJ, Devereux RB. Natural history of mitral valve prolapse. Am J Cardiol 75:1028–1032, 1995.

11

Three-Dimensional Echocardiographic Reconstruction of Normal Mitral Valve and Mitral Valve Prolapse

Jiefen Yao, MD
Natesa G. Pandian, MD
Jos R.T.C. Roelandt, MD

Introduction

The mitral valve apparatus, including mitral annulus, chordae tendineae, papillary muscles, and left ventricle, forms a three-dimensional integrity to allow unidirectional blood flow from the left atrium to the left ventricle. Mitral valve prolapse is a frequently encountered problem in clinical cardiology.[1] Though mild prolapse is usually nonsignificant clinically,[2–4] when more severe prolapse develops and is combined with significant mitral regurgitation, clinical manifestations such as symptoms of deteriorated cardiac function and complications including cardiac arrhythmia, infective endocarditis, cerebral embolism, and even sudden death may occur.[5–9] Surgical treatment of mitral valve prolapse uses either mitral valve repair or replacement. It is ideal for the surgeons to under-

From: Boudoulas H, Wooley CF. *Mitral Valve: Floppy Mitral Valve, Mitral Valve Prolapse, Mitral Valvular Regurgitation.* Second revised edition. ©Futura Publishing Company, Armonk, NY, 2000.

stand, before the surgery, the specific site (scallop) of the mitral valve that prolapses and the extension and severity of the prolapse in order to make a decision of how to operate. In the past two and half decades, echocardiography, by its unique imaging capabilities, has considerably improved our knowledge of the mitral valve apparatus.

M-mode echocardiography, a one-dimensional scanning of the mitral valve structures, was used mainly in the early 1970s. The diagnosis of mitral valve prolapse depends on displacement of one of the mitral leaflets posterior to the mitral closure line.[10] It is understandable that the diagnostic accuracy and sensitivity with this technique was not high. Two-dimensional echocardiography, which is able to deliver tomographic views

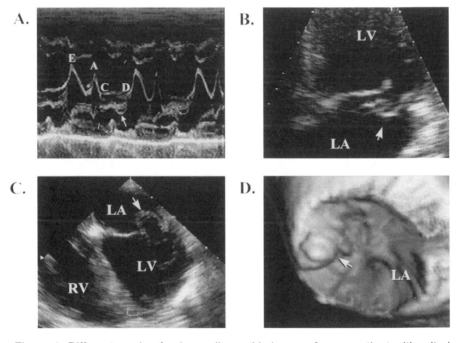

Figure 1. Different mode of echocardiographic images from a patient with mitral valve prolapse. **A**. M-mode echocardiogram. The diagnosis of mitral valve prolapse (arrow) is confirmed by disposition of the mitral leaflet posterior to the mitral closure line (C-D), but which leaflet prolapses cannot be determined. **B**. Transthoracic two-dimensional echocardiogram showing, in an apical four-chamber format, the superior displacement of posterior mitral leaflet (arrow). **C**. Transesophageal two-dimensional echocardiogram displaying clearly the prolapsing posterior mitral leaflet bulging into the left atrium (arrow) in a four-chamber view. **D**. Three-dimensional echocardiographic image obtained via transesophageal scanning portraying the accurate site, size, and extent of the mitral valve that is prolapsing into the left atrium in a surgeon's view (arrow). LA = left atrium; LV = left ventricle, RV = right ventricle.

of the heart with more information on the cardiac structures, improved the sensitivity for the diagnosis of mitral valve prolapse,[11] but confusion still exists in diagnostic standards due to the nonplanar (saddle) shape of the mitral annulus, which is designated as the landmark for defining superior displacement of mitral valve leaflets.[12,13]

Transesophageal echocardiography (TEE), although minimally invasive, yields superior images of the mitral valve apparatus and mitral regurgitant jet when combined with color flow imaging because of its optimal acoustic window and the use of the left atrial blood pool as an optimal ultrasound transmission medium. Nevertheless, the mitral valve apparatus is three-dimensional in both morphology and function. It is obvious that a technique with the ability of three-dimensional image display is preferable for accurate evaluation of the mitral valve and mitral valve prolapse. Different techniques of three-dimensional image reconstruction from two-dimensional echocardiography have evolved and, among them, volume-rendered three-dimensional echocardiography provides dynamic tissue-depicting images that also allow surgical views of the mitral valve (Fig. 1).[14,15] In this chapter, we will discuss the methodology of three-dimensional echocardiography and current clinical experience with its application in normal mitral valve and in mitral valve prolapse.

Techniques of Three-Dimensional Echocardiography

An ideal approach of three-dimensional echocardiography is online imaging of the cardiac structures in multiple dimensions. This, however, would require a special probe that has the ability of sampling a pyramidal volume of ultrasound signals from the heart and instantly processing the data. Such a prototype transducer is still in the experimental stage and has not yet been used clinically.[16]

Various approaches of three-dimensional echocardiography discussed here have been engaged in clinical and experimental studies.[14,16,17] Their common feature is to reconstruct the cardiac structures in three-dimension using images collected from two-dimensional echocardiography. Different methods are utilized for data acquisition, data processing, three-dimensional image reconstruction, and image display (Table 1).

Data Acquisition

Collection of multiple two-dimensional echocardiographic images is necessary for three-dimensional reconstruction. The following are two basic modes for image acquisition.

Table 1
Different Techniques of Three-Dimensional Echocardiography

	Wire-Frame	Volume-Rendered	Real-Time
Data acquisition			
image collection	random	sequential	on-line
temporal gating	no	ECG and respiration	—
Data processing			
image registration	spatial	spatial and temporal	—
space interpolation	no	yes	—
3D reconstruction			
image formation	manual tracing	digitized ultrasound signal	ultrasound signal
rendering	wire-frame or surface	surface or volume	volume
3D image display			
mode	static	static or dynamic	static or dynamic
secondary 2D images	no	yes	—

3D = three-dimensional; 2D = two-dimensional.

Random Data Acquisition

With random mode data acquisition, or free-hand imaging, a multitude of two-dimensional images of the heart are collected by moving the transducer freely at one acoustic window or at multiple acoustic windows. The location and orientation of the transducer are detected by positional sensor devices such as magnetic sensors, acoustic (spark gap) sensors, and goniometry. The acquired two-dimensional images are later realigned according to their spatial locations. This mode of acquisition is applied mainly to wire-frame or surface-rendered reconstruction and for volume or mass measurement of gross structures such as cardiac chambers. Reconstruction of three-dimensional images requires manual tracing of numerous two-dimensional images.[17]

Sequential Data Acquisition

For three-dimensional reconstruction of tissue-depicting images, small and regularly distributed gaps between two-dimensional echocardiographic samples are required. Sequential data acquisition uses different algorithms to collect two-dimensional images in computer-controlled predefined steps with ECG and respiratory gating. The currently used methods for sequential data acquisition are: parallel slicing, rotational imaging, and fan-like scanning (Fig. 2).

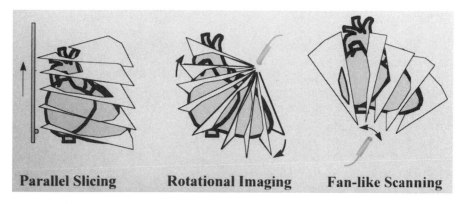

Parallel Slicing   **Rotational Imaging**   **Fan-like Scanning**

Figure 2. Schematics showing movement of the ultrasound transducer in parallel, rotational, and fan-like modes of three-dimensional data acquisition.

Parallel Slicing: The simplest algorithm for three-dimensional data acquisition is by moving the ultrasound probe in a linear direction while the heart is being imaged. With transthoracic echocardiography, a monitoring device controlled by the computer is mounted onto the probe. Precordial or subcostal windows can be used for this kind of imaging. With transesophageal echocardiography, a special TEE probe is attached to a sliding device controlled by the computer. The distal portion of the probe is enclosed in a casing carriage that can be straightened after the probe is introduced into the esophagus. The probe is then moved linearly in equal steps during collection of tomographic images of the heart.[18]

Rotational Imaging: This mode of data acquisition has become the most commonly used method in clinical studies because of the relatively smaller acoustic windows needed. Two-dimensional images are collected in equal-degree increments with the probe in a fixed site at either a transthoracic or a transesophageal window. Rotation of the imaging plane is realized by rotation of the transducer inside the probe with a computer controlled built-in motor (multiplane transthoracic or transesophageal transducer) or by rotation of the probe with an externally adapted motor device that is attached to the probe in transthoracic imaging and to the rotation knob in transesophageal approach.[19,20]

Fan-Like Scanning: With this method, the transducer is tilted in an arc in predefined equal steps while the ultrasound plane sweeps through the heart. With a motor device adapted to the ultrasound probe, the imaging plane is controlled by the computer with equal intervals. Precordial or subcostal windows have been used for this mode of data acquisition.[21]

Artifacts and Solutions

Many factors may cause artifacts in a three-dimensional data set. Major artifacts can be caused by patient or probe movement. The former can be prevented by explaining the procedure and asking the patient to stay relaxed and still. Great patience is needed for small children (except in sedated patients) and sometimes repeated procedures for acquisition are necessary. Probe movement can be avoided using mechanical arms to hold the probe or by experience accumulation after a learning curve for steadying the probe.

The heart is a highly dynamic organ and its dimensions, shape, and position change markedly during the cardiac cycle. ECG gating is used for synchronizing two-dimensional images acquired in different periods of a cardiac cycle and for rejecting images from irregular heart beats by monitoring and gating for ECG R-R intervals. Artifacts from respiration-related movements of the heart can be minimized by respiratory gating. Various methods have been used for respiration monitoring. A nasal thermometer is used to detect the temperature changes in the nasal cavity during respiration. The same ECG leads used for ECG gating can be used at the same time for detecting thoracic impedance changes during respiratory cycles. The stretch of the thoracic wall during respiration can also be sensed and used for gating purposes. Data acquisition is often gated to expiration phase, sometimes to inspiration (Fig. 3).

There are often artifacts derived from ultrasound signals. All kinds of artifacts that appear on two-dimensional echocardiography will result in the similar artifacts in three-dimensional echocardiography. These can be minimized by optimizing various control settings on the ultrasound machine during data acquisition.

Data Processing

After data acquisition, the collected two-dimensional images are calibrated and stored in a digital format. Images from different phases of the cardiac cycle and from different imaging planes are registered according to their spatial and temporal sequences (Fig. 3). For volume-rendered three-dimensional echocardiography, spaces between adjacent sampling slices are interpolated automatically by the computer and the pixel-rendered two-dimensional images are transferred into a voxel-based three-dimensional data set. The size of the three-dimensional data set can be diminished by defining and extracting a region of interest, or by extracting only one or a few phases out of the cardiac cycle. Noises in the three-dimensional data set can be diminished and image quality enhanced using various filtering algorithms by removing low-level noises, enhancing edges, and smoothing image signals.

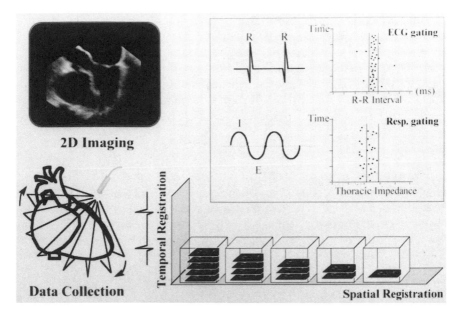

Figure 3. Schematic demonstration of spatial and temporal registration of sequentially acquired two-dimensional images with ECG and respiratory gating. Upper and lower left panels represent rotational data acquisition of two-dimensional images. Upper right panel shows gating set for ECG using R-R interval and gating for respiration using thoracic impedance. Expiration phase is selected in this example. Lower left and right panels demonstrate data collection (rotational) and temporal and spatial registration of acquired images. Images from different phases of the cardiac cycle are registered according to their temporal order in different ECG segments as represented on y axis. Images from different steps are registered according to their spatial order as shown on x axis. I = starting point of inspiration; E = starting point of expiration; resp. gating = respiration gating; 2D = two-dimensional.

Three-Dimensional Image Reconstruction

Different methods for three-dimensional echocardiographic image reconstruction have been developed in the past two and half decades. Earlier approaches with wire-frame reconstruction were used mainly in volume or mass quantification of the ventricles. A surface-rendering technique was later developed to add tissue-depiction to the reconstructed images. Recent achievement in volume-rendering reconstruction has provided both tissue-depicting pictures of normal and abnormal cardiac structures and accurate quantitative measurements of various cardiac indices.

Wire-Frame Formation: Three-dimensional image reconstruction with wire-frame formation needs manual tracing of the cardiac borders in numerous two-dimensional images acquired either randomly or sequentially. A semi-automatic border detection method has been tried to save the labor of tedious manual tracing but applied only to images with superior quality. The contours of the cardiac structures are demonstrated statically in a cage-like three-dimensional format without tissue depiction.[22]

Surface-Rendering Method: A surface can be applied to three-dimensional images reconstructed from either manual tracings or from ultrasound signals.[23] Provided with proper shading techniques, surface-rendered three-dimensional images can be tissue depicting and exhibit the depth of the objects. However, surface-rendered images give no additional information beyond the surface.

Volume-Rendering Technique: By digitization, interpolation and transformation of two-dimensional ultrasound signals, volume-rendered three-dimensional echocardiographic images enrich texture and depth display of cardiac structures. Tissues are differentiated from blood pool by adjusting threshold for uptaken signal strength and transparency of surface display. No manual tracing is needed for volume-rendered three-dimensional reconstruction. With appropriate shading, the reconstructed images display depth, texture, and natural sizes and shapes of the cardiac structures in cine mode with one cardiac cycle.[14]

One of the advantages of volume-rendering three-dimensional image reconstruction is that the three-dimensional data set can be electronically sectioned in any desired cutting plane and the cardiac structures can be demonstrated from various vantage points.[24] The roof or apex of the heart or part of the chamber walls can be removed directed by three orthogonal axes (α, β, γ) in the Cartesian coordinate system. The reconstructed image can also be turned around in any direction providing different projections.

Three different shading techniques have been used for three-dimensional image reconstruction.[25] Distance coding enhances tissue-depicting features of the image by application of different levels of gray scale according to the distance between the observer and the object (the further, the darker). Texture coding depends on ultrasound signal intensity of acquired two-dimensional images and represents tissue texture or density. Gray scale gradient shading illuminates the surface of the reconstructed image as if a light is held by the observer. A mixture of these three shading techniques gives a realistic three-dimensional image of the heart (Fig. 4).

Three-Dimensional Image Display

The reconstructed three-dimensional images can be displayed in various ways. A static image in any desired phase of the cardiac cycle is used to demonstrate the best view of a given structure or structures. Dynamic display of three-dimensional images provides in vivo pathophysiological anatomy of the heart. Multiple projections of the same image can be reconstructed and displayed as if the heart is turned around, providing more information than single-projection images. Three-dimensional echocardiographic images are usually displayed in gray scale. However, the reconstructed images can be encoded and demonstrated with pseudocolors according to the gray scale levels of the original ultrasound signals. A color-encoded display may assist in appreciation of cardiac tissue texture in a more realistic manner.[26]

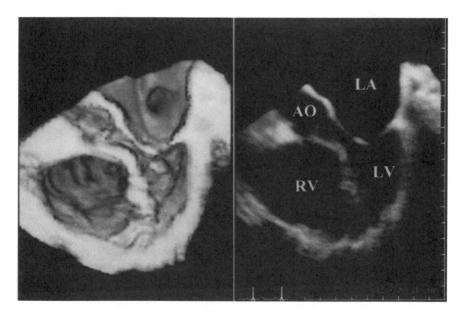

Figure 4. Volume-rendered three-dimensional image (left) using a mixture of various shading techniques in comparison with two-dimensional echocardiographic image (right) at the same cutting plane. It is readily observed that shaded three-dimensional reconstruction demonstrates not only the details but also the depth and texture of the cardiac structure. LA = left atrium; AO = aorta; RV = right ventricle; LV = left ventricle.

Multiplanar Review of Volume-Rendered Three-Dimensional Data Set

Volume-rendered three-dimensional data set can be sectioned arbitrarily to derive multiple secondary two-dimensional images (up to nine images including the reference image) at one time. With free manipulation of cutting planes guided by the Cartesian coordinate system, the heart can be viewed in any desired cross-sectional view. An unlimited number of novel views can be generated from the three-dimensional data set.[24] Several algorithms for obtaining multiplanar two-dimensional views have been used and are discussed as follows.

Anyplane Method: This is a basic method for acquiring secondary two-dimensional images from a three-dimensional data set. By first choosing an appropriate reference image, the cutting plane can be altered in the following ways: (a) defining the central point of the cutting plane; (b) rotating the cutting plane around any of the three axes (α, β and γ) of the Cartesian system, and; (c) moving the cutting plane in a parallel direction.

Paraplane Method: Once one cutting plane is defined using the anyplane method, a multitude of paraplane images can be realized automatically by the computer. This method is useful in quantitative volume measurement, selecting an optimal cutting plane and understanding spatial continuity of the cardiac structures.

Short-Axis and Long-Axis Methods: Two points can be given to a cardiac chamber or any specific structure to create an artificial "axis." Multiple "short-axis" views perpendicular to the axis or a cluster of "long-axis" views around the axis can be generated automatically by the computer. Distance between "short-axis" images and angle between "long-axis" images can be adjusted.

Main-Axis Method: By defining one cutting plane using the anyplane method, this algorithm will provide three orthogonal cutting planes perpendicular to each other with a common central point. These views may provide useful information on the spatial extent of cardiac abnormalities such as intracardiac masses.

Three-Dimensional Data Analysis

Three-dimensional echocardiography can be analyzed both qualitatively and quantitatively. Qualitative data analysis including appraisal of reconstructed three-dimensional images and review of the data set with secondary two-dimensional cutting planes is discussed in various related sections of this chapter. In this section, quantitative analysis of three-dimensional data is focused. The current available measurements directly on three-dimensional images or using secondary two-dimensional images are listed in Table 2.

It is an important advantage of three-dimensional echocardiography in direct distance measurement on reconstructed three-dimensional images. With direct viewing, distance between any two points can be measured accurately. Measurement of septal defect diameters and rims of the defect (width of tissue surrounding defect) could be facilitated for the ability of en face viewing of the defects otherwise impossible with other modalities. Similarly, better evaluation may also apply to measurements of the mitral or tricuspid annulus, papillary muscle or chordal lengths, and intercommissural distance.

Although, up to now, surface area cannot be measured directly on three-dimensional images (however, the algorithm is under active investigation), cross-sectional area measurement has been improved because of versatile cutting plane orientation and various multiplanar review abilities with the three-dimensional data set. Two-dimensional cutting plane placement can also be directed by three-dimensional image reconstruction such as in valve area measurement. The to-be-measured region can be traced manually or detected by the computer automatically using the gray level threshold method. Area and circumference of this area are computed automatically by the computer.

Volume of a given chamber or subject is measured by electronically sectioning the three-dimensional data set into multiple parallel slices with equal thickness. All of the slices are viewed with two-dimensional images derived either by the paraplane method or by the short-axis method. The area of interest is manually traced or automatically detected on each slice. With known thickness, volume of the area of inter-

Table 2
Quantitative Parameters That Can Be Derived from Three-Dimensional Echocardiography

	3D Images	Secondary 2D Images
Distance	+	+
Area	−	+
Circumference	−	+
Volume	−	+

Abbreviations are same as in Table 1.

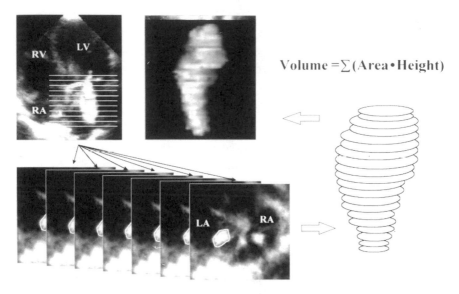

$$\text{Volume} = \sum (\text{Area} \cdot \text{Height})$$

Figure 5. Schematic demonstration of three-dimensional volume measurement of mitral regurgitant jet. Upper left is a reference image in a four-chamber format showing mitral regurgitant jet. Lines covering the regurgitant jet showing position of multiple parallel cutting planes used for volume measurement by tracing the jet area on each slice (lower left). The formula and schematics on the right show the volume calculation algorithm using the "summation of discs" method. The upper middle image is the reconstructed regurgitant jet extracted using the labeling system. RV = right ventricle; LV = left ventricle; RA = right atrium; LA = left atrium.

est on each slice and its total volume are calculated by the computer. By giving a special label to the traced object, it can be extracted from the rest of the three-dimensional data set and be reconstructed into three-dimensional images alone (Fig. 5).

Clinical Experience with Three-Dimensional Echocardiography of the Mitral Valve and Mitral Valve Prolapse

The mitral valve and mitral valve diseases have been the focuses of many three-dimensional echocardiographic studies either because of the morphologic and functional complexity or because of the susceptibility to various abnormalities.[13, 27–29] In this section, we will review some previous literature on mitral valve prolapse and introduce our own experience with normal mitral valve, mitral valve prolapse, and mitral regurgitation by three-dimensional echocardiography.

Image data acquisition for three-dimensional echocardiographic reconstruction can be realized via a transthoracic or a transesophageal window. It has been performed not only in echocardiographic laboratories, but also in various clinical settings including intensive care units, catheterization laboratories, and operating rooms.[30,31] Various cutting planes such as longitudinal, cross-sectional and, when necessary, oblique views can be selected for three-dimensional reconstruction and display of the mitral valve apparatus. Images of the mitral valve in longitudinal views can be reconstructed using four-chamber, two-chamber, or long-axis formats for comparative interpretation with two-dimensional echocardiography. With three-dimensional display, not only the cross-sectional image but also structures beyond the cutting plane is demonstrated in three dimensions (Fig. 4). Longitudinal images describe generally, besides mitral valve, sizes and shapes of the cardiac chambers and are also useful for studying the papillary muscles and chordae tendineae. Short-axis three-dimensional images of the mitral valve can be reconstructed by truncating the left ventricle (view from below) or left atrium (view from above) transversely. When viewed from below, as if the observer sits in the left ventricle looking up, the inferior surface of the mitral valve, its opening and closing movement, and left ventricular outflow tract are exhibited. The mitral valve area and mitral leaflet coaptation can be examined closely (Fig. 6).

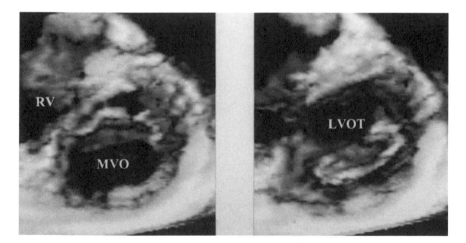

Figure 6. Three-dimensional images of a normal mitral valve viewed from below reconstructed from transthoracic parasternal data acquisition. During diastole (left), the opening of mitral valve, thickness of mitral leaflets, and the commissures are well seen. During systole (right), coaptation of mitral leaflets, the commissures, as well as left ventricular outflow tract are readily appraised. Dynamic images better display the movement and flexibility of the mitral valve. RV = right ventricle; MVO = mitral valve opening; LVOT = left ventricular outflow tract.

When the mitral valve is viewed from above, as if the roof of the left atrium is removed, the superior surface of the mitral leaflets, size, shape, and motion of the mitral annulus during diastole and systole, as well as the left atrial appendage are observed (Fig. 7). Two-dimensional images of the mitral valve and its apparatus derived from the three-dimensional data set can also be studied systematically using various multiplanar review methods.

Normal Mitral Valve

We observed, similar to anatomical results,[32] that the mitral valve acts like a gate between the left ventricle and the left atrium with the anterior mitral leaflet moving like a door and posterior leaflet more like the door frame with relatively less movement. The anterior leaflet lies anteromedially adjacent to the aortic valve. It is longer in height and shorter in width at the base, more or less in a semicircular shape. The posterior leaflet lies posterolaterally with a longer connection with the mitral annulus and is shorter in height. Indentations between leaflet scallops are sometimes seen.[27] The anteromedial and posterolateral commissures are also discernible. They tend to fold up when the mitral valve is closing. The coap-

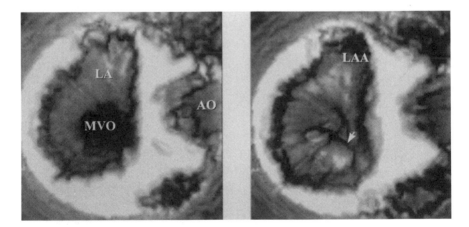

Figure 7. Diastolic (left) and systolic (right) images of the mitral valve viewed from above obtained from a patient with rheumatic mitral valve stenosis and prolapse. In diastole, the restricted mitral valve opening is clearly demonstrated. In systole, the superior surface of the mitral valve and the prolapsing portion of the posterior leaflet (arrow) is well portrayed. The left atrial appendage is also viewed. LA = left atrium; MVO = mitral valve opening; AO = aorta; LAA = left atrial appendage.

tation line of the mitral valve is a crescendo with the concave side medially positioned. The mitral annulus is nearly flat medially and more circular laterally in the shape of a saddle.[13,33] Its medial to lateral diameter is slightly shorter than the anterior to posterior diameter, with its anterior end about 1 cm higher than the posterior end. Normal chordae tendineae are hardly seen in three-dimensional images due to the fine features relative to lateral resolution of echocardiography, but major chordae (high-grade ones) are sometimes visible. Papillary muscles can be shown clearly and their movement appreciated. They usually bifurcate at their tips (Fig. 8).

Mitral Valve Prolapse

Dynamic volume-rendered three-dimensional echocardiography, for the first time, demonstrated live in vivo images of cardiac structures including the mitral valve in multidimensions.[14,15] The unique feature of mitral valve prolapse is that one portion of the mitral valve leaflet bulges or protrudes into the left atrium during systole (Fig. 9). When viewed from above, the scallop or scallops of the mitral valve leaflet involved in prolapse is best defined. This view is also called "surgeon's view" (Fig. 10). When viewed from the left ventricle, the prolapse portion of the mitral valve is like a spoon-shaped depression when the mitral valve is closed

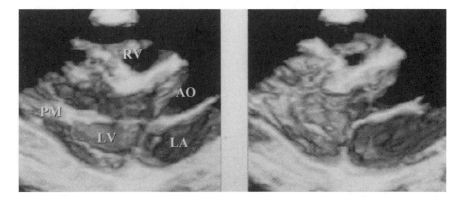

Figure 8. Three-dimensional images acquired via transthoracic rotational scanning demonstrating mitral apparatus. Left: diastolic image. Right: systolic image. The chamber sizes of left ventricle and left atrium, mitral valve, and subvalvular apparatus are well defined. RV = right ventricle; PM = papillary muscle; LV = left ventricle; LA = left atrium; AO = aorta.

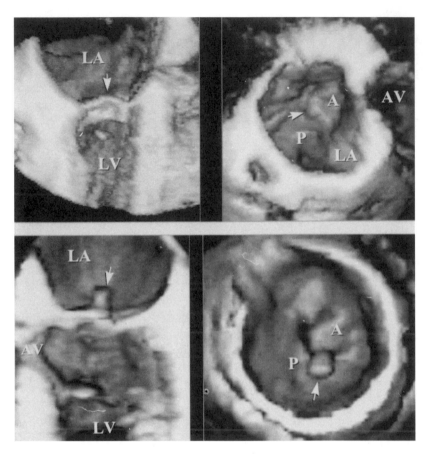

Figure 9. Longitudinal (left images) and surgical (right images) views of the mitral valve from two patients with mitral valve prolapse (arrows). The first patient had anterior mitral leaflet prolapse (middle portion). The second patient (lower images) also had anterior mitral leaflet flail as well as prolapsing. LA = left atrium; LV = left ventricle; A= anterior mitral leaflet; P= posterior mitral leaflet; AV = aortic valve.

(Fig. 11). During diastole, the mitral valve leaflet may show a fluffy movement and folds may be noticed at leaflet tips because of the enlarged size of the leaflet. In cases of chordal rupture or, rarely, papillary muscle rupture, the mitral valve may flail with the tip of the leaflet seen in the left atrium during systole (Fig. 12). The ruptured chordae tendineae can some-

---

Figure 11. Three-dimensional images from a patient with anterior mitral leaflet prolapse (arrows) viewed from the left ventricle (left panel) and the left atrium (right panel). The prolapse is shown as a depression on the ventricular side of the mitral valve and a protrusion on the atrial side. A = anterior mitral leaflet; P = posterior mitral leaflet.

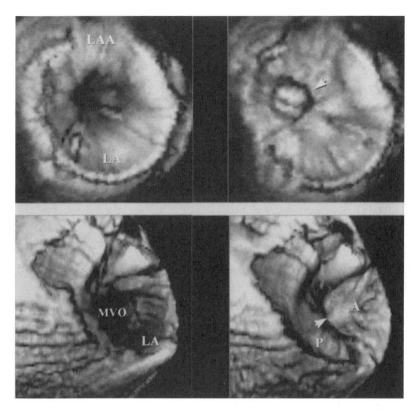

Figure 10. Surgical view of mitral valve prolapse (arrows) from two patients with diastolic images on the left and systolic images on the right. The location and extent of prolapse is well appreciated from this view. Diastolic frames show clearly the mitral annulus. LAA = left atrial appendage; LA = left atrium; MVO = mitral valve opening; A= anterior mitral leaflet; P = posterior mitral leaflet.

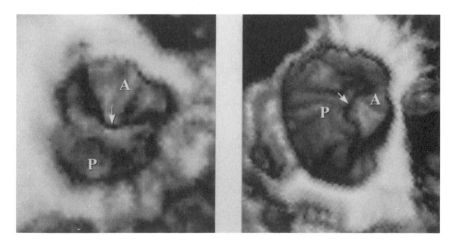

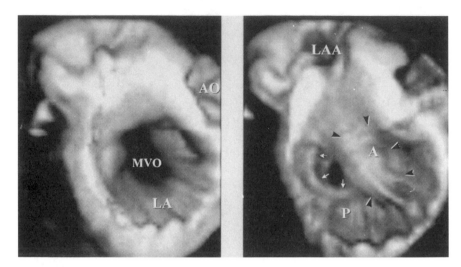

Figure 12. Diastolic (left) and systolic (right) three-dimensional images of the mitral valve obtained via transesophageal echocardiography in an operating room before surgery. This patient had myxomatous mitral valve with anterior leaflet prolapsing (black arrows) and posterior leaflet flail (white arrows). The normal mitral valve area in diastole and the regurgitant orifice in systole are well appreciated. The above observation of the mitral valve was confirmed during surgery, and mitral valve replacement was performed due to extensive involvement of both leaflets. AO = aorta; MVO = mitral valve opening; LA = left atrium; LAA = left atrial appendage; A = anterior mitral leaflet; P = posterior mitral leaflet.

times be detected as well.[34] The regurgitant orifice is sometimes visible and can be measured on two-dimensional anyplane images. While short-axis views aid in accurate estimation of the site and the extent of mitral valve that is involved in prolapse, longitudinal views may aid in appreciation of the depth of prolapse into the left atrium (Fig. 13). In addition to three-dimensional image display, two-dimensional multiplanar review of the three-dimensional data set also provides useful information for accurately evaluating the severity of mitral valve prolapse. The ability of three-dimensional echocardiography in offering accurate and incremental information on mitral valve prolapse provides essential information for preoperative planning and selection of surgical procedures for mitral valve repair or replacement.[27,28,35–37] Surgical views of the mitral valve, unobtainable with any other two-dimensional approaches so far, allows us to determine precisely which scallop of the mitral valve leaflet prolapses. Although much of this information can be obtained during surgery after the heart is open, preoperative diagnosis of the accurate location and extent of mitral valve prolapse may shorten the time needed for direct inspection of the mitral valve and, therefore, may reduce associated risks re-

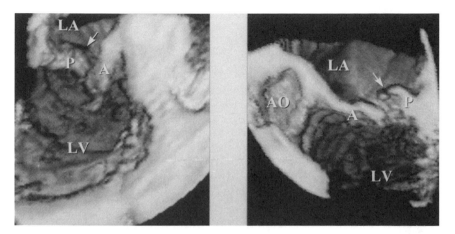

Figure 13. Longitudinal views of the mitral valve from two patients with different degrees of mitral valve prolapse (arrows). LA = left atrium; LV = left ventricle; AO = aorta; A = anterior mitral leaflet; P = posterior mitral leaflet.

lated to cardiopulmonary bypass. In addition, dynamic three-dimensional images of the mitral valve represent its in vivo status (e.g., shape and function) under complicated hemodynamic conditions that cannot be simulated during surgery. Three-dimensional echocardiographic reconstruction of the mitral valve immediately after surgery or later may also furnish postoperative evaluation of repaired or replaced mitral valve function.

Mitral Valve Regurgitation

An important factor affecting the outcome of mitral valve prolapse is mitral regurgitation. In many cases, the origin, direction, and shape of the jet are unpredictable, leading to difficulties in accurate estimation of the severity of mitral regurgitation. Three-dimensional echocardiography has also been applied successfully in reconstruction of intracardiac blood flows including mitral regurgitant jets acquired with color Doppler flow imaging.[38] The color Doppler signal can be transferred into gray scale format or retain the original colors in the three-dimensional data set. The instant jet volume can be quantified by three-dimensional echocardiography as well.[39] With dynamic three-dimensional images, the site of origin, direction of trajectory, shape and surface geometry of mitral regurgitant jet can be readily appreciated along with mitral valve prolapse. In addition, the proximal flow convergence region can be reconstructed into a three-dimensional image and viewed in different projections (Fig. 14). In preliminary observations in patients with mitral valve prolapse, various shapes of the proximal flow convergence region of mitral regurgitation have been

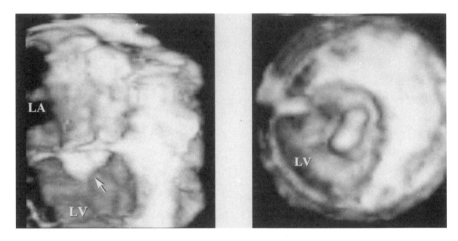

Figure 14. Three-dimensional images of mitral regurgitation obtained with two-dimensional and color Doppler imaging from a patient with mitral valve prolapse. The left panel demonstrates, in addition to cardiac chambers and mitral valve, the origin, morphology, and distribution of an eccentric mitral regurgitant jet. The proximal flow convergence region (arrow) is shown as well. The right panel displays the en face view of the proximal flow convergence zone of mitral regurgitation on the left ventricular side of the mitral valve. Its irregular shape in this case is noted. LA = left atrium; LV = left ventricle.

found. Thus, the PISA (proximal isovelocity surface area) method for quantifying mitral regurgitation using the assumption of a hemispheric flow convergence region is challenged. Three-dimensional estimation of mitral regurgitation using flow convergence is under investigation.[40,41] Another application of three-dimensional echocardiography in quantification of mitral regurgitation might be possible by measuring a cross-sectional area of the vena contracta of the mitral regurgitant jet.[42]

Conclusion

Three-dimensional echocardiography, especially with the volume-rendering technique, allows dynamic display of the anatomy and pathology of the mitral valve apparatus in its true appearance. The location and extension of mitral valve leaflets that prolapse can be precisely defined by three-dimensional echocardiography. Its ability of electronic removal and replacement of a given part of the heart (such as the mitral valve) also permits preoperative planning and rehearsal by the surgeons on the computer before surgery.[42] Rapid developments in computer techniques for faster and easier image collection, data processing, and three-dimensional image reconstruction strongly suggest that three-dimensional echocardiography has great potential in clinical diagnosis and management of mitral valve diseases such as mitral valve prolapse.

References

1. Levy D, Savage D. Prevalence and clinical feature of mitral valve prolapse. Am Heart J 113:1281–1290, 1987.
2. Barlow JB, Pocock WA: Billowing, floppy, prolapsed or flail mitral valves. Am J Cardiol 55:501–502, 1985.
3. Malkowski MJ, Boudoulas H, Wooley CF, Guo R, Pearson AC. Spectrum of structural abnormalities in floppy mitral valve echocardiographic evaluation. Am Heart J 132:145–151, 1996.
4. Boudoulas H, Kolibash AJ, Baker P, King BD, Wooley CF. Mitral valve prolapse and the mitral valve prolapse syndrome: A diagnostic classification and pathogenesis of symptoms. Am Heart J 118:796–818, 1989.
5. Panidis IP, McAllister M, Ross J, Mintz GS. Prevalence and severity of mitral regurgitation in the mitral valve prolapse syndrome: A Doppler echocardiographic study of 80 patients. J Am Coll Cardiol 7:975–981, 1986.
6. Devereux RB, Kramer-Fox R, Shear MK, Kligfield P, Pini R, Savage DD. Diagnosis and classification of severity of mitral valve prolapse: Methodologic, biologic, and prognostic considerations. Am Heart J 113:1265–1280, 1987.
7. Hickey AJ, MacMahon SW, Wilcken DEL. Mitral valve prolapse and bacterial endocarditis: When is antibiotic prophylaxis necessary? Am Heart J 109:431–435, 1985.
8. Kligfield P, Levy D, Devereux RB, Savage DD. Arrhythmias and sudden death in mitral valve prolapse. Am Heart J 113:1298–1307, 1987.
9. Philip AW, Sila CA. Cerebral ischemia with mitral valve prolapse. Am Heart J 113:1308–1315, 1987.
10. Dillon JC, Haine CL, Chang S, Feigenbaum H. Use of echocardiography in patients with prolapsed mitral valve. Circulation 43:503–507, 1971.
11. Gilbert BW, Schatz RA, Von Ramm OT, Behar VS, Kisslo JA. Mitral valve prolapse. Two-dimensional echocardiographic and angiographic correlation. Circulation 54:716–723, 1976.
12. Levine RA, Triulzi MO, Harrigan P, Weyman AE. The relationship of mitral annular shape to the diagnosis of mitral valve prolapse. Circulation 75:756–767, 1987.
13. Levine RA, Handschumacher MD, Sanfilippo AJ, Hagege AA, Harrigan P, Marshall JE, Weyman AE. Three-dimensional echocardiographic reconstruction of the mitral valve, with implications for the diagnosis of mitral valve prolapse. Circulation 80:589–598, 1989.
14. Pandian NG, Roelandt J, Nanda NC. Dynamic three-dimensional echocardiography: Methods and clinical potential. Echocardiography 11:237–259, 1994.
15. Schwartz SL, Cao QL, Azevedo J, Pandian NG. Simulation of intraoperative visualization of cardiac structures and study of dynamic surgical anatomy with real-time three-dimensional echocardiography. Am J Cardiol 73:501–507, 1994.
16. Feishman CE, Ota T, Li J, Bengur AR, Von Ramm O, Kisslo J. Real-time, three-dimensional echo: System improvements, scanning methods and normal cardiac anatomy. J Am Coll Cardiol 27(2) (Suppl A):149A, 1996.
17. King DL, Gopal AS, Sapin PM, Schroder KM, DeMaria AN. Three-dimensional echocardiography. Am J Card Imaging 7:209–220, 1993.
18. Kupferwasser I, Mohr-Kahaly S, Erbel R, Makowski T, Wittlich N, Kearney P,

Mumm B, Meyer J. Three-dimensional imaging of cardiac mass lesions by transesophageal echocardiographic computed tomography. J Am Soc Echocardiogr 7:561–570, 1994.

19. Ludomirsky A, Vermilion R, Nesser J, Marx G, Vogel M, Derman R, Pandian N. Transthoracic real-time three-dimensional echocardiography using the rotational scanning approach for data acquisition. Echocardiography 11:599–606, 1994.

20. Roelandt JRTC, Cate FJ, Vletter WB, Taams MA. Ultrasonic dynamic three-dimensional visualization of the heart with a multiplane transesophageal imaging transducer. J Am Soc Echocadiogr 7:217–229, 1994.

21. Delabays A, Pandian NG, Cao QL, Sugeng L, Marx G, Ludomirski A, Schwartz S. Transthoracic real-time three-dimensional echocardiography using a fan-like scanning approach for data acquisition: Methods, strength, problems, and initial clinical experience. Echocardiography 12:49–59, 1995.

22. Jiang L, Siu SC, Handschumacher MD, Guererro JL, Vazquez de Prada JA, King ME, Picard MH, et al. Three-dimensional echocardiography: In vivo validation for right ventricular volume and function. Circulation 89:2342–2350, 1994.

23. Gopal AS, King DL, Katz J, Boxt LM, King DL Jr, Shao MY. Three-dimensional echocardiographic volume computation by polyhedral surface reconstruction: In vitro validation and comparison to magnetic resonance imaging. J Am Soc Echocardiogr 5:115–124, 1992.

24. Roelandt J, Salustri A, Vletter W, Nosir Y, Bruining N. Precordial multiplane echocardiography for dynamic anyplane, paraplane and three-dimensional imaging of the heart. Thoraxcentre J 6(5):4–13, 1994.

25. Cao QL, Pandian NG, Azevedo J, Schwartz SL, Vogel M, Fulton D, Marx G. Enhanced comprehension of dynamic cardiovascular anatomy by three-dimensional echocardiography with the use of mixed shading techniques. Echocardiography 11:627–633, 1994.

26. Yao J, Cao QL, Marx G, Pandian NG. Three-dimensional echocardiography: Current development and future directions. J Med Ultrasound 4:11–19, 1996.

27. Salustri A, Becker AE, van Herwerden L, Vletter WB, Ten Cate FJ, Roelandt JRTC: Three-dimensional echocardiography of normal and pathologic mitral valve: A comparison with two-dimensional transesophageal echocardiography. J Am Coll Cardiol 27:1502–1510, 1996.

28. Cheng TO, Wang XF, Zheng LH, Li ZA, Lu P. Three-dimensional transesophageal echocardiography in the diagnosis of mitral valve prolapse. Am Heart J 128:1218–1224, 1994.

29. Gorman JH 3rd, Gupta KB, Streicher JT, Gorman RC, Jackson BM, Ratcliffe MB, Bogen DK, et al. Dynamic three-dimensional imaging of the mitral valve and left ventricle by rapid sonomicrometry array localization. J Thorac Cardiovasc Surg 112:712–726, 1996.

30. Marx G, Fulton DR, Pandian NG, Vogel M, Cao QL, Ludomirski A, Delabays A, et al. Delineation of site, relative size and dynamic geometry of atrial septal defects by real-time three-dimensional echocardiography. J Am Coll Cardiol 25:482–490, 1995.

31. Abraham TP, Warner JG, Kon ND, Fowle K, Kitzman DW. A feasibility trial of intraoperative three-dimensional transesophageal echocardiography in valve surgery. Circulation 94(8):I–211, 1996.

32. Ranganathan N, Lam JHC, Wigle ED, et al. Morphology of the human mitral valve: II. The valve leaflets. Circulation 41:459, 1970.

33. Pai RG, Tanimoto M, Jintapakorn W, Azevedo J, Pandian NG, Shah PM. Volume-rendered three-dimensional dynamic anatomy of the mitral annulus us-

ing a transesophageal echocardiographic technique. J Heart Valve Dis 4:623–627, 1995.

34. Hozumi T, Yoshikawa J, Yoshida K, Akasaka T, Takagi T, Yamamuro A. Assessment of flail mitral leaflets by dynamic three-dimensional echocardiographic imaging. J Am Cardiol 79:223–225, 1996.

35. Hozumi T, Yoshikawa J, Yoshida K, Akasaka T, Takagi T, Honda Y, Okura H. Dynamic three-dimensional imaging of mitral valve prolapse using multiplane transesophageal echocardiography. Circulation 92:I–720, 1992.

36. Kupferwasser I, Mohr-kahaly S, Dohmen G, Spieker M, Oelert H. Three-dimensional transesophageal echocardiographic determinants of successful repair in mitral valve prolapse. Circulation 92:I–191, 1992.

37. Fraser AG, van Herwerden LA. Surgical echocardiography of the native and reconstructed mitral valve. In Wells FC, Shapiro LM (eds): Mitral Valve Disease. UK, Butterworth-Heinemann Ltd,. 1996, pp 51–70.

38. Delabays A, Sugeng L, Pandian NG, Tsu TL, Ho SL, Chen CH, Marx GR, et al. Dynamic three-dimensional echocardiographic assessment of intracardiac blood flow jets. Am J Cardiol 76:1053–1058, 1995.

39. Yao J, Masani N, Acar P, Cao QL, Caldeira M, Zachistal J, Somerville S, et al. How well does three-dimensional echocardiographic volume measurement of mitral regurgitant jet reflects its severity? Comparison with other quantitative and semiquantitative methods. Circulation 94(8):I–335, 1996.

40. Sinclair BG, Teien D, Klas B, Derman R. Three-dimensional reconstruction of constrained flow convergence acceleration fields in an in vitro model of mitral valve prolapse. Circulation 92:I–797, 1995.

41. Franke A, Flachskampf FA, Steegers A, Paul R, Krebs W, Krüger S, Reul H, et al. Improved flow rate calculation by three-dimensional reconstruction of the proximal flow convergence field. J Am Coll Cardiol 27(2) (Suppl A):268A, 1996.

42. Delabays A, Shiota T, Teien D, Ge S, Sahn DJ, Pandian NG. Three-dimensional echocardiography allows accurate quantitation of the vena contracta and mitral regurgitation flow rates for asymmetric orifices: An in vitro validation study. Circulation 92(8):I–797, 1995.

43. Belohlavek M, Foley DA, Gerber TC, Kinter TM, Greenleaf JF, Seward JB. Three- and four-dimensional cardiovascular ultrasound imaging: A new era for echocardiography. Mayo Clin Proc 68:221–240, 1993.

Part VII

The Floppy Mitral Valve, Mitral Valve Prolapse, Mitral Valvular Regurgitation:
The Clinicians

The clinican takes a history, performs a physical examination, orders appropriate laboratory tests, and observes the clinical course. All along, he is endeavoring to synthesize his findings into a coherent hypothesis. At some point he begins to recognize a clinical syndrome and proceeds to make a diagnosis. Only then can he set a prognosis and prescribe a treatment. Although much is said about the art of medicine, this process of arriving at a diagnosis in actuality is a consumate scientific achievement.
—Alexander D. Langmuir, MD
1964

Introduction

The Floppy Mitral Valve, Mitral Valve Prolapse, Mitral Valvular Regurgitation:

The Clinicians

Charles F. Wooley, MD,
Harisios Boudoulas, MD, PhD

Clinical recognition of patients with the floppy mitral valve (FMV) came about in a circuitous manner. The path extends from the early 19th century cardiac physical diagnosis with cardiac auscultation and percussion to the introduction of clinical electrocardiography and phonocardiography in the early 20th century, culminating with cardiac catheterization, surgery, and imaging as the 20th century unfolded.

The cardiac physical examination provided clinicians with physical diagnostic cues and clues about valvular heart disease for almost 150 years. James Hope and his contemporary CJB Williams described the loud, widely transmitted apical systolic murmur of mitral valvular regurgitation (MVR) between 1830 and 1840. They related these loud apical systolic murmurs to mitral valve disease at autopsy, identified ruptured mitral chordae as a cause of severe MVR, presenting these findings in the journals and textbooks of the day. There was little controversy regarding these conclusions by the end of the 19th century.

The medical literature of the 19th century also contains a wealth of information about auscultation dealing with the clinical significance of systolic clicks, systolic gallop sounds, and apical mid- and late systolic murmurs. The interpretation of these auscultatory findings caused confusion, since authoritative figures in France declared these auscultatory phenomena to be extracardiac in origin, on occasion implicating pleuropericardial disease as the probable culprit. Despite reports from the United States de-

From: Boudoulas H, Wooley CF. *Mitral Valve: Floppy Mitral Valve, Mitral Valve Prolapse, Mitral Valvular Regurgitation*. Second revised edition. ©Futura Publishing Company, Armonk, NY, 2000.

scribing the rationale for classifying apical mid- and late systolic murmurs as evidence of mitral regurgitation of an unusual type, the die was cast. An additional factor was the association of these peculiar systolic clicks and apical systolic murmurs with individuals with "functional" cardiac disorders, i.e., individuals who did not have "organic" heart disease by the standards of the time. Since the individuals with functional heart disorders frequently had these cardiac auscultatory physical findings, it was reasoned that individuals with these physical findings must have functional cardiac disorders. These circular distortions in diagnostic logic persisted until the present time.

The clinicians eventually resolved these dilemmas in various ways, initially with cardiac auscultation and phonocardiography, and later with the use of hemodynamic and imaging techniques.

When the art of clinical auscultation was interpreted in light of clinical phonocardiography, a technology in which heart sounds and murmurs could be recorded, timed, and related to other events in the cardiac cycle, classic auscultatory tenets were challenged. These activities escalated at mid-20th century before and after the introduction of cardiac catheterization, cardiac surgery, and cardiac imaging, a time of great ferment in cardiac diagnosis.

Systolic ejection clicks arising from the aortic and pulmonary valves were distinguished from the apical systolic nonejection clicks that were shown to be related to the mitral or tricuspid valve with intracardiac phonocardiography. Interventional phonocardiography, with vasoactive maneuvers or drugs, showed that apical late systolic murmurs behaved as mitral regurgitant murmurs. Left ventricular cineangiography was used to document mild mitral regurgitation associated with prolapse of the mitral valve in individuals with apical mid- and late systolic murmurs, and to identify the distinctive features of the FMV.

John Reid in South Africa revived the postulate that the systolic clicks and apical late systolic murmurs were of mitral valve origin in 1961, suggesting the clicks arose from the mitral chordae and were in fact "chordal snaps." John Barlow (Fig. 1) had studied these auscultatory phenomena while in London in the late 1950s, and carried the quest with him to South Africa. Beginning in the early 1960s, and extending into the present time, Barlow and his colleagues presented a series of elegant correlative clinical studies. The late systolic murmurs responded to vasoactive maneuvers in a manner consistent with MVR, the response of the nonejection systolic clicks was compatible with intracardiac origin, and MVR was identified with left ventricular cineangiograms in four patients with late systolic murmurs. These reports from South Africa were prelude to further detailed sophisticated studies by Barlow and his associates that received worldwide recognition.

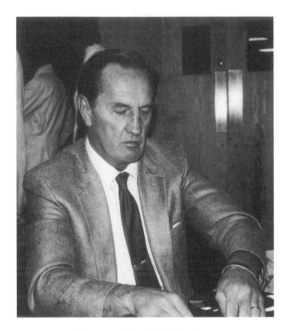

Figure 1. Dr. John Barlow.

The emphasis on the origins and significance of the nonejection systolic click or clicks, and the apical mid- and late systolic murmurs was the theme of multiple clinical correlative studies from the mid-1960s through the mid-1970s. Criley and associates provided the cineangiographic definition of the FMV morphology, relating and timing the cardiovascular auscultatory phenomena with "prolapse" of the FMV in 1966.

Intracardiac phonocardiography, a precursor of later cardiac Doppler studies, localized the clicks and murmurs to the left heart. The apical mid- and late systolic murmurs were recorded in the left atrium just above the FMV, associated with eccentric mitral regurgitant jets, while the systolic clicks were shown to originate from the FMV complex. These studies were performed in several institutions and the results were remarkably coherent. The murmur recorded in the left atrium was frequently earlier in onset, of longer duration, and greater intensity than the murmur recorded on the chest wall. Directional changes of the mitral regurgitant jet or jets were noted, features that would later be more precisely defined with echo Doppler techniques.

During this time the auscultatory, phonocardiographic, and angiographic characteristics of the floppy mitral valve provided the bases for mitral valve prolapse and MVR recognition and definition. When the dynamic changes in FMV function associated with changes in body posture and other vasoactive maneuvers were delineated, postural auscultation became an integral part of the diagnostic process.

This brief narrative summarizes a multitude of investigative studies and the clinical conclusions represent the work of numerous colleagues and investigators from around the world. Each set of original observations stimulated new approaches with departures from past dogma.

In the next chapter, our colleague Mary Elizabeth Fontana (Fig. 2), clinician–investigator whose studies identified the postural auscultatory complex in patients with the FMV/MVP/MVR triad, presents her approach to the clinical evaluation and the physical examination, vital steps in the diagnostic process. Her chapter and the one that follows, incorporate clinical wisdom based on the thinking clinician's approach to the individual patient.

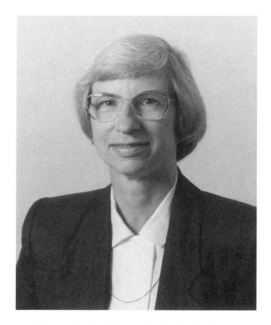

Figure 2. Dr. Mary Elizabeth Fontana.

12

Mitral Valve Prolapse and Floppy Mitral Valve:

Physical Examination

Mary Elizabeth Fontana, MD

Introduction

Before the 1960s, nonejection clicks and late systolic murmurs were thought to be extracardiac since no pathophysiological explanation could be determined. In the 1960s Reid, Barlow, and colleagues related the findings to the mitral valve,[1–5] with angiographic definition of mitral valve prolapse (MVP) by Criley.[6] The development of echocardiography and criteria defining MVP in the 1970s and 1980s, and further definition in the 1990s correlated with detailed pathologic studies and the clinical findings, have defined the broad pathologic and clinical spectrum of MVP[7–23]: how floppy the valve is, i.e., the degree of collagen abnormality and myxomatous degeneration of the leaflets and chordae, as well as annular dilatation, influences the clinical examination, particularly the auscultatory findings. The constellation of abnormalities seen in patients with MVP on physical examination can result in the diagnosis of a heritable disorder of connective tissue such as the Ehlers-Danlos or Marfan syndromes. The diagnosis of MVP can also raise suspicion of other diagnoses associated with MVP that may not have specific clinical clues on physical examination. Table 1

From: Boudoulas H, Wooley CF. *Mitral Valve: Floppy Mitral Valve, Mitral Valve Prolapse, Mitral Valvular Regurgitation.* Second revised edition. ©Futura Publishing Company, Armonk, NY, 2000.

Table 1
Conditions Associated with Mitral Valve Prolapse

Connective Tissue Disorders	Others—Genetic or Acquired
Marfan syndrome	Secundum atrial septal defect
Ehlers-Danles syndrome—types I–IV, VI, VIII, and X	Von Willebrand's disease
Adult polycystic kidney disease	Holt-Oram syndrome
Pseudoxanthoma elasticum	Myotonic dystrophy
Osteogenesis imperfecta	Duchenne muscular dystrophy
Cutis laxa	Wolff-Parkinson White syndrome
Larsen syndrome	Down syndrome
Stickler syndrome	Hyperthyrodism
Fragile X syndrome	Anorexia nervosa
	Systemic lupus erythematosis
	Relapsing polychondritis
	Polyarteritis nodosa

lists diagnoses that have been associated with MVP.[24–43] Diagnosing MVP, defining the severity of valve dysfunction, and determining associated disorders are invaluable in directing evaluation and treatment.

Physical Examination

Patients with MVP have skeletal features that suggest the diagnosis.[44–52] They tend to have a low body weight for their height, and an arm span greater than their height. Other features include a straight back, scoliosis, pectus excavatum, a high arched palate, and hyperextensible joints. Arachnodactyly, and upper segment–lower segment ratio less than 0.83 (Fig. 1) aid in the diagnosis of Marfan syndrome, up to 80% of whom have MVP.[24,53] Striae atrophica may be seen. Women dominate in the younger age groups and hypomastia is frequent. Manifestations typical of other associated heritable disorders of connective tissue include the blue sclera of osteogenesis imperfecta, abnormal joint mobility, and cigarette paper scars suggesting Ehlers-Danlos syndrome, angioid streaks on fundoscopic examination and redundant skin with a peau d'orange appearance and thickening at points of stress suggesting pseudoxanthoma elasticum, and abnormalities of neuromuscular function suggesting myotonic dystrophy. Examination of the eyes for the upward lens dislocation seen in Marfan syndrome is crucial to the diagnosis; however, slit-lamp examination is often required.

Patients with MVP tend to have a lower blood pressure than the normal population.[49] Orthostatic blood pressure measurements should be

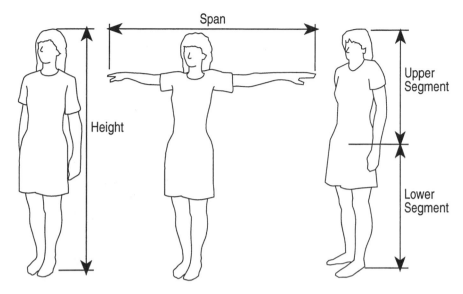

Figure 1. Measurement of height, arm span, upper segment (crown to pubis), and lower segment (pubis to floor) are important in the diagnosis of mitral valve prolapse and associated connective tissue disorders.

made, particularly in patients with orthostatic symptoms or syncope.[54] The resting pulse rate may be very rapid and increase dramatically on standing. The normal increase with standing is 10–12 beats per minute. Patients with MVP may increase their heart rate 30 or 40 beats per minute or more. There may not be an associated blood pressure drop.

Identifying the cardiac apex impulse is often easy because many patients have a long, slender thorax, straight back, pectus excavatum or scoliosis, as well as a low body weight, all of which facilitate palpation. At the mild end of the anatomic and functional spectrum, a systolic whoop or honk may cause the chest wall to vibrate, producing a palpable thrill. Systolic retractions may occur at the time of auscultatory clicks, the proposed mechanism being the prolapsing leaflets pulling the chordae and their papillary muscle attachments and therefore tugging on the ventricular wall.[55–57]

Auscultatory Findings: Mitral Valve Prolapse, Mild Regurgitation

A presence of one or more nonejection clicks in mid- or late systole with or without the mid- or late systolic murmur is characteristic of MVP.[58–61] The clicks occur at the time of maximum prolapse of the leaflets as demonstrated by phonocardiography with either cineangiography or echocardiography.[6-8] Tensing of redundant chordae has also been postulated as a cause.[59] The mitral valve is multiscalloped and therefore multiple nonejection clicks represent asynchronous maximum prolapse of different scallops (Fig. 2). The presence of multiple clicks may give the impression of a pericardial friction rub. A mitral valve click occurring early in systole may be confused with an ejection click arising from a congenitally abnormal semilunar valve or dilated great vessel. If maximum prolapse occurs synchronous with the first heart sound, the first heart sound may be accentuated. An early diastolic sound has been described in MVP[62-63] that has been ascribed to the prolapsing posterior leaflet abruptly returning toward the ventricle and slapping the anterior leaflet.[64] Other cardiac diagnoses producing extra sounds during systole or early diastole that may mimic nonejection clicks of MVP are listed in Table 2. Utilizing the apex impulse and carotid pulse as markers of systole assists in timing. Phonocardiography with pulse recordings and electrocardiogram is invaluable in timing events, but unfortunately not widely available in this age of imaging.

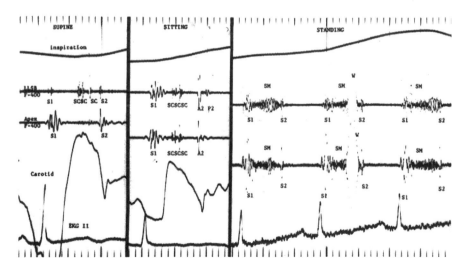

Figure 2. This phonocardiogram of a young woman with MVP demonstrates multiple nonejection clicks in the supine position best heard along the left sternal border (left panel). When she sits up, the clicks move toward the first sound (center panel). When she stands, the clicks merge with the first sound, a pansystolic murmur is present for the first time, and an intermittent systolic whoop is present (right panel). LLSB = lower left sternal border; S_1 = first heart sound; SC = systolic click; S_2 = second heart sound; A_2 = aortic second sound; P_2 = pulmonic second sound; SM = systolic murmur; W = whoop. (Reprinted from Fontana et al.,[60] with permission of the American Heart Association, Inc.)

Table 2
Auscultatory Mimics of Mitral Valve Prolapse

Nonejection Click	*Late Sytolic Murmur*
Pericardial knock of constrictive pericarditis	Tricuspid valve prolapse
Opening snap of mitral or tricuspid stenosis	Papillary muscle dysfunction
Widely split S_2 of RBBB	Hypertrophic cardiomyopathy
Fixed split S_2 of atrial septal defect	Ventricular septal defect
Ebstein's anomaly of the tricuspid valve	Severe valvular or infundibular pulmonic stenosis
Ejection clicks of semilunar valve stenosis	Coarctation of the aorta
Ejection clicks of aortic or pulmonary artery dilatation	
Pacemaker sounds	
Ventricular or atrial septal aneurysm	
Pleuropericardial adhesions	
Left-sided pneumothorax	
Mediastinal emphysema	
Xiphosternal crunch	
Splenic flexure syndrome	

S_2 = second heart sound; RBBB = right bundle branch block

The murmur of mitral regurgitation at the mild end of the anatomic spectrum of MVP begins in mid- or late systole and continues up to the aortic second sound (Fig. 3). The murmur can crescendo into the second sound or decrescendo prior to the second sound. It is most often blowing in character, but occasionally can be harsh, and is characteristically high pitched. Occasionally a whoop or a honk is present that may be audible to the patient (Fig. 2). The duration of the murmur may not be an exact indicator of the duration of mitral regurgitation. Intracardiac phonocardiography and echo Doppler studies have demonstrated that the regurgitation is often of greater duration than that which is clinically apparent, that small amounts of mitral regurgitation are seen in patients with no murmur, and no regurgitation may be seen in patients with a murmur.[59, 65–69]

The murmur is usually best heard at the apex. Radiation of the murmur up along the left sternal border to the aortic area may result in a misdiagnosis of left ventricular outflow tract obstruction (Fig. 4). Echocardiographic studies have demonstrated that prolapse of the posterior leaflet of the mitral valve directs the regurgitant jet medially

Supine   Standing   Squatting

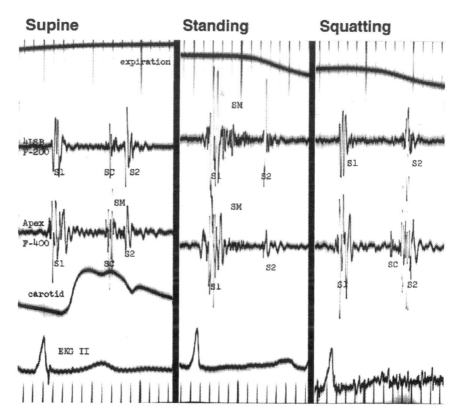

Figure 3. This phonocardiogram of a 20-year woman shows a prominent none-jection click followed by a late systolic murmur best recorded at the apex in the supine position (left panel). When she stands, the click has merged with the first heart sound and the murmur is pansystolic and recorded well at the apex and left sternal border (center panel). With prompt squatting, the click moves very late in systole, and the murmur is again later, similar to the supine position. 4 LSB = fourth intercostal space, left sternal border; S_1 = first heart sound; SC = systolic click; S_2 = second heart sound; SM = systolic murmur.

against the aortic root, therefore explaining the radiation pattern of the murmur.[14, 67–72] Prolapse of the anterior leaflet or both leaflets of the mitral valve generally results in the murmur being confined to the apex or, in the case of more severe regurgitation, radiating to the axilla and back. The murmur may occasionally spill over into early diastole due to regurgitation continuing as the prolapsed leaflets return toward the ventricle. Such a murmur could be confused with other early diastolic murmurs such as aortic or high pressure pulmonary regurgitation or a

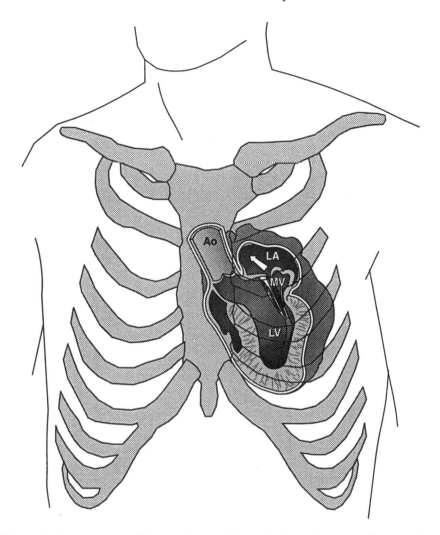

Figure 4. A prolapsed or flail posterior leaflet directs the mitral regurgitation jet toward the aortic root, which explains why the murmur can radiate up the left sternal border to the aortic area and be confused with the murmur of left ventricular outflow tract obstruction.

tricuspid valve flow murmur in a patient with atrial septal defect. The murmur could also be confused with a continuous murmur of a coronary or chest wall arteriovenous fistula or a ruptured sinus or Valsalva aneurysm. Late systolic murmurs without clicks may be due to diagnoses other than MVP (Table 2).

Postural Auscultatory Pattern of Mitral Valve Prolapse

Mitral valve prolapse has a characteristic auscultatory pattern with changes in posture that distinguish it from almost all other cardiac diagnoses. Barlow described the postural auscultatory pattern in the 1960s, but provided little documentation.[5] The author documented the changes in the clicks and murmurs by phonocardiographic recordings in a series of patients in the supine, left lateral, sitting, standing, and squatting positions in 1970.[60] The systolic clicks move toward the first heart sound with assumption of upright posture and new clicks may appear (Figs. 2, 3). The systolic murmur becomes longer, often louder and frequently pansystolic, especially in the standing position if there is excessive heart rate acceleration. Systolic whoops or honks are most often heard in the standing position (Fig. 2). The auscultatory findings may be minimal in the supine position. Therefore, postural auscultation is crucial to defining the presence of MVP in those patients at the mild end of the anatomic spectrum. Prompt squatting from a standing position results in the clicks and murmur returning to their late systolic positions similar to supine (Fig. 3). The left lateral position will increase the intensity of the auscultatory findings due to the heart being closer to the chest wall. Appreciation of the auscultatory changes is best when the auscultator does the stand-squat-stand maneuver with the patient, listening the entire time (Fig. 5). The heart rate acceleration from the squatting position to the standing position is often dramatic and the beat to beat changes in timing of the clicks and the murmurs are easily appreciated. The patient must be able to squat promptly and a reflex bradycardia should occur. If it does not, then the hemodynamic changes that result in movement of the clicks and murmur may not occur and the value of the maneuver is compromised.

Some patients may be unable to quickly perform the stand-squat-stand maneuver. The Valsalva maneuver is a useful alternative with the straining phase producing changes similar to standing and the post-release phase producing changes similar to squatting. If the auscultator is unable to do the stand-squat-stand maneuver, he or she can sit in a chair while the patient performs it (Fig. 5).

The intracardiac and extracardiac mimics of nonejection clicks and late systolic murmurs listed in Table 2 do not have this characteristic auscultatory pattern. The only exception is that of the murmur of hypertrophic obstructive cardiomyopathy. The murmur of hypertrophic cardiomyopathy tends to peak earlier in systole and to be better heard at the

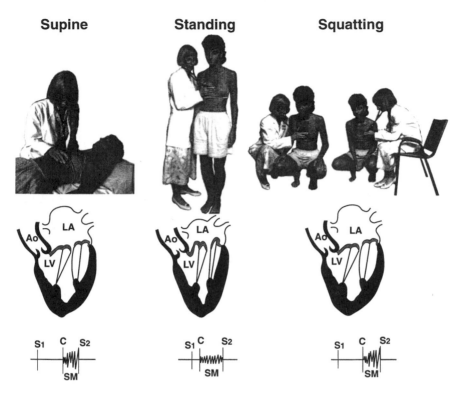

Figure 5. Postural auscultation and schematics of the mechanism of the postural auscultatory changes in MVP. On the left, the click and murmur are mid-late systolic in position, with the patient supine. A larger ventricular volume allows only mid-prolapse to occur late in systole. When the patient stands (center), the click and murmur move earlier because ventricular volume reduction allows earlier and greater prolapse and regurgitation. Prompt squatting (right) increases ventricular volume and the click and murmur move later, similar to the supine findings.

left sternal border rather than at the apex. Tricuspid valve prolapse may produce auscultatory findings similar to MVP, but may be distinguished by a later position of the clicks and murmurs with deep inspiration or any maneuver that increases venous return such as raising the legs. On standing from the squatting position, tricuspid valve auscultatory phenomena will change their position within a few beats in contrast to several beats for mitral valve phenomena. Tricuspid valve prolapse[73,74] invariably coexists with MVP making differentiation difficult. Table 3 outlines the auscultatory patterns of MVP with various maneuvers and interventions.

Table 3
Auscultatory Patterns of Mitral Valve Prolapse

Situation	Auscultatory Changes	Mechanism
Left lateral position	Click(s), murmur louder	Heart closer to chest wall
Sitting	Click(s) earlier, murmur longer, louder	Decreased venous return, decreased ventricular volume
Standing	Same as sitting	Same as sitting
Prompt squatting	Click, murmur late	Increase venous return, bradycardia, increased ventricular volume
Leg raising	Click, murmur late	Increased venous return increased ventricular volume
Post PVC beat	Click, murmur late	Long diastole, increased ventricular volume
Valsalva: strain	Click earlier, murmur longer, ± louder	Decreased venous return, increased heart rate, decreased ventricular volume
Valsalva: post release	Click, murmur later	Increased venous return, increased heart rate, decreased ventricular volume
Isometrics: handgrip, phenylephrine infusion	Click, murmur louder, later	Increased afterload, bradycardia, increased ventricular volume
Anxiety, exercise, sympathomimetic drugs	Clicks earlier, murmur longer, louder	Increased catecholamines, increased contractility and heart rate, decreased ventricular volume
Amyl nitrite	Click earlier, murmur longer, softer or same	Decreased venous return, increased heart rate, decreased ventricular volume
Beta blockade	Click later, murmur later, softer	Decreased heart rate and contractility, increased ventricular volume
Pregnancy	Same a beta-blocker therapy	Increased blood volume, increased ventricular volume

PVC = premature ventricular contraction.

Postural Changes In Ventricular and Valvular Dynamics

The major determinant of the postural changes in the auscultatory findings is a change in ventricular volume (Fig. 5). Any maneuver or drug that reduces ventricular volume exaggerates the prolapse and the auscultatory findings. A maneuver or drug that augments ventricular volume minimizes prolapse and the auscultatory findings. Upright posture reduces venous return, which reduces end-diastolic volume. With a smaller end-diastolic volume, the distance from the mitral annulus to the tips of the papillary muscles shortens. Therefore, the leaflets will be closer to a position of prolapse. During systole the smaller end-systolic volume allows earlier and greater prolapse, which can result in new or greater regurgitation. This explanation has been corroborated by cineangiographic (Fig. 6) and echocardiographic studies using upright tilt, amyl nitrite, and blood pressure cuffs to change ventricular volume.[75–77] The marked in-

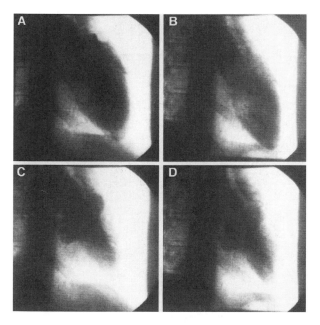

Figure 6. Frames from supine and upright cineangiograms demonstrating the reduction in ventricular volume and increase in prolapse in the upright position (60° head-up tilt) (frames B and D) compared with supine (frames A and C). Frame **A**: supine LVEDV = 98 mL/m^2; frame **B**: upright LVEDV = 78 mL/m^2; frame **C**: supine ESV = 34 mL/m^2, area under prolapsed leaflet 18.6 cm; frame **D**: upright ESV 27 mL/m^2, area under prolapsed leaflet 19.6 cm; LVEDV = left ventricular end-diastolic volume; ESV = end systolic volume. (See reference 75.)

crease in heart rate that occurs in some MVP patients on standing further reduces ventricular volume and markedly accentuates the postural changes. The excessive heart rate response may be a response to postural hypotension, autonomic dysfunction, or possibly the sequestration of volume under the prolapsing leaflets of a floppy mitral valve.

Prompt squatting increases venous return, which increases ventricular end-diastolic volume. The leaflets therefore prolapse less and later, and the clicks and murmurs move back to a later position similar to supine (Fig. 3). Peripheral resistance is increased by squatting, which results in a reflex bradycardia that is additive in augmenting ventricular volume. The increased afterload may result in the murmur and click being louder than in the supine position.

The increased intrathoracic pressure during the straining phase of the Valsalva maneuver reduces venous return, and if sustained will also reduce blood pressure. Amyl nitrite reduces venous return by venodilatation and also reduces afterload by arterial dilatation. Both of these modalities produce the expected movement of the clicks and murmurs earlier in systole similar to standing, but the murmur may actually soften because of the decreased afterload (Fig. 7). If a marked reflex tachycardia occurs in re-

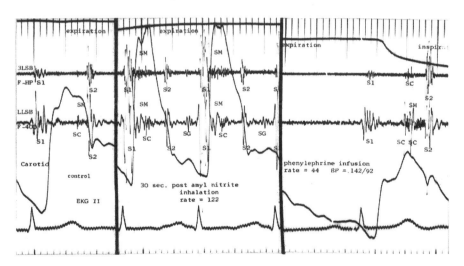

Figure 7. Phonocardiogram of a 30-year-old male with MVP. A late systolic click and apical late systolic murmur are recorded in the supine position (left panel). Within 30 seconds after beginning amyl nitrite inhalation, the click and murmur are earlier in systole (middle panel). During a phenylephrine infusion, the murmur is markedly accentuated compared with the baseline, but remains similar in timing (right panel). A second systolic click is recorded for the first time. 3 LSB = third intercostal space, left sternal border; LLSB = lower left sternal border; S_1 = first heart sound; SM = systolic murmur; S_2 = aortic second sound; SG = gallop; SC = systolic click.

sponse to the hypotension following amyl nitrite inhalation, the murmur may accentuate because of the inotropic effect of the tachycardia. The response to these two interventions helps to differentiate hypertrophic obstructive cardiomyopathy from MVP. In hypertrophic obstructive cardiomyopathy, the murmur usually markedly accentuates early after amyl nitrite inhalation or during the straining phase of the Valsalva maneuver. Other distinguishing features of hypertrophic obstructive cardiomyopathy include the marked accentuation of the murmur after a premature beat, whereas the click and murmur of MVP may move later, the presence of an S4 gallop by auscultation and palpation, and the presence of the spike and dome carotid pulse. In addition, the peripheral pulses will not augment normally on a post-extrasystolic beat in hypertrophic cardiomyopathy.

Increasing ventricular contractility with an increase in ejection fraction and smaller end-systolic volume will also move the clicks and murmurs to an earlier position. Endogenous catecholamine release such as in an anxious patient, exogenous administration of a catecholamine such as isoproterenol or sympathomimetic medications and exercise will change the timing and intensity of the findings of MVP similar to standing. Conversely, the administration of a beta-blocking drug will enlarge ventricular volume by reducing heart rate and contractility, so the murmurs and clicks occur later, or even disappear with very mild MVP. The increase in blood volume during pregnancy and the increase in afterload resulting from handgrip or infusing pleuylephrine have a similar effect (Table 3) (Fig. 7).

The auscultatory findings may vary from visit to visit, including fluctuation in the intrinsic level of catecholamine stimulation, change in heart rate and contractility, which will influence the number of clicks, the presence of the murmur and its intensity, and the changes produced by maneuvers. In general, however, on longitudinal follow-up of patients, the clinical examination in patients with clicks and late systolic murmurs tends to be reproducible. An anxious patient coming in to a physician's office for a first visit will often have more dramatic changes than the patient in a hospitalized setting or who is more comfortable with the physician. Patients already on beta-blocking agents at the time of referral may make diagnosing mild MVP very difficult. Confirming the diagnosis in individuals on beta blockers with no postural change in heart rate may require repeat examination off beta blockers. Echocardiography performed in the supine and left lateral positions may not demonstrate MVP in patients on beta blockers or in patients who have isolated clicks or minimal murmur. Also, all scallops of the mitral valve may not be adequately imaged. Therefore, if a patient has one or more nonejection clicks with or without a late systolic murmur and typical postural changes as described above, the diagnosis of MVP can be made even if the echocardiogram is negative. It is rare to see a thickened myxomatous floppy mitral valve on echocardiography when the postural auscultatory examination is normal.

The Floppy Mitral Valve and Progressive Mitral Regurgitation

Progression in valve dysfunction can be documented by physical examination. With pansystolic prolapse and moderate regurgitation, the clicks merge with the first heart sound, often increasing its intensity, and the murmur is pansystolic in all auscultatory positions. The murmur may still have late systolic accentuation in the supine and squatting positions and be louder throughout systole on standing. The intensity of the murmur does not correlate well with severity of regurgitation although grade II pansystolic murmurs usually indicate mild regurgitation and grades IV or V murmurs indicate moderate or severe regurgitaiton. The absence of findings associated with markedly increased left ventricular early diastolic filling (S3, early diastolic murmur, enlarged left ventricular apex) further identify regurgitation as mild or moderate. The physical findings in severe regurgitation differ according to whether the onset is acute, such as from chordal rupture or valve destruction from infective endocarditis, or chronic from progressive pathological changes rendering the valve more floppy.

In acute mitral regurgitation, the apex impulse is often hyperdynamic but not necessarily enlarged or displaced. A palpable parasternal heave in the midclavicular line may be present due to palpable left atrial V wave. An apical systolic thrill may be present. The first heart sound may be difficult to distinguish from the beginning of the loud high-pitched often harsh pansystolic murmur. The murmur may be decrescendo, since the regurgitant volume may diminish in late systole due to severe regurgitation elevating pressure in a normal or slightly enlarged left atrium (large V wave) (Fig. 8). The murmur is usually best heard at the apex, but may radiate up the sternal border to the base of the heart if the posterior leaflet is disrupted (Fig. 4). The pulmonic component of the second heart sound is usually accentuated due to secondary pulmonary hypertension. A palpable and easily audible S_3 gallop is frequent and an S_4 gallop may be heard, since a vigorous atrial contraction is usually maintained. The patient is usually tachycardic, so a loud summation gallop audible even with the diaphragm of the stethoscope may be present (Fig. 8). The patient will usually have signs of pulmonary congestion (orthopnea, increased respiratory rate, rales).

In chronic mitral regurgitation, the left atrium is markedly enlarged and may compress the right and left ventricles against the chest wall (Fig. 9). A left parasternal heave in this setting may be a "pseudo" right ven-

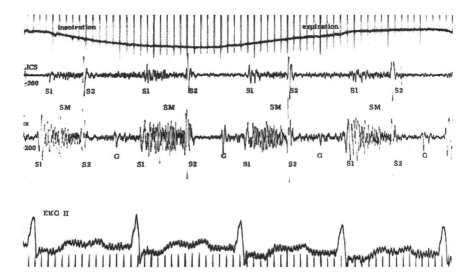

Figure 8. Phonocardiogram of a patient with acute severe mitral regurgitation illustrating the decrescendo of the pansystolic murmur (SM) and a prominent gallop (G) which could be an S_4 or a summation gallop since the patient has sinus tachycardia.

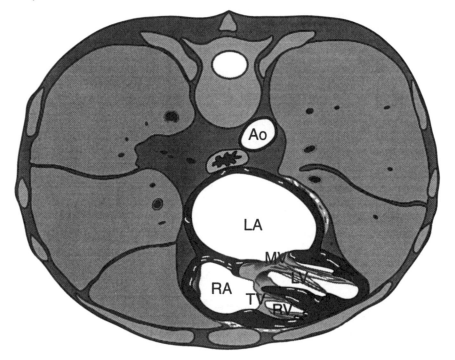

Figure 9. Schematic cross-section of the thorax illustrating the "pancaking" of the heart against the anterior chest wall by the markedly enlarged left atrium resulting in a "pseudo" right ventricular heave and overestimation of left ventricular size on palpation.

tricular heave since pulmonary hypertension and right ventricular hypertrophy are often absent or mild and the left atrial pressure is not significantly elevated. The left ventricular impulse is hyperdynamic, enlarged, and displaced to the left. The ventricle tends to feel much larger than it actually is because of the pancaking effect of the large left atrium (Fig. 9). Again, a systolic thrill may be present. The first heart sound may be obscured by the beginning of the murmur, but it also may be markedly increased in intensity because of early prolapse of the large floppy leaflets. The murmur is often of grade IV or grade V intensity, pansystolic, and may occasionally even run through the aortic component of the second sound. The radiation pattern is similar to that described in acute mitral regurgitation. With severe regurgitation, a prominent S_3 gallop is often followed by a short, intense, early diastolic rumble of much shorter duration than the diastolic rumble of mitral stenosis (Fig. 10). Most of these patients are in atrial fibrillation. An S_4 gallop is rarely heard, even if sinus rhythm is present, due to poor mechanical function of the large left atrium. More patients with severe, chronic mitral regurgitation are males over 60 years

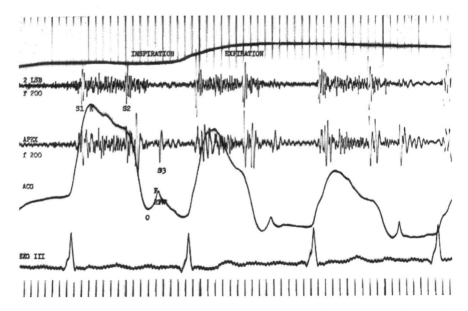

Figure 10. Phonocardiogram with apexicardiogram (ACG) from a patient with MVP with chronic, severe mitral regurgitation. The pansystolic murmur is similarly recorded at the apex and upper left sternal border, consistent with predominant posterior leaflet prolapse. A loud S_3 synchronous with a sharply peaked rapid filling wave of the apexcardiogram (RFW) and brief diastolic rumble are recorded at the apex. The murmur is of equal intensity with changing R-R intervals in atrial fibrillation, which helps differentiate mitral regurgitation from left ventricular outflow tract murmurs.

of age,[78-80] unless a heritable connective tissue disease is present. Those patients, male or female, may have floppy valves and severe regurgitation much earlier.

The postural auscultatory changes no longer occur once the floppy or disrupted mitral valve allows severe regurgitation. The ventricular volume is already increased and postural changes in volume are insufficient to change valve function. Prompt squatting may result in accentuation of the murmur because of the increase in afterload. It is therefore difficult to determine the etiology of severe mitral regurgitation by auscultation, although a very loud first heart sound may be an important clue and a systolic thrill is often associated with ruptured chordae.

Hemodynamic Evaluation

Hemodynamic studies were performed on patients with MVP in the 1960s and 1970s in an attempt to explain the associated symptom complex. In patients at the mild end of the anatomic spectrum intracardiac pressures, cardiac output, ejection fraction, and coronary anatomy are generally normal. At the present time, cardiac catheterization studies are not done in this population unless some other associated abnormality is suspected or unless the patient has protracted symptomatology. Diastolic dysfunction, coronary spasm, and abnormal coronary arteries can be demonstrated in some individuals.

Once a patient with MVP develops severe mitral regurgitation, the hemodynamic findings are determined by whether the severe regurgitation is acute or chronic. Acute chordal rupture in the setting of a previously mild regurgitation without significant atrial enlargement results in high left atrial pressure with large V waves and secondary pulmonary hypertension. The left ventricular end-diastolic pressure is often high and the cardiac output is low. The left ventricular ejection fraction is often in the high normal range. Chronic severe mitral regurgitation is characterized by a low cardiac output with modest left atrial and pulmonary artery pressure elevation. There is no large V wave because the large left atrium accommodates the regurgitant volume without raising pressure. The left ventricle is usually enlarged and ventricular function is well maintained in most cases. Any reduction of ejection fraction from the high normal range is a sign of left ventricular decompensation.

Summary

The physical examination in MVP and floppy mitral valve is valuable in ascertaining the degree of valvular dysfunction and in making important associations with disorders of connective tissue that affect the natural history and prognosis. When combined with a complete echo Doppler study, patients can be placed in the anatomic and functional spectrum of the floppy mitral valve and appropriate decisions regarding patient evaluation and management can be made.

References

1. Reid JVO. Midsystolic clicks. S Afr Med J 35:353–355, 1961.
2. Barlow JB, Pocock WA, Marchand P, Denny M. The significance of late systolic murmurs. Am Heart J 66:443–452, 1963.
3. Barlow JV. Conjoint clinic on the clinical significance of late systolic murmurs and non-ejection systolic clicks. J Chron Dis 18:665–673, 1965.
4. Barlow JV, Bosman CK. Aneurysmal protrusion of the posterior leaflet of the mitral valve. Am Heart J 71:166–178, 1966.
5. Barlow JB, Bosman CK, Pocock WA, Marchand P. Late systolic murmurs and non-jection mid-late systolic clicks. Br Heart J 30:203–218, 1968.
6. Criley JM, Lewis KB, Humphries JO'N, Ross RS. Prolapse of the mitral valve: Clinical and cine-angiocardiographic findings. Br Heart J 18:488–496, 1966.
7. Dillon JC, Haisse CL, Chang S, Feigenbaum H. Use of echocardiography in patients with prolapsed mitral valve. Circulation 43:503–508, 1971.
8. Kerber RE, Isaeff DM, Hancock EW. Echocardiographic patterns in patients with the syndrome of systolic click and late systolic murmur. N Engl J Med 284:691–693, 1971.
9. Marks AR, Choong CY, Chir MBB, et al. Identification of high-risk and low-risk subgroups of patients with mitral valve prolapse. N Engl J Med 320:1031–1036,1989.
10. Abbasi A, Cristonfano D, Anabtawi J, et al. Mitral valve prolapse: Comparative value of M-mode, two-dimensional and Doppler echocardiography. J Am Coll Cardiol 2:1219–1223,1983.
11. Coe PC, Riley MF, Carl VL, Nakao S. Pulsed Doppler echocardiographic evaluation of valvular regurgitation in patients with mitral valve prolapse: Comparison with normal subjects. J Am Coll Cardiol 8:1355–1364, 1986.
12. Panidis IP, McAllister M, Ross J, Mintz GS. Prevalence and severity of mitral regurgitation in the mitral valve prolapse syndrome: A Doppler echocardiographic study of 80 patients. J Am Coll Cardiol 7:975–981,1986.
13. Anthony P, Chandraratra H, Shah PM. Role of echocardiography and Doppler ultrasound in diagnosing mitral valve prolapse. In Boudoulas H, Wooley CF (eds): Mitral Valve Prolapse and the Mitral Valve Prolapse Syndrome. Mount Kisco, NY, Futura Publishng Co, Inc., 1988, pp 239–256.
14. Malkowski MJ, Boudoulas H, Wooley CF, Guo R, Pearson AC, Gray PG. Spectrum of structural abnormalities in floppy mitral valve echocardiographic evaluation. Am Heart J 132:145–151, 1996.
15. Langholz D, Mackin WJ, Wallis DE, Jacobs WR, Scanlon PJ, Louie EK. Transesophageal echocardiographic assessment of systolic mitral leaflet displacement among patients with mitral valve prolapse. Am Heart J 135:197–206, 1998.
16. Bailey OT, Hickam JB. Rupture of mitral chordae tendinae. Am Heart J 28:578–600, 1944.
17. Read RC, Thal AP, Wendt VE. Symptomatic valvular myxomatous transformation (the floppy valve syndrome). Circulation 32:897–910,1965.

18. Fernex M, Fernex C. La degerescence mucoide des valvules mitrales. Ses repercussions fonctionnelles. Helvetica Medica Acta 25:394–405, 1958.
19. Pomerance A. Ballooning deformity (mucoid degeneration) of atrioventricular valves. Br Heart J 31:343–351, 1969.
20. Davies MJ, Moore BP, Braimbridge MV. The floppy mitral valve: Study of incidence, pathology, and complications in surgical, necropsy and forensic material. Br Heart J 40:468–481,1978.
21. Becker AE, Davies MJ. Pathomorphology of mitral valve prolapse. In Boudoulas H, Wooley CF (eds): Floppy Mitral Valve, Mitral Valve Prolapse, Mitral Valvular Regurgitation, 2nd edition. Armonk, NY, Futura Publishing Co, 2000.
22. Baker PB, Boudoulas H, Wooley CF. The floppy mitral valve: Structural and Physical Characteristics. In Boudoulas H, Wooley CF (eds): Floppy Mitral Valve, Mitral Valve Prolapse, Mitral Valvular Regurgitation, 2nd edition. Armonk, NY, Futura Publishing Co, 2000.
23. Fontana ME, Sparks EA, Boudoulas H, Wooley CF. Mitral valve prolapse and the mitral valve prolapse syndrome. Curr Probl Cardiol 16:311–375, 1991.
24. Pyeritz RE. Genetics and cardiovascular disease. In Braunwald (ed): Heart Disease: A Textbook of Cardiovascular Medicine, 5th ed. Philadelphia, PA, WB Saunders, 1997, pp 1656–1663.
25. Pyeritz RE. Heritable disorders of connective tissue. In Boudoulas H, Wooley CF (eds): Mitral Valve Prolapse and the Mitral Valve Prolapse Syndrome. Mount Kisco, NY, Futura Publishng Co, Inc., 1988, pp 129–146.
26. McKusick VA. The cardiovascular aspects of Marfan's syndrome: A heritable disorder of connective tissue. Circulation 11:321–341, 1955.
27. Brown OR, DeMots H, Kloster FE, Roberts A, Menashe VD, Beals RK. Aortic root dilatation and mitral valve prolapse in Marfan's syndrome: An echocardiographic study. Circulation 53:651–657, 1975.
28. Pyeritz RE, Wappel MA. Mitral valve dysfunction in the Marfan syndrome. Am J Med 74:797–807, 1983.
29. Leier CV, Call TD, Fulkerson PK, Wooley CF. The spectrum of cardiac defects in the Ehler-Danlos syndrome: Types I and III. Ann Int Med 92:171–178, 1980.
30. Jaffe AS, Galtman EM, Rodey GE, Uitto J. Mitral valve prolapse: A consistent manifestation of type IV Ehlers-Danlos syndrome. Circulation 64:121–125, 1981.
31. Stickler GB, Belau PG, Farrell FL. Hereditary progressive arthro-ophthalmopathy. Mayo Clin Proc 40:433–455, 1965.
32. Ishikawa K. Cardiac involvement in progressive muscular dystrophy of the Duchenne type. Jpn Heart J 38:163–180, 1997.
33. Lebwohl MG, Distefano D, Prioleau PG, Uram M, Yannuzzi LA, Fleishmajer R. Pseudoxanthoma elasticum and mitral valve prolapse. N Engl J Med 307:228–231, 1982.
34. Sillence DO, Senn A, Danks DM. Genetic heterogeneity in osteogenesis imperfecta. J Med Genet 16:101–116, 1979.
35. Schwarz T. Gotsman MS. Mitral valve prolapse in osteogenesis imperfecta. Isr J Med Sci 17:1087–1088,1981.
36. Loehr JP, Sunhorst DP, Wolfe RR, Hagerman RJ. Aortic root dilatation and mitral valve prolapse in the fragile X syndrome. Am J Med Genet 23:189–194,1986.
37. Leier C, Baker P, Kilman J, Wooley CF. Cardiovascular abnormalities associated with adult polycystic kidney disease. Ann Intern Med 100:683–688,1984.

38. Goldhaber SZ, Brown WD, St. John Sutton MG. High frequency of mitral valve prolapse and aortic regurgitation among asymptomatic adults with Down's syndrome. JAMA 258:1793, 1987.
39. Noah MS, Sulimani RA, Famuyiwa FO, Al-Nozha M, Qaraqish A. Prolapse of the mitral valve in hyperthyroid patients in Saudi Arabia. Int J Cardiol 19:217–223, 1988.
40. Froom P, Margulis T, Grenadier E, Palant A, David M, Aghai E. Von Willebrand factor and mitral valve prolapse. Thromb Haemost 60:230–231, 1988.
41. Streib EW, Meyers DG, Sun SF. Mitral valve prolapse and myotonic dystrophy. Muscle Nerve 8:650–653,1985.
42. Comens SM, Alpert MA, Sharp GC, Pressly TA, Kelly DL, Hazelwood SE, Mukerji V. Frequency of mitral valve prolapse in systemic lumpus erthematosus, progressive systemic sclerosis and mixed connective tissue disease. Am J Cardiol 63:369–370,1989.
43. Johnson GL, Humphries LL, Shirley PB, Mazzoleni A, Noonan JA. Mitral valve prolapse in patients with anorexia nervousa and bulemia. Arch Int Med 146:1525–1529, 1986.
44. BonTempo CP, Ronan JA Jr, DeLeon AC Jr, Twigg HL. Radiographic appearance of the thorax in systolic click-late systolic murmur syndrome. Am J Cardiol 36:27–31, 1975.
45. Udoshi MB, Shah A, Fisher VJ, Dolgin M. Incidence of mitral valve prolapse in subjects with thoracic skeletal abnormalities: A prospective study. Am Heart J 97:303–311, 1979.
46. King B, Boudoulas H, Fontana ME, Wooley CF. Mitral valve prolapse syndrome: Anthropometric, sexual and clinical features (abstract). Am J Cardiol 45:443, 1980.
47. Salomon J, Shah PM, Heinle RA. Thoracic skeletal abnormalities in idiopathic mitral valve prolapse. Am J Cardiol 36:32–36, 1975.
48. Schutte JE, Gaffney FA, Blend L, Blomqvist CG. Distinctive anthropometric characteristics of women with mitral valve prolapse. Am J Med 71:533–538, 1981.
49. Devereux RD, Brown WT, Lutas EM, Kramer-Fox R, Laragh JH. Association of mitral valve prolapse with low body weight and low blood pressure. Lancet 2:792–795, 1982.
50. Chan FL, Chen WWC, Wong PHC, Chow JSF. Skeletal abnormalities in mitral valve prolapse. Clin Radiol 34:207–213, 1983.
51. Hirschfeld SS, Rudner C, Nash CL Jr, Nussbaum E, Brower EM. Incidence of mitral valve prolapse in adolescent scoliosis and thoracic hypokyphosis. Pediatrics 70:451–454, 1982.
52. Roman MJ, Devereux RB, Kramer-Fox R, Spitzer MC. Comparison of cardiovascular and skeletal features of primary mitral valve prolapse and the Marfan syndrome. Am J Cardiol 3:317–321, 1989.
53. Pyeritz RE, McKusick VA. The Marfan syndrome: Diagnosis and management. N Engl J Med 300:772–777, 1979.
54. Santos AD, Mathew PK, Hilal A, Wallace WA. Orthostatic hypotension: A commonly unrecognized cause of symptoms in mitral valve prolapse. Am J Med 71:746–750, 1981.
55. Kesteloot H, VanHoote O. On the origin of the telesystolic murmur preceded by a click. Acta Cardiol (Brux) 20:197–200, 1965.
56. Epstein EJ, Coulshed N. Phonocardiogram and apex cardiogram in systolic click-late systolic murmur syndrome. Br Heart J 35:260–275, 1973.

57. Spencer WH III, Behar VS, Orgain GS. Apex cardiogram in patients with prolapsing mitral valve. Am J Cardiol 32:276–282, 1973.
58. Barlow JB, Pocock WA. Mitral leaflet billowing and prolapse. In Barlow JB (ed): Perspectives on the Mitral Valve. Philadelphia, FA Davis, 1987, pp 45–112.
59. Weis AJ, Salcedo EE, Stewart WH, Lever HM, Klein AL, Thomas JD. Anatomic explanation of mobile systolic clicks: Implications for the clinical and echocardiographic diagnosis of mitral valve prolapse. Am Heart J 129: 314–320, 1995.
60. Fontana ME, Pence HL, Leighton RL, Wooley CF. The varying clinical spectrum of the systolic click-late systolic murmur syndrome: A postural auscultatory phenomenon. Circulation 41: 807–816, 1970.
61. Fontana ME, Kissel GL, Criley MJ. Functional anatomy of mitral valve prolapse. In Physiologic Principles of Heart Sounds and Mumurs. Dallas American Heart Association, 1970, pp 126–132.
62. Bonner AJ Jr, Noble RJ, Feigenbaum H, Tavel ME. Early diastolic sound associated with mitral valve prolapse. Arch Int Med 136:347–349, 1976.
63. Wei JY, Fortuin NJ. Diastolic sounds and murmurs associated with mitral valve prolapse. Circulation 63:559–564, 1981.
64. Criley JM, Siegel RJ. Functional anatomy and pathophysiology of mitral valve prolapse. In Boudoulas H, Wooley CF (eds): Mitral Valve Prolapse and the Mitral Valve Prolapse Syndrome. Mount Kisco, NY, Futura Publishing Co, Inc., 1988, pp 200.
65. Leighton RF, Page WL, Goodwin RS, Molnar W, Wooley CF, Ryan JM. Mild mitral regurgitation. Am J Med 41:168–182, 1966.
66. Leon DF, Leonard JJ, Kroetz FW, Page WL, Shaver JA, Lancaster JF. Late systolic murmurs, clicks and whoops arising from the mitral valve. Am Heart J 72:325–336, 1966.
67. Abbasi A, Cristofano D, Anabtawi J, Irvin L. Mitral valve prolapse: Comparative value of M-mode, two-dimensional and Doppler echocardiography. J Am Coll Cardiol 2:1219–1223, 1983.
68. Come PC, Riley MF, Carl LV, Nakao S. Pulsed Doppler echocardiographic evaluation of valvular regurgitation in patients with mitral valve prolapse: Comparison with normal subjects. J Am Coll Cardiol 8:1355–1364, 1986.
69. Panidis IP, McAllister M, Ross J, Mintz GS. Prevalence and severity of mitral regurgitation in the mitral valve prolapse syndrome: A Doppler echocardiographic study of 80 patients. J Am Coll Cardiol 7:975–981, 1986.
70. Yoshida K, Yoshikawa J, Yamaura Y, Hozumi T, Shakudo M, Akasaka T, Kato H. Value of acceleration flows and regurgitant jet direction by color Doppler flow mapping in the evaluation of mitral valve prolapse. Circulation 81: 879–885, 1990.
71. Pearson AC, St Vrain S, Mrosek D, Labovitz AJ. Color Doppler echocardiographic evaluation of patients with a flail mitral leaflet. J Am Coll Cardiol 16:232–239, 1990.
72. Ansari A, Maron BJ. Leaflet dependent spectrum of regurgitation jets in mitral valve prolapse. Circulation 97:805, 1998.
73. Gooch AS, Maranhao V, Scampardonis G, Cha SD, Yang SS. Prolapse of both mitral and tricuspid leaflets in systolic murmur-click syndrome. N Engl J Med 287:1218–1222, 1972.
74. Morganroth J, Jones RH, Chen CC, Naito M. Two dimensional echocardiography in mitral, aortic, and tricuspid valve prolapse. Am J Cardiol 46:1164–1177, 1980.
75. Fontana ME, Wooley CR, Leighton FR, Lewis RP. Postural changes in left ven-

tricular and mitral valvular dynamics in the systolic click-late systolic murmur syndrome. Circulation 51:165–173, 1975.

76. Mathey DG, Decoodt PR, Allen HN, Swan HJC. The determinants of mitral valve prolapse in the systolic click-late systolic murmur syndrome. Circulation 51:522–529, 1976.

77. Abinader EG, Oliven A. the effect of congesting cuffs on the echophonocardiographic findings in mitral valve prolapse. Chest 80:197–200, 1981.

78. Higgins CB, Reinke RT, Gosink BB, Leopold GR. The significance of mitral valve prolapse in middle aged and elderly med. Am Heart J 91:292–296, 1976.

79. Kolibash AJ, Bush CA, Fontana MB, Ryan JM, Kilman JW, Wooley CF. Mitral valve prolapse syndrome: Analysis of 62 patients aged 60 years and older. Am J Cardiol 52:534–539, 1983.

80. Kolibash AJ, Kilman JW, Bush CA, Ryan JM, Fontana ME, Wooley CF. Evidence for progression from mild to severe mitral regurgitation in mitral valve prolapse. Am J Cardiol 58:762–767, 1986.

13

The Floppy Mitral Valve, Mitral Valve Prolapse, Mitral Valvular Regurgitation:

Clinical Presentation, Diagnostic Evaluation, and Therapeutic Considerations

Harisios Boudoulas, MD, PhD
Charles F. Wooley, MD

Introduction

It is apparent today that the floppy mitral valve (FMV) is the central issue in the FMV, mitral valve prolapse (MVP), mitral valvular regurgitation (MVR) triad (Fig. 1).[1–4] The FMV is a common mitral valve abnormality with a broad spectrum of structural and functional changes. While the pathobiology of the FMV has been, and is being reexamined in contemporary terms, we are still dealing with gross structural and morphological characteristics at the clinical level. Distinguishing between the normal mitral valve with its minor variants and a mitral valve with an intrinsic structural derangement remains a difficult matter.[1–22]

The clinical presentation of patients with FMV, MVP, and MVR is

From: Boudoulas H, Wooley CF. *Mitral Valve: Floppy Mitral Valve, Mitral Valve Prolapse, Mitral Valvular Regurgitation.* Second revised edition. ©Futura Publishing Company, Armonk, NY, 2000.

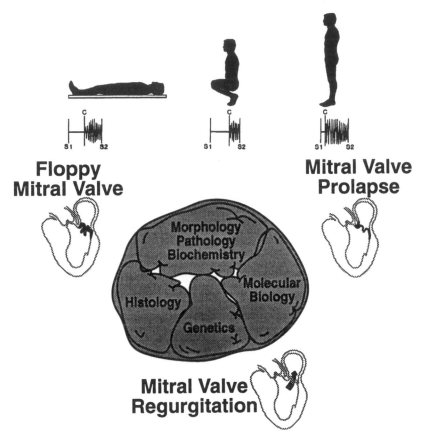

Figure 1. The floppy mitral valve/mitral valve prolapse/mitral valvular regurgitation triad (FMV/MVP/MVR). The FMV occupies the central role in the triad. Postural ausculatory phonocardiographic changes are illustrated at the top of the figure. (Used with permission from Wooley CF, et al.[2])

largely related to the progression of MVR and to complications secondary to FMV/MVP. Further, FMV/MVP may be associated with other cardiac or constitutional abnormalities, and in certain instances may be a part of well-recognized heritable disorders of connective tissue (see Chapter 7). All of these associated abnormalities obviously contribute to the clinical presentation of patients with FMV/MVP and will be discussed in this chapter.

Floppy Mitral Valve/Mitral Valve Prolapse: Prevalence

The prevalence of FMV/MVP has not been well defined. It is important to separate earlier studies that dealt solely with prolapse from those

Table 1
Floppy Mitral Valve/Mitral Valve Prolapse: Prevalence

Method	Number of Cases	FMV/MVP(%)
Auscultation	79,698	1.4–6.3
Echocardiogram	11,431	4.5–14.5
Necropsy	6,529	1.0–7.4

FMV = floppy mitral valve; MVP = mitral valve prolapse.

identifying individuals with FMV/MVP.[1,6,8,22–34] Published studies during the past four decades reflect the diagnostic techniques and the criteria applied for the diagnosis of FMV/MVP in different populations. All of the available diagnostic methods have intrinsic limitations, and the prevalence of FMV/MVP may be different among various ethnic groups. It appears, however, that the prevalence of clinically significant FMV/MVP ranges from 2% to 4%. Of interest, auscultatory and necropsy studies dealing with the prevalence of FMV/MVP have reached close agreement, while the prevalence of FMV/MVP based on earlier echocardiographic studies, especially in the Framingham study, has been reported to be much higher (Table 1).[6,8,22,29]

The prevalence of FMV/MVP increases with age (Fig. 2). Sakamoto, in a phonocardiographic study, found an incidence of MVP of 0.753% in

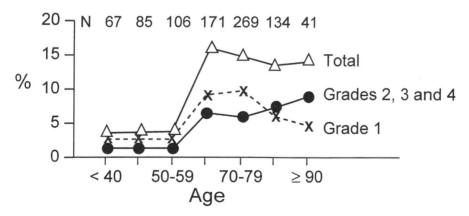

Figure 2. Incidence of floppy mitral valve/mitral valve prolapse (FMV/MVP) in females from a routine necropsy study. Grade 1 is mild, Grade 2 is moderate, Grade 3 is moderately severe, and Grade 4 is severe FMV/MVP. The total represents all patients with grades 1, 2, 3, and 4 FMV/MVP. Approximately same incidence and pattern were observed in males. (Figure constructed with data from Davies MJ, et al.[6] Figure is used with permission from Boudoulas H, et al.[5])

Japanese elementary school children, and 1.325% in the middle school children (see Chapter 22). Hickey and Wilcken[35] investigated the incidence of MVP in 6,887 consecutive patients referred for echocardiography and in 206 first-degree relatives of 65 patients with MVP. The incidence of MVP from ages 0 to 19 was 0.3%, from 20 to 39 was 2.0%, from 40 to 59 was 2.7%, and from 60 to 79 was 2.3%. The incidence of MVP in the first-degree relatives from ages 0 to 19 was 3%, from 20 to 39 was 15%, from 40 to 59 was 11%, and from 60 to 79 was 9%. Ohara et al.[30] studied the incidence of MVP by two-dimensional echocardiography in 4,328 children age from 1 day to 15 years. MVP was not seen in any of the 198 children ages 1 to 28 days; the incidence of MVP was 0.25% in 391 children ages from 6 to 18 months, 2.1% in 2,801 children ages 6 to 7 years, and 5.1% in 938 children ages 12 to 15 years. Significant MVR was present in 6 children (2 ages 6–7 years, and 4 ages 12–15 years). Greenwood evaluated 3,100 children with an age range from 1 month to 18 years and diagnosed MVP by auscultation in 154 children (4.97%). In another clinical auscultatory study Greenwood evaluated 6,168 children ages from 2 months to 21 years; MVP was present in 331 (6.37%), 175 boys and 156 girls.[31,33]

Floppy Mitral Valve/Mitral Valve Prolapse: Inheritance

As yet, genetic diagnostic testing for FMV/MVP has not entered clinical practice.[8,22,36–38] It is likely that FMV/MVP genetically is a heterogeneous group; in this case degeneration of the mitral valve may be the final pathway for several protein defects. At present, it appears that at least two forms of inheritance exist. One form is transmitted by an autosomal dominant manner with a different degree of penetration (most common form); the other form (less common) is X-chromosome-linked valvular disease with myxomatous degeneration (see Chapter 8). Further definition of genetic defects will allow better classification of this complex valvular abnormality. Such approaches open up diagnostic pathways that are not part of our current perspectives, but will be part of the 21st century cardiologist's armamentarium.

Floppy Mitral Valve/Mitral Valve Prolapse/Mitral Valvular Regurgitation: Association with Other Abnormalities

FMV/MVP/MVR may be associated with several other cardiovascular and noncardiovascular abnormalities (Table 2).[39–99] A secundum atrial septal defect is the most common congenital cardiac defect associated with

Table 2
Floppy Mitral Valve/Mitral Valve
Prolapse: Associated
Abnormalities

Skeletal abnormalities
Hypomastia
Cardiac abnormalities
 • Atrial septal defect
 • Tricuspid valve defect
 • Aortic valve prolapse
 • AV conduction defect
 • Accessory AV pathways
Other abnormalities or diseases
 • Grave's disease, thyroiditis
 • Sickle cell disease
 • Myotonia atrophica
 • Muscular dystrophy
 • Von Willbrand's disease
 • Neurological disorder
 • Pulmonary function abnormalities

FMV = floppy mitral valve; MVP = mitral
valve prolapse;
AV = atrioventricular.

FMV/MVP, but there are a variety of other congenital cardiac defects in which an association with FMV/MVP has been reported.[42] Floppy tricuspid valve with tricuspid valve prolapse coexists frequently with FMV/MVP (Fig. 3).[16,100–103] The precise incidence is uncertain; the sensitivity and specificity of diagnostic techniques for tricuspid valve prolapse remain to be defined. The coexistence of aortic valve prolapse or atrial septal aneurysm with FMV/MVP has also been reported.[41,46,100–101] Atrioventricular conduction defect and accessory atrioventricular pathways are more common in patients with FMV/MVP than in the general population (see Chapter 16).[72,97,98]

Earlier studies suggested that the incidence of FMV/MVP is greater in patients with hypertrophic cardiomyopathy compared to the general population. Other studies, however, involving large groups of patients with hypertrophic cardiomyopathy, indicated that the incidence of FMV/MVP in patients with hypertrophic cardiomyopathy was not greater than it was expected in the general population.[50] The presence of FMV/MVP, however, in patients with hypertrophic cardiomyopathy appeared to predispose such patients to atrial fibrillation. In one study the incidence of congenital abnormalities of the coronary arteries in patients with FMV/MVP was reported to be slightly greater compared to patients without FMV/MVP.[51]

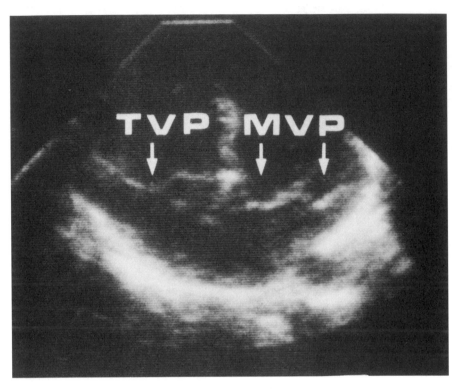

Figure 3. Apical four-chamber view demonstrating tricuspid valve prolapse (TVP) and mitral valve prolapse (MVP). (Used with permission from Boudoulas H, et al.[1])

An increased incidence of FMV/MVP in patients with Graves's disease and chronic thyroiditis, sickle cell disease, and myotonia atrophica has also been suggested.[43,44,92–94] FMV/MVP has also been reported in patients with von Willebrand's disease, muscular dystrophy, and a progressive neurological disorder characterized by external ophthalmoplegia, ataxia, and neuropathy. Pulmonary function abnormalities may be present in certain patients with FMV/MVP.[89]

Heritable Disorders of Connective Tissue

FMV/MVP occurs as a pleiotropic manifestation of several of the most common heritable disorders such as Marfan syndrome, Stickler syndrome, Ehlers-Danlos syndrome, and polycystic kidney disease in adults and children (see Chapter 7).[52–56,58–61] The precise relationship between FMV/MVP and heritable connective tissue disorders is being defined with basic genetic, molecular, and biochemical methods. Understanding the pathophysiology and natural history of FMV/MVP in these syndromes will improve understanding of the natural history of familial FMV/MVP.

Isolated FMV/MVP may be considered a cardiovascular abnormality of connective tissue origin, which in most instances does not fit within the presently recognized heritable disorders of connective tissue.[61] By virtue of its high frequency in the general population, FMV/MVP constitutes the largest group of patients with a connective tissue abnormality of the heart, and multiple surgical and autopsy studies have shown collagen disruption or dissolution to be the primary process in affected valves (see Chapter 5).[1,10,11,16,20]

Floppy Mitral Valve/Mitral Valve Prolapse: Diagnostic Evaluation

The FMV should be considered basic to the diagnosis of MVP (Fig. 1).[1-4] Auscultatory findings and imaging characteristics are directly related to the basic pathology and function of the mitral valve apparatus.

The diagnosis of FMV/MVP has been based on history, physical examination, echocardiographic–phonocardiographic studies, electrocardiogram, chest X-ray, imaging techniques, M-mode, two-dimensional, transesophageal, and three-dimensional echocardiography, cinecardioangiography, magnetic resonance imaging, Doppler studies, and hemodynamic measurements. Further, valve inspection at cardiac surgery, correlative intraoperative imaging studies and surgical pathology of excised valve tissue have provided important information (Table 3).

Table 3
Mitral Valve Prolapse:
Diagnostic Evaluation

History and physical examination
Phonoechocardiography
Electrocardiogram, chest x-ray
Echocardiography
  • M-mode
  • Two-dimensional
  • Transesophageal
  • Three-dimensional
  • Pulsed Doppler
  • Color Doppler
Magnetic resonance imaging
Cinecardioangiography
Hemodynamic evaluation
Surgical inspection
Dynamic postmortem examination

Medical History: Physical Examination

A medical history with particular emphasis on the family history, the patient's knowledge of a heart murmur, the nature of the cardiac symptoms (if present), coupled with a physical examination with emphasis on skeletal proportions, asthenic body habitus, joint mobility, skin integrity, thoracic skeletal abnormalities, and dynamic auscultation frequently represent the first steps toward the clinical diagnosis.[1-3] Family history provides important information since FMV/MVP may be inherited and may be associated with, or is the cardiac manifestation of, an inherited connective tissue disorder.[104-106] If the family history is suggestive or productive, development of a detailed pedigree is the next step.

General Inspection: Anthropometrics

The FMV has been defined as heritable in family studies in the absence of well-defined constitutional or systemic connective tissue disorders, and in individuals with an asthenic habitus, or hypomastia, that do not fit the specific criteria for presently recognized heritable connective tissue syndromes (see also Chapter 7).[1,61] Thus, many individuals with FMV/MVP are thinner than normal with a height to weight ratio greater than normal and an arm span greater than height (Fig. 4).[13,62,63,68,85,107,108]

Skeletal abnormalities have been reported in up to two-thirds of patients with FMV/MVP. Skeletal abnormalities of the chest and spine include scoliosis, narrow anteroposterior diameter, straight back, pectus excavatum, and pectus carinatum. Park et al.,[63] studied 87 children ages 1 month to 18 years, mean age 5.4 years, with pectus excavatum. Twenty of the 87 children (23%) had echocardiographic evidence of MVP; 11 of these had auscultatory findings of a non-ejection click or late systolic murmur and 4 had significant MVR. The authors concluded that the incidence of MVP is high in children with pectus excavatum; the incidence of MVP is higher when the pectus deformity is severe. A high, arched, or cathedral palate is another common finding in patients with FMV/MVP, especially if it is associated with other heritable connective tissue disorders. Crowding of the teeth may also occur. Similarly, MVP was four times more common in severe adolescent idiopathic scoliosis (13.6%) than in the normal adolescent population (3.2%), was associated with a lower body weight, and was persistent after corrective surgery.[65]

These studies suggest that a thorough clinical evaluation including a careful survey of the musculoskeletal system is mandatory. Since FMV/MVP may be associated with heritable disorders of connective tissue,

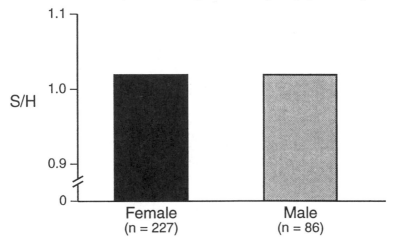

FMV/MVP:
Arm Span to Height Ratio (S/H) (n = 313)

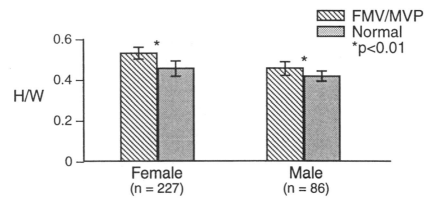

Height to Weight Ratio (H/W) (n = 313)

Figure 4. Upper panel: The arm span to height ratio in patients with floppy mitral valve (FMV), mitral valve prolapse (MVP) is usually greater than 1, which indicates that arm span is greater than height. Lower panel: The height-to-weight ratio in patients with FMV/MVP is greater compared with that of normals, which indicates that FMV/MVP patients are usually thinner than normal.

the extremities should be checked for arachnodactyly, dolicostenomelia (long limbs relative to trunk), characteristics of Marfan syndrome, and joint hypermobility, common in Ehlers-Danlos syndrome, and in certain patients with Marfan syndrome. The fingers, wrists, elbows, knees, hips, and ankles should also be evaluated (see Chapter 7).

Auscultation–Phonocardiography

Cardiac auscultation is the key to the clinical diagnosis of FMV/MVP/MVR (see Chapter 12). The first and second heart sounds (S_1 and S_2) usually are normal. When prolapse occurs early in systole, S_1 may be accentuated since it represents the summation of normal components of S_1 with a superimposed mitral systolic click.[109–115,117–123] Multiple clicks may be present when prolapse of different leaflet scallops occur at different times during ventricular systole.

The presence of nonejection systolic click(s) with or without late mitral systolic murmur constitutes the auscultatory criteria for the diagnosis of FMV/MVP. Multiple systolic clicks that occur in succession may sound like a pericardial friction rub or resemble the scratching sound produced by sandpaper on wood. The high-pitched mid- to late systolic murmur of MVR often is introduced by a click or may occur alone; the murmur may crescendo into the S_2. When the posterior mitral valve leaflet prolapses, the regurgitant flow may be directed anteriorly toward the aortic root; in this case the MVR murmur is heard at the apex, and may radiate along the left sternal border to the aortic area and mimic left ventricular (LV) outflow tract murmurs. In contrast, when the anterior mitral valve leaflet prolapses, the MVR murmur may radiate to the axilla and to the spine. Phonocardiography is an important adjunct to clinical auscultation and in certain cases may be used to confirm the auscultatory findings. Patients with redundant FMV and significant MVR may have holosystolic murmurs even in the supine position and click(s) may not be audible (Fig. 5).

Dynamic Auscultation

The most specific physical diagnostic criteria for the diagnosis of FMV/MVP/MVR are the characteristic changes of the systolic click(s) and/or the MVR murmur that occur with postural changes. The systolic click(s) moves toward the S_1 with upright posture, often merging with the S_1 if marked postural tachycardia occurs, and new clicks may appear. The systolic MVR murmur becomes longer in duration, often louder, and may become holosystolic if an exaggerated heart rate response occurs (Fig. 6A-C). An MVR murmur may be present only in the upright position. Rarely a systolic precordial honk or whooping sound may be heard with the MVR murmur; most of the time the systolic honk or whooping sounds are heard only in the sitting or standing positions. Precordial honks may be very transient and only heard for a few beats immediately after standing (see Chapter 12).[1,3,13,124–128]

The postural auscultatory changes occurring in patients with FMV/MVP/MVR are primarily related to changes in LV volume, myocar-

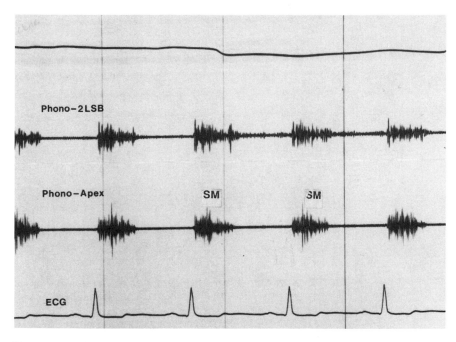

Figure 5. Holosystolic murmur in a patient with floppy mitral valve, mitral valve prolapse, and severe mitral valvular regurgitation. Note that the murmur is transmitted to the left sternal border (LSB). SM = systolic murmur; phono = phonocardiogram; ECG = electrocardiogram.

dial contractibility, and heart rate (Fig. 7). LV volume is decreased in the upright compared to the supine position. The position of the mitral leaflets at end-systole is determined by the distance from the mitral valve annulus to the attachment of the chordae to the papillary muscles. The reflex tachycardia that occurs in the upright position will further reduce LV volume. A decrease in LV volume will shorten the mitral annular–papillary muscle distance and, thus, the mitral valve leaflets will prolapse earlier at the onset of ventricular systole. Because the end-systolic volume is also smaller in the upright compared to the supine position, the mitral valve leaflets will prolapse more and earlier in systole and the click that usually occurs at the time of mitral valve leaflet prolapse will become earlier in systole. Likewise, MVR will occur earlier and the murmur will become longer in duration, become louder, or a new murmur may appear.

Adrenergic state, intravascular volume status, and pharmacological agents that affect the heart rate, the LV volume, and myocardial contractility may change the auscultatory findings especially in the upright position. Thus, β-blocking agents may markedly attenuate or abolish the auscultatory findings; it follows that lack of diagnostic auscultatory–postural

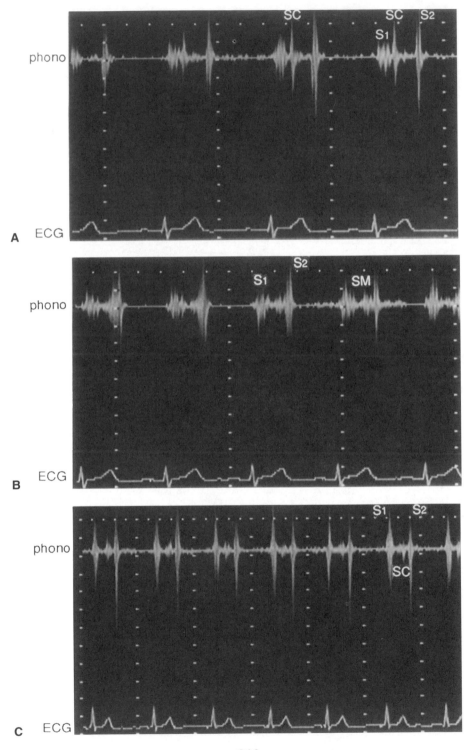

FMV/MVP/MVR: Dynamic Auscultation

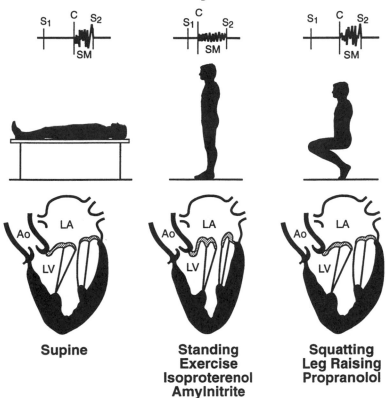

Supine

Standing
Exercise
Isoproterenol
Amylnitrite

Squatting
Leg Raising
Propranolol

Figure 7. Postural changes and auscultatory phenomena in patients with floppy mitral valve/mitral valve prolapse (FMV/MVP). Alterations of systolic click (C) and systolic murmur (SM) occur with postural changes. As the left ventricular (LV) volume decreases, the click moves toward the first heart sound (S1), and the murmur becomes more holosystolic. Ao = aorta; LA = left atrium.

findings for FMV/MVP in a patient receiving these agents does not exclude the diagnosis (Fig. 7).

Other maneuvers that change LV volume can be used in the diagnosis of FMV/MVP/MVR, such as elevating the legs, isometric handgrip exercise, tourniquets on the extremities, lower body negative pressure, Val-

---

Figure 6. Phonocardiogram from a patient with floppy mitral valve/mitral valve prolapse (FMV/MVP). **A.** Sitting position. First and second heart sounds (S_1, S_2) are shown. Note an early systolic click (SC). **B.** Standing position. A systolic murmur (SM) is present. **C.** Squatting position. The systolic murmur disappears and the click becomes late systolic.

salva maneuver, or amyl nitrite inhalation. None of these interventions, however, is as practical and helpful as a systematically performed postural dynamic auscultation.

Conditions with Auscultatory Findings that May Mimic FMV/MVP

Floppy tricuspid valve with tricuspid valve prolapse may coexist with FMV/MVP. Separation of the auscultatory phenomena of FMV/MVP from tricuspid valve prolapse by physical examination may be difficult. Systolic click(s) and systolic murmur moving later in systole immediately on deep inspiration, with leg raising, or with squatting may suggest tricuspid valve origin, since FMV/MVP click(s) and MVR murmur require several beats after the intervention to change timing. The jugular venous pulse generally is normal unless a sufficient degree of tricuspid regurgitation is present to produce a prominent C-V wave; such patients will have holosystolic murmur of tricuspid regurgitation. Confirming the diagnosis of tricuspid valve prolapse as the cause of the tricuspid regurgitation requires imaging techniques.[2,15,110]

Hypertrophic cardiomyopathy with dynamic LV outflow tract pressure gradient may produce dynamic auscultatory changes that may mimic the FMV/MVP/MVR postural auscultatory changes. Apical nonejection systolic clicks are not generally present in hypertrophic cardiomyopathy. Further, double or triple apex impulse and the spike and dome carotid arterial pulse favor the diagnosis of hypertrophic cardiomyopathy.[1,3,110]

Electrocardiogram (ECG)

Although patients with FMV/MVP may have normal ECGs, ECG abnormalities may be present. Common ECG changes include nonspecific ST and T wave changes and inverted T waves, especially in leads ll, III, and aVF. Diffuse T wave inversion has also been observed. T wave inversion may be complete or partial; prominent, upright U waves may also occur.[129-133] Spontaneous changes in the ECG may be noted, particularly with postural intervention. The T wave inversions may normalize after strenuous effort. Electrocardiographic changes during exercise consistent with an ischemic response have been reported and do not always correlate with the presence or absence of chest pain. A high incidence, up to 50%, of false positive exercise ECGs has been reported, with some patients having a greater than 2-mm ST-segment depression. Thus, the ECG response with exercise testing must be interpreted with care.

Chest X-Ray

The chest x-ray is of limited value in terms of specific diagnostic criteria; however, information about left atrial (LA) and LV size, pulmonary vasculature or congestion, and thoracic skeletal abnormalities may be of value. Straight-back syndrome, pectus excavatum, and mild scoliosis often are seen in patients with FMV/MVP.

Echocardiography–Doppler Echocardiography

Echocardiography is the most useful noninvasive test for the diagnostic evaluation of patients with FMV/MVP/MVR (see Chapter 10).[134–152] The echocardiogram will identify the presence and the magnitude of FMV, the thickness of the mitral valve leaflets, the mitral annulus size, the chordae tendineae length, and the LV and LA size and function (Fig. 8). Further, associated cardiac abnormalities (Table 2) can be defined. It should be emphasized, however, that echocardiography is a tomographic cross-sectional technique, and thus, no single view should be considered as diagnostic. The parasternal long-axis view permits visualization of medial aspect of the anterior and middle scallop of the posterior mitral valve leaflets. If prolapse, however, is localized to the lateral scallop of the posterior mitral valve leaflet, then it would be best visualized by the apical four-chamber view. Since FMV/MVP may be focal this view should not be ignored. All available echocardiographic views should be utilized with a provision that the anterior mitral valve leaflet sagging alone in the four-chamber view is not an evidence of FMV/MVP. A displacement of the posterior leaflet or the coaptation point in any view, however, including the apical views, should suggest the diagnosis of FMV/MVP. The diagnosis of FMV/MVP by echocardiography must be based on firm criteria dealing with structural changes, such as leaflet thickening, redundancy, increasing surface area, annular dilatation, and chordal elongation. The diagnostic accuracy of echocardiography improved using a constellation of findings, which include structural as well as functional changes. It should also be emphasized that the FMV pathologic process may also involve more than one valve. The introduction of three-dimensional echocardiography in clinical practice provides additional and more precise information related to the structure and function of FMV (see Chapter 11). Echocardiography and especially transesophageal echocardiography can define potential embolic sources on the mitral valve or in cardiac chambers in patients with focal neurological signs and symptoms.

Doppler and color Doppler echocardiography are useful for the detection and quantitation of MVR. MVR jet, magnitude, and direction can also be defined. Patients with late systolic murmurs usually have no more

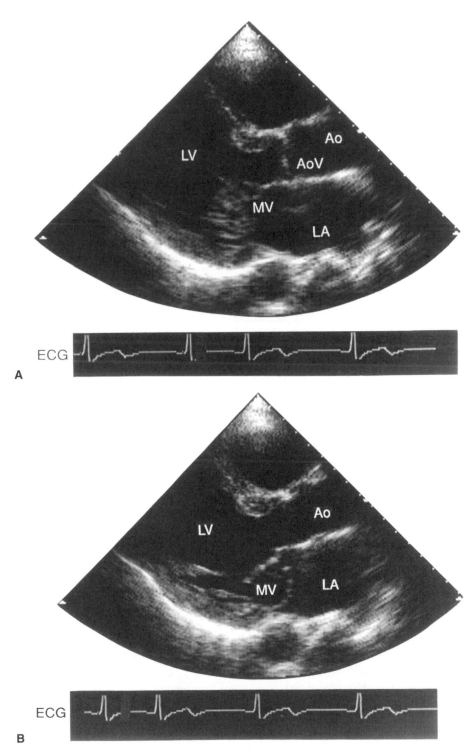

than mild or mild to moderate MVR by Doppler echocardiography. Postural echo Doppler studies will be of great value in patients with the FMV/MVP/MVR triad. However, to date, there are no detailed reports.

The diagnostic features of M-mode echocardiography are summarized in Table 4. A sharp mid- to late systolic posterior displacement of the mitral valve is a highly characteristic finding in patients with known FMV/MVP (Fig. 9) but has low sensitivity (40–50%). Early systolic prolapse may also occur; this consists of posterior displacement of a mitral valve leaflet, immediately after the closure of the mitral valve. Holosystolic posterior displacement (hammocking) of the mitral valve, although

---

Table 4
Floppy Mitral Valve/Mitral Valve Prolapse: Echocardiographic
Findings

M-Mode Echocardiogram
- Mid- to late systolic posterior mitral valve displacement
- Early systolic posterior mitral valve displacement
- Holosystolic posterior mitral valve displacement (>2 mm)
- Thickened MV leaflet(s)–multilayered mitral valve echoes
- Increased mitral valve excursion

2-D Echocardiogram
- Systolic displacement of mitral valve into left atrium
- Thickened mitral valve leaflets with redundant tissue
- Mitral annular dilatation

Floppy Mitral Valve/Mitral Valve Prolapse/Flail Mitral Valve
Leaflet: Echocardiographic Findings

M-Mode Echocardiogram
- Anterior diastolic motion of posterior leaflet
- Chaotic (course) diastolic fluttering of mitral valve leaflet
- Systolic fluttering of mitral valve leaflet
- Mitral valve leaflet into left atrium during systole

2-D Echocardiogram
- Absence of leaflet coaptation of free margin
- Sudden whipping motion of a leaflet from left ventricle to left atrium
- Prolapse of a leaflet beginning in presystole

Figure 8. Echocardiogram from a patient with floppy mitral valve/mitral valve prolapse (FMV/MVP), significant mitral valvular regurgitation; thick floppy mitral valve (MV) is shown. **A.** Diastolic frame: Note the thickness of the MV. LA = left atrium; LV = left ventricle; Ao = aorta; ECG = electrocardiogram. Continued.**B.** Systolic frame: Mitral valve (MV) is prolapsing into the left atrium (LA). LV = left ventricle; Ao = aorta; ECG = electrocardiogram.

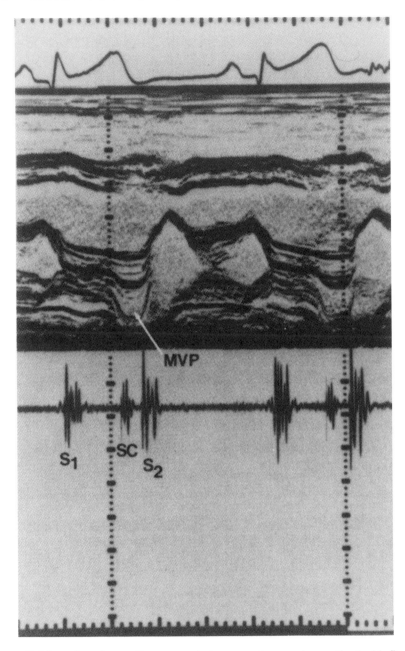

Figure 9. M-mode echocardiogram and phonocardiogram in a patient with floppy mitral valve (FMV), mitral valve prolapse (MVP). Note the timing of MVP with the systolic click (SC). S_1, S_2 = first and second heart sounds.

often seen in patients with FMV/MVP, is not specific; it has been suggested that posterior displacement greater than 2 mm should be a diagnostic requirement. A thickened mitral valve leaflet with normal or increased excursion of the mitral valve is a finding of FMV/MVP but also is nonspecific. Multilayered mitral valve echoes may suggest thickening of the leaflets.

The diagnostic features of two-dimensional echocardiography of FMV/MVP include thickened mitral valve leaflets with redundant tissue of one or both leaflets or dilatation of the mitral annulus (Table 4). A systolic displacement of a leaflet into the left atrium beyond the mitral annular plane in the parasternal long-axis and apical two-chamber views is characteristic of FMV/MVP. MVP may be seen in the apical four-chamber view but in this view false positive MVP has been reported (see Chapters 10 and 11).

The diagnostic features of two-dimensional echocardiography in a flail mitral valve leaflet include the absence of leaflet coaptation at the tips of free margins, the sudden, whipping motion of a leaflet from the LV to the LA, prolapse of a leaflet or a portion of one leaflet into the LA beginning in presystole after the end of the P wave of the electrocardiogram and continuing during ventricular systole. A presystolic prolapse is highly characteristic of a flail leaflet and is not observed in the other forms of FMV/MVP (Table 4). Transesophageal echocardiogram at present is the test of choice to define flail leaflet in patients with FMV/MVP/MVR (see Chapter 19).

Transesophageal echocardiography should be performed in patients prior to and in the operating room during reconstructive mitral valve surgery. Chordae tendineae length, mitral valve leaflet length and thickness, mitral anulus size, leaflet(s), and isolated scallop(s) prolapse can be precisely defined by transesophageal echocardiography (see Chapter 19).

Three-dimensional echocardiography (see Chapter 11), although not in routine clinical use, provides important information and details related to mitral valve annulus, chordae tendineae, mitral valve leaflets, and scallops and may be very helpful in the preoperative evaluation of patients prior to reconstructive surgery.

Clinical–Echocardiographic Correlates

FMV patients with echocardiographic criteria of MVP without evidence of thickened redundant leaflets require thoughtful analysis. If such patients have typical auscultatory findings, then the echocardiogram usually confirms the clinical diagnosis.[151,152] A patient with typical auscultatory findings and phonocardiographic confirmation but with a negative echocardiogram probably has FMV/MVP, but is at one end of the spectrum not detectable by routinely performed echocardiography. One explanation for this discrepancy could be that echocardiography is routinely done in the supine and left lateral positions, when LV volume is maximal, while the auscultatory findings of FMV/MVP are more evident in the upright positions (see dynamic auscultation and Chapter 12).

The likelihood of finding FMV/MVP using echocardiography in patients with or without symptoms who have negative, carefully performed dynamic auscultation is extremely low. The issue is whether patients with symptoms, negative auscultatory findings and nonspecific FMV/MVP findings on echocardiogram should be labeled as having FMV/MVP and their symptoms ascribed to FMV/MVP. We favor *not* labeling these patients with diagnosis of FMV/MVP. In certain cases repeat examination and/or echocardiograms over a couple of years may be necessary (Fig. 10). Family history may be useful in such cases since FMV/MVP may be inherited.

Generally, the diagnosis of FMV/MVP is reliable when it is based on the auscultatory postural complex with confirmatory echo-phonocardiographic and Doppler findings (Fig. 11). Diagnosis based on a subjective interpretation of auscultatory systolic click without echocardiographic con-

Floppy Mitral Valve / Mitral Valve Prolapse / Mitral Valvular Regurgitation (FMV/MVP/MVR): Diagnostic Steps

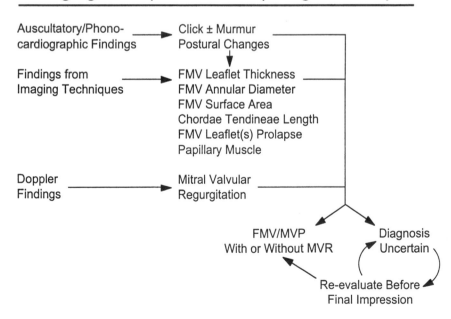

Figure 10. Diagnostic steps for the diagnosis of FMV/MVP/MVR.

Medical History, Physical Examination, Laboratory

Diagnostic Tick-Tac-Toe

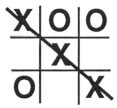

Multi-Dimensional Approach to FMV, MVP, MVR Diagnosis

Figure 11. Multidimensional approach is necessary for the diagnosis of floppy mitral valve (FMV), mitral valve prolapse (MVP), and mitral valvular regurgitation (MVR).

firmation, or on nonspecific echocardiographic findings without other clinical correlates contributed to exaggeration of the incidence of FMV/MVP and resulted in an epidemic of FMV/MVP due to overdiagnosis. FMV/MVP on occasion, however, may be present without auscultatory findings; thus, typical FMV/MVP on echocardiogram should not be ignored.

Cardiac Catheterization/Ventriculography

The indications for cardiac catheterization have changed with the development of increasingly sophisticated imaging techniques.[102,115,153–157] Ventriculography can demonstrate the characteristic appearance of the mitral valve that resulted from the systolic prolapse of one or both or portions of the mitral valve leaflets into the left atrium (Fig. 12). Systolic prolapse of the mitral valve is in part the result of an exaggerated inflation of the posterior leaflet; thus, the enlarged leaflet assumed the shape of an incomplete doughnut seen on edge in the right anterior oblique projection. In the left anterior oblique projection, the bulging leaflet projected over the atrioventricular annulus, while the convex atrial aspect of the anterior leaflet developed a potbellied appearance as the point of leaflet apposition was displaced posterolaterally. MVR, if present, usually becomes evident in mid- to late systole (see Chapter 9).

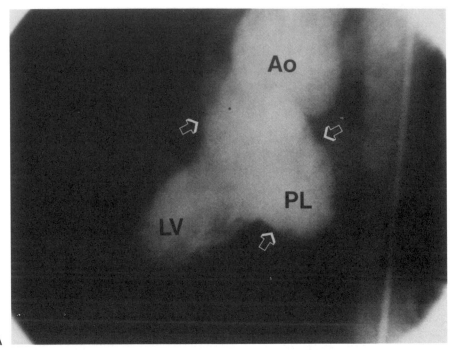

A

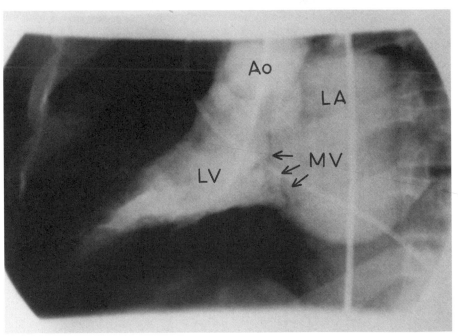

B

Cardiac catheterization studies are useful in those patients with protracted symptoms unresponsive to simple therapeutic measures, where hemodynamic measurements may be of benefit, and to evaluate associated conditions (e.g., atrial septal defect, coronary artery anomalies). Cineangiography and coronary arteriography may be important prior to decisions regarding surgical intervention in symptomatic FMV/MVP patients with significant MVR, a history of angina pectoris, myocardial infarction, or evidence of myocardial ischemia.

Hemodynamic findings in patients with mild to moderate FMV/MVP at rest usually are normal. A decreased LV diastolic volume and cardiac output in the upright posture may be present in symptomatic patients with FMV/MVP without significant MVR (see also Chapter 24).

Decreased cardiac output, increased LV diastolic volume and pressure, and increased LA volume and pressures with prominent V waves may occur in patients with FMV/MVP and significant MVR.

Magnetic Resonance Imaging

Magnetic resonance imaging techniques have not been widely used in clinical practice in the diagnostic evaluation of patients with FMV/MVP. Data, however, suggest that this method could be applied to follow patients with FMV/MVP/MVR since it is the best available method to follow changes in LV size, LV mass, and the severity of MVR.[158] The role of cine-computer-assisted tomography for the evaluation of patients with FMV/MVP/MVR is incompletely defined at this time.

Electrophysiologic Testing

The indications for electrophysiologic testing in patients with FMV/MVP are similar to those in general clinical practice.[98,159,160] Electrophysiologic studies are necessary in patients with supraventricular tachycardia, since accessory atrioventricular pathways are more common in patients with FMV/MVP compared to the general population. Electrophysiologic studies in this subset of patients is important, since radiofrequency ablation can be used during the same procedure for management of such patients. Upright tilt studies with monitoring blood pres-

---

Figure 12. A. Ventriculogram in a patient with floppy mitral valve and mitral valve (MV) prolapse without mitral valvular regurgitation. Ao = aorta; LV = left ventricle; LA = left atrium; arrows = posterior mitral valve leaflet prolapse. **B.** FMV/MVP with severe MVR. Ao = aorta; LV = left ventricle; PL = posterior leaflet; MV = mitral valve. Note, the posterior mitral valve leaflet prolapse (in Figure 12A, arrows) and the thickness of the mitral valve leaflets (in Figure 12B, arrows).

sure and cardiac rhythm may be valuable in patients with lightheadedness or syncope when neurocardiogenic syncope is suspected.

Surgical Inspection

Surgical inspection of the mitral valve complex at the time of cardiovascular surgery has contributed to many of the etiological, pathophysiological, and imaging principles already mentioned and provided the basis for new types of in vivo clinical pathological correlates. In turn, the surgical observations have stimulated the development of surgical procedures emphasizing tissue conservation and valve reconstruction (see Chapter 18). The limitations of the method are related to changes in hemodynamics, cardiac rhythm, and intravascular volume associated with anesthesia and the particular surgical approach.

Postmortem Examination

A dynamic postmortem examination with inspection of the mitral valve from the left atrium before opening the ventricle and observation of mitral valve dynamics following ventricular filling has provided postmortem observations that parallel imaging studies and surgical observations (see Chapter 4). The characteristic macroscopic appearance of the FMV is easily recognized, and inspection of the closed mitral valve from the left atrium allows identification of cusp prolapse. After the left ventricle is opened, the mitral annulus circumference and mitral valve surface area may be measured, and the chordae tendineae examined for tortuosity, elongation, thinning, or rupture. When chordal rupture is present, the posterior cusp is most commonly involved; specific papillary muscle abnormalities have not yet been identified. Mitral valves excised from patients with severe FMV/MVP/MVR have large mitral valve surface areas and the mitral annulus size may vary from normal to grossly abnormal. This morphology differs significantly from normal mitral valves (Fig. 13). The most specific, fundamental, and characteristic histologic change is col-

→

Figure 13. **A.** Floppy mitral valve (FMV), atrial view, from a patient with severe mitral valvular regurgitation (MVR). The surface area of the valve is increased, with increased folding of the valve surface. The widths of the anterior leaflet (AL) and the posterior leaflet (PL) are almost equal. Individual scallops of the posterior leaflet are enlarged and redundant. **B.** Comparison of an excised FMV from a patient with FMV/MVP (top) with a normal mitral valve from a patient who died of noncardiac cause (bottom), showing the increased surface area of both anterior leaflets (AL) and posterior leaflets (PL) of the FMV with enlarged and redundant posterior leaflet scallops, enlarged mitral annulus, elongated chordae tendineae. PCS = posteromedial commissural scallop; MS = middle scallop; ACS = anterolateral commissural scallop. (Used with permission from Boudoulas H, et al.[5])

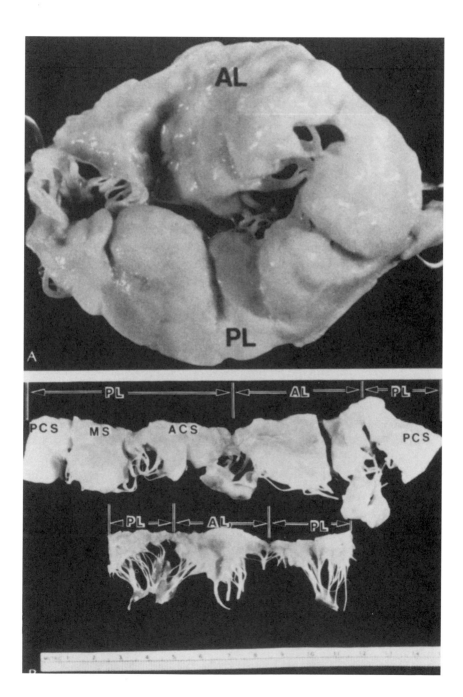

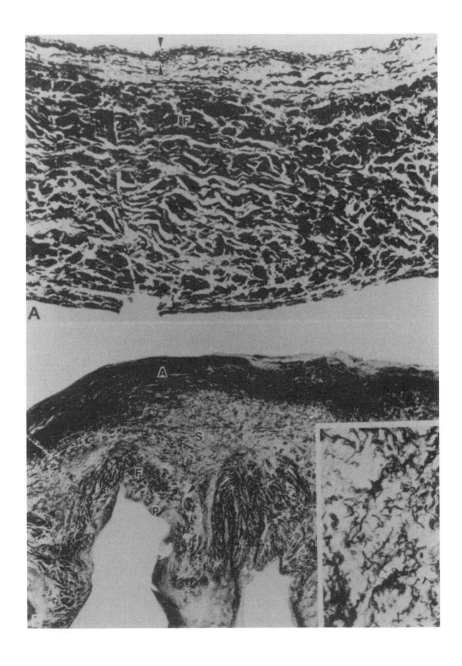

lagen dissolution and disruption in the pars fibrosa of the mitral valve leaflets (Fig. 14). There is also a replacement of the dense collagenous fibrosa by loose myxomatous connective tissue with high acid mucopolysaccharide content. Similar histologic abnormalities have been observed in chordae tendineae (Fig. 15).

Scanning electron photomicrographs demonstrated surface folds and focal loss of endothelial cells on mitral valve leaflets obtained from patients with severe FMV/MVP and significant MVR (Fig. 16). These surface abnormalities may predispose to thromboembolic complications and/or to infective endocarditis. Continuous pressure and stress due to LV systole on the mitral valve leaflets and chordae tendineae contribute to gradual progression of these histologic changes.[1]

Floppy Mitral Valve/Mitral Valvular Prolapse: Diagnostic Considerations (Table 5)

Diagnosis and Clinical Classification

The diagnosis of FMV/MVP is generally reliable when based on the auscultatory postural complex with confirmatory echocardiographic findings (Fig. 11).[1,3] In cases where mitral valve involvement is minimal, there may be a systolic click or characteristic late systolic murmur, but no definite echocardiographic abnormality. Conversely, because echocardiographic and cineangiographic studies have shown that FMV/MVP may occur without auscultatory phenomena, some diagnostic flexibility may be exercised. New developments in three-dimensional echocardiography will provide better definition of the FMV and the mitral valve apparatus (see Chapter 11). In certain cases, multiple valvular prolapse may occur (Fig. 3).

Figure 14. **A.** A normal mitral valve cusp. The histologic zones are represented in a cross-section. The atrialis is a thin zone of dense collagen immediately below the inflow surface (between arrowheads). The next zone, the spongiosa (S), consists of loose connective tissue, and the remainder of the cusp, composed of dense collagen, is the fibrosa (F). (Jones' silver stain; original magnification x25.) **B.** Floppy mitral valve cusp. The cusp has a large expanded central zone of myxomatous connective tissue with focal thickening and disruption of the fibrosa (arrow). The dense layer seen at the top just below the inflow surface is the markedly thickened atrialis (**A**). Fibrous connective tissue pads are seen on the ventricular surface. (Jones' silver stain; original magnification x40.) The lower right inset is a high magnification view of the myxomatous area showing disoriented, separated collagen bundles. A Mowry's colloidal iron stain demonstrated abundant accumulation of acid mucopolysaccharides in this area. (Jones' silver stain; original magnification x100.) (Used with permission from Boudoulas H, et al.[3])

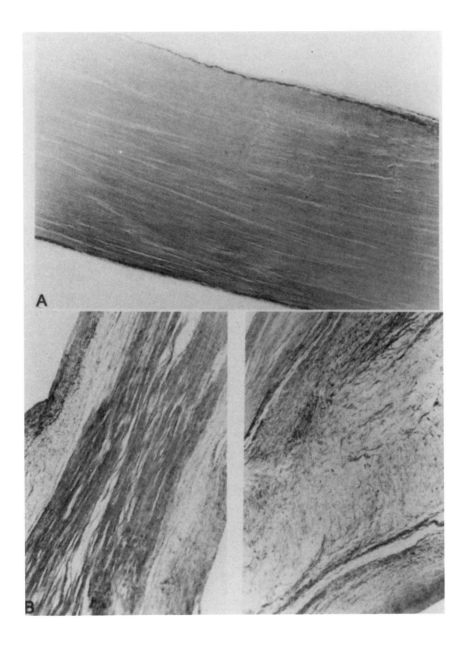

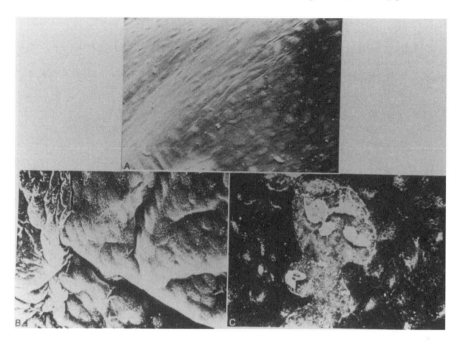

Figure 16. A. Normal mitral valve. Scanning electron photomicrograph (original magnification x280) shows smooth valve cusp surface covered by endothelial cells. **B.** Mitral valve from a patient with floppy mitral valve (FMV), mitral valve prolapse (MVP), and severe mitral valvular regurgitation (MVR). Scanning electron photomicrograph (original magnification x400) shows an irregular surface with deep infolding. **C.** Mitral valve from a patient with FMV/MVP and severe MVR. Scanning electron photomicrograph (original magnification x600) shows an area of denuded endothelium exposing the underlying collagen. (Used with permission from Boudoulas H, et al.[1])

Figure 15. A. Normal mitral valve chordae tendineae. This chordae has a dense central collagenous core surrounded by a thin zone of compact, dark-staining elastic fibers. This histological appearance was uniformly seen in normal mitral valve chordae (Weigert's elastic stain, original magnification x40). **B.** Floppy mitral valve chordae tendineae. These chordae show two patterns of histopathological alterations. The chordae on the left shows myxomatous expansion of the peripheral connective tissue with loss of the distinct elastic layer. The chordae on the right has severe separation and attenuation of collagen in the central core while the peripheral elastic layer remains intact. Mowry's colloidal iron stain demonstrated abundant acid mucopolysaccharide accumulation in both chordae (Weigert's elastic stain, original magnification x25). (Used with permission from Boudoulas H, et al.[3])

Table 5
Floppy Mitral Valve/Mitral Valve Prolapse: Diagnostic
Considerations

Diagnosis of floppy mitral valve/mitral valve prolapse (FMV/MVP)
Severity of mitral valve abnormalities
Anthropometric characteristics and associated abnormalities
FMV/MVP in recognized heritable disorders of connective tissue
Complications/symptoms related to FMV/MVP
  • Infective endocarditis
  • Thromboembolism
  • Cardiac arrhythmias
  • Syncope
  • Cardiac arrest
  • Progressive mitral valvular regurgitation
  • Congestive heart failure
  • Chest pain
Special considerations
  • Childhood
  • Pregnancy
  • Athletics

Based on our experience and that of others, we proposed the following classification of patients with FMV/MVP.

FMV/MVP refers to patients with FMV/MVP with a wide spectrum of mitral valve abnormalities from mild to severe (Table 6, Fig. 17). The term floppy mitral valve comes from surgical and pathologic studies and refers to the expansion of the area of the mitral valve leaflets with elongated chordae tendineae, frequently with a dilated mitral annulus. Symptoms and physical and laboratory findings in these patients are directly related to mitral valve dysfunction and progressive MVR.

FMV/MVP syndrome refers to the occurrence of symptoms resulting from neuroendocrine or autonomic dysfunction in patients with FMV/MVP in whom the symptoms cannot be explained on the basis of the valvular abnormality alone (see Chapter 24).[1,3]

This classification is clinically useful because it separates patients with FMV/MVP and symptoms related to mitral valve dysfunction from those whose symptoms may be secondary to autonomic dysfunction.

The Severity of Mitral Valve Abnormalities

FMV/MVP occurs in a heterogeneous group of patients with a wide spectrum of mitral valve involvement and hemodynamic abnormalities. Thus, it is important in each case to establish not only the diagnosis of

---

Table 6
Classification of Floppy Mitral Valve–Mitral Valve Prolapse*

Floppy Mitral Valve (FMV), Mitral Valve Prolapse (MVP), Mitral Valvular Regurgitation (MVR)	*Floppy Mitral Valve/ Mitral Valve Prolapse Syndrome*
• Common mitral valve abnormality with a spectrum of structural and functional changes, mild to severe The basis for: • Systolic click; mid-late systolic murmur • Mild or progressive mitral valve dysfunction • Progressive mitral valvular regurgitation, atrial fibrillation, congestive heart failure • Infective endocarditis • Embolic phenomena • Characterized by long natural history • May be heritable, or associated with heritable disorders of connective tissue • Conduction system involvement possibly leading to arrhythmias and conduction defects • FMV/MVP/MVR postsurgical intervention	• Patients with FMV/mitral valve prolapse • Symptom complex: palpitations, fatigue, exercise intolerance, dyspnea, chest pain, postural phenomena, syncope-presyncope, neuropsychiatric symptoms. • Neuroendocrine or autonomic dysfunction (high catecholamines, catecholamine regulation abnormality, β-adrenergic receptor abnormality, hyperresponsive to adrenergic stimulation, parasympathetic abnormality, baroreflex modulation abnormality, renin-aldosterone regulation abnormality, decreased intravascular volume, decreased left ventricular volume with upright posture, atrial natriuretic factor secretion abnormality) may provide explanation for symptoms. • Floppy mitral valve/mitral valve prolapse - a possible marker for autonomic dysfunction.

*From ref. 1.

FMV/MVP, but also to define within the spectrum of mitral valve abnormalities the severity of mitral valve abnormalities (Tables 7 and 8). Auscultatory findings should be described in detail (i.e., click, multiple clicks, murmur, etc.); phonocardiographic confirmation of auscultatory findings may be valuable in certain circumstances and may contribute to more precise auscultatory conclusions. The echocardiographic interpretation (M-mode, two-dimensional, three-dimensional, transesophageal) should include the type of prolapse (late systolic, holosystolic, anterior, posterior leaflet, etc.), the thickness of mitral valve leaflets, the size of the mitral annulus, and the left ventricular and left atrial structure and function. Doppler analysis should include the presence, severity, and timing of MVR. Cinecardioangiographic analysis should include the size of mi-

FMV/MVP/MVR:
Dynamic Spectrum & Natural Progression

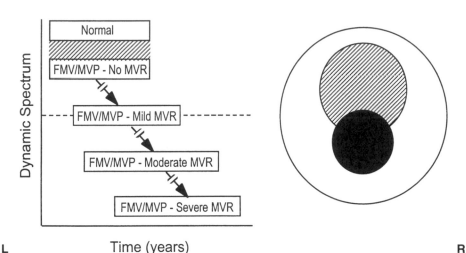

L   Time (years)   R

Figure 17. Left. The dynamic spectrum, time in years, and the progression of floppy mitral valve (FMV) and mitral valve prolapse (MVP) are shown. A subtle gradation (cross-hatched area) exists between the normal mitral valve and valves that produce mild FMV/MVP without mitral valvular regurgitation (MVR). Progression from the level FMV/MVP–no MVR to another level may or may not occur. Most of the patients with FMV/MVP–syndrome occupy the area above the dotted line, while patients with progressive mitral valve dysfunction occupy the area below the dotted line. **Right.** The large circle represents the total number of patients with FMV/MVP. Patients with FMV/MVP may be symptomatic or asymptomatic. Symptoms may be directly related to mitral valve dysfunction (black circle), or to autonomic dysfunction (cross-hatched circle). Certain patients with symptoms directly related to mitral valve dysfunction may present and continue to have symptoms secondary to autonomic dysfunction. (Used with permission from Boudoulas H, et al.[1])

tral valve leaflets, the presence of prolapse, the severity of MVR and LV size, function, and contraction pattern. The presence and severity of hemodynamic findings should also be given in detail.

Complications Related to Floppy Mitral Valve/Mitral Valve Prolapse

Patients with FMV/MVP are at risk for certain well-defined complications (Fig. 18). Prevention of these complications should be the primary approach.

Table 7
Floppy Mitral Valve/Mitral Valve Prolapse: Assessment of Severity of
Mitral Valve Abnormalities

Auscultation:	Systolic, nonejection, single or multiple clicks
	Murmur (mid-late systolic, holosystolic)
	Postural phenomena
Phonocardiogram:	Confirmation of auscultatory findings
Electrocardiogram:	Normal
	Nonspecific changes
Echocardiogram:	Thickened mitral valve leaflets, increased surface
(M-mode,	area
2-dimensional,	Large mitral annulus
transesophageal,	MVP (late systolic, early systolic, holosystolic)
3-dimensional)	-anterior or posterior or both leaflets
	Flail mitral leaflet
	LV, LA structure and function
Doppler:	No MVR
	MVR (late systolic, early systolic, holosystolic)-
	mild, moderate, severe
Chest x-ray:	Normal
	Skeletal abnormalities
	Cardiac enlargement
	Pulmonary congestion
Magnetic resonance	Abnormal mitral leaflet tissue
imaging:	Severity of MVR
	LV-LA structure and function
Cinecardioangiography:	MVP (anterior or posterior or both leaflets)
	MVR (mild, moderate, severe)
	LV size and function
	LV contraction pattern
Hemodynamic findings:	Normal
	Increased LV diastolic and LA pressures; LA-PVW,
	large V waves
	Decreased cardiac output
	Pulmonary hypertension
	Regurgitant fraction

FMV = floppy mitral valve; MVP = mitral valve prolapse; MVR = mitral valvular
regurgitation; LV = left ventricle; LA = left atrium; PVW = pulmonary venous wedge.

Infective Endocarditis

FMV/MVP patients are at higher risk for infective endocarditis.[161–169] The diagnosis, recognition, treatment, and prophylaxis of infective endocarditis is described in Chapter 14. It should be emphasized that short-term therapy with antibiotics may alter or obscure the clinical picture of infective endocarditis. It is suggested, therefore, that before patients with

Table 8
Floppy Mitral Valve/Mitral Valve Prolapse: Spectrum of Mitral Valve Abnormalities

Terminology	Mitral Valve Anatomy and Pathology	Echocardiogram	Auscultatory Findings	Hemodynamic Findings	Cineangiography	Doppler
Normal valve	Normal	Normal	Normal	Normal	Normal	Normal
FMV/MVP/no MR	Large mitral leaflets, long chordae tendineae	Large mitral leaflets, long chordae tendineae probable prolapse	Nonejection click	Normal	Probable prolapse	Normal
FMV/MVP/mild MR	Large mitral leaflets, long chordae tendineae Disruption of leaflet edge apposition	Large mitral leaflets, long chordae tendineae probable prolapse;	Nonejection click or murmur	Usually normal	Probable prolapse; mitral reguritation	MR
FMV/MVP/severe MR (floppy valve)	Voluminous leaflets; chordae tendineae elongation	Floppy mitral valve; probable prolapse; probable LV and LA enlargement	Systolic murmur, may be holosystolic; probably non-ejection click	Increased LV diastolic and LA pressure; prominent V waves	Mitral regurgitation; probable prolapse; probable LV and LA enlargement	MR
Flail valve	Chordae tendineae rupture; grossly elongated chordae	Flail mitral valve; LV enlargement; probable LA enlargement	Systolic murmur	Increased LV diastolic and LA pressure; markedly prominent V waves	Severe mitral regurgitation; flail mitral valve; LV enlargement; probable LA enlargement	MR

FMV = floppy mitral valve; MVP = mitral valve prolapse; MR = mitral regurgitation; LV = left ventricle; LA = left atrium.
From Boudoulas and Wooley,[5] with permission.

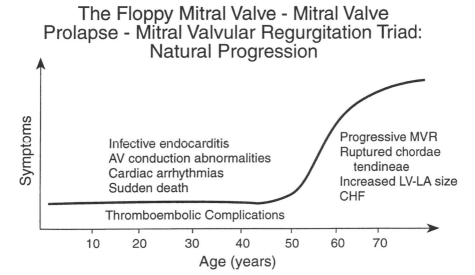

The Floppy Mitral Valve - Mitral Valve
Prolapse - Mitral Valvular Regurgitation Triad:
Natural Progression

Figure 18. Floppy mitral valve (FMV), mitral valve prolapse (MVP), and mitral valvular regurgitation (MVR). Symptoms are plotted against patient age in years. Increased symptoms occurred after age 50 and are related to progressive MVR, atrial fibrillation, left atrial (LA), and left ventricular (LV) dysfunction, and congestive heart failure (CHF). Thromboembolic complications, infective endocarditis, and cardiac arrhythmias have been reported at a wide range of ages. (Modified with permission from Boudoulas H.[13])

FMV/MVP are treated with antibiotics, the diagnosis of infective endocarditis should be considered and blood cultures obtained.

Thromboembolic Complications

Patients with FMV/MVP may be at risk for embolic events (see Chapter 15),[170–178] the embolic source presumably being the surface of the FMV; platelet aggregation phenomena may also be involved. In patients with chronic or paroxysmal atrial fibrillation, intra-atrial thrombosis may be responsible for thromboembolic complications.

Patients with FMV/MVP who experience thromboembolic complications may have abnormal platelet survival time, platelet functional test abnormalities, and increased platelet aggregation, and decreased survival time may be partially related to high adrenergic tone. Thus, in these patients platelet functional tests and urinary and plasma catecholamine measurements may help to define the underlying mechanism or prothrombotic coagulation defects. Further, definition of the mitral valve size, mitral valve leaflet thickness, the severity of MVR, and left ventricle and left atrial size and the possible presence of mitral annular or aortic valvular calcification (particularly in the older patients or those with hereditary connective tissue disorders) should be defined.

Cardiac Arrhythmias/Syncope/Cardiac Arrest

Cardiac arrhythmias may constitute a major problem in patients with FMV/MVP.[133,179–188] Identification and characterization may be difficult in some patients because of the transient nature of the arrhythmias. Patients with cardiac arrhythmias may be asymptomatic or may have a wide range of symptoms including nonspecific complaints, palpitations, syncope, or presyncope, and, rarely, sudden death.

Several studies have suggested that the incidence of cardiac arrhythmias in patients with FMV/MVP is greater compared to the general population. The incidence of FMV/MVP among patients referred for electrophysiologic studies and the incidence of electrophysiologic abnormalities in symptomatic patients with FMV/MVP who had electrophysiologic studies at The Ohio State University Medical Center were analyzed. During the period 1976 to 1986, 1,856 patients were referred for electrophysiologic studies; 271 patients (14.6%) had FMV/MVP without significant MVR. One or more electrophysiologic abnormalities were found in 220 patients with FMV/MVP (81.2%). Assuming that the prevalence of FMV/MVP in the general population is 2–4%, our data suggest that the incidence of symptomatic arrhythmias in patients with FMV/MVP is greater than that of the general population. A higher incidence of arrhythmias has also been reported in the younger age group.[130,131]

The incidence of ventricular arrhythmias and sudden death is also higher in the FMV/MVP group (see Chapters 16 and 17). The most common cause of sudden death in FMV/MVP is ventricular fibrillation.

The cause of ventricular arrhythmias in patients with FMV/MVP appears to be multifactorial (Table 9).[130] Papillary muscle traction in

---

Table 9
Floppy Mitral Valve/Mitral Valve Prolapse: Possible Cause of Ventricular Arrhythmias

Likely multifactorial
Endocardial friction lesions
Platelet aggregation – fibrin deposits (emboli of coronary arteries)
Papillary muscle traction/ventricular stretch
QT dispersion
Mechanical stimulation of myocardium by leaflets
Abnormal innervation of floppy mitral valve
Autonomic dysfunction ($\uparrow$norephinephrine$\rightarrow$ $\downarrow$K$\dagger$, postural phenomena)
Myocardial fibrosis

FMV/MVP may be responsible for ventricular arrhythmias. Membrane depolarization is caused by both gradual and rapid ventricular stretch, but premature ventricular depolarizations are more readily elicited by rapid stretch.[189,190] Recent studies have demonstrated the existence of stretch-activated membrane channels in ventricular myocardium; these may contribute to ventricular ectopy under conditions of differential ventricular loading as in FMV/MVP. Echocardiographic data demonstrated that, in normal subjects, the distance between the papillary muscle tips and the mitral annulus during systole remains relatively constant. In contrast, in patients with FMV/MVP, mitral valve leaflet displacement into the left atrium results in papillary muscle displacement that causes traction of the muscle (Fig. 19).[130]

Endocardial friction lesions resulting from friction between the chordae and LV myocardium have been reported at autopsy studies in patients

Floppy Mitral Valve/Mitral Valve Prolapse: Cardiac Arrhythmias

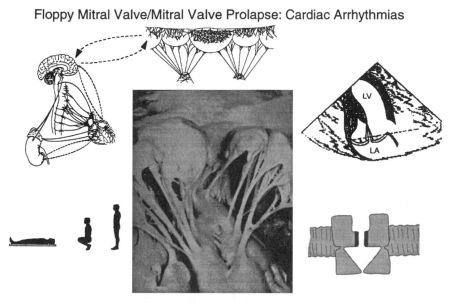

Figure 19. The cause of cardiac arrhythmias in floppy mitral valve/mitral valve prolapse is multifactorial. Autonomic dysfunction-neurohormonal abnormalities, papillary muscle traction/ventricular stretch-stretch receptors activation, orthostatic phenomena, innervation of the mitral valve, and mechanical stimulation of myocardium by mitral valve leaflets are contributory factors. Floppy mitral valve is shown in the middle. (Used with permission from Edwards JE. Circulation 43:606–612, 1971.) Above, the mitral valve innervation of the mitral valve is shown schematically; upper right, papillary muscle tension during ventricular systole; lower right, stretch-activated receptor is shown schematically. Left upper part shows schematically interactions between the brain-heart-kidneys and adrenals. Lower left part shows schematically orthostatic phenomena. LV = left ventricle; LA = left atrium. (Used with permission from Ohara N, et al.[130])

with FMV/MVP who died suddenly.[191–193] It is possible that this pathology may be responsible for, or contribute to the development of, ventricular arrhythmias. Platelet aggregation, hemorrhage, and fibrin deposits have been observed in the angle between the left atrium and the posterior mitral leaflet, and microembolism from these deposits may involve the coronary circulation, with subsequent myocardial ischemia and ventricular arrhythmias.

Innervation of the mitral valve may also contribute to the genesis of cardiac arrhythmias in FMV/MVP.[130,194] Human cardiac valves have distinct patterns of innervation that comprise both primary sensory and autonomic components. The presence of distinct nerve terminals suggests a neural basis for interactions between the central nervous system and the mitral valve. The subendocardial surface on the atrial aspect at the middle portion of the mitral valve is rich in nerve endings, including afferent nerves; mechanical stimuli from this area caused by abnormal coaptation in FMV/MVP may cause abnormal autonomic nerve feedback between the central nervous system and mitral valve nervous system (see Chapter 21).

Autonomic dysfunction may initiate, precipitate, or contribute to arrhythmias in symptomatic patients with FMV/MVP.[195–205] Increased adrenergic activity, catecholamine regulation abnormality, and adrenergic hyperresponsiveness have been observed in certain patients with FMV/MVP. Altered vagal tone or baroreceptor activity may also play a role in the pathogenesis of cardiac arrhythmias in certain patients. Increased adrenergic activity associated with FMV/MVP in some instances may be associated with hypokalemia which, in turn, may contribute to cardiac arrhythmias. Autonomic dysfunction and stretch-activated mechanoreceptors may contribute to QT dispersion, which may cause ventricular arrhythmias in some patients with FMV/MVP. As a general rule, the duration of the QT interval is normal in patients with FMV/MVP. The incidence of QT dispersion, however, has been reported to be higher in patients with MVP compared to the general population.[130]

Patients with FMV/MVP often present with postural phenomena such as orthostatic decreases in cardiac output, orthostatic hypotension, tachycardia, and symptoms related to alterations in heart rate, blood pressure, and cardiac output.[206,207] Orthostatic phenomena are multifactorial in origin. Decreased intravascular volume, an abnormal renin-aldosterone response to volume depletion, a baroreflex modulation abnormality, a hyperadrenergic state, or a parasympathetic abnormality may partially account for these phenomena. Further, the development of the third chamber when prolapse occurs and the inability to maintain normal LV diastolic volume in the upright posture will contribute to orthostatic phenomena (see also Chapter 24).

In general, sudden death in patients with FMV/MVP without significant MVR has been almost exclusively reported in symptomatic patients with FMV/MVP. Patients with a history of recurrent syncope, a history of complex ventricular arrhythmias, or a family history of cardiac sudden death appear to be at higher risk for sudden death.[130]

We reported nine cases of resuscitated survivors of sudden death in patients with FMV/MVP, only one of whom had significant MVR. All patients but one were symptomatic before the cardiac arrest; eight had long histories of palpitations with documented ventricular arrhythmia, and three of the eight had recurrent syncope. Electrocardiographic ST segment and T wave changes are frequently present in patients with FMV/MVP and sudden death or ventricular fibrillation (see Chapter 17).[131]

Patients with FMV/MVP who are currently classified to the incompletely defined high-risk category (Table 10) should have further diagnostic studies such as ambulatory monitoring, exercise testing, transtelephonic electrocardiography, or electrophysiologic studies in order to identify the potential for serious arrhythmias. Appropriate therapy would depend on the outcome of such testing and is subject to the same limitations and potential benefit of individualized antiarrhythmic therapy. Patients with significant MVR should undergo valve reconstruction or replacement when indicated, to prevent irreversible ventricular damage (see Chapter 18).

The prognosis of patients with cardiac arrhythmias, in general, is related to the nature of the arrhythmias (atrial vs. ventricular) and to the presence and severity of cardiac disease (the severity of MVR, left ventricular and left atrial structure and function, coexisting coronary artery disease, accessory atrioventricular pathways). Diagnostic studies directed at identifying the underlying cardiac pathology are of obvious clinical importance while a search for other possible factors known to aggravate or initiate arrhythmias, such as metabolic–electrolyte abnormalities, psychotropic or sympathomimetic drugs, caffeine or alcohol excess, and heavy smoking, should be pursued assiduously.

Syncope, or presyncope, is among the most difficult of symptoms to evaluate. While in many patients syncope is neurocardiogenic and is not

---

Table 10
Floppy Mitral Valve/Mitral Valve Prolapse: Ventricular
Arrhythmias; The High-Risk Patient

Past history compatible with cardiac arrhythmias (palpitations, premature
  ventricular beats, syncope)
Family history of sudden death
Autonomic dysfunction (orthostatic phenomena, syncope)
QT dispersion

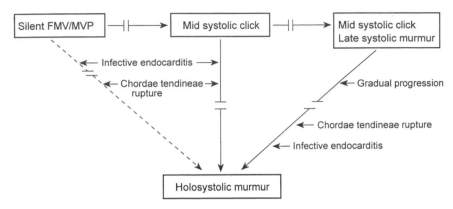

Figure 20. Progression of floppy mitral valve (FMV), mitral valve prolapse (MVP) is associated with changes in auscultatory findings. Infective endocarditis and chordae tendineae rupture may abruptly exaggerate the progression from one level to the other or the progression may be gradual.

associated with severe circulatory disease, or a poor prognosis, occasionally it may be a harbinger of sudden death (see Chapter 17).[131,179]

Progressive Mitral Valvular Regurgitation–Congestive Heart Failure

The progression of MVR through the spectrum of mild to severe in patients with FMV/MVP is generally gradual, and the entire process accelerates after a prolonged asymptomatic interval.[208–221] The average age at which severe symptoms develop is 60 years. Progressive MVR is related to various combinations of annular dilatation, elongation of the chordae tendineae, or frank chordal rupture. When chordal rupture occurs, MVR may be further accentuated (Fig. 20). In certain cases, chordae tendineae rupture may lead to acute MVR (see Chapter 20).

Individuals with thick mitral valve leaflets (i.e., with FMV) and mitral systolic murmur are at higher risk of developing complications; men and those older than 50 years are at particularly high risk (Table 11, Fig. 21). LV

Table 11
Floppy Mitral Valve/Mitral Valve
Prolapse: The High-Risk Patient

Men, age >50
Mitral systolic murmur
Thick redundant mitral valve leaflets
Left ventricular–left atrial enlargement
Combinations of the above

FMV/MVP/MVR: The High Risk Patient

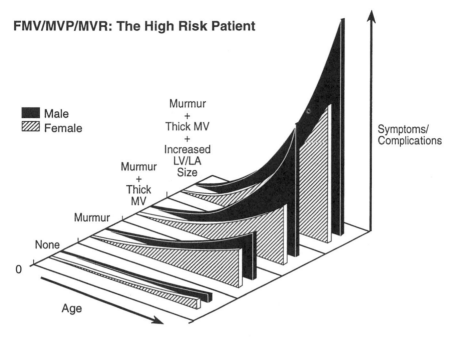

Figure 21. Patients with floppy mitral valve (FMV), mitral valve prolapse (MVP), and systolic murmur, thick, redundant mitral valve (MV) leaflets; men over age 50 are at higher risk of developing complications. Left ventricular (LV) enlargement in patients with FMV/MVP predicts the need for mitral valve surgery. Presence of two or more of the above abnormalities markedly increases the likelihood of complications. Absence of all three of these features identifies patients with FMV/MVP at extremely low risk. LA = left atrium. (Used with permission from Boudoulas H, et al.[9])

enlargement in patients with FMV/MVP is a good predictor of the subsequent need for mitral valve surgery. When two or more of the above abnormalities coexist, the possibility of complications is increased. In contrast, the absence of all of these features identifies patients with MVP at exceedingly low risk. Aortic function has also been suggested to be an important factor related to progression of MVR (see Chapter 21).

Progression of MVR usually is associated with LV dysfunction and/or congestive heart failure. Cardiac catheterization and cardioangiography are indicated in patients with congestive heart failure to help define the ventricular function and hemodynamics, the severity of MVR, and the coronary anatomy. At the present time, we recommend cardiac catheterization for patients being considered as candidates for mitral valve surgery.

For chest pain, see chapters and sections on mitral valve prolapse syndrome.

Table 12

Floppy Mitral Valve/Mitral Valve Prolapse: Therapeutic Considerations

---

Associated abnormalities
FMV/MVP in recognized heritable disorders of connective tissue
Severity of mitral valve abnormalities
Complications/Symptoms
 • Infective endocarditis
 • Thromboembolism
 • Arrhythmias (syncope, cardiac arrest)
 • Progressive mitral valvular regurgitation
 • Congestive heart failure
 • Chest pain
Special considerations
 • Childhood
 • Pregnancy
 • Athletics
 • Insurance

FMV = floppy mitral valve; MVP = mitral valve prolapse.

For special considerations related to childhood, pregnancy, athletics, and aviation, see Chapter 25).

Therapeutic Considerations (Table 12)

Associated Lesions

FMV/MVP may be associated with other cardiovascular and noncardiovascular abnormalities. These abnormalities should be appropriately recognized and treated if clinical indications exist.

Floppy Mitral Valve/Mitral Valvular Prolapse in Recognized Heritable Disorders of Connective Tissue

FMV/MVP may occur in patients with recognized heritable disorders with or without aortic root dilatation and/or aortic regurgitation, such as Marfan syndrome, Ehlers-Danlos syndrome, and polycystic kidney disease. The recognition of FMV/MVP as a part of these syndromes should prompt appropriate therapy (see Chapter 7).

Severity of Mitral Valve Abnormalities

In our opinion, it is important to define as precisely as possible where the individual with FMV/MVP fits within the spectrum of mitral valve abnormality or dysfunction, and to diagnose any associated abnormalities in order to determine a prognosis and to avoid or recognize complications related to FMV/MVP (Tables 7 and 8).

Diagnostic definition and categorization, followed by a careful explanation to the patient, along with a program for medical follow-up where indicated may be sufficient in the asymptomatic or mildly symptomatic patient or in patients with mild MVR. A knowledge of the extent of family involvement may be of prognostic value and serve as a basis for long-term management. This is particularly true when dealing with families with overt or subtle hereditary connective tissue disorders.

Complications/Symptoms

Infective Endocarditis

In general, patients with FMV/MVP should receive antibiotic prophylaxis for diagnostic and therapeutic procedures where predictable bacteremia is a risk (Tables 13 and 14).[169,222–227] Recommended antibiotic regimens for dental, respiratory tract, gastrointestinal, and genitourinary procedures are summarized in Tables 15 and 16. Infective endocarditis

---

Table 13
Procedures With Risk for Infective Endocarditis

Definite
- Dental procedures known to induce gingival or mucosal bleeding, including professional cleaning
- Tonsillectomy and/or adenoidectomy
- Surgical operations that involve intestinal or respiratory mocusa
- Bronchoscopy with a rigid bronchoscope
- Sclerotherapy for esophageal varices
- Esophageal stricture dilatation
- Endoscopic retrograde cholangiography with biliary obstruction
- Gallbladder surgery
- Cystoscopy
- Urethral dilatation
- Urethral catheterization if urinary tract infection is present*
- Urinary tract surgery if urinary tract infection is present*
- Prostatic surgery
- Incision and drainage of infected tissue*
- Vaginal delivery in the presence of infection*
- Endodontia
- Endoaortic instrumentation or surgery

---

* In addition to a prophylactic regimen for genitourinary procedures, antibiotic therapy should be directed against the most likely bacterial pathogen.

Table 14
Procedures Which Entail Risk for Infective Endocarditis

Uncertain*
- Alveolar ridge incision in denture patients without preexistent ulcerations
- Various crown and bridge procedures
- Nasal septoplasty
- Ear piercing
- Acupuncture
- Dermatologic procedures (involving acneiform lesions)
- Inguinal herniorraphy
- Lithotripsy
- Transrectal prostatic biopsy
- Transesophageal echocardiography

* These are just a few of the many miscellaneous other procedures that raise questions in this regard but where "official" recommendations have not been issued or widely accepted. In such situations, patient-specific judgments are required. In some cases (such as those procedures involving the nasal mucosa), the best approach probably includes collection of "survey cultures" which then dictate chemoprophylaxis decisions and selections.

Table 15
Prophylactic Regimens for Dental, Oral, Respiratory Tract, or Esophageal Procedures

Situation	Agent	Regimen*
Standard general prophylaxis	Amoxicillin	Adults: 2.0 g; children 50 mg/kg orally 1 hour before procedure
Unable to take oral medications	Ampicillin	Adults: 2.0 g intramuscularly (IM) or intravenously (IV); children: 50 mg/kg IM or IV within 30 min before procedure
Allergic to penicillin	Clindamycin or	Adults: 600 mg; children: 20 mg/kg orally 1 hour before procedure
	Cephalexin† or cefadroxil† or	Adults: 2.0 g; children: 15 mg/kg orally 1 hour before procedure
	Azithromycin or clarithromycin	Adults: 500 mg; children: 15 mg/kg orally 1 hour before procedure
Allergic to penicillin and unable to take oral medications	Clindamycin or	Adults: 600 mg; children: 20 mg/kg IV within 30 min before procedure
	Cefazolin†	Adults: 1.0 g; children: 25 mg/kg IM or IV within 30 min before procedure

* Total children's dose should not exceed adult dose.
† Cephalosporins should not be used in individuals with immediate-type hypersensitivity reaction (urticaria, angioedema, or anaphylaxis) to penicillin.
From ref. 222.

Table 16
Prophylactic Regimens for Genitourinary Gastrointestinal (Excluding Esophageal) Procedures*

Situation	Agent*	Regiment†
High-risk patients	Ampicillin plus gentamicin	**Adults:** ampicillin 2.0 g intramuscularly (IM) or intravenously (IV) plus gentamicin 1.5 mg/kg (not to exceed 120 mg) within 30 min of starting the procedure; 6 hours later, ampicillin 1 g IM/IV or amoxicillin 1 g orally **Children:** ampicillin 50 mg/kg IM or IV (not to exceed 2.0 g) plus gentamicin 1.5 mg/kg within 30 min of starting the procedure; 6 hours later, ampicillin 25 mg/kg IM/IV or amoxicillin 25 mg/kg orally
High-risk patients allergic to ampicillin/ amoxicillin	Vancomycin plus gentamicin	**Adults:** vancomycin 1.0 g IV over 1–2 hours plus gentamicin 1.5 mg/kg IV/IM (not to exceed 120 mg); complete injection/infusion within 30 min of starting the procedure **Children:** vancomycin 20 mg/kg IV over 1–2 hours plus gentamicin 1.5 mg/kg IV/IM; complete injection/infusion within 30 min of starting the procedure
Moderate-risk	Amoxicillin or ampicillin	**Adults:** amoxicillin 2.0 g orally 1 hour before procedure, or ampicillin 2.0 g IM/IV within 30 min of starting the procedure **Children:** amoxicillin 50 mg/kg orally 1 hour before procedure, or ampicillin 50 mg/kg IM/IV within 30 min of starting the procedure
Moderate-risk patients allergic to ampicillin/ amoxicillin	Vancomycin	**Adults:** vancomycin 1.0 g IV over 1–2 hours; complete infusion within 30 min of starting the procedure **Children:** vancomycin 20 mg/kg IV over 1–2 hours; complete infusion within 30 min of starting the procedure

* Total children's dose should not exceed adult dose.
† No second dose of vancomycin or gentamicin is recommended.
* From ref. 222.

prophylaxis in general is currently a matter of considerable debate, as well as the subject of changing attitudes and recommendations. Patients should be encouraged to maintain the best possible oral hygiene to reduce potential sources of bacterial seeding since poor dental hygiene, periodontal or periapical infections, or irritations caused by ill-fitting dentures may induce bacteremia without dental manipulation or procedures.

The management of infective endocarditis is outlined in Chapter 14. Patients with FMV/MVP complicated by infective endocarditis who develop progressive valvular dysfunction, acute congestive heart failure, recurrent emboli, conduction system abnormalities, or manifest evidence of persistent infection may require surgical intervention as part of their overall therapy.

Thromboembolic Complications (see also Chapter 15)

Certain young women with FMV/MVP and a history of thromboembolic complications may be at increased risk for thromboembolic disease, and if it seems otherwise reasonable following a general medical evaluation, we think it wise to avoid oral contraceptives until the pathogenesis of embolic phenomena has been more precisely defined. Individuals who have had clinical manifestations of retinal, cerebral, or peripheral emboli should discontinue oral contraceptives, abstain from chronic cigarette smoking, and have a careful cardiovascular and hematological evaluation before long-term anticoagulant or antiplatelet therapy is considered. Chronic anticoagulation should be considered in patients with chronic atrial fibrillation, with or without embolic phenomena.

Cardiac Arrhythmias/Syncope/Sudden Death

A detailed discussion of therapy is presented in Chapters 16 and 17. A few general principles may be stated. First, precipitating or initiating factors should be considered. Caffeine or other stimulants such as alcohol, smoking, and sympathomimetic drugs should be avoided in FMV/MVP patients with tachyarrhythmias.[130,179] Supraventricular tachycardia can be suppressed by digitalis, antiarrhythmic agents, β-blocking drugs, calcium channel blocking agents, or combinations. The primary goal in patients with atrial fibrillation (if refractory to conversion) is control of the ventricular rate (70–80 beats/min at rest) in order to maximize overall LV performance. Anticoagulation therapy should be considered and individualized in patients with MVR and chronic atrial fibrillation.

Patients with ventricular arrhythmias require individual assessment; those at high risk for severe complications (presyncope, syncope, sudden death) should be identified as described above. LV dysfunction, coexistent myocardial ischemia, prolonged electrical systole, or electrical systole greater than electromechanical systole (QT > QS), QT dispersion, frequent and complex premature ventricular beats, ventricular tachycardia, and a history of ventricular fibrillation constitute high-risk factors and necessitate more aggressive management (see Chapters 16 and 17).

In some cases, when recurrent tachyarrhythmias are refractory to antiarrhythmic drugs or the patient is intolerant to therapy, various mechanical devices may be helpful. Automatic defibrillator implantation may be required to control ventricular arrhythmias in selected patients who have survived cardiopulmonary regurgitation. Catheter ablation plays a role in a variety of conditions including the Wolff-Parkinson-White syndrome. Mitral valve surgery in patients with ventricular arrhythmias associated with severe MVR and congestive heart failure may result in improvement in the arrhythmias in certain patients. Although mitral valve reconstruction has been reported to provide the relief of symptoms including syncope and ventricular fibrillation, these studies involved relatively few, highly selected patients and should not be extrapolated to the general high-risk population. Infrequent premature ventricular beats in patients with normal LV function without evidence of ischemia are usually benign and no specific therapy is indicated.

The wide variety of disorders that can result in syncope makes it clear that effective treatment demands accurate diagnosis. Therapy for the patient with syncope varies from simple maneuvers, such as avoiding precipitating factors to more direct forms of therapy including potent antiarrhythmic drugs or cardiac pacemakers.

Patients with FMV/MVP and a history of cardiac arrest (a survivor following cardiopulmonary resuscitation for ventricular fibrillation or asystole) should undergo a thorough evaluation to define the mechanisms and most appropriate therapy for the cardiac arrhythmias.

Progressive Mitral Valvular Regurgitation

Asymptomatic patients with isolated mitral systolic clicks usually have FMV/MVP of limited clinical significance. The prevention of infective endocarditis is the major consideration in these patients (Fig. 22).

Patients with mitral systolic click or clicks, mid- to late systolic, murmurs, and increased mitral valve surface area and annulus size represent FMV/MVP with mild to moderate MVR, with a greater potential for progression. Therapeutic considerations in these patients include preventing infective endocarditis, and recognizing and preventing progressive MVR. It is important to recall that at present very little, if anything, is known about the effects of usual life activities such as heavy labor or physical exercise on the progression of MVR.

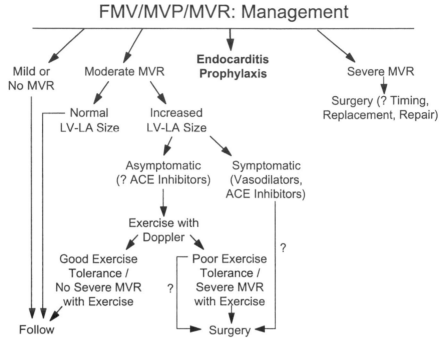

Figure 22. Management of patients with floppy mitral valve (FMV), mitral valve prolapse (MVP), mitral valvular regurgitation (MVR). Prophylaxis for infective endocarditis is indicated in all patients with FMV/MVP. LV = left ventricle; LA = left atrium; ACE = angiotensin-converting enzyme.

Progressive MVR with the development of congestive heart failure is usually associated with left atrial enlargement progressing to left atrial failure, with the development of chronic atrial fibrillation. Data suggest that therapy with angiotensin-converting enzyme inhibitors in patients with significant MVR may slow the natural progression of the disease.[40,116,228] More acute or subacute forms of MVR may be the result of ruptured chordae tendineae occurring in the presence of preexisting mild or moderately severe MVR (see Chapter 20). In most patients with significant MVR and symptoms related to MVR, surgical therapy should be considered (see Chapters 18 and 20). Judgments about the necessity for mitral valve surgery, either mitral valve reconstructive surgery or mitral valve replacement, are best made following appropriate diagnostic studies.[229–241]

Congestive Heart Failure

Chronic congestive heart failure in patients with FMV/MVP usually results from the progression of MVR with left atrial and left ventricular dysfunction. Acute and subacute forms of congestive heart failure may be coincident with, or associated with, the recent onset of atrial fibrillation and/or ruptured chordae tendineae. Attempts should be made to convert to sinus rhythm with antiarrhythmic drugs or cardioversion in patients with a recent onset of atrial fibrillation. If atrial fibrillation persists, and significant MVR is present, surgical intervention should be considered.

Chest pain is discussed in Chapter 24.

Special considerations related to childhood, pregnancy, and athletics, are discussed in Chapter 25.

Floppy Mitral Valve/Mitral Valve Prolapse: Individual Patient Analysis

The individual patient analysis presents a logical approach to the diagnostic process. Emphasis should be placed on the diagnostic process and the individual patient profile (Figs. 23 and 24).[22]

Diagnostic methods vary. Much depends on the physician's experience, diagnostic facilities, and available technology. Diagnostic facilities vary from institution to institution, from country to country, and definitely will change dramatically in years to come. Thus, specific definition of the anatomic lesions(s), physiologic state, and the pathophysiologic abnormalities for the individual patient should remain as the ultimate standards.

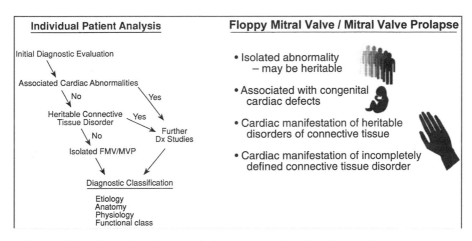

Figure 23. Individual patient analysis. Incorporates the diagnostic steps necessary to develop a diagnostic classification. FMV = floppy mitral valve; MVP = mitral valve prolapse; Dx = diagnostic.

Individual Patient Analysis

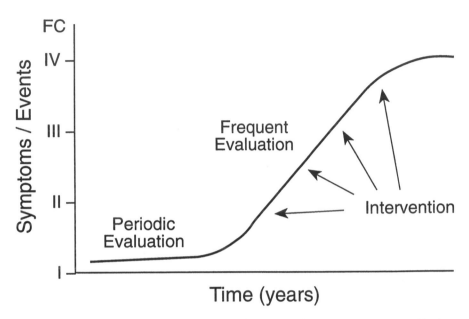

Figure 24. Periodic evaluation is replaced by more frequent evaluation with the development of symptoms or events. Intervention indicated by multiple arrows, may involve medical therapy or surgical procedure at varying times during the course of the disease.

References

1. Boudoulas H, Wooley CF (eds). Mitral Valve Prolapse and the Mitral Valve Prolapse Syndrome. NY, Mount Kisco, Futura Publishing Co., 1988.
2. Wooley CF, Sparks EA, Boudoulas H. The floppy mitral valve-mitral valve prolapse-mitral valvular regurgitation triad. ACC Current J Rev July/August 1994, pp 25–26.
3. Boudoulas H, Kolibash AJ, Baker P, King BD, Wooley CF. Mitral valve prolapse and the mitral valve prolapse syndrome: A diagnostic classification and pathogenesis of symptoms. Am Heart J 118:796–818, 1989.
4. Wooley CF, Baker PB, Kolibash AJ, Kilman JW, Sparks EA, Boudoulas H. The floppy, myxomatous mitral valve, mitral valve prolapse and mitral regurgitation. Prog Cardiovasc Dis 33:397–433, 1991.
5. Boudoulas H, Wooley CF. Mitral valve prolapse and the mitral valve prolapse syndrome. In Yu PN, Goodwin JF (eds): Prog in Cardiovasc Dis 14:275–309, 1986.
6. Davies MJ, Moore BP, Brainbridge MV. The floppy mitral valve: Study of incidence, pathology, and complications in surgical, necropsy and forensic material. Br Heart J 40:468–481, 1978.

7. Wooley CF, Boudoulas H. Mitral valve prolapse. In Rakel RE (ed): Conn's Current Therapy. Philadelphia, W.B. Saunders Co., 1999, pp 289–293.
8. Boudoulas H. Valvular Disease. American College of Cardiology Self-Assessment Program (ACCSAP) 2000, in press.
9. Boudoulas H, Kolibash AH, Wooley CF. Mitral valve prolapse: A heterogeneous disorder. Primary Cardiol 17:29–43, 1991.
10. King BD, Clark MA, Baba N, et al. 'Myxomatous' mitral valves: Collagen dissolution as the primary defect. Circulation 66:288–296, 1982.
11. Baker PB, Bansal G, Boudoulas H, Kolibash AJ, Kilman J, Wooley CF. Floppy mitral valve chordae tendineae: Histopathologic alterations. Human Pathol 19:507–512, 1988.
12. Boudoulas H, Kolibash AJ, Wooley CF. Mitral valve prolapse: The high-risk patient. Practical Cardiol 17:15–31, 1991.
13. Boudoulas H. Mitral valve prolapse and the mitral valve prolapse syndrome. In Toutouzas P, Boudoulas H (eds): Cardiac Diseases, Parissianos Medical and Scientific Editions, Athens, 1991, 2:135–156.
14. Malkowski MT, Boudoulas H, Wooley CF, Guo R, Pearson AC. The spectrum of structural abnormalities in the floppy mitral valve: Echocardiographic evaluation. Am Heart J 132:145–151, 1996.
15. Boudoulas H, Wooley CF. Mitral valve disorders. Curr Opinion Cardiol 5:162–170, 1990.
16. Pomerance A. Ballooning deformity (mucoid degeneration) of atrioventricular valves. Br Heart J 31:343–351, 1969.
17. Lucas RV Jr, Edwards JE. The Floppy Mitral Valve. Chicago, Year Book Med Publ., 1982, pp 1–48.
18. Freed LA, Levy D, Levine RA, Larson MG, Evans JC, Fuller DL, Lehman B, et al. Prevalence and clinical outcome of mitral valve prolapse. N Engl J Med 341:1–7, 1999.
19. Gilon D, Buonanno FS, Joffe MM, Leavitt M, Marshall JE, Kistler JP, Levine RA. Lack of evidence of an association between mitral valve prolapse and stroke in young patients. N Engl J Med 341:8–13, 1999.
20. Cole WG, Chan D, Hickey AJ, Wilcken DEL. Collagen composition of normal and myxomatous human mitral heart valves. Biochem J 219:451–460, 1984.
21. Becker AE. Acquired heart valve pathology. Herz 23:415–419, 1998.
22. Boudoulas H, Wooley CF. The floppy mitral valve, mitral valve prolapse, mitral valvular regurgitation. In Moss, Adams (eds): Heart Disease in Infants, Children and Adolescents. 6th ed. in press.
23. Procacci PM, Savran SV, Schreiter SL, et al. Prevalence of clinical mitral valve prolapse in 1169 young women. N Engl J Med 294:1086–1088, 1976.
24. Markiewicz W, Stoner J, London E, et al. Mitral valve prolapse in 100 presumably healthy young females. Circulation 53:464–473, 1976.
25. Hickey AJ, Wolfers J, Wilcken DEL. Mitral valve prolapse: Prevalence in an Australian population. Med J Austr 1:31–33, 1981.
26. Wanns LS, Grove JR, Hess TR, et al. Prevalence of mitral valve prolapse by two-dimensional echocardiography in healthy young women. Br Heart J 49:334–340, 1983.
27. Savage DD, Garrison RJ, Devereux RB, et al. Mitral valve prolapse in the general population. In: Epidemiologic features: The Framingham study. Am Heart J 106:571–576, 1983.
28. Bryhn M, Persson S. The prevalence of mitral valve prolapse in healthy men and women in Sweden: An echocardiographic study. Acta Med Scand 215:157–160, 1984.

29. Savage DD, Devereux RB, Garrison RJ, et al. Mitral valve prolapse in the general population. In: Clinical features: The Framingham Study. Am Heart J 106:577–581, 1983.
30. Ohara N, Mikajima T, Takagi J, Kato H. Mitral valve prolapse in childhood: The incidence and clinical presentations in different age groups. Acta Paediatr Jpn 33:467–475, 1991.
31. Greenwood RD. Mitral valve prolapse: Incidence and clinical course in a pediatric population. Clin Pediatr 23:318–320, 1984.
32. Ohara N, Mikajima T, Takagi J, Kato H. Mitral valve prolapse in childhood: The incidence and clinical presentation in different age groups. Acta Paediatr Jpn 4:467–475, 1991.
33. Greenwood RD. Mitral valve prolapse in childhood. Hosp Pract August: 41–42, 1986.
34. Warth DC, King ME, Cohen JM, Tesoriero VL, Marcus E, Weyman AE. Prevalence of mitral valve prolapse in normal children. J Am Coll Cardiol 5:117, 1985.
35. Hickey AJ, Wilcken DEL. Age and the clinical profile of idiopathic mitral valve prolapse. Br Heart J 55:582–586, 1986.
36. Devereux RB, Brown WT, Kramer-Fox R, Sachs I. Inheritance of mitral valve prolapse: Effect of age and sex on gene expression. Ann Int Med 97:826–832, 1982.
37. Rizzon P, Biasco G, Brindicci G, Mauro F. Familial syndrome of midsystolic click and late systolic murmur. Br Heart J 35:245–259, 1973.
38. Malcolm AD. Mitral valve prolapse associated with other disorders. Casual coincidence, common link, or fundamental genetic disturbance? Br Heart J 53:353–562, 1985.
39. Stickler GB, Belau PG, Farrell FL. Hereditary progressive arthro-ophthalmopathy. Mayo Clin Proc 40:433–455, 1965.
40. Levine AB, Muller C, Levine TB. Effects of high-dose lisinopril-isosorbide dinitrate on severe mitral regurgitation and heart failure remodeling. Am J Cardiol 82:1299–1300, 1998.
41. Barbosa MM, Pena JL, Motta MM, Fortes PR. Aneurysms of the atrial septum diagnosed by echocardiography and their associated cardiac abnormalities. Int J Cardiol 29:71–78, 1990.
42. Takahashi H, Sakamoto T, Hada Y, et al. Mitral valve prolapse in patients with surgically-closed atrial septal defect. J Cardiol 19:893–900, 1989.
43. Piraino P, Zura ML, Loureiro O, Andrade A. Mitral valve prolapse associated with Basedow's disease and active hyperthyroidism. Preliminary report. Rev Med Chil 118: 649–652, 1991.
44. Kontopoulos AG, Harsoulis P, Adam K, Papadopoulos G, Polymenidis Z, Boudoulas H. Frequency of HLA antigents in Graves hyperthyroidism and mitral valve prolapse. J Heart Valve Dis 5:543–545, 1996.
45. Bastianon V, Pasquino AM, Giglioni E, et al. Mitral valve prolapse in Turner syndrome. Eur J Pediatr 148:533–534, 1989.
46. Rahko PS, Xu QB. Increased prevalence of atrial septal aneurysm in mitral valve prolapse. Am J Cardiol 66:235–237, 1990.
47. Morales AR, Romanelli R, Boucek RJ, Tate LG, Alvarez RT, Davis, JT. Myxoid heart disease: An assessment of extravalvular cardiac pathology in severe mitral valve prolapse. Hum Pathol 23:129–137, 1992.
48. Pellegrino MJ, Van Fossen D, Gordon C, Ryan JM, Waylonis GW. Prevalence of mitral valve prolapse in primary fibromyalgia: A pilot investigation. Arch Phys Med Rehab 70:541–543, 1989.

49. Toriello HV, Higgins JV, Malvitz T, Waterman DF. Two siblings with Tel Hashomer camptodactyly and mitral valve prolapse. Am J Med Genet 36:398–403, 1990.
50. Petrone RK, Klues HG, Panza JA, Peterson EE, Maron BJ. Coexistence of mitral valve prolapse in a consecutive group of 528 patients with hypertrophic cardiomyopathy assessed with echocardiography. J Am Coll Cardiol 20: 55–61, 1992.
51. Tuzcu EM, Moodie DS, Chambers JL, Keyser P, Hobbs RE. Congenital heart diseases associated with coronary artery anomalies. Cleveland Clin J Med 57:178–180, 1990.
52. Bowen J, Boudoulas H, Wooley CF. Cardiovascular disease of connective tissue origin. Am J Med 82:481–488, 1987.
53. Lebwohl MG, Distefano D, Prioleau PG, et al. Pseudoxanthoma elasticum and mitral valve prolapse. N Engl J Med 307:228–231, 1982.
54. Schwarz T, Gotsman MS. Mitral valve prolapse in osteogenesis imperfecta. Isr J Med Sci 17:1087–1088, 1981.
55. Loehr JP, Synhorst DP, Wolfe RR, et al. Aortic root dilatation and mitral valve prolapse in the fragile X syndrome. Am J Med Genet 23:189–194, 1986.
56. Leier C, Baker P, Kilman J, et al. Cardiovascular abnormalities associated with adult polycystic kidney disease. Ann Intern Med 100:683–688, 1984.
57. Donnelly TJ, Wooley CF, Boudoulas H. Mitral valve prolapse: Aortic dimensions may reflect a connective tissue disorder. Am J Noninvas Cardiol 5:47–51, 1991.
58. Leier CV, Call TD, Fulkerson PK, et al. The spectrum of cardiac defects in the Ehlers-Danlos syndrome, types I & III. Ann Int Med 92:171–178, 1980.
59. Jaffe AS, Geltman EM, Rodey GE, et al. Mitral valve prolapse: A consistent manifestation of type IV Ehlers-Danlos syndrome. Circulation 64:121–125, 1981.
60. Tayel S, Kurczynski TW, Levine M, et al. Marfanoid children. Etiologic heterogeneity and cardiac findings. Am J Dis Child 145:90–93, 1991.
61. Glesby MJ, Pyeritz RE. Association of mitral valve prolapse and systemic abnormalities of connective tissue: A phenotypic continuum. JAMA 262: 523–528, 1989.
62. Devereux RB, Brown WT, Lutas EM, et al. Association of mitral valve prolapse with low body weight and low blood pressure. Lancet 2:792–795, 1982.
63. Park JM, Varma SK. Pectus excavatum in children: Diagnostic significance for mitral valve prolapse. Indian J Pediatr 57:219–222, 1990.
64. Seliem MA, Duffy CE, Gidding SS, Berdusis K, Benson DW Jr. Echocardiographic evaluation of the aortic root and mitral valve in children and adolescents with isolated pectus excavatum: Comparison with Marfan patients. Pediatr Cardiol 13:20–23, 1992.
65. Kumar UK, Sahasranam KV. Mitral valve prolapse syndrome and associated thoracic skeletal abnormalities. J Assoc Physicians India 39:536–539, 1991.
66. Udoshi MB, Shah A, Fisher VJ, et al. Incidence of mitral valve prolapse in subjects with thoracic skeletal abnormalities: A prospective study. Am Heart J 97:303–311, 1979.
67. Salomon J, Shah PM, Heinle RA. Thoracic skeletal abnormalities in idiopathic mitral valve prolapse. Am J Cardiol 36:32–36, 1975.
68. Schutte JE, Gaffney FA, Blend L, et al. Distinctive anthropometric characteristics of women with mitral valve prolapse. Am J Med 71:533–538, 1981.
69. BonTempo CP, Ronan JA Jr, DeLeon AC Jr. Radiographic appearance of the

thorax in systolic click-late systolic murmur syndrome. Am J Cardiol 36:27–31, 1975.

70. Boudoulas H. Mitral valve prolapse: Serious or not? Hospital Med September, 34–62, 1992.

71. Boudoulas H, King BD, Wooley CF. Mitral valve prolapse: A marker for anxiety or overlapping phenomenon? Psychopathology 17:98–106, 1984.

72. Sorbo MD, Buja GF, Miorelli M, Nistri S, Perrone C, Manca S, Grasso F, et al. The prevalence of the Wolff-Parkinson-White syndrome in a population of 116,542 young males. G Ital Cardiol 25:681–687, 1995.

73. Horvath M. Association of hiatal hernia with mitral valve prolapse. Eur J Pediatr 156:35–36, 1997.

74. Pueschel SM, Werner JC. Mitral valve prolapse in persons with Down syndrome. Research in developmental disabilities 15:91–97, 1994.

75. Malkowski MT, Boudoulas H, Wooley CF, Guo R, Pearson AC. Abnormal elastic properties of the aorta in mitral valve prolapse. Circulation 92(Suppl I):I–357, 1995.

76. Ivy DD, Shaffer EM, Johnson AM, Kimberling WJ, Dobin A, Gabow PA. Cardiovascular abnormalities in children with autosomal dominant polycystic kidney disease. J Am Soc Nephrol 5:2032–2036, 1995.

77. Dhuper S, Ehlers KH, Fatica NS, Byridakis DJ, Klein AA, Friedman DM, Levine DB. Incidence and risk factors for mitral valve prolapse in severe adolescent idiopathic scoliosis. Pediatr Cardiol 18:425–428, 1997.

78. Cordas TA, Rossi EG, Grinberg M, et al. Mitral valve prolapse and panic disorder. Arq Bras Cardiol 56:139–142, 1991.

79. Raj A, Sheehan DV. Mitral valve prolapse and panic disorder. Bull Menninger Clin 54:199–208, 1990.

80. Wooley CF, Sparks EH, Hirata K, Boudoulas H. The aortapathy of heritable cardiovascular disease. In Boudoulas H, Toutouzas PK, Wooley CF (eds): Functional Abnormalities of the Aorta. Armonk, NY, Futura Publishing Co, 1996, pp 312–313.

81. Katerndahl DA. Panic and prolapse. Meta-analysis. J Nerv Ment Dis 11:539–544, 1993.

82. Bon Tempo CP, Ronan JA Jr, deLeon AC JR, Twigg HL. Radiographic appearance of the thorax in systolic click-late systolic murmur syndrome. Am J Cardiol 36:27–36, 1975.

83. Schutte JE, Gaffney FA, Blend L, Blomqvist CG. Distinctive anthropometric characteristics of women with mitral valve prolapse. Am J Med 71:533–538, 1981.

84. Rippe JM, Sloss LJ, Angoff G, Alpert JS. Mitral valve prolapse in adults with congenital heart disease. Am Heart J 97:561–573, 1979.

85. Rosenberg CA, Derman GH, Grabb WC, Buda AJ. Hypomastia and mitral valve prolapse. N Engl J Med 309:1230–1232, 1983.

86. Chandraratna PAN, Nimalasuriya A, Kawanishi D, Duncan P, Rosin B, Rahimtoola SH. Identification of the increased frequency of cardiovascular abnormalities associated with mitral valve prolapse by two-dimensional echocardiography. Am J Cardiol 54:1283–1285, 1984.

87. Lippman SM, Ginzton LE, Thigpen T, Tanaka KR, Laks MM. Mitral valve prolapse in sickle cell disease. Arch Int Med 145:435–438, 1985.

88. Swartz MH, Herman MV, Teichholz LE. Dermatoglyphic patterns in patients with mitral valve prolapse: A clue to pathogenesis. Am J Cardiol 38:58–92, 1976.

89. ZuWallack R, Sinatra S, Lahiri B, Godar TJ, Liss JP, Jeresaty RM. Pulmonary function studies in patients with prolapse of the mitral valve. Chest 7:17–20, 1979.

90. Devereux RB, Brown WT, Lutas EM, Kramer-Fox R, Laragh JH. Association of mitral valve prolapse with low bodyweight and low blood pressure. Lancet October 9:792–795, 1982.

91. McKay R, Yacoub M. Acute aortic dissection and medical degeneration in patients with 'floppy' mitral valves. Thorax 31:49–54, 1976.

92. Channick BJ, Spann JF. Hyperthyroidism and mitral valve prolapse. Primary Cardiol Oct:73–84, 1983.

93. Marks AD, Channick BJ, Adlin EV, Kessler RK, Braitman LE, Denenberg BS. Chronic thyroiditis and mitral valve prolapse. Ann Int Med 102:479–483, 1985.

94. Brauman A, Algom M, Gilboa Y, Ramot Y, Golik A, Stryjer D. Mitral valve prolapse in hyperthyroidism of two different origins. Br Heart J 53:374–377, 1985.

95. Handler CE, Child A, Light ND, Dorrance DE. Mitral valve prolapse, aortic compliance, and skin collagen in joint hypermobility syndrome. Br Heart J 54:501–508, 1985.

96. Lebwohl MG, Distefano D, Prioleau PG, Uram M, Yannuzzi LA, Fleischmajer R. Pseudoxanthoma elasticum and mitral valve prolapse. N Engl J Med 307:228–231, 1982.

97. DeSilva RA, Shubrooks SJ Jr. Mitral valve prolapse with atrioventricular and sinoatrial node abnormalities of long duration. Am Heart J 93:772–775, 1977.

98. Ware JA, Magro SA, luck JC, Mann DE, Nielsen AP, Rosen KM, Wyndham CRC. Conduction system abnormalities in symptomatic mitral valve prolapse: An electrophysiologic analysis of 60 patients. Am J Cardiol 53: 1075–1078, 1984.

99. Deliagin VM, Pil'kh AD, Bashenova LK. Echocardiographic study of the heart in children with mitral valve prolapse and connective tissue dysplasia. Pediatriia (1)52–58, 1990.

100. Suzuki K, Murakami Y, Mori K, Mimori S. Four boys with multiple floppy valves involving all cardiac valves and hyperextensive joints. J Cardiol 21:161–172, 1991.

101. Suzuki K, Murakami Y, Mori K, et al. Multiple floppy valves with all cardiac valves prolapsing: clinical course and treatment. Pediatr Cardiol 12:110–113, 1991.

102. Gooch AS, Maranhao V, Scampardonis G, Cha SD, Yang SS. Prolapse of both mitral and tricuspid leaflets in systolic murmur-click syndrome. N Engl J Med 24:1218–1222, 1972.

103. Kasper W, Meinertz T, Weber T, Geibel A, Just H. Incidence of tricuspid valve prolapse. Z Kardiol 80:333–337, 1991.

104. Allen HD. Mitral valve prolapse: Back to the basics. AJDC 145:1095–1096, 1991.

105. Cooper MJ, Abinader EG. Family history in assessing the risk for progression of mitral valve prolapse: Report of a kindred. Am J Dis Child 135(7):647–649, 1981.

106. Zuppiroli A, Roman MJ, O'Grady M, Devereux RB. A family study of anterior mitral leaflet thickness and mitral valve prolapse. Am J Cardiol 82:823–826, 1998.

107. Rodriguez Y, Petersen F, Villarreal A, Esquirel J, Reyes PA. Caracteristicas clinicas en el prolapso valvular mitral idiopatico. Arch Inst Cardiol Mex 61:587–591, 1991.

108. Hirata K, Triposkiadis F, Sparks E, Bowen J, Boudoulas H, Wooley CF. The Marfan syndrome: Cardiovascular physical findings and diagnostic correlates. Am Heart J 123:743–752, 1992.
109. Barlow JB, Pocock WA. Mitral leaflet billowing and prolapse. In: Barlow JB (ed): Perspectives on the Mitral Valve. Philadelphia, FA Davis Company, 1987, pp 45–112.
110. Fontana ME, Sparks EA, Boudoulas H, Wooley CF. Mitral valve prolapse and the mitral valve prolapse syndrome. Curr Probl Cardiol 16:311–375, 1991.
111. Fontana ME, Pence HL, Leighton R, et al. The varying clinical spectrum of the systolic click-late systolic murmur syndrome. Circulation 41:807–816, 1970.
112. Mathey DG, Decoodt PR, Allen HN, et al. The determinants of mitral valve prolapse in the systolic click-late systolic murmur syndrome. Circulation 53:872–878, 1976.
113. Akasaka T, Yoshikawa J, Yoshida K, Yamaura Y, Hozumi T. Temporal resolution of mitral regurgitation in patients with mitral valve prolapse: A phonocardiographic and Doppler echocardiographic study. J Am Coll Cardiol 13:1053–1061, 1989.
114. Tofler OB, Tofler GH. Use of auscultation to follow patients with mitral systolic clicks and murmurs. Am J Cardiol 66:1355–1358, 1990.
115. Criley JM, Lewis KB, Humphries J O'N, et al. Prolapse of the mitral valve: Clinical and cine-angiocardiographic findings. Br Heart J 28:488–496, 1986.
116. Schon HR, Schroter G, Barthel P, Schomig A. Quinapril therapy in patients with chronic mitral regurgitation. J Heart Valve Dis 3:303–312, 1994.
117. Rokicki W, Krzystolik-Ladzinska J, Goc B. Clinical characteristics of primary mitral valve prolapse syndrome in children. Acta Cardiologica 1:147–153, 1995.
118. Barlow JB, Pocock WA, Marchand P, Denny M. The significance of late systolic murmurs. Am Heart J 66:443–452, 1963.
119. Tei C, Shah PM, Cherian G, Wong M, Ormiston JA. The correlates of an abnormal first heart sound in mitral valve prolapse syndromes. N Engl J Med 307:334–339, 1982.
120. Mathey DG, Decoodt PR, Allen HN, Swan HJC. The determinants of onset of mitral valve prolapse in the systolic click-late systolic murmur syndrome. Circulation 53:872–878, 1976.
121. Criley JM, Kissel GL. Prolapse of the mitral valve: The click and late systolic murmur syndrome. Progr Cardiovasc Dis 4:23–36, 1975.
122. Yokota Y, Kumaki T, Miki T, Fukuzaki H. Clinical and exercise echocardiographic findings in patients with mitral valve prolapse. Jpn Circ J 54:62–70, 1990.
123. Nutter DO, Wickliffe C, Gilbert CA, Moody C, King SB III. The pathophysiology of idiopathic mitral valve prolapse. Circulation 52:297–309, 1975.
124. Fontana ME, Wooley CR, Leighton RF, et al. Postural changes in left ventricular and mitral valvular dynamics in the systolic click-late systolic murmur syndrome. Circulation 51:165–173, 1975.
125. Winkle RA, Goodman DJ, Popp RL. Simultaneous echocardiographic-phonocardiographic recordings at rest and during amyl nitrite administration in patients with mitral valve prolapse. Circulation 51:522–529, 1976.
126. Sukumaran TU, Manjooran RJ, Thomas K. A clinical profile of mitral valve prolapse syndrome. Indian J Pediatr 57:771–773, 1990.
127. Olive KE, Grassman ED. Mitral valve prolapse: Comparison of diagnosis by physical examination and echocardiography. South Med J 83:1266–1269, 1990.
128. Jeresaty RM. Mitral valve prolapse. JAMA 254:793–795, 1985.

129. Engle MA. The syndrome of apical systolic click, late systolic murmur, and abnormal T waves. Circulation 39:1–5, 1969.
130. Boudoulas H, Schaal SF, Wooley CF. Floppy mitral valve/mitral valve prolapse: Cardiac arrhythmias. In Cardiac Arrhythmias, Pacing, and Electrophysiology. Vardas PE (ed): Great Britain, Kluwer Academic Publisher, 1998, pp 89–95.
131. Boudoulas H, Schaal SF, Stang JM, et al. Mitral valve prolapse: Cardiac arrest with long-term survival. Int J Cardiol 26:37–44, 1990.
132. Swartz MH, Teichholz LE, Donoso E. Mitral valve prolapse: A review of associated arrhythmias. Am J Med 62:377–389, 1977.
133. Campbell RWF, Godman MG, Fiddler GI, Marquis RM, Julian DG. Ventricular arrhythmias in syndrome of balloon deformity of mitral valve. Definition of possible high risk group. Br Heart J 38:1053–1057, 1976.
134. Grayburn PA, Berk MVR, Spain MG, Harrison MVR, Smith MD, DeMaria AN. Relation of echocardiographic morphology of the mitral apparatus to mitral regurgitation in mitral valve prolapse: Assessment by Doppler color flow imaging. Am Heart J 119:1095–1102, 1990.
135. Levine RA, Handschumacher MD, Sanfilippo AJ, et al. Three-dimensional echocardiographic reconstruction of the mitral valve, with implications for the diagnosis of mitral valve prolapse. Circulation 80:589–598, 1989.
136. ACC/AHA Task Force Report. ACC/AHA Guidelines for the Management of Patients with Valvular Heart Disease. A Report of the American College of Cardiology/American Heart Association Task Force on Practice Guidelines (Committee on Management of Patients with Valvular Heart Disease). JACC 32:1486–1588, 1998.
137. Sanfilippo AJ, Weyman AE, Levine RA. The problem of echocardiographic detection of mitral valve prolapse and determination of its true prevalence. Herz 13:284–292, 1988.
138. Panidis IP, McAllister M, Ross J, et al. Prevalence and severity of mitral regurgitation in the mitral valve prolapse syndrome: A Doppler echocardiographic study of 80 patients. J Am Coll Cardiol 7:975–981, 1986.
139. You-Bing D, Takenaka K, Sakamonto T, et al. Follow-up in mitral valve prolapse by phonocardiography, M-mode and two-dimensional echocardiography and Doppler echocardiography. Am J Cardiol 65:349–354, 1990.
140. Deliagin VM, Pil'kh AD, Bazhenova LK. Echocardiographic study of the heart in children. Pediatrica (1):52–58, 1990.
141. Tokuyama, A. Continuity from normal to prolapsed mitral valves: Two-dimensional and color Doppler echocardiographic investigations. J Cardiol 21:403–413, 1991.
142. Salustri A, Becker AE, van Herwerden L, Vletter WB, Ten Cate FJ, Roelandt JR. Three-dimensional echocardiography of normal and pathologic mitral valve: A comparison with two-dimensional transesophageal echocardiography. J Am Coll Cardiol 27:1502–1510, 1996.
143. Shah PM, Pravin M. Update of mitral valve prolapse syndrome: When is echo prolapse a pathological prolapse? Echocardiography 1:87–95, 1984.
144. Garcia-Fernandez MA, Grana N, Blanco E, Banuelos F. Two-dimensional echocardiography and Doppler findings in mitral valve prolapse: Evaluation of causes of mitral insufficiency. J Cardiovasc Ultrasonogr 3:339–344, 1984.
145. Come PC, Riley MF, Carl LV, Nakao S. Pulsed Doppler echocardiographic evaluation of valvular regurgitation in patients with mitral valve prolapse: Comparison with normal subjects. J Am Coll Cardiol 8:1355–1364, 1986.

146. Weiss AN, Mimbs JW, Ludbrook PA, Sobel BE. Echocardiographic detection of mitral valve prolapse: Exclusion of false-positive diagnosis and determination of inheritance. Circulation 52:1091–1096, 1975.
147. Yamamoto M, Fukuda N, Asai M, et al. Phase analysis of mitral regurgitation in mitral valve prolapse: Comparison of pulsed Doppler echocardiography with phonocardiography. J Cardiogr 13:467–481, 1983.
148. Gutgesell HP, Bricker JT, Colvin EV, Latson LA, Hawkins EP. Atrioventricular valve anular diameter: Two-dimensional echocardiographic-autopsy correlation. Am J Cardiol 53:1652–1655, 1984.
149. Devereux RB, Kramer-Fox R, Brown WT, et al. Relation between clinical features of the mitral prolapse syndrome and echocardiographically documented mitral valve prolapse. J Am Coll Cardiol 8:763–772, 1986.
150. Hozumi T, Yoshikawa J, Yoshida K, Akasaka T, Takagi T, Yamamuro A. Assessment of flail mitral leaflets by dynamic three-dimensional echocardiographic imaging. Am J Cardiol 79:223–224, 1996.
151. Winkle RA, Goodman DJ, Popp RL. Simultaneous echocardiographic-phonocardiographic recordings at rest and during amyl nitrite administration in patients with mitral valve prolapse. Circulation 51:522, 1973.
152. Hung J, Otsuki Y, Handschumacher MD, Schwammenthal E, Levine RA. Mechanism of dynamic regurgitant orifice area variation in functional mitral regurgitation: Physiologic insights from the Proximal Flow Convergence Technique. J Am Coll Cardiol 33:538–545, 1999.
153. Scampardonis G, Yang SS, Maranhao V, Goldberg H, Gooch AS. Left ventricular abnormalities in prolapsed mitral leaflet syndrome. Review of eighty-seven cases. Circulation 48:287–297, 1973.
154. Cipriano PR, Kline SA, Baltaxe HA. An angiographic assessment of left ventricular function in isolated mitral valvular prolapse. Invest Radiol 15:293–298, 1980.
155. Cobbs BW Jr, King SB III. Ventricular buckling: A factor in the abnormal ventriculogram and peculiar hemodynamics associated with mitral valve prolapse. Am Heart J 93:741–758, 1977.
156. Ranganathan N, Silver MD. Idiopathic prolapsed mitral leaflet syndrome: Angiographic-clinical correlations. Circulation 54:707–723, 1976.
157. Tebbe U, Schicha H, Neumann P, Voth E, Emrich D, Neuhaus KL, Kreuzer H. Mitral valve prolapse in the ventriculogram: Scintigraphic, electrocardiographic, and hemodynamic abnormalities. Clin Cardiol 8:341–347, 1985.
158. Bennell DJ. The contribution of MRI in the evaluation of cardiac function. ACC Current J Review May/June 1999, 70–72.
159. Dobmeyer DJ, Stine RA, Leier CV, Schaal SF. Electrophysiologic mechanisms of provoked atrial flutter in mitral valve prolapse syndrome. Am J Cardiol 56:602–604, 1985.
160. Boudoulas H, Geleris P, Schaal SF, Leier CV, Lewis RP. Comparison between electrophysiologic studies and ambulatory monitoring in patients with syncope. J Electrocardiol 16:91–96, 1983.
161. Lachman AS, Bramwell-Jones DM, Lakier JB, et al. Infective endocarditis in the billowing mitral leaflet syndrome. Br Heart J 37:236–330 1975.
162. Kincaid DT, Botti RE. Subacute bacterial endocarditis in a patient with isolated, nonejection systolic click but without a murmur. Chest 66:88–89, 1974.
163. LeBauer EJ, Perloff JK, Keliher TF. The isolated click with bacterial endocarditis. Am Heart J 73(4):534–537, 1967.
164. Danchin N, Briancon S, Mathieu P, et al. Mitral valve prolapse as a risk factor for infective endocarditis. Lancet April:743–745, 1989.

165. Sandor GK, Vasilakos SS, Vasilakos JS. Mitral valve prolapse: A review of the syndrome with emphasis on current antibiotic prophylaxis. J Can Dent Assoc 57:321–325, 1991.

166. MacMahon SW, Hickey AJ, Wilcken DEL, et al. Risk of infective endocarditis in mitral valve prolapse with and without precordial systolic murmurs. Am J Cardiol 59:105–108, 1987.

167. Lachman AS, Bramwell-Jones DM, Lakier JB, Pocock WA, Barlow JB. Infective endocarditis in the billowing mitral leaflet syndrome. Br Heart J 37:326–330, 1975.

168. Ringer M, Feen DJ, Drapkin MS. Mitral valve prolapse: Jet stream causing mural endocarditis. Am J Cardiol 45:383–385, 1980.

169. Strom BL, Abrutyn E, Berlin JA, Kinman JL, Feldman RS, Stolley PD, Levison ME, et al. Dental and cardiac risk factors for infective endocarditis: A population-based, case-control study. Ann Intern Med 129:761–769, 1998.

170. Barnett HJM, Jones MW, Boughner DR, et al. Cerebral ischemic events associated with prolapsing mitral valve. Arch Neurol 33:777–782, 1976.

171. Boughner DR, Barnett HJM. The enigma of the risk of stroke in mitral valve prolapse. Stroke 16:175–177, 1985.

172. Barletta GA, Gagliardi R, Benvenuti L, Fantini F. Cerebral ischemic attacks as a complication of aortic and mitral valve prolapse. Stroke 16:219–223, 1985.

173. Jones HH Jr, Nagger CZ, Seljan MP, et al. floppy mitral valve, mitral valve prolapse and cerebral ischemic events. Stroke 13:451–456, 1982.

174. Steele P, Weily H, Rainwater J, et al. Platelet survival time and thromboembolism in patients with mitral valve prolapse. Circulation 60:43–47, 1979.

175. Zuppiroli A, Cecchi F, Ciaccheri M, et al. Platelet function and coagulation studies in patients with mitral valve prolapse. Clin Cardiol 9:487–492, 1986.

176. Walsh PN, Kansu TA, Corbett JJ. Platelets, thromboembolism and mitral valve prolapse. Circulation 63:552–559, 1981.

177. Elam MB, Viar MJ, Ratts TE, Chesney CM. Mitral valve prolapse in women with oral contraceptive-related cerebrovascular insufficiency. Arch Int Med 146:73–77, 1986.

178. Boughner Dr. Mitral valve prolapse as a cause of transient ischemic attack and stroke. Practical Cardiol 8:143–149, 1982.

179. Boudoulas H, Nelson SD, Schaal SF, Lewis RP. Diagnosis and management of syncope. In Alexander RW, Schlant RC, Fuster V, O'Rourke RA, Roberts R, Sonnenblick EH (eds): Hurst's The Heart, 9th ed, New York, McGraw-Hill, 1988, pp 1059–1080.

180. Wei JY, Bulkey BH, Schaeffer AH, et al. Mitral valve prolapse syndrome and recurrent ventricular tachyarrhythmias: A malignant variant refractory to conventional drug therapy. Ann Int Med 89:6–9, 1978.

181. Babuty D, Cosnay P, Breuillac JC, Charniot JC, Delhomme C, Fauchier L, Fauchier JP. Ventricular arrhythmia factors in mitral valve prolapse. Pacing Clin Electrophysiol 6:1090–1099, 1994.

182. Kavey REW, Blackman MS, Sondheimer HM, Byrum CJ. Ventricular arrhythmias and mitral valve prolapse in childhood. J Pediatr 105:885–890, 1984.

183. Berry FA, Lake CL, Johns RA, Rogers BM. Mitral valve prolapse: Another cause of intraoperative dysrhythmias in the pediatric patient. Anesthesiology 62:662–664, 1985.

184. Bobkowski W, Siwinska A, Gorzna H, Niedbalski R, Paluszak W, Maciejewski J. Dysrhythmias documented by 48-hour electrocardiographic monitoring in children with mitral valve prolapse. Pediatr Pol 71:493–497, 1996.

185. Nowak A, Czerwionka-Szaflarska M. Arrhythmias in children with mitral valve prolapse syndrome. Pediatr Pol 71:499–504, 1996.
186. Ritchie J, Hammermeister KE, Kennedy JW. Refractory ventricular tachycardia and fibrillation in a patient with the prolapsing mitral leaflet syndrome: Successful control with overdrive pacing. Am J Cardiol 37:314–316, 1976.
187. Winkle RA, Lopes MG, Popp RL, Hancock EW. Life-threatening arrhythmias in the mitral valve prolapse syndrome. Am J Med 60:961–967, 1976.
188. LaVecchia L, Centofante P, Varotto L, et al. Arrhythmic profile, ventricular function, and histomorphometric findings in patients with idiopathic ventricular tachycardia and mitral valve prolapse: Clinical and prognostic evaluation. Clin Cardiol 21:731–735, 1998.
189. Sanfilippo AJ, Harrigan P, Popvic AD, et al. Papillary muscle tension in mitral valve prolapse: Quantitation by two-dimensional echocardiography. J Am Coll Cardiol 19:564–571, 1992.
190. Franz MR, Cima R, Wang D, Proffit D, Kuntz R. Electrophysiological effects of myocardial stretch and mechanical determinants of stretch-activated arrhythmias. Circulation 86:968–978, 1992.
191. Farb A, Tang AL, Atkinson JB, McCarthy WF, Virmani R. Comparison of cardiac findings in patients with mitral valve prolapse who die suddenly to those who have congestive heart failure from mitral regurgitation and to those with fatal noncardiac conditions. Am J Cardiol 70:234–239, 1992.
192. Dollar AL, Roberts WC. Morphologic comparison of patients with mitral valve prolapse who died suddenly with patients who died from severe valvular dysfunction or other conditions. J Am Coll Cardiol 17:921–931, 1991.
193. Chesler E, King RA, Edwards JE. The myxomatous mitral valve and sudden death. Circulation 67:632–639, 1983.
194. Marron K, Yacoub MH, Polak JM, et al. Innervation of human atrioventricular and arterial valves. Circulation 94:36–75, 1996.
195. Boudoulas H, Reynolds JC, Mazzaferri E, et al. Metabolic studies in mitral valve prolapse syndrome. Circulation 61:1200–1205, 1980.
196. Gaffney FA, Bastian BC, Lane LB, et al. Abnormal cardiovascular regulation in the mitral valve prolapse syndrome. Am J Cardiol 52:316–320, 1983.
197. Coghlan HC, Phares P, Crowley M, et al. Dysautonomia in mitral valve prolapse. Am J Med 67:236–244, 1979.
198. Davies AO, Su CJ, Balasubramanyam A, Codina J, Birnbaumer L. Abnormal guanine nucleotide regulatory protein in FMV/MVP dysautonomia: Evidence from reconstitution of Gs. J Clin Endocrinol Metab 72:867–875, 1991.
199. Balasubramanyam A, Davies AO, Codina J, Birnbaumer L. Abnormal Gs function in mitral valve prolapse dysautonomia is not associated with abnormal alpha S cDNA sequence. Life Sci 48:789–793, 1991.
200. Whinnery FE. Acceleration tolerance of asymptomatic aircrew with mitral valve prolapse. Aviat Space Environ Med October:986–992, 1986.
201. Davies AO, Mares A, Pool JL, et al. Mitral valve prolapse with symptoms of β-adrenergic hypersensitivity: β-Adrenergic receptor supercoupling with desensitization of isoproterenol exposure. Am J Med 82:193–201, 1987.
202. Gaffney AF, Karlsson ES, Campbell W, et al. Autonomic dysfunction in women with mitral valve prolapse syndrome. Circulation 59:894–901, 1979.
203. Anwar A, Kohn SR, Dunn JF, et al. Altered β-adrenergic receptor function in subjects with symptomatic mitral valve prolapse. Am J Med Sci 302:9–97, 1991.

204. Zdrojewski TR, Wyrzykowski B, Krupa-Wojciechowska B. Renin-aldosterone regulation during upright posture in young men with mitral valve prolapse syndrome. J Heart Valve Dis 4:236–241, 1995.

205. Zdrojewski TR, Purzycki Z, Rynkiewicz A, Kubasik A, Wyrzykowski B, Krupa-Wojciechowska B. QT/QS2 ratio in mitral valve prolapse syndrome, hyperthyroidism and borderline hypertension: Possible indication of dysautonomia. Am J Noninvas Cardiol 7:19–22, 1993.

206. Bashore TM, Grines C, Utlak D, Boudoulas H, Wooley CF. Postural exercise abnormalities in symptomatic patients with mitral valve prolapse. J Am Coll Cardiol 11:499–507, 1988.

207. Santos AD, Mathew PK, Hilal H. Orthostatic hypotension: A commonly unrecognized cause of symptoms in mitral valve prolapse. Am J Med 71:746–750, 1981.

208. Bisset GS III, Schwartz DC, Meyer RA, et al. Clinical spectrum and long-term follow-up of isolated mitral valve prolapse in 119 children. Circulation 62:423–429, 1980.

209. Nishimura RA, McGoon MD, Shub C, et al. Echocardiographically documented mitral valve prolapse: Long-term follow-up of 237 patients. N Engl J Med 313:1305–1309, 1985.

210. Wilcken DEL, Hickey AJ. Lifetime risk for patients with mitral valve prolapse of developing severe valve regurgitation requiring surgery. Circulation 78:10–14, 1988.

211. Duren DR, Beeker AE, Dunning AJ. Long-term follow-up of idiopathic mitral valve prolapse in 300 patients: A prospective study. J Am Coll Cardiol 11:42–47, 1988.

212. Kolibash AJ, Kilman JW, Bush CA, et al. Evidence for progression from mild to severe mitral regurgitation in mitral valve prolapse. Am J Cardiol 58:762–767, 1986.

213. Marks AR, Choong CY, Chir MBB, et al. Identification of high-risk and low-risk subgroups of patients with mitral valve prolapse. N Engl J Med 320:1031–1036, 1989.

214. Enriquez-Sarano M, Tajik AJ. Natural history of mitral regurgitation due to flail leaflets. Eur Heart J 18:705–707, 1997.

215. Boudoulas H, Boudoulas D, Sparks EA, Pearson AC, Nagaraja HN, Wooley CF. Left atrial performance indices in chronic mitral valve disease. J Heart Valve Dis 4(Suppl 2):S242–247, 1995.

216. Mills P, Rose J, Hollingsworth J, Amara I, Craige E. Long-term prognosis of mitral valve prolapse. N Engl J Med 297:13–21, 1977.

217. Wilcken DEL, Hickey AJ. The lifetime risk of mitral valve prolapse subjects developing severe mitral regurgitation. Circulation 74(Suppl 2):453, 1986.

218. Ronan JA, Steelman RB, DeLeon AC Jr, Waters TJ, Perloff JK, Harvey WP. The clinical diagnosis of acute severe mitral insufficiency. Am J Cardiol 27:284–90, 1971.

219. Roberts WC, Braunwald E. Acute severe mitral regurgitation secondary to ruptured chordae tendineae. Circulation 33:58–70, 1966.

220. Jeresaty RM, Edwards JE, Chawla SK. Mitral valve prolapse and ruptured chordae tendineae. Am J Cardiol 55:138–142, 1985.

221. Salisbury PF, Cross CE, Rieben PA. Chorda tendinea tension. Am J Physiol 205(2):385–392, 1963.

222. Dajani AS, Taubert KA, Wilson W, et al. Prevention of bacterial endocarditis: Recommendations by the American Heart Association. JAMA 277:1794–1801, 1997.

223. Dental and cardiac risk factors for infective endocarditis. A population-based, case-control study. Ann Intern Med 129:761–769, 1998.
224. Hickey AJ, MacMahon SW, Wilcken DE. Mitral valve prolapse and bacterial endocarditis: When is antibiotic prophylaxis necessary? Am Heart J 109:431–435, 1985.
225. Normand J, Bozio A, Etienne J, Sassolas F, Le Bris H. Changing patterns and prognosis of infective endocarditis in childhood. Eur Heart J 16(Suppl B):28–31, 1995.
226. Delahaya F, et al. Infective endocarditis: Results of a French study suggest a lack of compliance with management guidelines. J Am Coll Cardiol 33:788–793, 1999.
227. Clemens JD, Horwitz RI, Jaffe CC, et al. A controlled evaluation of the risk of bacterial endocarditis in persons with mitral valve prolapse. N Engl J Med 397(13):776–781, 1982.
228. Host U, Kelbaek H, Hildebrandt P, Skagen K, Aldershvile J. Effect of ramipril on mitral regurgitation secondary to mitral valve prolapse. Am J Cardiol 80:655–658, 1997.
229. Cohn LH. Surgery for mitral regurgitation. JAMA 260:2883–2887, 1988.
230. Oda T. Handgrip-induced reduction in left ventricular ejection fraction and contractility in pediatric patients with mitral valve prolapse syndrome as evaluated by relation of fiber shortening velocity to end-systolic wall stress. Am J Noninvas Cardiol 6:168–172, 1992.
231. Krishnan US, Welton M, Gersony MD, Berman-Rosenzweig E, Apfel HD. Late left ventricular function after surgery for children with chronic symptomatic mitral regurgitation. Circulation 96:4280–4285, 1997.
232. Stoddard MF, Prince CR, Dillon S, Longaker RA, Morris GT, Liddell NE. Exercise-induced mitral regurgitation is a predictor of morbid events in subjects with mitral valve prolapse. J Am Coll Cardiol 25:693–699, 1995.
233. Cohn LH, Couper GS, Aranki SF, Rizzo RJ, Kinchla NM, Collins JJ Jr. Long-term results of mitral valve reconstruction for regurgitation of the myxomatous mitral valve. J Thorac Cardiovasc Surg 107:143–150, 1994.
234. Skoularigis J, Sinovich V, Joubert G, Sareli P. Evaluation of the long-term results of mitral valve repair in 254 young patients with rheumatic mitral regurgitation. Circulation 90:II167–174, 1994.
235. Lee EM, Shapiro LM, Wells FC. Superiority of mitral valve repair in surgery for degenerative mitral regurgitation. Eur Heart J 1:655–663, 1997.
236. Enriquez-Sarano M, Schaff HV, Frye RL. Early surgery for mitral regurgitation. The advantages of youth. Circulation 96:4121–4123, 1997.
237. Gottdiener JS, Borer JS, Bacharach SL, Green MV, Epstein SE. Left ventricular function in mitral valve prolapse: Assessment with radionuclide cineangiography. Am J Cardiol 47:7–19, 1981.
238. Gaffney FA, Wohl AJ, Blomqvist CG, Parkey RW, Willerson JT. Thallium-201 myocardial perfusion studies in patients with the mitral valve prolapse syndrome. Am J Med 64:21–26, 1978.
239. Kuruma T, Nagashima R, Maruyama T, Kaji Y, Kanaya S, Fujino T. Effects of exercise on mitral regurgitation in healthy subjects. J Cardiol 27(Suppl II):51–55, 1996.
240. Tischler MD, Battle RW, Ashikaga T, Niggel J, Rowen M, LeWinter MM. Effects of exercise on left ventricular performance determined by echocardiography in chronic, severe mitral regurgitation secondary to mitral valve prolapse. Am J Cardiol 77(5):397–402, 1996.
241. Hermann DD, Greenberg BH. Vasodilator therapy in left heart valvular regurgitation. ACC Current J Rev 27–29, January/February 1998.

Part VIII

Floppy Mitral Valve:
Surface Complications

Introduction

The Floppy Mitral Valve, Mitral Valve Prolapse, Mitral Valvular Regurgitation:
Infective Endocarditis

Charles F. Wooley, MD, Harisios Boudoulas, MD, PhD

> *The possibility of infective endocarditis should be considered in any cardiac patient who becomes mysteriously unwell, develops heart failure, arrhythmia, heart block, or, most obvious of all, a new cardiac murmur.*
> —JF Goodwin, 1985[1]

Infective endocarditis has an old and honorable lineage as a classic disease, rich with eponyms derived from descriptions by famous personages in the remote past. Certain time-honored pathological and clinical observations have roots in the 19th and early 20th centuries when the disease was debilitating, incurable, and uniformly fatal. Although the 21st century version of infective endocarditis shares certain characteristics with the classic form of the disease, the substantive changes in all facets of the disease process—etiology, pathogenesis, diagnosis and management—are such that clinicians must continually reexamine the basic tenets of the modern versions of the disease.

Infective endocarditis is also a disease that cuts across specialty lines, through the basic sciences, dental sciences, and the clinical sciences including internal medicine, infectious disease, cardiovascular disease, and cardiovascular surgery. The medical literature dealing with infective en-

From: Boudoulas H, Wooley CF. *Mitral Valve: Floppy Mitral Valve, Mitral Valve Prolapse, Mitral Valvular Regurgitation.* Second revised edition. ©Futura Publishing Company, Armonk, NY, 2000.

docarditis reflects this diversity, and, as a result, is not as sharply focused as the literature dealing with clinical entities that fit neatly into specific specialty disease categories.

Several themes run through the infective endocarditis literature during the past two decades. Guidelines have been established for the management of patients with valvular heart disease, the more precise diagnosis of infective endocarditis, and for antibiotic prophylaxis for cardiac patients at risk. Major innovations in diagnosis and therapy include the appropriate use of imaging technology in the diagnosis of infective endocarditis, and the surgical approach to valve destruction resulting from prior, ongoing, or acute valvular infection. And yet there are fundamental gaps between these insights and the translation to clinical practice.

Patients with cardiac disease, even those who are well informed, face significant obstacles understanding and applying the various guidelines and recommendations. Clinicians also face hurdles in the application of the conventional wisdom about infective endocarditis to clinical practice. The entire issue of antibiotic prophylaxis to prevent infective endocarditis is necessarily imprecise, given the magnitude of the population at risk and the uncertainties about pathogenesis of the disease. Once established, the prognosis of the disease remains severe despite the medical and surgical advances.

Infective endocarditis is a great mimic. Patients present with a variety of symptoms, and diagnosis requires careful assessment by a thinking clinician. An inadequate initial clinical evaluation and the failure to consider infective endocarditis as a primary diagnosis frequently delay diagnosis. Failure to use blood cultures in cardiac patients with fever, or who are unwell, or the use of inappropriate antibiotic therapy prior to establishing a precise diagnosis are common mistakes in this patient population.

Most patients with uniformly fatal diseases receive their care under the supervision of qualified specialists who deal with the specific disorder. However, infective endocarditis patients are not handled in a uniform manner in many hospitals, and the mode of clinical management or supervision may not always be in the patient's best interests. Infective endocarditis is a malignant disease that requires specialty care involving cardiology, infectious disease, microbiology, and cardiovascular surgery.

Surprisingly, there are few data dealing with critical appraisal of the quality of management of patients with infective endocarditis. A detailed report from Delahaye et al.[2] is a humbling profile listing multiple inadequacies and compliance failures, emphasizing that the gaps noted above may instead be chasms. Their suggestions include increased individual patient responsibility, including carrying a prophylaxis card, similar to what is done with surveillance of anticoagulant treatment, advising patients at risk to go for blood cultures when fever lasts for more than 3 days without having to consult with their physician.

Turning from these general considerations about infective endocarditis, let us consider the patients with the FMV/MVP/MVR triad, the basis for FMV surface complications, and the infective endocarditis interface.[3] Our basic premise is that patients with the FMV are at increased risk for infective endocarditis by virtue of the particular properties of the FMV described in Chapter 13.

Simply stated, patients with FMVs should receive infective endocarditis prophylaxis. This posture is similar to the recommendations for patients with a bicuspid aortic valve, ventricular septal defect, or persistent ductus arteriosus. The controversies in the earlier literature about MVP and infective endocarditis prophylaxis recommendations are a carryover from the era when "prolapse" was dissociated from the FMV diagnosis, a topic discussed at length earlier in the text. Precision in the diagnosis of the FMV obviates most of the earlier controversy.

The selection of appropriate antibiotic coverage is well documented in the recommendations based on the type of procedure being contemplated and the presumed source and nature of the bacteremia.

Our respected colleague in the Department of Internal Medicine, Susan L. Koletar, MD, provides her perspectives from the infectious disease viewpoint in the following chapter.

References

1. Goodwin JF. The challenge and the reproach of infective endocarditis. Br Heart J 54:115–118, 1985.
2. Delahaye F, Rial MO, Gevigney G, Ecochard R, Delaye JA. Critical appraisal of the quality of the management of infective endocarditis. J Am Coll Cardiol 33:788–793, 1999.
3. Eykyn SJ. Infective endocarditis: Some popular tenets debunked? Heart 77:191–193, 1997.

14

Mitral Valve Prolapse and Infective Endocarditis

Susan L. Koletar, MD

Introduction

The association between infective endocarditis (IE) and mitral valve prolapse (MVP) has been the subject of controversy and investigation since MVP was first described. In the initial report that angiographically linked late systolic murmurs (often associated with mid-systolic clicks) to mitral insufficiency, Barlow et al. prophetically suggested that such patients "should be regarded as potential candidates for subacute bacterial endocarditis."[1] Since then, much attention has been directed toward determining whether the relationship between infective endocarditis and MVP is more than coincidental. This chapter will review the epidemiology, clinical and pathological manifestations, diagnosis and management, and prophylaxis recommendations for IE and the prolapsed mitral valve.

Epidemiology

Mitral valve prolapse is a common finding in the general adult population with prevalence estimates of 4–22%.[2–12] The wide range reflects variations in the criteria used to define MVP (i.e., clinical, echocardiographic, or pathological specimens) and on the composition of the study population. These same factors also bias the interpretation of IE data in

From: Boudoulas H, Wooley CF. *Mitral Valve: Floppy Mitral Valve, Mitral Valve Prolapse, Mitral Valvular Regurgitation.* Second revised edition. ©Futura Publishing Company, Armonk, NY, 2000.

MVP. A brief review of the age and sex distribution of MVP helps place IE in MVP in better perspective.

In younger age groups (<40 years old) who are evaluated by clinical and echocardiographic means, the preponderance of subjects with documented MVP is female.[2–5,10,13] When similar methods are applied to older populations (>60 years), this male to female ratio becomes more equal,[14–16] or reverses to a male predominance.[17,18] One of the best summaries of this epidemiological trend continues to be the Framingham study;s6 of MVP (Fig. 1A). There was: (1) an overall prevalence of MVP of 5%; (2) a noted female predominance of 17% in the second decade that markedly declined with age; (3) a prevalence of MVP of <5% in males, that was similar in all age groups; and (4) a slightly greater percentage of males versus females in the >80-year old group.

Using pathological (either surgical or autopsy) specimens to define MVP[19–23] further substantiated the male preponderance in older age groups. The potential implication of these findings is that this subset may have more complications, thus allowing for pathological evaluation.

In contrast to the relatively common occurrence of MVP, the incidence of IE overall is seemingly low. For example, a baseline age- and sex-adjusted incidence rate of 4.9 cases/100,000 person-years has been reported in two population-based cohorts.[24] More recently reported incidences of IE have varied from 1.3 cases/100 person-years in HIV-in-

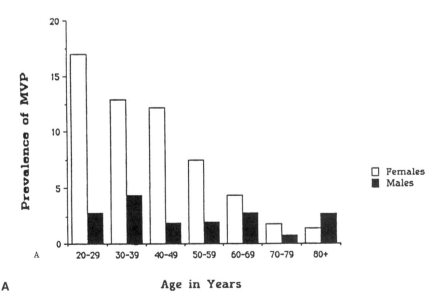

A

Age in Years

Figure 1. A. Prevalence of MVP by age and sex in the Framingham study.[6]

fected injecting-drug users[25] to 5.9/100,000 persons per year in a 5-year prospective study in an urban population in Sweden.[26] As with defining MVP, the variability of the incidence statistics depends on the composition of the study population (e.g., injecting drug use, native versus prosthetic valves, community versus nosocomially acquired) and the criteria used to define the disease. Until recently, it was the latter factor that had the most significant impact on assessing the true incidence of IE. The very strict case definition of IE proposed by von Reyn et al .in 1981,[27] categorized as few as 20% of clinically diagnosed cases as "definite" because pathological specimens were required for confirmation. In 1994, a group of investigators at Duke University proposed a new strategy that allowed for the categorization of definite cases of IE based on the presence of defined clinical and echocardiographic findings.[28] The validity of the "Duke criteria" has subsequently been demonstrated.[29–34] Consequently, it is impractical to compare historical incidence data with current trends. A noteworthy epidemiological characteristic pertinent to infection in MVP, however, is the increased risk that has been documented in older age groups, with a significant gender bias toward males.[24,35,36]

The probability of developing IE as a complication of MVP is, therefore, a function of a relatively common phenomenon (MVP) and a relatively uncommon disease (IE). In short, the risk of infection is small, but the population at risk is large.

Over the past two decades, two major phenomena have highlighted the relationship between MVP and IE. First, the decreased incidence of rheumatic heart disease, at one time a major risk factor for the development of IE, has resulted in the aforementioned upward shift in the age distribution of all IE patients. This trend is particularly evident in the MVP population with IE in which there is a preponderance of older males,[8,17,37–40] and is graphically depicted in Figure 1B. Second, the widespread availability and increased use of cardiac imaging techniques, particularly transthoracic and transesophageal echocardiography, have allowed for increased recognition and better definition of both MVP[13,41,42] and IE.[33,43,44]

Although mitral regurgitation due to MVP was recognized in the early 1960s, the first case report of endocarditis complicating MVP was not published until 1967 by LeBauer and associates.[45] Before 1975 there were only 22 cases of IE complicating the "billowing mitral leaflet" syndrome in the literature.[46] While most of these cases occurred in patients with audible regurgitant murmurs (with or without a click), there have been a few cases in which the only manifestation of the MVP syndrome was an isolated click.[45–47]

The nature of the MVP–IE association has been the subject of a number of retrospective analyses and follow-up series. Reviews of docu-

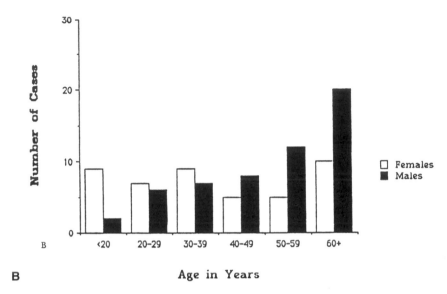

Figure 1. B. Age and sex distribution of reported patients with MVP and IE. Used with permission of Drs. Baddour and Bisno, University of Tennessee, Memphis. 38,38

mented endocarditis cases have consistently shown MVP to be the underlying defect in nearly one-third of the cases.[37–40,48,49] On the contrary, the incidence of IE complicating known MVP has varied widely in follow-up studies. This variance is best explained by differences in diagnostic criteria, study populations, and duration of follow-up. For example, one of the earliest reports of long-term follow-up (mean 25 years) of 69 patients with systolic clicks (with or without late systolic murmurs) showed that none developed IE.[50] This low incidence in patients with isolated clicks has been confirmed by others.[51,52]

At the other end of the spectrum, a 6–8% incidence of IE has been reported in association with MVP.[53–56] Studies showing this increased incidence of infection involved patients with systolic murmurs as opposed to isolated clicks. MacMahon and colleagues[57] demonstrated the increased risk of developing IE in patients with preexisting murmurs compared to those without murmurs in a case-control study, supporting the contention that IE is more frequently seen in MVP with murmurs than isolated clicks.

Case-control studies designed to assess the significance of MVP as a risk factor for IE have been the most helpful in clarifying the relationship between these two entities. The prevalence of MVP was ascertained primarily by echocardiographic criteria in cases (those with documented IE), and controls (two or three matched patients without infection). The findings of four studies, summarized in Table 1, clearly demonstrated an in-

Table 1
Summary of Case-Control Studies Assessing the Risk of Infective
Endocarditis in Patients with Mitral Valve Prolapse

| Reference [No.] | No. with MVP total No. (%) | | Matched Odds Ratio (95% C.I.) |
	Cases	Controls	
Hickey et al. [8]	11/56 (20)	7/168 (4)	5.3 (2.0–14.4)
Devereaux et al. [17]	11/67 (16)	3/134 (2)	6.7 (2.0–22.9)
MacMahon et al. [40]	21/111 (19)	16/222 (7)	2.9 (1.3–6.1)
Clemens et al. [58]	13/15 (25)	10/153 (7)	8.2 (2.4–28.4)

MVP = mitral valve prolapse.

creased risk of IE in persons found to have MVP.[8,17,40,58] When analyzed collectively, there is an approximately five times greater risk in persons with MVP for developing endocarditis compared to those without this valvular abnormality, validating Barlow's original prediction.

Pathogenesis

The pathogenesis of infective endocarditis complicating MVP is similar to that for other endomyocardial defects. Hemodynamic factors lead to endothelial surface damage. The injured endothelium then becomes infected during the transient bacteremias that occur in all individuals. The roles of complement, circulating immune complexes, and various cytokines in the pathogenesis and subsequent clinical manifestations of endocarditis are areas of ongoing study.[59]

In MVP, mechanical stresses, turbulent blood flow, and regurgitant jet streams may injure the endocardial surface, resulting in exposed collagen and the consequential deposition of platelets and fibrin. When transient bacteremias occur, microorganisms may adhere to the nonspecific "sterile" thrombus resulting in microbial colonization. Some factors influencing infection of the injured endothelium include the intensity and duration of bacteremia, the surface characteristics of the specific infecting organism, and the presence of agglutinating antibodies.[60] Once colonization is established within the thrombus, vegetations enlarge by a continual cycle of bacterial replication and platelet-fibrin deposition.

In MVP, as in other forms of mitral regurgitation, the characteristic site of infection is the atrial surface of the valve. This pattern of bacterial deposition results from a Venturi effect, which occurs as a result of blood flow from a high-pressure zone (i.e., the left ventricle) to a low-pressure

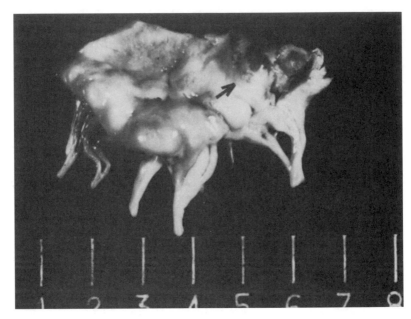

Figure 2. Surgical specimen of infected, prolapsed mitral valve showing redundant deformity of anterior cusp, thickened chordae tendineae, and evident vegetation (arrow) near the posteromedial commissure. Photograph courtesy of Dr. Peter Baker, Ohio State University, Department of Pathology.

sink (i.e., the left atrium). The maximal microbial colony distribution is predictably found just beyond the valve opening on the atrial side of the leaflet.[61] In addition, regurgitant jet streams may traumatize the atrial mural endocardium, allowing the establishment of another focus of infection.

The pathogenetic mechanisms are corroborated by studies that have examined surgical or autopsy specimens from patients with MVP and active endocarditis (Fig. 2). Pathological vegetations have been found to involve primarily the mitral valve leaflets,[36,62,63] and commonly occur in conjunction with other atrial wall vegetations.[63,64] Additionally, there is one case report whose only site of infection was a left atrial wall lesion.[65]

Pathology

The gross and histological characteristics of MVP have been well described and reviewed elsewhere in this book.[19–22,64,66–69] Common macroscopic features include: doming of the valve cusps toward the left atrium; voluminous, redundant leaflets; elongation and thinning of the chordae tendineae; and mitral annular dilatation. Histological examinations consistently show myxomatous degeneration of the fibrosa layer of the valve leaflets. These fibrosal changes may explain the predisposition of patients with MVP to develop IE. Transformation from a normal dense collagen matrix to loose myxomatous tissue may allow for stretching of the valve cusps by normal intraventricular pressure changes. The overlying endocardium would then likewise be subject to tension changes with potential disruption of endothelial continuity and consequent fibrin deposition. Pomerance supported this hypothesis with pathology specimens from 10 cases, all of whom had sterile "fibrinous" endocarditis.[61]

The pathology of bacterial vegetations in IE complicating MVP is similar to other cases of IE. As already noted, the vegetations occur in areas of erosive endothelial damage. They consist of fibrin-platelet aggregates and contain large numbers of bacteria (10^8 to 10^{10} cfu/g). Polymorphonuclear leukocytes are rare within the vegetations because they are usually unable to penetrate the fibrin matrix. This absence of phagocytic cells in the vegetation helps to explain the need for prolonged bactericidal therapy.

Clinical Features

The clinical manifestations of IE in MVP are the result of four basic pathophysiological mechanisms: (1) the effect of the inflammatory process on the infected endocardial tissue, (2) embolization, (3) metastatic infection, and (4) deposition of abnormal globulins.[60]

The typical case of IE complicating MVP follows a subacute course. The onset of symptoms is usually insidious and nonspecific. Fevers, sweats, fatigue, anorexia, and general malaise are among the common complaints. At the time of presentation, physical findings may be localized to extracardiac sites. Classic peripheral stigmata of subacute bacterial endocarditis (petechiae, splinter hemorrhages, Roth spots, Janeway lesions, Osler's nodes) may be present, but are usually indicative of a prolonged infection. As previously mentioned, auscultatory findings in IE complicating MVP show that systolic murmurs (with or without an associated click) are very common, whereas isolated clicks are documented much less frequently.

Diagnosis and Management

The aforementioned signs and symptoms, when occurring in the appropriate clinical setting, are suggestive but not definitive of endocarditis. In a minority of patients, the establishment of a diagnosis of IE is assured when pathologic specimens with positive histology and/or culture are available. For the majority who do not require acute surgical intervention (or die from their disease and have available autopsy results), the current approach to clinical diagnosis of IE is based on the Duke criteria.[28] Using this schema, a definite diagnosis of IE can be made by meeting the two major criteria: (1) persistently positive blood cultures with an organism typical for causing IE, and (2) evidence of endocardial involvement.

The variety and frequency of etiological agents causing infection in MVP are similar to those of other native valve IE[37,39] with viridans streptococci accounting for almost half of the cases. In addition to the viridans streptococci, other gram-positive organisms commonly found as causes for IE include enterococci, *Streptococcus bovis*, and staphylococci.[35] Fastidious gram-negative bacilli comprise 5–10% of cases of native valve IE[70]; these are collectively known as the HACEK group (*Haemophilus* sp., *Actinobacillus actinomycetemcomitans, Cardiobacterium hominis, Eikenella corrodens*, and *Kingella kingae*). In all cases of IE, including those complicating MVP, the continuous and low-grade bacteremia allow for recovery of the etiological agent more than 90% of the time from the first two blood cultures. Antibiotic therapy ideally should be based on the microbiological findings, with high doses of bactericidal agents being optimal.[71]

Echocardiography is the primary means of demonstrating endocardial involvement. The first report demonstrating the capability of this diagnostic modality to show bacterial vegetations was in 1973 by Dillon et al.[72] With subsequent qualitative technical improvements and experienced operators, echocardiography has become standard in the diagnostic and prognostic evaluation of patients suspected of having IE.

While the specificity for detecting vegetations using any form of echocardiography is high, the sensitivity can range between 40% and 80%, depending on various factors.[73–77] Of note, good anatomic correlation has been demonstrated between echocardiographically detected vegetations and surgical and autopsy specimens.[73,78,79]

Both image quality and sensitivity are improved using transesophageal echocardiography (TEE) compared with transthoracic (TTE) techniques,[43,44] and the utility of a negative TEE as an aid for excluding the diagnosis of IE has been demonstrated.[76,80] In one of these studies, TEE was 100% sensitive in visualizing mitral valve vegetations versus 50% for TTE.[44] In addition to improved sensitivity in detecting vegetations, TEE also has demonstrated utility in diagnosing complications of IE, such as perivalvular leaks, abscesses, fistulae, or leaflet perforations,[44,76,77] which may be important determinants in the management and ultimate outcome.

The prognostic value of echocardiography is further underscored by the mere detection of vegetations, which may put patients at increased risk for developing complications such as peripheral embolization or cardiac decompensation.[73,81]

There are, however, some inherent limitations of the application of echocardiography to IE complicating MVP. The most important is that the usual echocardiographic presentation of uncomplicated MVP reflects localized cusp thickening and redundancy that can potentially be confused with endocarditic vegetations.[79,82,83] In addition, as with all IE, echocardiograms have not been found to be useful in differentiating active from healed disease.[72,82-84]

The majority of patients with MVP and IE can do well with medical management alone. In a small study comparing MVP endocarditis to other IE, all 10 patients with MVP responded to antibiotic therapy alone, and the majority had no or only minor complications.[48] On the other hand, there is no evidence that endocarditis in MVP is a more benign disease than other IE. Serious complications, including worsening mitral insufficiency, congestive heart failure, and major embolic episodes, whether acute or delayed, do occur.[37,39,54] These complications and/or findings of unremitting bacteremia dictate the need for surgical intervention. Progressive mitral regurgitation with unmanageable congestive heart failure is the primary reason for mitral valve replacement in patients with MVP and IE.

Prophylaxis

Recommendations for antibiotic prophylaxis prior to dental and some surgical procedures in patients with MVP have been a matter of ongoing controversy. On the one hand, patients with MVP have a small but significantly increased risk of developing IE. Since the pathogenesis and clinical features of IE in MVP are similar to IE involving other endocardial defects, logical reasoning would support the use of prophylaxis. On the other hand, there is minimal information regarding the actual risk/benefit ratios of antimicrobial prophylaxis in MVP. This is due in part to uncertainty regarding the risks of prophylaxis, most notably allergic reactions, and in part to a paucity of controlled studies documenting the efficacy of endocarditis prophylaxis in general. One small case-control study demonstrated an impressive 91% protective efficacy of antibiotic prophylaxis; in this study, three of the eight case patients had MVP as their underlying cardiac lesion.[85] In contrast, a recent study suggests that while valvular abnormalities such as MVP are strong risk factors for the development of IE, dental treatments per se posed minimal, if any risk. The main conclusion of this study was that even with 100% efficacy, antibiotic prophylaxis prior to dental manipulations would prevent very few cases of IE.[86]

Recommendations for antibiotic prophylaxis specifically for patients with MVP continue to evolve. The earliest reports[45-47] suggested that all patients with clinically detectable MVP (clicks, murmurs, or both) should receive prophylaxis prior to dental and surgical procedures. While this opinion was supported by subsequent studies,[42,49,87] questions regarding the risk/benefit ratio of widespread prophylaxis have been raised. One study, by Bor and Himmelstein,[88] specifically addressed the possibility of allergic reactions. Using published epidemiological data and physician surveys, they calculated, from best-estimate analyses, the benefits and risks of antibiotic prophylaxis in patients with MVP undergoing dental procedures. Their extrapolations suggested that fatal anaphylactic reactions from standard penicillin prophylaxis were greater than mortality due to IE in patients receiving either no or erythromycin prophylaxis.

While acknowledging the controversy surrounding the use of prophylaxis in MVP, the most current consensus statement from the American Heart Association,[89] includes "mitral valve prolapse with valvular regurgitation and/or thickened leaflets" among the cardiac conditions that warrant endocarditis prophylaxis. These recommendations are based on an analysis of the spectrum of clinical presentations of MVP and the available literature (discussed in previous sections). In addition, recent favorable cost-benefit analyses have also supported the use of prophylaxis in patients with MVP, particularly those with evidence of regurgitation.[90,91]

The focal point of the decision to use prophylaxis is the detection of mitral regurgitation. If there is an audible murmur, prophylaxis is recommended. If mitral regurgitation cannot be determined by auscultatory examination, more evaluation is warranted, often requiring echocardiographic or Doppler demonstration. Of interest, a recent study showed that echocardiography performed on patients referred specifically for evaluation of MVP infrequently impacted the use of antibiotic prophylaxis, in part because "high-risk" MVP was found in only 5% of those with no history or minimal clinical suspicion of MVP.[92] Guidelines for the clinical application of echocardiography have been published by the American College of Cardiology in conjunction with the American Heart Association.[93]

The cumulative evidence over the past five decades has defined subsets within the large population of patients with MVP who are at increased risk for developing IE. These include patients with evidence of regurgitation, advancing age, and male gender. Antibiotic prophylaxis should be most strongly recommended for those with consistently documented regurgitant murmurs and particularly for older males. Antibiotic prophylaxis for other patients should be individualized and should include consideration of clinical conditions, antibiotic allergies, and the potential intensity of the anticipated bacteremia. Efforts directed toward further clarifying risks/benefit and cost/benefit ratios as well as the mechanisms and efficacy of antibiotic prophylaxis should continue.

References

1. Barlow JB, Pocock WA, Marchand P, Denny M. The significance of late systolic murmurs. Am Heart J 66(4):443–452, 1963.
2. Brown OR, Kloster FE, DeMots H. Incidence of mitral valve prolapse in the asymptomatic normal. Circulation (Suppl 2)51:77, 1975.
3. Markiewicz W, Stoner J, London E, Hunt SA, Popp RL. Mitral valve prolapse in one hundred presumably healthy young females. Circulation 53:464–473, 1976.
4. Procacci PM, Savran SV, Schreiter SL, Bryson AL. Prevalence of clinical mitral valve prolapse in 1169 young woman. N Engl J Med 294(20):1084–1088, 1976.
5. Sbarbaro JA, Mehlman DJ, Wu L, Brooks HL. A prospective study of mitral valvular prolapse in young men. Chest 75:555–559, 1979.
6. Savage DD, Garrison RJ, Devereux RB, Castelli WP, Anderson SJ, Levy D, McNamara PM, et al. Mitral valve prolapse in the general population. I: Epidemiologic features: The Framingham study. Am Heart J 106(3):571–576, 1983.
7. Cheitlin ND, Byrd RC. Prolapsed mitral valve: The commonest disease? Curr Prob Cardiol 8(10):1–54, 1984.
8. Hickey AJ, MacMahon SW, Wilcken DE. Mitral valve prolapse and bacterial endocarditis: When is antibiotic prophylaxis necessary? Am Heart J 109: 431–435, 1985.
9. Jeresaty RM. Mitral valve prolapse. JAMA 254(6):793–795, 1985.
10. Retchin SM, Fletcher RH, Earp J, Lamson N, Waugh RA. Mitral valve prolapse: Disease or illness? Arch Int Med 146:1081–1084, 1986.
11. Cheng TO, Barlow JB. Mitral leaflet billowing and prolapse: Its prevalence around the world. Angiology 40(2):77–87, 1989.
12. Zua MS, Dziegielewski SF. Epidemiology of symptomatic mitral valve prolapse in black patients. J Natl Med Assoc 87(4):273–275, 1995.
13. Malkowski MJ, Boudoulas H, Wooley CF, Guo R, Pearson AC, Gray PG, Spectrum of structural abnormalities in floppy mitral valve echocardiographic evaluation. Am Heart J 132(Pt 1):145–151, 1996.
14. Naggar CZ, Pearson WN, Seljan MP: Frequency of complications of mitral valve prolapse in subjects aged 60 years and older. Am J Cardiol 58:1209–1212, 1986.
15. Kolibash AJ, Bush CA, Fontana MB, Ryan JM, Kilman J, Wooley CF. Mitral valve prolapse syndrome: Analysis of 62 patients aged 60 years and older. Am J Cardiol 52:534–539, 1983.
16. Gardin JM, Henry WL, Savage DD, Epstein SE. Echocardiographic evaluation of an older population without clinically apparent heart disease. Am J Cardiol 39:277, 1977.
17. Devereux RB, Hawkins I, Kramer-Fox R, Lutas EM, Hammond IW, Spitzer MC, Hochreiter C, et al. Complications of mitral valve prolapse. Am J Med 81(5):751–758, 1986.
18. Kolibash AJ, Kilman JW, Buch CA, Ryan JM, Fontana ME, Wooley CF. Evidence for progression from mild to severe mitral regurgitation in mitral valve prolapse. Am J Cardiol 58:762–767, 1986.
19. McKay R, Yacoub MH. Clinical and pathological findings in patients with "floppy" valves treated surgically. Circulation (Suppl 3) 47:63–73, 1973.
20. Rippe J, Fishbein MC, Carabello B, Angoff G, Sloss L, Collins JJ, Alpert JS. Primary myxomatous degeneration of cardiac valves. Br Heart J 44:621–629, 1980.

21. Waller BF, Morrow AG, Maron BJ, Del Negro AA, Kent KM, McGrath FJ, Wallace RB, et al. Etiology of clinically isolated, severe, chronic, pure mitral regurgitation: Analysis of 97 patients over 30 years of age having mitral valve replacement. Am Heart J 104(2):276–288, 1982.

22. Tresch DD, Doyle TP, Boncheck LI, Siegel R, Keelan MH, Olinge GN, Brooks HL. Mitral valve prolapse requiring surgery. Am J Med 78:245–250, 1985.

23. Higgins CB, Reinke RT, Gosink BB, Leopold GR. The significance of mitral valve prolapse in middle-aged and elderly men. Am Heart J 91(3):292–296, 1976.

24. Steckelberg JM, Melton LJ, Ilstrup DM, Rouse MS, Wilson WR. Influence of referral bias on the apparent clinical spectrum of infective endocarditis. Am J Med 88(6):522–528, 1990.

25. Spijkerman IJ, van Ameijden EJ, Mientjes GH, Coutinho RA, van den Hoek A. Human immunodeficiency virus infection and other risk factors for skin abscesses and endocarditis among injection drug users. J Clin Epidemiol 49(10):1149–1154, 1996.

26. Hogevik H, Olaison L, Andersson R, Lindberg J, Alestig K. Epidemiologic aspects of infective endocarditis in an urban population: A 5–year prospective study. Medicine 74(6):324–339, 1995.

27. Von Reyn CF, Levy BS, Arbeit RD, Friedland G, Crumpacker CS. Infective endocarditis: An analysis based on strict case definitions. Ann Int Med 94: 505–518, 1981.

28. Durack DT, Lukes AS, Bright DK and the Duke Endocarditis Service. New criteria for diagnosis of infective endocarditis: Utilization of specific echocardiographic findings. Am J Med 96:200–209, 1994.

29. Bayer AS, Ward JI, Ginzton LE, Shapiro SM. Evaluation of new clinical criteria for the diagnosis of infective endocarditis. Am J Med 96:211–222, 1994.

30. Olaison L, Hogevik H. Comparison of the von Reyn and Duke criteria for the diagnosis of infective endocarditis. Scand J Infect Dis 28:399–406, 1996.

31. Dodds GA III, Sexton DJ, Durack DT and the Duke Endocarditis Service. Negative predictive value of the Duke criteria for infective endocarditis. Am J Cardiol 77:403–407, 1996.

32. Heiro M, Nikoskelainen J, Hartiala JJ, Saraste MK, Kotilainen PM. Diagnosis of infective endocarditis: Sensitivity of the Duke vs von Reyn criteria. Arch Intern Med 158:18–24, 1998.

33. Gagliardi JP, Nettles RE, McCarty DE, Sanders LL, Corey GC, Sexton DJ. Native valve infective endocarditis in elderly and younger adult patients: Comparison of clinical features and outcomes with use of the Duke criteria and the Duke endocarditis data base. Clin Inf Dis 26:116–168, 1998.

34. Bayer AS, Bolger AF, Taubert KA, Wilson W, Steckelberg J, Karchmer AW, Levison M, et al. Diagnosis and management of infective endocarditis and its complications. Circulation 98:2936–2948, 1998.

35. Van der Meer JTM, Thompson J, Valkenburg HA, Michel MF. Epidemiology of bacterial endocarditis in the Netherlands. Arch Intern Med 152:1863–1868, 1992.

36. Goldman ME, Fisher EA, Winters S, Reichstein R, Stavile K, Gorlin R, Fuster V. Early identification of patients with native valve infectious endocarditis at risk for major complications by initial clinical presentation and baseline echocardiography. Int J Cardiol 52(3):257–264, 1995.

37. Corrigall D, Bolen J Hancock EW, Popp RL. Mitral valve prolapse and infectious endocarditis. Am J Med 63:215–222, 1977.

38. Baddour LM, Bisno AL. Mitral valve prolapse: Multi-factorial etiologies and variable prognosis. Am Heart J 112(6):1359–1362, 1986.
39. Baddour LM, Bisno AL. Infective endocarditis complicating mitral valve prolapse: Epidemiologic, clinical , and microbiologic aspects. Rev Infect Dis 8(1):117–137, 1986.
40. MacMahon SW, Roberts JK, Kramer-Fox R, Zucker DM, Roberts RB, Devereaux RB. Mitral valve prolapse and infective endocarditis. Am Heart J 113: 1291–1298, 1987.
41. Hershman WY, Moskowitz MA, Marton KI, Balady GJ. Utility of echocardiography in patients with mitral valve prolaspe. Am J Med 87:371–376, 1989.
42. Marks, AR, Choong CY, Sanfilippo AJ, Ferre M, Weyman AE. Identification of high-risk and low-risk subgroups of patients with mitral valve prolapse. N Engl J Med 320:1031–1036, 1989.
43. Lindner JR, Case A, Dent JM, Abbott RD, Scheld WM, Kaul S. Diagnostic value of echocardiography in suspected endocarditis. Circulation 93:730–736, 1996.
44. Birmingham GD, Rahko PS, Ballantyne F III. Improved detection of infective endocarditis with transesophageal echocardiography. Am Heart J 123:774–781, 1992.
45. LeBauer EJ, Perloff JK, Kerliher TF. The isolated click with bacterial endocarditis. Am Heart J 73:534–537, 1967.
46. Lachman AS, Bramwell-Jones DM, Lakier JB, Pocock WA, Barlow JB. Infective endocarditis in the billowing mitral leaflet syndrome. Br Heart J 37:326–330, 1975.
47. Kincaid DT, Botti RE. Subacute bacterial endocarditis in a patient with isolated, nonejection systolic click but without a murmur. Chest 66:88–89, 1974.
48. Nolan CM, Kane JJ, Grunow WA. Infective endocarditis and mitral prolapse. Arch Int Med 141:447–450, 1981.
49. McKinsey DS, Ratts TE, Bisno AL. Underlying cardiac lesions in adults with infective endocarditis. Am J Med 82:681–688, 1987.
50. Appelblatt NH, Willis PW, Lenhart JA, Schulman JI, Walton JA. Ten to 40 year follow-up of 69 patients with systolic click with or without apical systolic murmur. Am J Cardiol 35:119, 1975.
51. Koch FH, Hancock EW. Ten year follow-up of forty patients with the mid-systolic click syndrome. Am J Cardiol 37:149, 1976.
52. Retchin SM, Fletcher RH, Waugh RA. Endocarditis and mitral valve prolapse: What is the "risk"? Int J Cardiol 5:653–659, 1984.
53. Allen H, Harris A, Leatham A. Significance and prognosis of an isolated late systolic murmur: A 9–22 year follow-up. Br Heart J 36:525–532, 1974.
54. Mills P, Rose J, Hollingsworth J, Amara I, Craige E. Long-term prognosis of mitral valve prolapse. N Engl J Med 297:13–18, 1977.
55. Belardi J, Lardani H, Shedlon W. Idiopathic prolapse of the mitral valve: Follow-up study of 136 patients studied by angiography. Am J Cardiol 47:426, 1981.
56. Duren DR, Becker AE, Dunning AJ. Long-term follow-up of idiopathic mitral valve prolapse in 300 patients: A prospective study. J Am Coll Cardiol 11:42–47, 1988.
57. MacMahon SW, Hickey AJ, Wilcken DEL, Wittes JT, Fenely MP, Hickie JB. Risk of infective endocarditis in mitral valve prolapse with and without precordial systolic murmurs. Am J Cardiol 58:105–108, 1986.
58. Clemens JD, Horwitz RI, Jaffe CC, Feinstein AR, Stanto BF. A controlled evaluation of the risk of bacterial endcarditis in persons with mitral valve prolapse. N Engl J Med 307(13):776–781, 1982.

59. Brown M, Griffin GE. Immune responses in endocarditis. Heart 79:1–2, 1998.
60. Weinstein L, Schlesinger JJ. Pathoanatomic, pathophysiologic and clinical correlations in endocarditis. N Engl J Med 291(6):832–837, 1974.
61. Robard S. Blood velocity and endocarditis. Circulation 27:18–28, 1963.
62. Arnett EN, Roberts WC. Acute infective endocarditis: A clinicopathologic analysis of 137 necropsy patients. Curr Prob Cardiol 1:1–76, 1976.
63. Lucas R, Edwards JE: The floppy mitral valve. Curr Prob Cardiol 7(4):5–48, 1982.
64. Pomerance A. Ballooning deformity (mucoid degeneration) of atrioventricular valves. Br heart J 31:343–351, 1969.
65. Ringer M, Feen DJ, Drapkin MS. Mitral valve prolapse: Jet stream causing mural endocarditis. Am J Cardiol 45:383–385, 1980.
66. Davies MJ, Moore BP, Braimbridge MV. The floppy mitral valve: Study of incidence, pathology, and complications in surgical, necropsy, and forensic material. Br Heart J 40:468–481, 1978.
67. Olsen EGJ, Al-Rufaie HK. The floppy mitral valve: Study on pathogenesis. Br Heart J 44:674–683, 1980.
68. Aslam PA, Eastridge CE, Bernhardt H, Pate JW. Myxomatous degeneration of cardiac valves. Chest 57(6):535–539, 1970.
69. Kolibash AJ, Bush CA, Kilman J, Ryan JM, Wooley CF. Myxomatous mitral valves, mitral valve prolapse and progressive mitral regurgitation. JACC 3(2):559, 1984.
70. Geraci JE, Wilson WR. Symposium on infective endocarditis, III: Endocarditis due to gram-negative bacteria, report of 56 cases. Mayo Clinic Proc 57:145–148, 1982,
71. Wilson WR, Karchmer AW, Dajani AS, Taubert KA, Bayer A, Kaye D, Bisno AL, et al. Antibiotic treatment of adults with infective endocarditis due to streptococci, enterococci, staphylococci, and HACEK microorganisms. JAMA 274:1706–1713, 1995.
72. Dillon JC, Feigenbaum H, Konecke LL, Davis RH, Chang S. Echocardiographic manifestations of valvular vegetations. Am Heart J 86(5):698–704, 1973.
73. Mintz GS, Kotler MN, Segal BL, Parry WR. Comparison of two-dimensional and M-mode echocardiography in the evaluation of patients with infective endocarditis. Am J Cardiol 43:738–744, 1979.
74. Wann LS, Hallam CC, Dillon JC, Weyman AE, Feigenbaum H. Comparison of M-mode and cross-sectional echocardiography in infective endocarditis. Circulation 60(4):728–733, 1979.
75. Mugge A, Daniel WG, Frank G, Lichtlen PR. Echocardiography in infective endocarditis: Reassessment of prognostic implications of vegetation size determined by the transthoracic and the transesophageal approach. J Am Coll Cardio 14:631–638, 1989.
76. Shively BK, Gurule FT, Roldan CA, Leggett JH, Schiller NB. Diagnostic value of transesophageal compared with transthoracic echocardiography in infective endocarditis. J Am Coll Cardio 18:391–397, 1991.
77. Shapiro SM, Young E, DeGuzman S, Ward J, Chiu CY, Ginzton LE, Bayer AS. Transesophageal echocardiography in diagnosis of endocarditis. Chest 105:377–382, 1994.
78. Brandenburg RO, Giuliani ER, Wilson WR, Geraci JE. Infective endocarditis: A 25 year overview of diagnosis and therapy. J Am Coll Cardiol 1:280–291, 1983.
79. Popp RL. Echocardiography and infectious endocarditis. Current Clinical Topics in Infectious Diseases. In Remington JS, Swartz MN (eds), New York, McGraw-Hill, 1983, pp 98–110.

80. Sochowski RA, Chan K-L. Implication of negative results on a monoplane transesophageal echocardiographic study in patients with suspected infective endocarditis. J Am Coll Cardiol 21:216–221, 1993.
81. Davis RS, Strom JA, Frishman W, Becker R, Matsumoto M, LeJemtel TH, Sonnenblick EH, et al. The demonstration of vegetations by echocardiography in bacterial endocarditis. Am J Med 69:57–63, 1980.
82. Wann LS, Dillon JC, Weyman AE, Feigenbaum H. Echocardiography in bacterial endocarditis. N Engl J Med 295(3):135–139, 1976.
83. Chandraratna PAN, Langevin E. Limitations of the echocardiogram in diagnosing valvular vegetation in patients with mitral valve prolapse. Circulation 56:436–438, 1977.
84. Roy P, Tajik AJ, Giuliani ER, Schattenberg TT, Gau GT, Frye RL. Spectrum of echocardiographic findings in bacterial endocarditis. Circulation 53(3): 474–482, 1976.
85. Imperiale TF, Horwitz RI. Does prophylaxis prevent postdental infective endocarditis? A controlled evaluation of protective efficacy. Am J Med 88: 131–136, 1990.
86. Strom BL, Abrutyn E, Berlin JA, Kinman JL, Feldman RS, Stolley PD, Levison ME, et al. Dental and cardiac risk factors for infective endocarditis: A population-based, case-control study. Ann Int Med 129:761–769, 1998.
87. Nishimura RA, McGoon MD, Shub C, Miller FA, Ilstrup DM, Tajik AJ. Echocardiographically documented mitral valve prolapse. Long-term follow up of 237 patients. N Engl J Med 313:1305–1309, 1985.
88. Bor DH, Himmelstein DU. Enndocarditis prophylaxis for patients with mitral valve prolapse. Am J Med 76:711–717, 1984.
89. Dajani AS, Taubert KA, Wilson W, Bolger AF, Bayer A, Ferrieri P, Gewitz MH, et al. Prevention of bacterial endocarditis. JAMA 277(22):1794–1801, 1997.
90. Frary CJ, Devereaux RB, Kramer-Fox R, Roberts RB, Ruchlin HS. Clinical and health care cost consequences of infective endocarditis in mitral valve prolapse. Am J Cardiol 73:263–267, 1994.
91. Devereaux RB, Frary CJ, Kramer-Fox R, Roberts RB, Ruchlin HS. Cost-effectivenes of infective endocarditis prophylaxis for a mitral valve prolapse with or without a mitral regurgitant murmur. Am J Cardiol 74:1024–1029, 1994.
92. Heidenreich PA, Bear J, Browner W, Foster E. The clinical impact of echocardiography on antibiotic prophylaxis use in patients with suspected mitral valve prolapse. Am J Med 102:337–343, 1997.
93. Cheitlin MD, Alpert JS, Armstrong WF, Aurigemma GP, Beller GA, Bierman, FZ, Davidson TW, et al. ACC/AHA guidelines for the clinical application of echocardiography: A report of the American College of Cardiology/American Heart Association Task Force on Practice Guidelines (Committee on Clinical Application of Echocardiography). Circulation 95:1686–1744, 1997.

Part IX

Floppy Mitral Valve:
Thromboembolic Complications

Introduction

The Floppy Mitral Valve, Mitral Valve Prolapse, Mitral Valvular Regurgitation:
Thromboembolic Phenomena

Charles F. Wooley, MD,
Harisios Boudoulas, MD, PhD

Neurologists came to recognize the floppy mitral valve/mitral valve prolapse/mitral valvular regurgitation (FMV/MVP/MVR) triad as a potential cause of stroke in the 1970s, and MVP now appears on most lists of potential sources of cardiac emboli, particularly in young individuals. Our neurological colleagues present their perspectives based on clinical studies and their personal experiences with MVP, cerebral ischemia, and stroke. Their explanations about the difficulties in establishing causal relationships between the FMV and cerebral events reflect the current state of knowledge and are pertinent to the FMV/MVP/MVR story.

The medical literature dealing with patients with FMV/MVP/MVR triad who experience thromboembolic phenomena reflects a variety of clinical experiences set against the background of changing cardiovascular and neurological nosology, investigative methods, and diagnostic criteria. As attention is directed toward the recognition of the many cardiovascular thromboembolic causes of cerebral ischemia, stroke, and systemic phenomena, and refined imaging techniques are used in prospective clinical studies, traditional concepts are constantly refined.

Our early clinical experiences in the 1960s and 1970s with FMV/MVP patients included several young patients with retinal vessel occlusive events that our neuro-ophthalmologists thought were embolic in nature. These early experiences were examples of what might be referred to as "smoking gun" phenomena, i.e., FMV patients who had retinal embolic

From: Boudoulas H, Wooley CF. *Mitral Valve: Floppy Mitral Valve, Mitral Valve Prolapse, Mitral Valvular Regurgitation.* Second revised edition. ©Futura Publishing Company, Armonk, NY, 2000.

events in the absence of other clear-cut cause and effect relationships. Our histopathological studies, and those of our colleagues, suggested that valve surface phenomena might be the basis for such events. However, there were confounding factors, such as oral contraceptive therapy and cigarette smoking, and decisions about therapy were necessarily empirical, based on clinical judgment with little supportive data.

Some time later, one of our senior ophthalmologists with FMV presented with a "blue toe syndrome"; after a nondiagnostic evaluation by the peripheral vascular surgeons, he came for a cardiac evaluation. Interestingly, after careful questioning, he reviewed his office daybooks, and recalled a remote retinal vascular event three decades earlier that resulted in a field cut confirmed by objective testing. Over the subsequent three decades he had three TIA episodes that defied precise neurological or hematological explanation. Therapy aimed at inhibition of platelet aggregation provided long-term benefit. However, as often happens in real life, during the next two decades he developed mitral annular calcification, paroxysmal atrial fibrillation, and most recently, thickening and irregularities of the lumen of the ascending thoracic aorta, all potential causes of thromboemboli.

The clinical events described above are examples of the difficulties facing clinicians when multiple confounding phenomena prevent a neat explanation as to cause and effect relationships between the FMV and thromboembolic phenomena. Reviewing the earlier medical literature requires discernment, since the earlier studies based on M-mode echocardiography placed emphasis on "prolapse" of the mitral valve rather than dealing with the consequences of the FMV/MVP/MVR triad.

When patients with the FMV/MVP/MVR triad present with peripheral or cerebral vascular thromboembolic events, clinicians are faced with a cascade of potential causes requiring a global approach to individual patient analysis (Table 1).

FMV surface characteristics may predispose to endothelial disruption with platelet aggregation, infective endocarditis, or nonbacterial thrombotic endocarditis (NBTE), clinical entities associated with thromboembolic phenomena.

The development of left atrial enlargement, left atrial myopathy, paroxysmal, or chronic atrial fibrillation in clinical course of patients with FMV/MVP/MVR may result in thromboemboli.

The list of cardiovascular structural abnormalities with the potential for thromboemboli has expanded during the imaging era. Structural abnormalities include patent foramen ovale, atrial septal aneurysms, atrial septal defects; mitral annular calcification; and atherosclerotic aortic and carotid disease. When these defects coexist with the FMV, the differential diagnosis of the source for thromboemboli is further expanded.

Table 1
The Floppy Mitral Valve and
Thromboembolic Phenomena

Surface Phenomena
  Endothelial disruption
  Nonbacterial thrombotic endocarditis
  Infective endocarditis
FMV/MVP/MVR with LAE
  Left atrial myopathy
  Paroxysmal/chronic atrial fibrillation
Coagulation Disorders
  Platelet disorders
  Platelet activation associated with MVR
  Prothrombotic disorders
Coexisting Structural Abnormalities
  Patent foramen ovale
  Atrial septal defect
  Atrial septal aneurysm
  Mitral annular calcification
  Aortic/carotid origin

Coagulation abnormalities, prothrombotic disorders, and platelet dysfunction, either inherited or acquired, are recognized with increasing frequency in patients experiencing thromboembolic events. Detection requires sophisticated testing and has important consequences in terms of specific therapy and family testing.

In other words, a simple cause-and-effect approach to the FMV/MVP/MVR triad and the occurrence of thromboembolic events is no longer appropriate. Rather, when patients or families with the FMV/MVP/MVR triad present with a history of thromboemboli or experience thromboembolic events, thoughtful clinical analysis involves particular attention to the potential overlap or coexisting phenomena described above.

In addition, the approach to a specific diagnosis should be corrected for age and family history to a certain extent. Thromboemboli in the infant, child, and young adult suggest coexisting prothrombotic disorders, while in the adult and elderly patient, thromboemboli may be a consequence of FMV dysfunction, atrial enlargement, atrial fibrillation, or mitral annular calcification. The structural abnormalities noted above should be considered in all age groups. A history suggesting a familial thromboembolic disorder requires development of a pedigree and sophisticated hematologic evaluation.

Clinical assessment based on the history and physical examination remains pertinent but is imprecise in determining the origin of thromboemboli in general as well as in patients with FMVs. Strict diagnostic criteria, cardiovascular and neurologic imaging studies, and sophisticated hematologic laboratory assessment are necessary to insure diagnostic precision.

Precision in diagnosis always precedes rationale therapy. Since the range of potential therapies in patients experiencing thromboembolic phenomena is extensive, therapeutic decisions involving hematologic, neurologic, vascular, electrophysiologic, or cardiovascular surgical interventions must be preceded by thoughtful individual patient analysis.

15

Cerebral Ischemia in Mitral Valve Prolapse

Andrew P. Slivka, MD
Elizabeth T. Walz, MD

Introduction

Approximately 15% of all ischemic strokes are of cardioembolic etiology. This percentage is somewhat higher, about 30%, in young patients presenting with ischemic stroke.[1] Barnett was the first to suggest mitral valve prolapse (MVP) as a cause for stroke in 1974, when he reported four patients with stroke and MVP documented by cardiac angiography.[2] All of these patients were less than 50 years old and had no atherosclerotic risk factors and normal cerebral angiograms. Since then other clinical series and pathological studies have supported a potential etiologic role for MVP in stroke or transient ischemic attacks (TIAs). In this chapter we will discuss the association of MVP and stroke including natural history and treatment options. The work-up of patients with MVP and stroke or TIA, with emphasis on younger patients, will also be outlined.

Prevalence

Most longitudinal studies of patients with MVP demonstrate a low stroke risk.[3–7] One study in particular deserves mention because of the

From: Boudoulas H, Wooley CF. *Mitral Valve: Floppy Mitral Valve, Mitral Valve Prolapse, Mitral Valvular Regurgitation.* Second revised edition. ©Futura Publishing Company, Armonk, NY, 2000.

large number of patients included and the study design. Orencia et al. reported on follow-up of 1,079 patients with MVP and without prior stroke or TIA diagnosed over a 14-year period.[7] There was a twofold increased incidence of stroke relative to an age- and sex-matched reference population, but this was attributed to the presence of several accompanying clinical conditions using multivariant analysis. For those with an auscultatory diagnosis of MVP as the only indication for echocardiography, the stroke risk relative to the reference population was 1.0. In this population-based study, the age at first stroke in MVP patients was similar to that reported in an unselected population and no strokes occurred in 4,169 patient years in patients less than 45 years of age.

MVP is identified in approximately 5–10% of patients with stroke or TIA, although several studies report a higher prevalence (Table 1).[8–13] Other identifiable mechanisms of stroke are found in as many as 60–70% of patients with MVP, particularly in the elderly.[10,14] Most series of patients less than 45 years old with stroke or TIA find MVP to be an uncommon cause in the absence of other risk factors, [8,9,12,13] suggesting that alternative causes of cerebral ischemia should be excluded before implicating MVP.[15]

The experience at Ohio State University is similar to that reported in the literature. Data on hospitalized patients with acute ischemic stroke and TIA are entered into the Ohio State University Stroke database. Demographic and historical information, physical examination, laboratory, radiographic, and echocardiographic results are included for each patient. The etiology of each patient's TIA or stroke is classified using published criteria.[16] From January 1994 to December 1996, 438 patients with TIA or stroke had been entered into the database. Of the total, 97 had transesophageal echocardiography, and in 71 the ischemic event was classified as cardioembolic. Ten patients had MVP and in nine patients another echocardiographic abnormality was found including mitral valve thickening, mitral valve strands, patent foramen ovale, valvular vegetation, or atherosclerosis of the aorta while the single patient with isolated MVP also had atrial fibrillation. In six of the 10 patients with MVP the TIA or stroke was classified as cardioembolic. Only one patient with MVP and a cardioembolic TIA or stroke had MVP as the only potential cardiac source. Of the other five patients with MVP three also had mitral valvular vegetations, one had atrial fibrillation, and one had a patent foramen ovale and mitral valve strands.[17,18]

In summary, the risk of stroke or TIA from MVP appears to be low and not much greater than in an age- and sex-matched population. In patients with stroke or TIA, MVP is identified in about 5–10% of patients, which is approximately the incidence of MVP in the general population. Furthermore, many of these patients have other identifiable mechanisms of cerebral ischemia.

Table 1
Clinical Series of Patients with Stroke or TIA

	Barnett et al.[10]	Barnett et al.[10]	Jones et al.[4]	Bogousslasky et al.[11]	Bevan et al.[12]	Urbinati et al.[8]	Carolei et al.[13]	Adams et al.[5]
No. of patients	60	141	43*	41	48	125	333	329
Male/female ratio	6:5	11:5	—	3:5	3:2	3:2	1:1	6:5
Age (range)	6–45 yr	49–87 yr	—	16–29 yr	15–45 yr	16–45 yr	15–44 yr	15–45 yr
MVP diagnosis	M-mode echo	M-mode echo	echo	2-D echo	M-mode or 2-D echo	2-D echo	M-mode or 2-D echo	2-D or transesophageal echo
Inclusion criteria:								
stroke	+							+
stroke/TIA		+	+	+	+	+	+	
No. with MVP (%)	24 (40%)	8 (6%)	9 (21%)	13 (32%)	2 (4%)	7 (6%)	28 (8%)	5 (2%)
No. with MVP as likely source of embolus (%)	18 (30%)	2 (1%)	—	12 (29%)	—	—	—	—

*43 patients without carotid disease of obvious cardiac source of emboli selected from population of 401 patients with stroke or TIA.
TIA = transient ischemic attack.

Mechanisms

Emboli from valvular thrombi are the presumed mechanism of stroke or TIA in patients with MVP. Platelet or fibrin thrombi free of inflammatory cells have been identified on the surface of prolapsed mitral valves at autopsy in numerous reports.[19–23] In one series gross thrombi on the mitral valve were identified in 33% of valves when careful examination was performed.[24] Valves without gross lesions frequently had microscopic thrombi although these were often of insufficient size to occlude a major cerebral artery.[24] Localized echo densities on the anterior and posterior leaf of the mitral valve consistent with thrombi have also been seen on echocardiography in patients with MVP.[25–28]

Only four autopsies in patients with MVP and stroke have been reported.[29–32] Of the four patients, two had atrial fibrillation and MVP [31,32] and one had mitral valve vegetations in the setting of adenocarcinoma of the lung,[29] so drawing conclusions about the etiologic role of MVP in producing stroke in these cases is difficult. The fourth case was a 21-year-old black male who died 5 days after the onset of a right hemispheric stroke.[30] He had no risk factors associated with stroke. Postmortem examination revealed a thickened posterior mitral valve leaflet with fine granular friable yellow fibrin thrombus on the atrial surface. Histologic examination of the posterior leaflet revealed myxomatous degeneration without inflammatory cells and an intact endothelium over the valve. Fibrin emboli were seen in the small intracerebral arteries of the right frontal lobe as well as in the coronary and intrarenal arteries. This case provides compelling evidence that MVP can cause stroke by an embolic mechanism.

Several other diseases associated with MVP such as atrial fibrillation, subacute bacterial endocarditis, and migraine[33] are potential causes of stroke independent of MVP. Other cardiac arrhythmias, which may also occur in patients with MVP, are a rare cause of focal cerebral ischemia.[34,35]

Stroke Risk Stratification

Because the risk of stroke in MVP is low, attempts have been made to look for associated factors that may put an individual at increased risk. No demographic features have been identified that separate high-risk from low-risk patients.[36]

Data on echocardiographic features that may predispose patients with MVP to stroke or TIA are limited, with the exception of mitral valve thickening. The presence of thickened or redundant mitral valve alone has not been associated with an increased stroke risk.[6,7,37–40]

Single studies have shown an increased risk of stroke in those with multiple valve prolapses and associated myxomatous changes, mitral annulus abnormalities, atrial septal aneurysm, and the combination of a patent foramen ovale and MVP.[37,41,42] As these associated echocardiographic features have to date been reported in single series with small numbers of patients, none can be said to reliably predict those with an increased risk of stroke or TIA.

Diagnostic Evaluation

In patients with previously diagnosed MVP and recent stroke or TIA, an extensive evaluation searching for other sources is warranted, since often other identifiable etiologies for stroke exist, as described in case 1 (see Case Reports at the end of the chapter). A CT or MR scan is necessary to rule out mass lesions, which may present like acute cerebral ischemic events. MR is the preferred imaging study in younger patients since multiple sclerosis may also present acutely and MR is more sensitive than CT in identifying demyelinating lesions. Complete blood count, platelet count, prothrombin time, partial thromboplastin time, sedimentation rate, electrolytes, and glucose are ordered to identify potential metabolic sources of focal neurological symptoms. An electrocardiogram is helpful in documenting arrhythmias and ischemic or hypertensive heart disease.

In young patients, cerebral angiography or MR angiography of the head and neck are performed routinely to identify vascular etiologies of stroke such as premature atherosclerosis, fibromuscular dysplasia, or arterial dissection. Echocardiography is done to determine whether other potential cardiac sources of emboli exist, particularly those with greater embolic potential than MVP such as atrial, ventricular, or valvular thrombus. Transesophageal echocardiography is recommended in young patients since it is more sensitive in detecting cardioembolic sources. Finding abnormalities in antithrombin III, protein C, protein S, or antiphospholipid antibodies may alter treatment options and so are also obtained. In selected instances cerebral spinal fluid studies and Holter monitoring are also done.

An alogorithm for evaluation of patients older than 55 years is outlined in Figure 1. Transthoracic echocardiography is generally used as a screen with transesophageal echocardiography being reserved for patients with a history suggestive of other cardioembolic sources or to clarify abnormalities seen on the thoracic study. MRI of the neck and head are done in selected cases when finding intracranial or vertebrobasilar atheromatous disease may alter therapy.

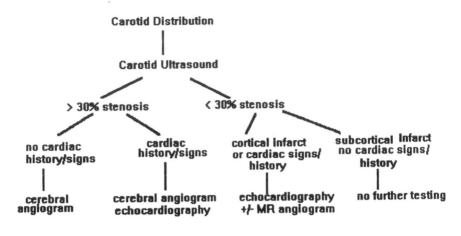

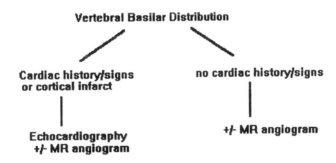

Figure 1. Algorithm for evaluation of patients older than 55 years.

Treatment

Given the low incidence of stroke or TIA in patients with MVP, treatment to prevent cerebral ischemia is not recommended in an asymptomatic patient. If future studies are able to consistently demonstrate echocardiographic, demographic, or laboratory features that predict an increased risk of stroke, then primary preventative treatment may be warranted.

Since no treatment trials have been done on patients with MVP and TIA or stroke, treatment is empiric. A treatment approach is outlined in the alogorithm in Figure 2. Antiplatelet agents are the first line of therapy, as described in case 2, because of the low recurrence rate in patients with MVP.[43,44] When an etiology for stroke or TIA other than MVP is identified, that condition should be treated accordingly, as discussed in case 3.

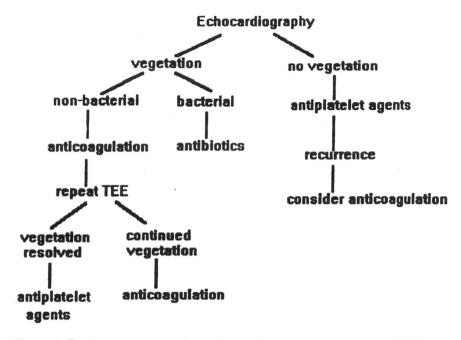

Figure 2. Treatment approach for patients with mitral valve prolapse (MVP) and stroke/transient ischemic attacks (TIA).

Prognosis

Data on the rate of recurrent cerebral ischemia in patients with MVP and stroke or TIA are limited and other mechanisms of stroke are identified in a significant number of these patients, which may influence recurrence risk.

Wolf and Sila reviewed six case series of patients with MVP and stroke collected from 1977 to 1985.[43] Of the total 114 patients, 32% presented with TIA alone and 66% had a stroke. A significant neurological deficit after the presenting event occurred in 32% of patients but most resolved completely. Approximately 20% of patients suffered recurrent cerebral ischemic events. These recurrences were often months to years after the first event and were more often transient rather than permanent.

Jackson et. al. reported 32 patients less than 45 years of age of whom 44% had ischemic recurrences at the time of the diagnosis of MVP.[44] Half of these prior recurrent events were TIAs and half were strokes. During a mean follow-up of 8 years, only 16% had recurrences (6.8/100 patient years), with the majority of these events being TIAs. Of those with stroke only 9% had any residual deficit. At the time of follow-up 50% of patients were taking antiplatelet agents and 8% were taking anticoagulants. As mentioned previously, older individuals with MVP and stroke or TIA often have other mechanisms for cerebral ischemia. In the elderly population with MVP and TIA or stroke, there is no increased risk of recurrent stroke compared with age- and sex-adjusted rates of recurrent stroke in the community.[45]

In summary, the risk of recurrent cerebral ischemic events in patients with MVP and stroke or TIA appears to be low. These recurrences are frequently TIAs, and when strokes occur they are rarely associated with significant deficits.

Summary

MVP does not appear to increase the risk for stroke compared to the general population. However, autopsy data suggest MVP may be a cause of stroke in individual patients. Treatment of patients with MVP and stroke or TIA is empiric since no treatment trials have been done. Antiplatelet agents are used as initial therapy because of the low risk of recurrent ischemic events, specifically stroke.

Case Reports

Case #1

A 48-year-old female had a 20-minute episode of dysarthria, left upper extremity weakness, and numbness that resolved completely without residual deficit. Her past history was significant for mitral valve prolapse and Hodgkin's lymphoma stage IA diagnosed 7 years previously for which she received radiation therapy to the mediastinum and cervical region.

Laboratory evaluation, including complete blood count, platelet count, prothrombin time, partial thromboplastin time, electrolytes and glucose, was normal as was an ECG and CT scan. Transthoracic echocardiography was repeated and confirmed the mitral valve prolapse. No other abnormalities were identified. Cerebral angiography including the aortic arch and a selective right carotid injection revealed an occlusion of the proximal right internal carotid artery. This was attributed to radiation vasculopathy and she was treated with aspirin 325 mg/day.

Case #2

A 43-year-old male presented with global aphasia, a right field deficit, and right hemiplegia. The past medical history was significant for insulin-dependent diabetes mellitus. Over the next 2–3 days, the right-sided weakness resolved and the patient was able to comprehend though he still had limited speech output. Over the next week language function normalized except for mild word-finding problems. His only residual was a mild right field deficit, which resolved over the subsequent month.

Initial laboratory evaluation, including complete blood count, platelet count, prothrombin time, partial thromboplastin time, and electrolytes, was normal as was an ECG and CT scan. His glucose was 167 mg/dL. An MR scan done 2 days after the onset of symptoms revealed a left occipital infarction. Cerebral angiography including an arch study and selective left carotid and vertebral injections was normal. Transesophageal echocardiography revealed mitral valve prolapse and a diffusely thickened mitral valve. He was treated with aspirin 325 mg/day and has had no recurrences after 1 year of follow-up.

Case #3

A 44-year-old female presented with a 5-hour episode of diplopia, dysarthria, gait ataxia, and confusion. Neurological examination was normal after the episode. Her past history was significant for venous thrombosis following a minor surgical procedure.

Laboratory evaluation, including complete blood count, platelet count, prothrombin time, partial thromboplastin time, electrolytes, and glucose, was normal as was an ECG and MR scan. Cerebral angiography including an arch study and selective vertebral injection was normal. Transesophageal echocardiography revealed a patient foramen ovale with spontaneous right to left shunting, mitral valve prolapse, tricuspid valve prolapse, and mitral valve strands. A bilateral extremity venous duplex scan revealed a small amount of thrombus along the walls of the right common femoral vein. Antithrombin III, plasminogen, protein C, and protein S levels were normal and antiphospholipid antibodies were negative. She did have resistance to activated protein C due to a mutation in the gene for factor V.

After the work-up was completed, she was treated with intravenous heparin and then switched to warfarin. Because of the recent cerebral ischemic event, presumed to be due to a paradoxical embolus, the past history of deep venous thrombosis, and the factor V mutation she was maintained on long-term anticoagulation. She has had no recurrent ischemic events after 3 months of follow-up.

References

1. Cerebral Embolism Task Force. Cardiogenic brain embolism: The second report of the cerebral embolism task force. Arch Neurol 46:727–743, 1989.

2. Barnett HJM. Transient cerebral ischemia: Pathogenesis, prognosis and management. Ann R Cell Phys Surg Can 7:153–173, 1974.
3. Mills P, Rose J, Hollingsworth J, Amara I, Craige E. Long-term prognosis of mitral valve prolalpse. N Engl J Med 297:13–18, 1977.
4. Jones HR, Naggar CZ, Seljan MP, Downing LL. Mitral valve prolapse and cerebral ischemic events: A comparison between a neurology population with stroke and a cardiology population with mitral valve prolapse observed for five years. Stroke 13:451–453, 1982.
5. Sandok BA, Giuliani ER. Cerebral ischemic events in patients with mitral valve prolapse. Stroke 13:448–450, 1982.
6. Nishimura RA, McGoin MD, Shub C, Miller FA, Ilstrup DM, Tajik AJ. Echocardiographically documented mitral valve prolapse: Long-term follow-up of 237 patients. N Engl J Med 313:1305–1309, 1985.
7. Orencia AJ, Petty GW, Khandheria BK, Annegers JF, Ballard DJ, Sicks JD, O'Fallon WM, et al. Risk of stroke with mitral valve prolapse in population-based cohort study. Stroke 26:7–13, 1995.
8. Urbinati S, DiPasquale G, Andreoli A, Lusa A, Manini G, Lanzino G, Grazi P, et al. Role and indication of two-dimensional echocardiography in young adults with cerebral ischemia: A prospective study in 125 patients. Cerebrovasc Dis 2:14–21, 1992.
9. Adams HP, Kapelle J, Biller J, Gordon DL, Love B, Gomez F, Heffner M. Ischemic stroke in young adults. Experience in 329 patients enrolled in the Iowa registry of stroke in young adults. Arch Neurol 52:491–495, 1995.
10. Barnett HJM, Boughner DR, Taylor DW, Cooper PE, Kostuk WJ, Nichol PM. Further evidence relating mitral-valve prolapse to cerebral ischemic events. N Engl J Med 302:139–144, 1980.
11. Bogousslavsky J, Regli F. Ischemic stroke in adults younger than 30 years of age. Cause and prognosis. Arch Neurol 44:479–482, 1987.
12. Bevan H, Sharma K, Bradley W. Stroke in young adults. Stroke 21:382–386, 1990.
13. Carolei A, Marini C, Ferranti E, Frontoni M, Prencipe M. Fieschi C, National Research Council Study Group. A prospective study of cerebral ischemia in the young: Analysis of pathogenic determinants. Stroke 24:362–367, 1993.
14. Petty GW, Orencia AJ, Khandheria BK, Whisnant JP. A population-based study of stroke in the setting of mitral valve prolapse: Risk factors and infarct subtype classification. Mayo Clin Proc 69:632–634, 1994.
15. Bogousslavsky J, Pierre P. Ischemic stroke in patients under age 45. Neurol Clin 10:113–124, 1992.
16. Adams HP, Bendixen BH, Kapelle LJ, Biller J, Love BB, Gordon DL, Marsh EE, and the Toast Investigators. Classification of subtype of acute ischemic stroke: Definitions for use in a multicenter clinical trial. Stroke 24:35–41, 1993.
17. Tice FD, Slivka AP, Walz ET, Orsinelli DA, Pearson AC. Mitral valve strands in patients with focal cerebral ischemia. Stroke 27:1183–1186, 1996.
18. Di Tullio M, Sacco RL, Gopal A, Mohr JP, Homma S. Patent foramen ovale as a risk factor for cryptogenic stroke. Ann Int Med 117:461–465, 1992.
19. Hanson MR, Conomy JP, Hodgman JR. Brain events associated with mitral valve prolapse. Stroke 11:499–506, 1980.
20. McKay R, Yacoub MH. Clinical and pathological findings in patients with "floppy" valves treated surgically. Circulation 47(Supp III):III-63 -III-73, 1973.
21. Chesler E, King RA, Edwards JE. The myxomatous mitral valve and sudden death. Circulation 67:632–639, 1983.

22. Lucas R, Edwards JE. The floppy mitral valve. Curr Prob Cardiol 7(4):1–48, 1982.
23. Kostuk WJ, Boughner DR, Barnett HJM, Silver MD. Strokes: A complication of mitral-leaflet prolapse? Lancet 2:313–316, 1977.
24. Pomerance A, Davies MJ. Strokes: A complication of mitral-leaflet syndrome. Lancet 2:1186, 1977.
25. Nichol P, Kertesz A. Two dimensional echocardiographic (2 DE) detection of left atrial thrombus in patients with mitral valve prolapse and strokes. Circulation 60(Suppl II):II-18, 1979.
26. Rothbard RL, Nanda NC, Fleck G, Heinle RA. Mitral valve prolapse and stroke: Detection of potential emboli by real time two-dimensional echocardiography. Circulation 60(Suppl II):II-99, 1979.
27. Saffro R, Talano JV. Transient ischemic attack association with mitral systolic clicks. Arch Intern Med 139:693–694, 1979.
28. Donaldson RM, Emanuel RW, Earl CJ. The role of two-dimensional echocardiography in the detection of potentially embolic intracardiac masses in patients with cerebral ischemia. J Neurol Neurosurg Psych 44:803–809, 1981.
29. Bramlet DA, Decker EL, Floyd WL. Nonbacterial thrombotic endocarditis as a cause of stroke in mitral valve prolapse. South Med J 75:1133–1135, 1982.
30. Geyer SJ, Franzini DA. Myxomatous degeneration of the mitral valve complicated by nonbacterial thrombotic endocarditis with systemic embolization. Am J Clin Pathol 72:489–492, 1979.
31. Schnee MA, Bucal AA. Fatal embolism in mitral valve prolapse. Chest 83:285–287, 1983.
32. Cook AW, Bird TD, Spence AM, Pagon RA, Wallace JF. Myotonic dystrophy, mitral valve prolapse, and stroke. Lancet 1:335–336, 1978.
33. Spence JD, Wong DE, Melendez LJ, Nichol PM, Brown JD. Increased prevalence of mitral valve prolapse in patients with migraine. Can Med Assoc J 131:1457–1460, 1984.
34. Walter PF, Reid SD, Wenger NK. Transient cerebral ischemia due to arrhythmia. Ann Int Med 72:471–474, 1970.
35. Reed RL, Siekert RG, Merideth J. Rarity of transient focal cerebral ischemia in cardiac dysrhythmia. JAMA 223:893–895, 1973.
36. Davidsen B, Egeblad H, Pietersen A. Thromboembolism in patients with advanced mitral valve prolapse. J Int Med 226:433–436, 1989.
37. Barletta GA, Gagliardi R, Benvenuti L, Fantini F. Cerebral ischemic attacks as a complication of aortic and mitral valve prolapse. Stroke 16:213–219, 1985.
38. Zenker G, Bone G, Ladumer G, Lechner H. The myxomatous mitral valve: A risk factor for ischemic stroke in young patients? Eur Neurol 24:82–84, 1985.
39. Marks AR, Choong CY, Chir MBB, Sanfilippo AJ, Ferre M, Weyman. Identification of high-risk and low risk subgroups of patients with mitral valve prolapse. N Engl J Med 320:1031–1036, 1989.
40. Naggar CZ, Pearson WN, Seljan MP. Frequency of complications of mitral valve prolapse in subjects aged 60 years and older. Am J Cardiol 58:1209–1212, 1986.
41. Cheng TO. Atrial septal aneurysm as a "newly discovered" cause of stroke in patients with mitral valve prolapse. Am J Cardiol 67:327–328, 1991.
42. Lechtat P, Mas JL, Lascault G, Loron P, Theard M, Klimazac M, Drobirski G, et al. Prevalence of patent foramen ovale in patients with stroke. N Engl J Med 318:1148–1152, 1988.

43. Wolf PA, Sila CA. Cerebral ischemia with mitral valve prolapse. Am Heart J 113:1308–1315, 1987.
44. Jackson AC, Goughner DR, Barnett HJM. Mitral valve prolapse and cerebral ischemic events in young patients. Neurology 34:784–797, 1984.
45. Orencia AJ, Petty GW, Khandheia BK, O'Fallon WM, Whisnant JP. Mitral valve prolapse and the risk of stroke after initial cerebral ischemia. Neurology 45:1083–1086.

Part X

The Floppy Mitral Valve, Mitral Valve Prolapse, Mitral Valvular Regurgitation:

Arrhythmias and Sudden Death

Introduction

The Floppy Mitral Valve, Mitral Valve Prolapse, Mitral Valvular Regurgitation–Cardiac Arrhythmias:

The Interface with Circulatory Phenomena

Charles F. Wooley, MD,
Harisios Boudoulas, MD, PhD

Patients with the floppy mitral valve/mitral valve prolapse/mitral valvular regurgitation (FMV/MVP/MVR) triad may experience cardiac arrhythmias. The frequency and significance of cardiac arrhythmias in this setting is a topic that has stimulated a wide range of opinions during the past four decades.

Within the FMV/MVP/MVR triad, arrhythmias occupy an interface area with a broad range of clinical expression. While palpitations may be due to inappropriate sinus tachycardia, significant atrial and ventricular arrhythmias may present with similar symptoms. Episodes of syncope may be related to arrhythmias, volume depletion, autonomic nervous system dysfunction, or combinations therein. Sudden cardiac death, while rare, is a devastating event that occurs in relatively young individuals with an arrhythmia substrate.

As with the medical literature dealing with the imaging characteristics of the FMV/MVP/MVR triad, the tone and focus of the published studies dealing with cardiac arrhythmias has changed considerably since the earlier reports in the 1960s. The initial studies of cardiac arrhythmias in patients with FMVs dealt with clinical recognition and attempts to iden-

From: Boudoulas H, Wooley CF. *Mitral Valve: Floppy Mitral Valve, Mitral Valve Prolapse, Mitral Valvular Regurgitation.* Second revised edition. ©Futura Publishing Company, Armonk, NY, 2000.

tify causative mechanisms. However, during the time of spurious diagnostic criteria based on "prolapse" and concerns about selection bias, the significance of cardiac arrhythmias was downgraded. When FMV/MVP/MVR patients experiencing arrhythmias were compared with "control" populations, attention was directed away from the basic problem, i.e., what type of arrhythmias did these patients have, and what were the mechanisms and significance?

We analyzed the incidence of electrophysiological abnormalities in symptomatic patients with FMV/MVP studied during the period from 1976 to 1986. Of 1,856 patients referred for electrophysiological studies, 271 patients (14.6%) had FMV/MVP without significant MVR. One or more electrophysiological abnormalities were found in 220 of the FMV/MVP patients (81.2%). Although interpretation of these data is dependent on FMV/MVP prevalence figures, we interpreted these data to suggest that the incidence of significant symptomatic arrhythmias was greater than that of the general population. As detailed in Chapter 16, a higher incidence of arrhythmias has also been reported in the younger age groups by multiple investigators.

Current published studies aimed at answering the arrhythmia questions emphasize precision in arrhythmia detection; definition of arrhythmogenic myocardial or electrophysiological substrate and mechanisms; correlation with conduction system, atrial and ventricular pathophysiology, and dysfunction; and targeted antiarrhythmia therapy.

Clinicians are faced with multiple diagnostic concerns when dealing with FMV/MVP/MVR patients with arrhythmias. The age of the patient, the description of symptoms, overall clinical assessment, and the clinical stage of the cardiac disorder are important considerations in the initial assessment. Appropriate use of basic electrocardiography, arrhythmia monitoring, electrophysiological testing, and echo Doppler studies provide the markers that help in the identification of patients at risk for the presence of, or development of, intermittent, paroxysmal, or chronic atrial or ventricular arrhythmias.

Those individuals with the FMV/MVP/MVR triad who are sensitive or responsive to the stresses imposed by postural alterations, sustained exercise, G-forces, weightlessness, intravascular volume depletion, neuroendocrine activation, or pharmacological agents may manifest their responsiveness with the development of arrhythmias, orthostatic intolerance, syncope, or collapse. The interrelations among these clinical responses are complex, and clarification requires careful clinical and laboratory evaluation.

The occurrence, coexistence, or association of atrioventricular bypass tracts, ventricular preexcitation, prolonged Q-T interval syndromes, or recurrent ventricular tachycardia in patients with the FMV/MVP/MVR triad may confound clinical assessment, however, proper identification is necessary in order to clarify therapeutic decisions.

Discussions of sudden death in individuals with the FMV/MVP/MVR triad have been more controversial and emotional than similar discussions about sudden death in patients with aortic stenosis or hypertrophic cardiomyopathy. When our group presented a paper on cardiac arrest with long-term survival in nine patients with FMV/MVP at the national cardiology meetings in 1986, the response was mixed. At the time, the MVP diagnostic criteria were still yielding exaggerated incidence figures, and the conventional wisdom stated that "MVP" was a benign entity best managed with reassurance. The specific critiques about the sudden death presentation centered on the significance of small numbers of FMV/MVP patients who experienced cardiac arrest with survival. In addition, concern was expressed that discussions of sudden death would alarm the postulated vast numbers of MVP patients. When we submitted the manuscript for publication, reviewers cited selection bias and the alarm factor as bases for rejection. In fact, the experience was merely the clinical counterpart of several excellent pathological studies from diverse sources.

All of the concerns listed above, and the pertinent references, are addressed in the following chapters dealing with cardiac arrhythmias and sudden cardiac death. Most importantly, the therapeutic approaches tend to avoid generalizations, and emphasize the wisdom of the individual patient analysis.

16

Mitral Valve Prolapse:

Cardiac Arrhythmias and Electrophysiological Correlates

Stephen F. Schaal, MD

Introduction

The descriptions of arrhythmic disorders many years ago as soldier's heart, neurocirculatory asthenia, and DaCosta's syndrome were likely some of the first descriptions of rhythm abnormalities occurring in the setting of mitral valve prolapse (MVP).[1] Early observations often focused on the potential for sudden death associated with MVP.[2,3] In general, while MVP is a commonly found abnormality with a strikingly high likelihood of arrhythmias, the condition is considered quite benign.[4,5]

The Incidence of Arrhythmias Disorders

Tachyarrhythmias

The reported incidence of rhythm disorders associated with MVP has varied. Most investigators have found the incidence of rhythm abnormalities higher than in control populations. De Maria et al.[6] reported 16% of 31 patients with MVP to be free of all arrhythmias noted on 10-hour Holter monitoring compared with 60% of 40 normals. The results of 24-hour am-

From: Boudoulas H, Wooley CF. *Mitral Valve: Floppy Mitral Valve, Mitral Valve Prolapse, Mitral Valvular Regurgitation.* Second revised edition. ©Futura Publishing Company, Armonk, NY, 2000.

bulatory monitoring in 61 subjects with MVP were compared with those of 179 controls in the Framingham study.[7] While supraventricular and ventricular arrhythmias were more common in patients with MVP, the differences did not reach statistical significance because of the high incidence of arrhythmias in the control group. When the number of subjects was increased by adding black female patients over 40 years of age, a significant excess of arrhythmias was found in those patients with MVP as compared to those without MVP. In a group of 40 consecutive males over the age of 50 years in whom MVP was diagnosed unequivocally by echocardiogram, Higgins et al.[8] found significant arrhythmias consisting of frequent atrial or paroxysmal atrial tachycardia, atrial flutter, or atrial fibrillation in 19. Atrial fibrillation was the most common arrhythmia, occurring in 14 of these patients. Of this group, 15 were asymptomatic, 21 had cardiomegaly, and 19 had left atrial enlargement.

In a symptomatic group of 24 patients evaluated by Winkle et al.,[9] atrial arrhythmias were present in 63%, and 21% of those had paroxysmal supraventricular tachycardia (SVT). Summarizing the cases of SVT associated with MVP reported to 1975, Swartz et al.[10] found 54.8% of 589 patients to have atrial premature depolarizations (APDs) or ventricular premature depolarizations (VPDs).

The incidence of VPDs found by ambulatory electrocardiographic monitoring in adult populations with MVP has been reported to range from 49% to 85%.[7,11] In Winkle's symptomatic patients, 75% were found to have VPDs, 42% had multiform VPDs, 50% had ventricular couplets, and 21% ventricular tachycardia.[9] The prevalence of complex ventricular arrhythmias was reported to vary between 43% and 56% as summarized by Kligfield and Devereux in 1985.[12] Excluding patients with hemodynamically important mitral regurgitation, Kramer et al.[13] found 63% to have VPDs, with multiform VPDs in 43%, VPD couplets in 6%, and ventricular tachycardia in 5% of the patients. Only 40% of this group of patients were symptomatic. Exercise testing appears to increase the incidence of arrhythmias in the MVP population. While 50% of 24 patients with MVP had arrhythmias present on the resting ECG, Gooch et al.[14] reported that 75% were found to have arrhythmias with treadmill exercise testing.

The increased incidence of tachyarrhythmias has been reported in the younger age group as well. Kavey et al.[15] evaluated a group of 103 children between the ages of 6 and 18 years in whom MVP had been detected by auscultation and confirmed by echocardiography. Only 25% of those patients had been evaluated because of symptoms. Ambulatory electrocardiography demonstrated 38% to have VPDs with multiform VPDs or sequential VPDs in 9% of patients.

While the prevalence of tachyarrhythmias in patients with MVP appears to be high, the lack of control groups, with the exception of the studies reported by Savage et al.[7] and De Maria et al.,[6] makes the results difficult to interpret. Kramer et al.,[13] in an attempt to match populations with regard to symptomatic state, compared 63 MVP patients with 28 symptom-matched control patients. The frequency of APDs and VPDs did not differ between the groups. The control group included seven patients whose initial echocardiograms were suggestive of prolapse, six with symptoms suggestive of MVP, and eight recruited as relatives of probands with MVP. This study confuses boundaries of patient populations by using echocardiography as the final determinant of MVP. One of their control patients had a click, one had a click and murmur, and nine had a systolic murmur. While echocardiography tends to be used as the sine qua non for the diagnosis of prolapse, it occasionally does not confirm MVP when MVP is identified by clinical and angiographic assessment. Also, this assumes that this genetically determined syndrome requires MVP as an all-or-none marker. Arrhythmia prevalence studies in the general population have shown a VPD incidence of 50% in young men[16] and 54% in young women.[17] Hinkle et al.[18] reported a 62% incidence of VPDs and a 3% incidence of ventricular tachycardia in men with a median age of 55 years. Thus, the prevalence of tachyarrhythmias in symptomatic patients with MVP is high; the prevalence in a population of normals appears to be less than in the MVP population although adequate comparisons are not possible at this time.

The presence of significant mitral regurgitation in patients with MVP likely influences the prevalence of tachyarrhythmias. Kligfield et al.[19] found a higher percentage of VPDs, VPD complexity, APDs, and atrial fibrillation in 17 MVP patients with mitral regurgitation compared with 63 MVP patients without mitral regurgitation. The patients without mitral regurgitation tended to be younger with a higher percentage of males; neither difference reached statistical significance. The same methods demonstrated similar prevalences of complex tachyarrhythmias in patients with comparable mitral regurgitation regardless of the presence of MVP. However, De Maria et al.[6] and Kavey et al.[15] found no increase in tachyarrhythmias in MVP patients with mitral regurgitation.

Bradyarrhythmias and Conduction Defects

Bradycardiac rhythms reported in association with MVP have included sinoatrial and atrioventricular (AV) conduction abnormalities. De Maria et al.[6] found a 24% incidence of bradyarrhythmias in a group of 31 patients with MVP. Two patients in this group had sinus bradycardia, two had episodes of sinoatrial pause, six had marked sinus arrhythmia, and two had wandering atrial pacemakers. Gulotta et al.[20] reported four patients with AV conduction defects, including two with sinus bradycardia. Seven patients with AV node conduction abnormalities were described by Greenspon et al.[21] One of these patients had sinoatrial exit block in addition to AV conduction abnormality. Leichtman et al.[22] reported a family prone to marked sinus bradycardia and syncope associated with MVP. Of the seven patients with sinus bradycardia, five had MVP on echocardiograph. In a group of 60 symptomatic patients with MVP, Ware et al.[23] found eight patients with spontaneous second- or third-degree AV block, 19 with persistent sinus bradycardia, and one with sinoatrial exit block. The reported AV conduction abnormalities in association with MVP have been primarily localized to the AV node, although Andre-Fouet et al.[24] described one patient with AV block due to His bundle sclerosis. Additionally, bundle branch block appears to be common in patients with MVP. Ware et al.[23] found 10 of their 60 symptomatic patients to have bundle branch block. We reported 25 bundle branch block in eight patients of a series of 58 patients with MVP documented by auscultation and echocardiography. In a group of 55 consecutive patients with MVP, Chandraratra et al.[26] reported three with bundle branch block and five with a prolonged PR interval. Of 52 patients with MVP, Tartini et al.[27] found a 22.5% incidence of bundle branch block.

The bradycardic rhythms, notably sinus bradycardia, sinus exit block, and AV conduction defects, have usually been described in symptomatic patients, most notably those with syncope. The prevalence of AV conduction defects in this population of relatively young MVP patients is quite marked, making MVP the most frequently found diagnosis in the younger patient with AV conduction disease. The need for pacemaker therapy in this group has not been common.

Sudden death in the setting of MVP is discussed in Chapter 17. Additional comments appear in the next section of this chapter.

Electrophysiological Studies in Mitral Valve Prolapse

A number of reports have detailed the results of electrophysiological study (EPS) in patients with MVP. Ware et al.[23] reported on a series of 60 symptomatic patients, Rosenthal et al.[28] on a series of 20 patients with documented ventricular arrhythmias, Engel et al.[29] on a series of 14 patients with ventricular arrhythmias, Morady et al.[30] on a group of 36 patients with MVP, Josephson et al.[31] on a group of 12 patients with paroxysmal SVT, and Levy et al.[32] on a group of 18 patients with MVP.

Electrophysiological Findings in Mitral Valve Prolapse

Over the past 10 years we have studied 264 patients with echocardiographic or angiographic as well as physical findings (click, murmur) of MVP in our electrophysiologic laboratory.[33] These patients were referred for EPS for a variety of reasons: syncope or near-syncope, 107 (40.5%); proven or suspected SVT, 52 (19.7%); palpitations, 22 (8.3%); premature ventricular depolarizations, 17 (6.4%); ventricular tachycardia, 30 (11.4%); ventricular fibrillation or history of sudden death, 19 (7.1%); and brady-cardic events (sinus bradycardia, pauses, or AV block), 24 (13.6%). The great majority of these patients had MVP without significant mitral regur-gitation, without left atrial or left ventricular enlargement, and without left ventricular dysfunction. Thus, this tended to be a group of relatively young patients with an average age of 37.6 years who were primarily symptomatic from dysrhythmias or suspected dysrhythmias.

Bradycardia

Sinoatrial abnormalities were found in 19 patients. The average age was 37.7 years (range 16–69); 15 were female. Fourteen presented with syncope and four with presyncope (Table 1). Sinus bradycardia and/or si-nus pauses were present in nine patients. Sinoatrial abnormalities (pro-longed sinus node recovery time or sinoatrial conduction time, or both) were found in 13 patients; two of these also had abnormal AV node con-duction. Ten patients demonstrated prolonged asystolic pauses (greater than 6 seconds), usually demonstrated during upright tilt or catheter in-duction. Neither sinoatrial abnormalities nor pauses were found in nine patients who presented with syncope plus sinus bradycardia or pauses. Not included in the bradycardia group were an additional two patients who had vasodepressor syncope with profound hypotension without bradycardia during upright tilt study. The incidence of abnormal blood

Table 1
Mitral Valve Prolapse: Electrophysiological Results and History in Patients with Sinoatrial Dysfunction

EPS Results	Patients
Total	19
Asystole pauses >6 sec	10
Prolonged CSNRT or SACT*	13
History	
Syncope or near-syncope	18
Sinus bradycardia or sinus pause	9
Sinus bradycardia or sinus pause with nega-tive EPS results	9

CSNRT = corrected sinus node recovery time; SACT = sinoatrial conduction time.

pressure responses to upright tilt in this group of patients is not apparent from these studies.

Atrioventricular Conduction Disorders

Symptoms of syncope or presyncope were present in 20 patients and were the most common reasons for EPS in this group of 32 patients found to have AV conduction abnormalities (Table 2). The conduction was abnormal at the AV node in all 32 patients as defined by a prolonged AH interval and AV node Wenckebach at an atrial pacing rate of less than 120 beats/minute. Spontaneous AV block (Wenckebach and 2:1 block) was often present during the EPS. Seventeen of this group had a prolonged PR interval, and 14 had spontaneous AV block found on routine ECG or prolonged electrocardiographic monitoring. In addition to abnormal AV conduction, 10 patients demonstrated other EPS abnormalities: sinoatrial conduction abnormalities in three, SVT in seven, and ventricular flutter in one. The average age of this group was 33.4 years (range 16–71); 17 of 32 were male. One patient who demonstrated spontaneous paroxysmal AV block on ambulatory monitoring was found to have normal AV conduction at EPS.

Supraventricular Tachycardia

Excluding atrial fibrillation and flutter, which will be discussed in the next section, AV nodal reentry tachycardia (29 of 51 patients) was the most common type of SVT detected (Table 3). Three of this group had a short

---

Table 2
Mitral Valve Prolapse: Electrophysiological Results
and History in Patients with Atrioventricular
Conduction Abnormalities

EPS Results	Patients
AV conduction delay	32
Sinoatrial abnormality	3
Atrial flutter/fibrillation or SVT	7
History	
Syncope or near-syncope	20
Spontaneous atrioventricular block	14
Prolonged PR internal	17

EPS = electrophysiological study; AV = atrioventricular; SVT = supraventricular tachycardia.

Table 3
Mitral Valve Prolapse: Electrophysiological
Results in Patient with Inducible
Supraventricular Tachycardia

SVT Type	Patients
AV node reentry	29
Accessory pathway reentry	15
Atrial reentry	4
Sinoatrial reentry	2
Junctional (automatic)	1
Total	*51**

SVT = supraventricular tachycardia; AV = atrioventricular.
*SVT documented previously in 26 patients; syncope or near-syncope in 18 patients.

AH interval. Seven patients had Wolff-Parkinson-White syndrome with AV reentry tachycardia via an accessory pathway; an additional eight patients had concealed accessory pathways. Other patients with SVT included four who had atrial reentry, one who demonstrated sinoatrial reentry, and one with junctional tachycardia. Twenty-four of the 48 patients had previously documented SVT by ECG. Syncope was historically present in 14 patients, nondescriptive tachycardia or palpitations in five, "ventricular tachycardia" in two, and sudden death in one. Supraventricular tachycardia had been diagnosed clinically in seven patients in whom either atrial flutter (three patients) or ventricular tachycardia (two patients), or no SVT other than sinus tachycardia (two patients) was found. In addition to the reproducible SVT in these patients, six had sustained atrial flutter provokable, four had AV conduction abnormalities, and one had sinoatrial reentry tachycardia. The average age of this group of patients was 39.5 years (range 16–80 years). Seven of the 46 were male.

Atrial Flutter and Fibrillation

Sustained atrial flutter or fibrillation, flutter-fibrillation, or both flutter and fibrillation at different moments were reproduced in 75 patients (Table 4). Of this group, 24 patients had previously documented SVT, 11 had undefined tachycardia, 32 had a history of syncope, and seven a history of near-syncope. Caffeine was historically important in four patients with the production of flutter or fibrillation only after caffeine challenge in the laboratory. The ventricular rate in most patients was rapid (140 beats/min or higher) and as high as 280 and 289 beats/min in two patients

Table 4
Mitral Valve Prolapse: Electrophysiological
Results and History in Patients with Inducible
Atrial Flutter/Fibrillation

EPS Results	Patients
Atrial flutter	43
Atrial fibrillation	11
Atrial flutter/fibrillation	12
Total	66
Short AH interval	11
AV node conduction abnormal	4
Sinoatrial abnormalities	3
History	
Syncope or near-syncope	37
Atrial flutter/fibrillation	27

EPS = electrophysiological; AV = atrioventricular.

with short AH intervals. Nine other patients had short AH intervals allowing rapid ventricular rate responses. Head-up tilt to 60° was performed in most instances during atrial flutter or fibrillation for a better assessment of the symptomatic state and the potential acceleration of the ventricular rate. In addition to flutter-fibrillation, four patients had AV node reentry tachycardia, four had AV node conduction abnormalities, and three had concomitant sinoatrial disease.

Ventricular Tachycardia

A total of 34 patients had ventricular arrhythmias provoked (Table 5). Paroxysmal ventricular tachycardia was the referral diagnosis in 40 patients. Of the 43 patients in whom ventricular tachycardia had been observed, nine had sustained ventricular tachycardia reproduced (requiring interruption because of symptomatic difficulty or duration longer than 30 seconds), 10 had nonsustained ventricular tachycardia provoked, and two had ventricular fibrillation provoked. Two patients had torsades de pointes ventricular tachycardia; one of these had a similar nonsustained rhythm reproducibly provoked. Of those patients in whom antecedent ventricular tachycardia had not been documented, syncope or near-syncope (nine patients) was the most common reason for EPS study. The tachycardia tended to be rapid and symptom producing (usually lightheadedness), particularly if produced in the upright tilt position. Frequent ventricular ectopy or ventricular ectopy plus syncope or near-syncope

Table 5
Mitral Valve Prolapse: Electrophysiological Results in
Patients with a History of, or Inducible, Ventricular
Tachyarrhythmia

EPS Results	Patients
VT (sustained)	11
VT (nonsustained)	21
Ventricular fibrillation	2
No inducible tachycardia with history of VT	18
VT without history of tachycardia	10

EPS = electrophysiological study; VT = ventricular tachycardia.

were indications for study in 54 patients. Of this group, nonsustained ventricular tachycardia was reproducibly provokable in 11. Ventricular flutter deteriorating to ventricular fibrillation was provoked in one patient who presented with syncope and ventricular couplets.

Ventricular Fibrillation

Twelve patients with documented ventricular fibrillation and four with a history of sudden collapse with resuscitation were studied (Table 6). Provokable rhythms were ventricular fibrillation in three, nonsus-

Table 6
Mitral Valve Prolapse: Electrophysiological
Results in Patients with History of "Sudden
Death" or Ventricular Fibrillation

History	Patients
"Sudden death"	4
Ventricular fibrillation	12
EPS Results	
VT (sustained)	1
VT (nonsustained)	6
Ventricular fibrillation	3
*No inducible tachycardia	6

*Two or six receiving antiarrhythmic drugs at time of
study; two patients studied with normokalemia while
"sudden death" occurred during hypokalemia.
EPS = electrophysiological study; VT = ventricular
tachycardia.

tained ventricular tachycardia in six, and sustained ventricular tachycardia in one. Two patients in whom significant repetitive responses could not be induced had profound hypokalemia present at the time of "sudden death." An additional two patients with no provokable tachycardia were receiving maintenance quinidine at the time of study.

Electrophysiological Studies in Patients with Mitral Valve Prolapse: A Review

Programmed electrical stimulation yields a high percentage of reproducible tachyarrhythmias and conduction defects in symptomatic patients with MVP. Similar to the findings of Ware et al.,[23] who reported eight of a total group of 60 patients to have sinoatrial abnormalities and eight to have a prolonged PR interval, we found a 7% incidence of sinoatrial abnormalities and a 12% incidence of AV node conduction abnormalities. In addition, 10 patients with syncope or near-syncope had prolonged asystolic pauses or profound hypotensive responses to upright tilt in the setting of normal sinoatrial and AV conduction. The incidence of hypotension and rhythm abnormalities with upright posture during EPS is not known because tilting studies in MVP patients have not been routinely performed. Ware et al.[23] compared characteristics of their 60 MVP patients studied electrophysiologically with those of a group of 101 patients who underwent EPS for similar indications and were individually matched to the patients in the MVP group by age, sex, documented prestudy arrhythmias, and structural heart disease other than MVP. While the patients in the control group tended to be older (mean age 45 versus 36), the only rhythm or conduction abnormalities more prevalent in the MVP patients were tachycardia-bradycardia syndrome (18% and 3% for MVP and control groups, respectively), dual AV pathways, and functional bundle branch block. Spontaneous AV block was present in 13% of MVP patients and in 5% of controls although the differences were not statistically significant. Levy et al.[32] compared 18 MVP patients who had EPS with a group of 20 control patients presumed normal. The MVP group had an increased incidence of abnormal AV node conduction, while the sinus node function was not different between the groups.

Supraventricular tachycardia mechanisms have been assessed in MVP patients with discordant results. Josephson et al.[31] found seven of 12 patients studied to have accessory AV bypass tracts as the mechanism for SVT. Of these seven all were left-sided, and four of the patients demonstrated only retrograde conduction over the accessory pathway. Of the 15 patients with reproducible SVT reported by Ware et al.,[23] 10 had AV node reentry and five had accessory pathway reentry. Twenty-four patients (40%) of their total group studied demonstrated dual AV nodal pathways.

This compared with 24% with dual AV node pathways in their control group. Accessory pathway reentry was demonstrated in 15 of our total of 51 patients with MVP in whom sustained SVT could be reproducibly provoked. Eight of these 15 patients had concealed accessory pathways. Of the 29 patients with AV node reentry SVT, indications for study included 20 with documented tachycardia prior to study, eight with syncope, and one with "sudden death." Our results in the MVP patient population with SVT are similar to those reported by Ware et al.[23] and are also similar to our findings of an approximate 65% incidence of AV node reentry in the general population of patients with SVT. It is noteworthy that in those patients in whom SVT was the only significant finding, 11 patients had syncope, six had presyncope, and one had a history of "sudden death."

Paroxysmal atrial flutter or fibrillation was reported by Ware et al.[23] in 11 patients before EPS and reproduced in a total of 17 patients. A total of 74 patients had reproducible sustained atrial flutter or fibrillation in our study. Sixteen of these patients had previously documented atrial flutter or fibrillation and an additional 11 had "tachycardia" of undefined type. Thirty-two of the patients were studied because of syncope, seven because of near-syncope. A short AH interval with the demonstration of a rapid ventricular response during tachycardia (four at 240 beats/min or faster) was found in 13 patients, five of whom had previously documented atrial flutter or fibrillation.

A number of studies have detailed the results of ventricular stimulation in patients with MVP and ventricular arrhythmias. Engle et al.[29] initially reported ventricular stimulation of 14 patients with MVP, only three of whom were symptomatic with ventricular tachyarrhythmias. Tachycardia was provokable only in the three patients with previously documented ventricular tachycardia.

Programmed ventricular stimulation was reported by Naccarelli et al.[34] to induce nonsustained ventricular tachycardia in five of 13 patients with a history of nonsustained tachycardia. Of the five patients with sustained ventricular tachycardia, three had inducible sustained and two had inducible nonsustained tachycardia. Morady et al.[30] performed ventricular stimulation with three extrastimuli in 36 patients with MVP and normal left ventricular function. Patients who were asymptomatic and without previously documented sustained ventricular tachycardia did not have provokable sustained ventricular tachycardia or ventricular fibrillation. Of 20 patients with recurrent syncope of presyncope and frequent VPDs or nonsustained ventricular tachycardia, provokable rhythms were unimorphic, with sustained ventricular tachycardia in two and nonsustained polymorphic tachycardia in eight. Three patients had previous ventricular fibrillation or sustained ventricular tachycardia; unimorphic ventricular tachycardia was provoked in all. Ware et al.[23] were able to reproduce sustained ventricular tachycardia in nine of 14 patients presenting with same. Six of 10 patients presenting with nonsustained ventricular tachycardia had nonsustained tachycardia provoked.

The Mechanisms of Arrhythmias in Mitral Valve Prolapse

The bradycardic abnormalities found in association with MVP have not been studied extensively from a pathological basis. Bharati et al.[35] described marked fatty infiltration in the approaches to the sinoatrial and AV nodes in the region of the atrial preferential pathways in a patient with MVP and a history of nonsustained ventricular tachycardia who died suddenly. They also found compression of the AV node by an enlarged left atrium or mitral orifice or by the invasion of calcium in the abnormally formed central fibrous body. Pathological study of a patient with MVP, Wolff-Parkinson-White syndrome, and AV block demonstrated His bundle sclerosis.[24] Bharati et al.[36] also described sinoatrial node artery thrombosis in one young patient who died suddenly with documented MVP.

Autonomic reflexes may play a role in the bradycardic arrhythmias. On return the supine position after tilt and following the Valsalva maneuver, Coghlan et al.[37] found prolonged bradycardia. Gaffney et al.[38] found attenuated heart rate responses to phenylephrine infusion as well as a reduced heart rate change in response to the diving reflex in patients with MVP. These responses suggest diminished vagal responsiveness, although sympathetic withdrawal in patients with elevated levels of catecholamines may be important.

The mechanism of SVT in many of the MVP patients is related to dual AV node pathways and accessory AV pathways. Whether patients with MVP are more likely to demonstrate such pathways has not been determined. Of the patients with AV node or accessory pathway reentry tachycardia studied in our institution over a 10-year span, 23% had MVP. This compares with an overall incidence of 13.8% of patients studied with a diagnosis of MVP over this same period. Electrophysiological characterizations by Ware et al.[23] and by us suggest that the incidence of accessory pathways in patients with MVP is similar to the overall incidence of accessory pathways responsible for SVT. Josephson et al.[31] reported a higher incidence of accessory pathways in patients with MVP than in the general population with SVT. Dual AV node pathways were found more commonly in patients with MVP than in controls as reported by Ware et al.[23]

The striking incidence of spontaneous and extrastimulus-provokable atrial flutter and atrial fibrillation in patients with MVP may be partially explained by the pathological findings of dense laminated collagen-containing elastic tissue in the atrial endocardium and fibrous nodules in the left atrial wall demonstrated by Chesler et al.[39] and the findings of fatty infiltration in the approaches to both the sinoatrial and the AV nodes by Bharati et al.[35] The potential for the mitral valve leaflets per se to be involved in atrial tachyarrhythmias was suggested by the studies of Wit et al.[40] Anterior mitral valve leaflet tissue from a human cardiac transplant recipient demonstrated spontaneous automatic impulses at a slow rate. Epinephrine accelerated the rate of spontaneous depolarization, produced delayed after depolarizations, and caused sustained triggered rhythmic activity. While prolonged intra- and interatrial conduction are the electrophysiological hallmarks of atrial flutter and fibrillation, such prolongation of atrial conduction has not been found in MVP patients with paroxysmal atrial flutter or fibrillation and normal atrial size. We have found differences in atrial refractoriness in patients with MVP and reproducible atrial flutter compared with normal subjects.[41] This alteration in atrial refractoriness between high and low right atrium might be explained by differences in the autonomic influence of these areas. Patients with atrial enlargement caused by mitral regurgitation would be expected to have the same increased propensity to atrial flutter and fibrillation as that seen with other pathological entities producing atrial enlargement with its attendant fibrosis.

With regard to ventricular arrhythmias, Bharati et al.[35] described scattered areas of fibrosis throughout the anterior left ventricular wall in a patient with nonsustained ventricular tachycardia and sudden death. Endocardial friction lesions were found at autopsy in 12 of the 14 patients with MVP studied by Chesler et al.[39] It is of note that none of the 14 patients described by Chesler et al. appeared to have extensive left ventricular disease and left ventricular enlargement as would be expected with mitral regurgitation. Right ventricular endomyocardial biopsies performed in 14 symptomatic patients with primary MVP by Mason et al.[42] demonstrated abnormal endocardial and interstitial fibrosis in 57% and a high frequency of myocyte and mitochondrial degeneration, nuclear chromatin clumping, and intracellular edema in MVP patients compared with controls. Eight of their 14 patients had palpitations and syncope or presyncope and only one had mitral regurgitation with left ventricular dysfunction.

Ventricular fibrosis, which appears to be present in a high percentage of symptomatic patients and patients who have died suddenly, is a possible mechanistic cause for the ventricular ectopy commonly found in these patients. Other mechanisms proposed have included chordae traction by the redundant prolapsing leaflets rendering the leaflets ischemic[43] and mechanical stimulation of the endocardium by redundant leaflets.[44] These hypotheses would require marked redundancy of leaflets, a finding not commonly observed in patients with MVP and significant ventricular ectopy, nor found in patients with sudden death studied at autopsy. Gornick et al.[45] in a study of the electrophysiological effects of papillary muscle traction in the intact dog found no change in myocardial blood flow. However, these investigations found that late diastolic traction tended to cause an earlier local ventricular activation in the area of traction and relative prolongation of the ventricular functional refractory period in the area of traction. These findings support the concept that abnormal ventricular wall motion as achieved with papillary muscle traction could be responsible for the induction or exacerbation of ventricular ectopic activity. Additionally, "stretch-activated" arrhythmias have been demonstrated by both rapid and gradual stretch of the ventricular myocardium.[46] Echocardiography has shown that the distance between papillary muscle tips and the annulus remains rather constant in normals while the mitral leaflet displacement into the left atrium results in papillary muscle displacement causing traction in patients with MVP.[47] Vectorcardiographic localization of premature ventricular contractions in patients with MVP has demonstrated that such originate in the posterobasal segments of the left ventricle, which would include areas in the region of the mitral apparatus.[48] The ventricular dilatation and stretch associated with mitral regurgitation would increase myocardial wall strain resulting in ventricular ectopy.[49]

Mechanosensitive atrial ATP-sensitive potassium channels have been demonstrated.[50] These channels may be important in the production of or contribute to contraction–excitation feedback in rhythms such as atrial flutter and other atrial tachycardias.[51]

The importance of ventricular repolarization abnormalities and prolonged QT interval in patients with ventricular ectopy is not clear. The Framingham study reported no evidence of QT prolongation associated with MVP.[52] Additionally, Cowan and Fye compared 100 younger women with MVP, of whom 60% were symptomatic, to 100 healthy age-matched controls with the finding of no significant differences in corrected QT interval between the groups.[53] A small proportion of patients with MVP associated with ventricular ectopy in all reported series have prolonged QT intervals. While the QT corrected for heart rate (QT_c) is not necessarily prolonged in a high percentage of MVP patients, Puddu et al.[54] found the QT_c to be statistically longer than that of controls in 10 of 15 symptomatic MVP patients and definitely prolonged (greater than 440 msec) in the other five patients. These patients also demonstrated elevated total serum catecholamine levels in the standing and supine positions compared with controls. Comparing 56 patients with MVP to 62 controls, Bekheit et al.[55]

found the QT_c to be significantly prolonged in the MVP population. Boudoulas et al.[56] demonstrated that patients with MVP had a greater increase in heart rate than controls during isoproterenol infusion and that electrical systole (QT interval) increased relative to electromechanical systole (QS_2) interval during isoproterenol infusion more markedly in patients with MVP than controls. This dynamic increase in the QT interval as seen with isoproterenol infusion has occasionally been noted during ambulatory monitoring in patients with MVP and could be important in the genesis of ventricular ectopic activity and tachycardia by promoting local differences in the recovery of excitability. Studies by Boudoulas et al.[56] showing parallel responses of the 24-hour urine catecholamine secretion to the frequency of ventricular premature depolarizations also highlight the importance of catecholamine responsiveness in the production of ventricular arrhythmias. Comparing groups of MVP patients with and without ventricular arrhythmias, Gaffney et al.[57] found significantly higher heart rate responses to venous pooling produced by lower body negative pressure. The striking reduction in ventricular ectopic frequency noted with beta-blocker therapy underlines the arrhythmogenesis of catecholamine effects in patients with MVP.

The importance of mitral regurgitation contributing to the prevalence of ventricular arrhythmias has been highlighted by Kligfield et al.[19] They found 41% of patients with mitral regurgitation to have frequent ventricular ectopy compared with only 3% of patients without mitral regurgitation. These results are in contrast to those reported by De Maria et al.,[6] who found no correlation between the presence of arrhythmias and the severity of MVP or mitral regurgitation. They noted "serious" premature ventricular depolarizations (frequency of greater than five per minute, multifocal, occurring in pairs or more, repetitive beating, or occurring on the T wave of the preceding beat) in 16 or 31 patients. Of the 36 patients studied with programmed electrical stimulation by Morady et al.,[30] 27 had complex ventricular ectopy and only three patients had significant mitral regurgitation. Among MVP sudden death survivors, mitral regurgitation does not appear commonly present. Boudoulas et al.[58] reported one of nine post-sudden-death patients to have significant mitral regurgitation; two of seven patients reported by Winkle et al.[3] had mitral regurgitation; none of the patients reported by Wei et al.[59] had mitral regurgitation; and only three of the 19 patients studied electrophysiologically by us had significant mitral regurgitation. Thus, while the presence of mitral regurgitation likely is associated with an increased incidence of significant ventricular ectopy, the incidence of ventricular arrhythmias without mitral regurgitation, particularly in symptomatic patients, appears to be only modestly increased.

Mitral Valve Prolapse: Arrhythmias and Electrophysiological Correlates

Evaluating Arrhythmias in Patients with Mitral Valve Prolapse

The patient with MVP, whether symptomatic or asymptomatic, deserves initially a careful examination with particular attention to the presence or absence of mitral regurgitation, left ventricular abnormalities, and orthostatic hypotension. The initial echocardiogram is important, particularly for the assessment of left atrial size, ventricular size, and function. A baseline ECG is necessary to screen for prolonged QT interval as well as AV, other conduction defects, short PR interval, or preexcitation.

Patients with MVP who are symptomatic with palpitations, light-headedness, or syncope should have a resting ECG, ambulatory monitoring for identifying potential arrhythmias, and exercise testing for arrhythmia surveillance during stress. The identification of mitral regurgitation and the contractile function and size of the left ventricle are important. If the symptomatic complex does not occur during ambulatory monitoring or exercise testing, repeat monitoring or ECG event recording should be attempted in an effort to view an electrocardiographic recording during the symptomatic difficulty. The incidence of postural hypotension and sinus tachycardia as significant causes of tachycardia, palpitations, and light-headedness is quite appreciable in patients with MVP.

The patient who is symptomatic during tachycardia and remains undefined, or the patient with syncope, should undergo tilt studies as well as EPS to assess the potential for neurocardiogenic syncope, sinoatrial node dysfunction, AV conduction defects, and various supraventricular or ventricular tachyarrhythmias. Once identified, the rhythm abnormalities can be analyzed with regard to drug efficacy in the laboratory as well as the definition and direction of rhythm-specific therapy, such as ablation or pacemaker therapy. Patients who have survived an episode of ventricular fibrillation should undergo EPS. If ventricular tachycardia or fibrillation is inducible, optimization of antiarrhythmic therapy is possible; an intracardiac defibrillating device may be required.

Still others who may require EPS are those patients who are not particularly symptomatic but who have episodes of ventricular tachycardia, either sustained or nonsustained. The inducibility of sustained ventricular tachycardia defines a patient who requires therapy. In the patient with inducible nonsustained ventricular tachycardia, the need for an electrophysiological definition of ventricular vulnerability is less clear. Morady et al.[30] did not treat any of the six asymptomatic patients with frequent VPDs, couplets, or triplets of whom three had inducible 7- to 15-beat runs of ventricular tachycardia; all have remained well in short-term follow-up.

The role of EPS assistance in the evaluation of the patient with VPDs but without ventricular tachycardia is unclear at this time. We studied 48 patients with VPDs, seven of whom had couplets, with the finding of inducible nonsustained ventricular tachycardia in 10 patients; ventricular fibrillation was induced in one patient who had couplets and a history of syncope. Four patients who were asymptomatic except for palpitations and occasional to frequent VPDs had inducible nonsustained ventricular tachycardia. Thus, the patient without syncope or near-syncope who has VDPs but no ventricular tachycardia does not likely benefit from electrophysiological evaluation.

Follow-up evaluation requires careful attention to symptomatic difficulty, with continued monitoring of orthostatic blood pressure and heart rate changes and rhythm surveillance by means of ambulatory ECG recording during symptoms and, occasionally, repeat exercise testing.

Therapy for Arrhythmias in Patients with Mitral Valve Prolapse

Abinader[60] administered oral propranolol to 35 patients with systolic murmur and nonejection clicks confirmed by phonocardiography to examine the electrophysiological abnormalities attending this syndrome. With regard to nonspecific ST and T wave abnormalities, six patients showed normalization, 22 demonstrated improvement, six showed no change, and one showed increased ST-T changes in response to propranolol therapy. Abinader suggested that the ECG changes may be due to an autonomic imbalance resulting in "sympathetic overactivity." A beneficial effect of propranolol was also noted by Sloman et al.[61] In a study of seven patients with palpitations, six noted improvement with propranolol. Winkle et al.[62] also assessed the effect of propranolol on the symptoms and rhythm of patients with MVP. Six of 12 patients with palpitations noted a decrease in their frequency; six noted no change in palpitations after propranolol. Propranolol produced an average 90% reduction in VPD frequency in five of nine patients with frequent VPDs on ambulatory electrocardiographic recording. Three patients showed no change in ventricular ectopic frequency with propranolol therapy and one had an increase in frequency. Propranolol abolished paroxysmal ventricular tachycardia in three of four patients and controlled ventricular couplets completely in four of nine patients. Of the four patients demonstrating frequent atrial ectopics, propranolol effected a 73% average reduction in total APDs. Propranolol did not control the frequency of paroxysmal SVT, although the type of SVT was not mentioned.

Beta-blockade also appears to be effective in the control of life-threatening ventricular arrhythmias. Reporting on a group of seven patients with ventricular fibrillation or ventricular tachycardia causing syncope of requiring cardioversion, Winkle et al.[3] found propranolol to be effective therapy in a follow-up of four patients, propranolol plus quinidine effective in one, and potassium replacement plus intermittent propranolol in another. Beta-blockade remains the therapy of choice in patients with ventricular arrhythmias because of its likelihood of reducing ventricular ectopy without usually causing significant side effects or aggravating the arrhythmia. However, the drug therapy must be individualized with careful attention to symptoms and documentation of effects with electrocardiographic monitoring, exercise testing, or even EPS in the patient with potentially lethal ventricular arrhythmias.

Particular attention should be paid to the baseline QT interval as well as the QT interval after therapy. A small percentage of patients with MVP will demonstrate QT prolongation. This group of patients deserves careful evaluation because of their potential for sudden death. Beta-blockade should be administered in the setting of ventricular arrhythmias and prolonged QT interval. Some of these patients require an automatic implantable cardioverter-defibrillator (AICD) as well. The potential benefit of beta-blockade administered prophylactically for prolonged QT without ventricular arrhythmias has not been established. Avoidance of drugs that prolong the QT interval is essential in the patient with ventricular arrhythmias and a prolonged QT interval.

As with any patient prone to dysrhythmias, attention to maintenance of a normal serum potassium is very important. Of the seven patients with life-threatening ventricular arrhythmias, Winkle et al.[3] reported profound hypokalemia in one and the intermittent use of diuretics in another and KCl withdrawal before arrest in a third. We found hypokalemia to be an important contributor to ventricular fibrillation in two of our 19 patients with "sudden death." Patients with MVP may be more prone to hypokalemia because of the hyperadrenergic state shown to be present in some studies.[56]

Therapy for ventricular tachyarrhythmias usually commences with beta-blockade. The Class IA antiarrhythmics need to be used with caution because of QT prolongation and proarrhythmic events. These drugs have not often been found effective in the control of ventricular arrhythmias associated with MVP. Pratt et al.[63] reported a series of 17 patients with MVP and drug-resistant ventricular arrhythmias. Fourteen of these patients had failed beta-blocker therapy and 13 had failed at least one Class IA antiarrhythmic drug. Compared with placebo, these patients had an overall 90% reduction in VPDs, a 96% reduction in ventricular couplets, and a 99% reduction in runs of ventricular tachycardia during therapy with moricizine. We have used flecainide successfully in five of seven patients with drug-resistant, symptomatic ventricular tachycardia.

Therapy for SVT requires defining the specific tachycardia. AV node reentry tachycardia or accessory pathway tachycardia is usually cured with ablation therapy. Atrial flutter and atrial fibrillation are effectively treated with Class IC or Class III agents. Caution is again required with regard to QT interval prolongation. While frequent APDs do not usually require therapy, Winkle et al.[54] found propranolol effective in a high percentage of patients.

Patients with the bradyarrhythmias, particularly sinoatrial and AV node dysfunction, have occasionally required pacemaker therapy. Because these patients have coexisting tachycardia, correlating periods of bradycardia with symptomatic difficulty is important before pacemaker implantation.

Therapy for patients with MVP and arrhythmic disorders will continue to improve as further understanding of the electrophysiological, autonomic, and pathological abnormalities becomes available.

References

1. Wooley CF. Where are the diseases of yesteryear? DaCosta's syndrome, soldier's heart, the effort syndrome, neurocirculatory asthenia–and the mitral valve prolapse syndrome. Circulation 53:749–751, 1976.
2. Shappell SD, Marshall CE, Brown RE, Bruce TA. Sudden death and the familial occurrence of mid-systolic click, late systolic murmur syndrome. Circulation 48:1128–1134, 1973.
3. Winkle RA, Lopes MG, Popp RL, Hancock EW. Life-threatening arrhythmias in the mitral valve prolapse syndrome. Am J Med 60:961–967, 1976.
4. Allen H, Harris A Leatham A. Significance and prognosis of an isolated late systolic murmur. Br Heart J 36:525–532, 1974.
5. Nishimura RA, McGoon MD, Shub C, Miller FA Jr, Ilstrup DM, Tajik AJ. Echocardiographically documented mitral valve prolapse. N Engl J Med 313:1305–1309, 1985.
6. DeMaria AN, Amsterdam EA, Vismara LA, Neumann A, Mason DT. Arrhythmias in the mitral valve prolapse syndrome. Ann Int Med 84:656–660, 1976.
7. Savage DD, Levy D, Garrison RJ, Castelli WP, Kligfield P, Devereux RB, et al. Mitral valve prolapse in the general population. 3. Dysrhythmias: The Framingham study. Am Heart J 106:582–586, 1983.
8. Higgins CB, Reinke RT, Gosink BB, Leopold GR. The significance of mitral valve prolapse in middle-aged and elderly men. Am Heart J 91:292–296, 1976.
9. Winkle RA, Lopes MG, Fitzgerald JW, Goodman DJ, Schroeder JS, Harrison DC. Arrhythmias in patients with mitral valve prolapse. Circulation 52:73–81, 1975.
10. Swartz MH, Teichholz LE, Donoso E. Mitral valve prolapse: A review of associated arrhythmias. Am J Med 62:377–389, 1977.
11. Kreisman K, Kleiger R, Schad N. Arrhythmia in prolapse of the mitral valve. Circulation 43(Suppl 2):137, 1971.
12. Kligfield P, Devereux RB. Arrhythmias in mitral valve prolapse. Clin Progr Electrophysiol Pacing 3:403–418, 1985.

13. Kramer HM, Kligfield P, Devereux RB, Savage DD, Kramer-Fox R. Arrhythmias in mitral valve prolapse: Effect of selection bias. Arch Int Med 144:2360–2364, 1984.
14. Gooch AS, Vicencio F, Maranhao V, Goldberg H. Arrhythmias and left ventricular asynergy in the prolapsing mitral leaflet syndrome. Am J Cardiol 29:611–620, 1972.
15. Kavey RW, Blackman MS, Sondheimer HM, Byrum CJ. Ventricular arrhythmias and mitral valve prolapse in childhood. J Pediatr 105:885–890, 1984.
16. Brodsky M, Wu D, Denes P, Kanakis C, Rosen KM. Arrhythmias documented by 24-hour continuous electrocardiographic monitoring in 50 male medical students without apparent heart disease. Am J Cardiol 39:390–395, 1977.
17. Sobotka PA, Moyer JH, Bauernfeind RA, Kanakis C, Rosen KM. Arrhythmias documented by 24-hour continuous ambulatory electrocardiographic monitoring in young women without apparent heart disease. Am Heart J 101:753–758, 1981.
18. Hinkle LE, Carver ST, Stevens M. The frequency of asymptomatic disturbances of cardiac rhythm and conduction in middle-aged men. Am J Cardiol 24:629–650, 1969.
19. Kligfield P, Hochreiter C, Kramer H, Devereux RB, Niles N, Kramer-Fox R, Borer JS. Complex arrhythmias in mitral regurgitation with and without mitral valve prolapse: Contrast to arrhythmias in mitral valve prolapse without mitral regurgitation. Am J Cardiol 55:1545–1549, 1985.
20. Gulotta SJ, Gulco L, Padmanabhan V, Miller S. The syndrome of systolic click, murmur and mitral valve prolapse: A cardiomyopathy? Circulation 49:717–728, 1974.
21. Greenspon AJ, Schaal SF. AV node dysfunction in the mitral valve prolapse syndrome. PACE 3:600–604, 1980.
22. Leichtman D, Nelson R, Gobel FL, Alexander CS, Cohn JN. Bradycardia with mitral valve prolape. Ann Int Med 85:453–457, 1976.
23. Ware JA, Magro SA, Luck JC, Mann D, Nielsen AP, Rosen KM, Wyndham CR. Conduction system abnormalities in symptomatic mitral valve prolapse: An electrophysiologic analysis of 60 patients. Am J Cardiol 53:1075–1078, 1984.
24. Andre-Fouet X, Tabib A, Jean-Louis P, Anne D, Dutertre P, Gayet C, de Mahenge AH, et al. Mitral valve prolapse, Wolff-Parkinson-White syndrome, His bundle sclerosis and sudden death. Am J Cardiol 56:700, 1985.
25. Schaal SF, Fontana MB, Wooley CF. Mitral valve prolapse: Spectrum of conduction defects and arrhythmias. Circulation 50(Suppl 3):97, 1974.
26. Chandraratna PA, Ribas-Meneclier C, Littman BB, Samet P. Conduction disturbances in patients with mitral valve prolapse. J Electrocardiol 10:233–236, 1977.
27. Tartini R, Moccetti T, Riva A, Belli C. Electrocardiographic changes and arrhythmias in Barrow's syndrome. Arch Mal Coeur Vaiss 73/9:1063–1074, 1980.
28. Rosenthal ME, Hamer A, Gang ES, Oseran DS, Mandel WJ, Peter T. The yield of programmed ventricular stimulation in mitral valve prolapse patients with ventricular arrhythmias. Am Heart J 110:970–976, 1985.
29. Engel TR, Meister SG, Frankl WS. Ventricular extrastimulation in the mitral valve prolapse syndrome. Evidence for ventricular reentry. J Electrocardiogr 11:137–142, 1978.
30. Morady F, Shen E, Bhandari A, Schwartz A, Scheinman MM. Programmed ventricular stimulation in mitral valve prolapse: Analysis of 36 patients. Am J Cardiol 53:135–138, 1984.

31. Josephson ME, Horowitz LN, Kastor J. Paroxysmal supraventricular tachycardia in patients with mitral valve prolapse. Circulation 57:111–115, 1978.
32. Levy PS, Blanc A, Clementy J, Dallocchio M, Bricaud H. Prolapsus valvulaire mitral: Les troubles du rhythme ont-ils un substratum electrophysiologique? Arch Mal Coeu 75:671–676, 1982.
33. Boudoulas H, Schaal SF, Wooley CF. Floppy mitral valve/mitral valve prolapse: Cardiac arrhythmias. In Vardas PE (ed.) Cardiac Arrhythmias. Great Britain, Pacing and Electrophysiology, Kluwer Academic Publishers, 1998, pp 89–95.
34. Naccarelli GV, Prystowsky EN, Jackman WM, Heger JJ, Rahilly GT, Zipes DP. Role of electrophysiologic testing in managing patients who have ventricular tachycardia unrelated to coronary artery disease. Am J Cardiol 50:165–171, 1982.
35. Bharati S, Granston AS, Liebson PR, Loeb HS, Rosen KM, Lev M. The conduction system in mitral valve prolapse syndrome with sudden death. Am Heart J 101:667–670, 1981.
36. Bharti S, Rosen KM, Miller LB, Strasberg B, Lev M. Sudden death in three teenagers. Circulation 64(Suppl 4):71, 1981.
37. Coghlan HC, Phares P, Cowley M, Copley D, James TN. Dysautonomia in mitral valve prolapse. Am J Med 67:236–244, 1979.
38. Gaffney FA, Bastian BC, Lane LB, Taylor WF, Horton J, Schutte JE, Graham RM, et al. Abnormal cardiovascular regulation in the mitral valve prolapse syndrome. Am J Cardiol 52:316–320, 1983.
39. Chesler E, King RA, Edwards JE. The myxomatous mitral valve and sudden death. Circulation 67:632–639, 1983.
40. Wit AL, Fenoglio JJ, Hordof AJ, Reemtsma K. Ultrastructure and transmembrane potentials of cardiac muscle in the human anterior mitral valve leaflet. Circulation 59:1284–1292, 1979.
41. Dobmeyer DJ, Stine RA, Leier CV, Schaal SF. Electrophysiologic mechanisms of provoked atrial flutter in mitral valve prolapse syndrome. Am J Cardiol 56:602–604, 1985.
42. Mason JW, Koch FH, Billingham ME, Winkel RA. Cardiac biopsy evidence for a cardiomyopathy associated with symptomatic mitral valve prolapse. Am J Cardiol 42:557–562, 1978.
43. Barlow JB, Boxman CK. Aneurysmal protrusion of the posterior leaflet of the mitral valve: An auscultatory-electrocardiographic syndrome. Am Heart J 71:166–178, 1966.
44. Zeilenga DW, Criley JM. Mitral valve dysfunction: A possible cause of arrhythmias in the prolapsed posterior leaflet syndrome. Clin Res 21:243, 1973.
45. Gornick CC, Tobler HG, Pritzker MC, Tuna IC, Almquist A, Benditt DG. Electrophysiologic effects of papillary muscle traction in the intact heart. Circulation 73:1013–1021, 1986.
46. Franz MR, Cima R, Wang D, Profitt D, Kurz R. Electrophysiologic effects of myocardial stretch and mechanical determinants of stretch-activated arrhythmias. Circulation 86:968–978, 1992.
47. Sanfilippo AJ, Harrigan P, Popovic AD, Weyman AE, Levine RA. Papillary muscle traction in mitral valve prolapse: Quantitation by two-dimensional echocardiography. J Am Coll Cardiol 19:564–571, 1992.
48. Lichstein E. Site of origin of ventricular premature beats in patients with mitral valve prolapse. Am Heart J 100:450, 1980.

49. Hansen DE, Craig CS, Hondeghem LM. Stretch-induced arrhythmias in the isolated canine ventricle. Circulation 81:1094–1105, 1990.
50. Van Wagoner DR. Mechanosensitive gating of atrial ATP-sensitive potassium channels. Circ Res 72:973–983, 1993.
51. Yamasheta T, Oikawa N, Marakama Y, Nakajima T, Omata M, Inone H. Contraction-excitation feedback in atrial reentry: Role of velocity of mechanical stretch. Am J Physiol 267(Heart Circ Physiol 36):H1254–H1262, 1994.
52. Levy D, Savage D. Prevalence and clinical features of mitral valve prolapse. Am Heart J 113:1281–1289, 1987.
53. Cowan M, Fye W. Prevalence of QT_c prolongation in women with mitral valve prolapse. Am J Cardiol 63:133–134, 1989.
54. Puddu PE, Pasternac A, Tubau JF, Krol R, Farley L, de Champlain J. QT interval prolongation and increased plasma catecholamine levels in patients with mitral valve prolapse. Am Heart J 105:422–428, 1983.
55. Bekheit SG, Ali AA, Deglin SM, Jain AC. Analysis of QT interval in patients with idiopathic mitral valve prolapse. Chest 81:620–625, 1982.
56. Boudoulas H, Reynolds JC, Mazzaferri E, Wooley CF. Mitral valve prolapse syndrome: The effect of adrenergic stimulation. J Am Coll Cardiol 2:638–644, 1983.
57. Gaffney FA, Karlsson ES, Campbell W, Schutte JE, Nixon JV, Willerson JF, Blomqvist CG. Autonomic dysfunction in women with mitral valve prolapse syndrome. Circulation 59:894–901, 1979.
58. Boudoulas H, Schaal SF, Stang JM, Fontana MB, Kolibash AJ, Wooley CF. Mitral valve prolapse–sudden death with long-term survival. Int J Cardiol 26:37–40, 1990.
59. Wei JY, Bulkley BH, Schaeffer AH, Greene HL, Reid PR. Mitral-valve prolapse syndrome and recurrent ventricular tachyarrhythmias. Ann Int Med 89:6–9, 1978.
60. Abinader EG. Adrenergic beta blockade and ECG changes in the systolic click murmur syndrome. Am Heart J 91:297–302, 1976.
61. Sloman G, Stannard M, Hare WSC, Goble AJ, Hunt D. Prolapse of the posterior leaflet of the mitral valve. Isr J Med Sci 5:727–731, 1969.
62. Winkle RA, Lopes MG, Goodman DJ, Fitzgerald JW, Schroeder JS, Harrison DC. Propranolol for patients with mitral valve prolapse. Am Heart J 93:422–427, 1977.
63. Pratt CM, Young JB, Wierman AM, Borland RM, Seals AA, Leon CA, Raizner A, Quinones MA, Roberts R. Complex ventricular arrhythmias associated with the mitral valve prolapse syndrome. Am J Med 80:626–632, 1986.

17

Floppy Mitral Valve/Mitral Valve Prolapse:

Sudden Death

Harisios Boudoulas, MD, PhD,
Charles F. Wooley, MD

Introduction

The floppy mitral valve (FMV) with mitral valve prolapse (MVP) and mitral valvular regurgitation (MVR) is a dynamic valvular abnormality. The MVR may progress from mild to severe (Fig. 1).[1–10] Symptoms and complications (including sudden death) may be related to the degree of valvular dysfunction; sequelae of progressive MVR, including left ventricular (LV) and left atrial (LA) dilatation and dysfunction;[11] autonomic nervous system function or dysfunction; and other abnormalities associated with FMV/MVP.

Major predictors of sudden death in most forms of heart disease, regardless of the specific cardiac pathology, include the presence and extent of LV dysfunction, coupled with electrophysiological propensity for "electrical instability" that may lead to lethal arrhythmia.[12] Repetitive ventricular ectopy or complex ventricular arrhythmias, including ventricular tachycardia, are strong indicators of the electrical instability that may lead to sudden death in the presence of LV dysfunction and ischemia. The presence of a prolonged electrical systole corrected for heart rate (QT$_c$ or QTI),

From: Boudoulas H, Wooley CF. *Mitral Valve: Floppy Mitral Valve, Mitral Valve Prolapse, Mitral Valvular Regurgitation*. Second revised edition. ©Futura Publishing Company, Armonk, NY, 2000.

FMV/MVP: Sudden Death

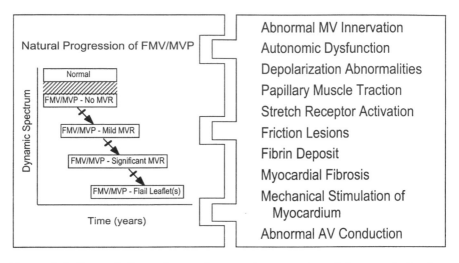

Figure 1. Left panel. Dynamic spectrum and progression of floppy mitral valve (FMV) and mitral valve prolapse (MVP). A subtle gradation exists between a normal mitral valve and minimal to mild FMV/MVP. Progression from one level of valvular dysfunction to a more severe form may occur. MVR = mitral valvular regurgitation; MV = mitral valve. Right panel. Factors that may produce or aggravate "electrical instability."

or electrical systole greater than electromechanical systole $QT>QS_2$), atrioventricular (AV) conduction abnormalities (i.e., different degrees of AV block and/or accessory AV pathways), and intraventricular conduction defects are other findings suggestive of electrical instability.[13,14] Factors that may aggravate the electrical instability include myocardial ischemia, pharmacological agents, metabolic and electrolytic abnormalities, autonomic dysfunction, and stimulants that alter autonomic function such as phosphodiesterase inhibitors (caffeine, aminophylline), other cyclic AMP stimulants (ephedrine-like drugs), cigarette smoking, and drug abuse (cocaine, heroin, marijuana, etc.). All of these factors should be taken into consideration in any study of cardiac sudden death regardless of the underlying cardiac pathology. Thus, it is reasonable to suggest that these influences, alone or in combination, may affect mortality in patients with FMV/MVP.

The incidence of sudden death in patients with FMV/MVP who have severe MVR and LV dysfunction is higher than in patients with FMV/MVP and normal LV performance. The same is true, however, for patients with coronary artery disease and other forms of valvular heart disease. Thus, the association between FMV/MVP and sudden death in patients who have developed significant valvular regurgitation, LV or LA dilatation, and dysfunction cannot be attributed to FMV/MVP alone. For this reason, only sudden death in FMV/MVP without significant MVR will be discussed in this chapter.

Floppy Mitral Valve/Mitral Valve Prolapse Without Significant Mitral Valvular Regurgitation: Sudden Death

Sudden death may occur in patients with FMV/MVP in the absence of hemodynamically significant MVR, but it is rare. Autopsy studies have shown that mitral annular circumference, anterior and posterior mitral valve leaflet lengths, posterior mitral valve thickness, and endocardial friction lesions were greater in hearts from patients with FMV/MVP and sudden death when compared to hearts from patients with other causes of death and incidental FMV/MVP. Clinical studies have shown that sudden death occurred almost exclusively in patients with thick mitral valve leaflets, changes that can be defined with echocardiographic techniques.[15-40]

In general, sudden death in patients with FMV/MVP without significant MVR has been reported almost exclusively in symptomatic patients (Table 1).[15] Patients with a history of recurrent syncope, a history of sustained supraventricular arrhythmias or complex ventricular arrhythmias,

Table 1
Floppy Mitral Valve/Mitral Valve Prolapse–Cardiac Arrest: Symptoms Prior to Cardiac Arrest*

Pt.	Age/Sex	Palpitations	Syncope	Other
1	66/M	25–30 years	No	No
2	22/M	5–10 years	No	Mild sleep apnea
3	26/F	10–15 years	No	Migraine
4	29/F	Many years	3 episodes (10 years)	Fatigue
5	36/F	No	No	No
6	25/F	Many years	5 episodes (10 years)	No
7	31/F	Many years	No	No
8	28/F	10 years	No	No
9	36/F	15–20 years	15 years	Dyspnea, chest pain, orthostatic symptoms

Pt. = patient; M = male; F = female
* Modified from Boudoulas H, et al.[15]

or a family history of cardiac sudden death appear to be at higher risk for sudden death.

In a study from The Ohio State University Medical Center, we reported nine cases of resuscitated survivors of patients with FMV/MVP and cardiac arrest, only one of whom had significant MVR. All but one of the patients were symptomatic before cardiac arrest; eight had long histories of palpitations with documented ventricular arrhythmias, and three of the eight had a history of recurrent syncope.[15]

Clinical characteristics in the eight patients without significant MVR include the auscultatory findings and laboratory descriptors shown in Table 2.[15] All eight patients had systolic clicks; six also had systolic murmurs. Electrocardiogram (available in four patients before and in all survivors after cardiac arrest) was normal in two, showed left axis deviation in one, prolonged electrical systole and electrical systole greater than electric mechanical systole ($QT>QS_2$) in one, inverted T waves in the inferolateral leads in one, sinus bradycardia in one, premature ventricular beats in one, premature ventricular beats and premature atrial beats in one. Chest x-rays available in four patients before, and in all survivors after cardiac arrest showed mild scoliosis in one, and were normal in seven. M-mode echocardiograms were available in three patients before and in all survivors after cardiac arrest demonstrated mitral valve prolapse in all.

Cardiac catheterization was performed in seven patients; six had cardiac catheterization after and one before cardiac arrest; FMV/MVP was demonstrated in all; all seven had normal coronary artery anatomy. Six patients had normal left ventricular size and systolic function; one patient had normal LV size (101 cm^3/ cm^2) with borderline systolic function (ejection fraction 50%).

A summary of arrhythmias and electrophysiological studies for each patient is presented in Table 3.[15] Electrocardiographic monitoring was performed before cardiac arrest in four patients and after cardiac arrest in four patients. Electrophysiological studies were performed in two patients before and in five patients after cardiac arrest. Five patients were treated with β-blocking drugs during the time when electrophysiological studies were performed.

The location in which the cardiac arrest occurred, the arrhythmias detected, and the therapy at the time of cardiac arrest for all eight patients are shown in Table 4.[15] Four patients collapsed at their work place. Three patients collapsed at work (two performing work with minimal physical exertion, one while teaching her students). Two patients collapsed at home during their routine physical activities. One patient collapsed at home during routine daily activities; it was initially thought that she had "seizure disorders"; ventricular fibrillation was documented several minutes later, but her physician attributed the arrhythmias to the seizure dis-

Table 2

Floppy Mitral Valve/Mitral Valve Prolapse–Cardiac Arrest: Auscultatory, Electrocardiographic (ECG), Chest X-Ray, Echocardiographic (Echo), and Cardiac Catheterization (Cath) Findings*

Pt.	Auscultatory	ECG	Chest X-Ray	Echo	Cath
1	Loud systolic click, no murmur	Normal	Normal	Normal LV size and function, normal LA, MVP	EDVI 101 cm, EF 50% MVP, no MVR, normal LV pressures, normal coronary arteries
2	Systolic click, no murmur	LAD	Mild scoliosis, otherwise normal	Normal LV size and function, normal LA, MVP	Normal LV size and function, MVP, normal coronary arteries
3	Systolic click plus murmur	Prolonged QT; QT > QS$_2$	Normal	Normal LV size and function, normal LA, MVP	Normal LV size and function, MVP, normal coronary arteries
4	Systolic click plus murmur, systolic "honk"	Inverted T waves in leads II III, aVF, V$_5$, V$_6$	Normal	Normal LV size and function, normal LA, MVP	Normal LV size and function, MVP, normal LV pressures, normal coronary arteries
5	Systolic click plus murmur	Sinus bradycardia	Normal	Normal LV size and function, normal LA, MVP	Normal LV size and function, MVP, mild MR, normal LV pressures, normal coronary arteries
6	Systolic click plus murmur	PVBs	Normal	Normal LV size and function, normal LA, MVP	Normal LV size and function, MVP, mild MVR, normal LV pressures, normal coronary arteries
7	Systolic click plus murmur	Normal	Normal	Normal LV size and function, normal LA, MVP	Not performed
8	Systolic click plus murmur	PVBs PABs	Normal	Normal LV size and function, normal LA, MVP	Normal LV size and function, MVP, MVR, normal LV pressures, normal coronary arteries

LAD = left axis deviation; QT = electrical systole; QS$_2$ = electromechanical systole; PVBs = premature ventricular beats; PABs = premature atrial beats; LV = left ventricle; LA = left atrium; MVP = mitral valve prolapse; EDVI = end-diastolic volume index; MVR = mitral valvular regurgitation; TVP = tricuspid valve prolapse; TR = tricuspid regurgitation; EF = ejection fraction.
* Modified from Bondoulas H, et al.[15]

Table 3
Floppy Mitral Valve/Mitral Valve Prolapse–Cardiac Arrest: Arrhythmias and Electrophysiological Studies*

Pt.	Electrocardiographic Monitoring	Electrophysiological Studies
1	Frequent PVBs and PABs, runs of SVT	Mobitz type I AV block at rate 110/minute, No VT or SVT
2	Frequent PVBs, short runs of VT	Slightly prolonged SA recovery time, Mobitz type I AV block at rate 120/minute, easily induced atrial flutter, no VT
3	Frequent PVBs	Nonsustained VT
4	Frequent PVBs, short runs of VT	Infra-His block, no VT or SVT
5	Frequent PVBs	Nonsustained VT
6	Frequent PVBs, PABs, bradycardia	Normal
7	Frequent multiformed PVBs	Not performed
8	SVT, PVBs with couplets, PABs	Normal

PVBs = premature ventricular beats; PABs = premature atrial beats; SVT = supraventricular tachycardia; VT = ventricular tachycardia; AV = atrioventricular; SA = sinoatrial.
* Modified from Boudoulas H, et al.[15]

order and initiated therapy with dilantin and phenobarbital. One year later she collapsed while she was walking in a store; ventricular fibrillation was also documented at that time. One patient collapsed in the hospital after she was admitted for evaluation of palpitations and another patient collapsed on the street while she was walking with her husband and her

Table 4
Floppy Mitral Valve/Mitral Valve Prolapse–Cardiac Arrest: Location, Arrhythmia Detected and Therapy at the Time of Cardiac Arrest*

Pt.	Location	Arrhythmia	Cardiopulmonary Resuscitation	Therapy at Event
1	Home	Ventricular fibrillation	Successful	None
2	Home	"Seizure" ventricular fibrillation	Successful	Dilantin, phenobarbital
3	Home	Ventricular tachycardia/ ventricular fibrillation	Successful	Digitalis, propranolol
4	Work	Ventricular fibrillation	Successful	None
5	Work	Ventricular fibrillation	Successful	None
6	Hospital	Ventricular fibrillation	Successful	None
7	Street	Unknown	Unsuccessful	Propranolol
8	Work	Ventricular fibrillation	Unsuccessful	Propranolol

* Modified from Boudoulas H, et al.[15]

child. Thus, none of the patients were performing unusual physical activities at the time of cardiac arrest.

Four of the patients were treated for their symptoms prior to cardiac arrest. One was treated with dilantin and phenobarbital for "seizure disorders"; one was treated with digitalis plus propranolol; two other patients were treated with propranolol. Thus, it seems unlikely that pharmacologic agents contributed to cardiac arrest.

Ventricular fibrillation was documented by the emergency squad personnel or in a hospital setting in seven patients. When the emergency squad arrived, there was no cardiac electrical activity found in one patient who had collapsed in the street. Cardiopulmonary resuscitation with defibrillation was successful in seven and unsuccessful in two patients.

Autopsy was performed in one of the two patients with unsuccessful resuscitation. The postmortem examination showed a prolapsing mitral valve with redundant mitral valve leaflets, myxomatous changes of mitral valve, with nodularity of the mitral valvular cusps. Microscopic examination of the mitral valve leaflets showed myxomatous changes and areas of mucoid degeneration. The other heart valves were normal. The anterior descending branch of the left coronary artery showed minimal atherosclerosis. All of the coronary arteries were patent; there was no evidence of myocardial infarction, inflammation, or fibrosis. There were no significant abnormalities of the brain. Blood cultures and a toxicology screen were negative.

The therapy the patients received after cardiac arrest and the subsequent clinical course are shown in Table 5. Patient #1 has been treated with

Table 5
Floppy Mitral Valve/Mitral Valve Prolapse–Cardiac Arrest: Therapy and Clinical Course after Cardiac Arrest*

Pt.	Years After Cardiac Arrest	Therapy	Symptoms
1	3	Atenolol	None
2	14	Digitalis, propranolol	Palpitations
3	3.5	Propranolol	None
4	3	Pacemaker, propranolol, quinidine, florinef	Orthostatic hypotension, near syncope, chest pain, palpitations
5	8	Metoprolol	None
6	13	Propranolol, procainamide	Palpitations

* Modified from Boudoulas H, et al.[15]

atenolol; 3 years post cardiac arrest he was asymptomatic. Patient #2 has been treated with digitalis and propranolol; she complained of palpitations and remained alive 14 years after cardiac arrest. Patients #2 and #5 have been treated with propranolol; both were asymptomatic and alive 3.5 and 8 years after cardiac arrest. Patient #4 has been treated with quinidine for cardiac arrhythmias and florinef for orthostatic phenomena; a permanent pacemaker was implanted for infra-His block; she was alive 3 years after cardiac arrest but continued to have orthostatic phenomena and palpitations. Patient #6 has been treated with propranolol and procainamide; she complained of palpitations and was alive 13 years after cardiac arrest.[15] It should be noted that the therapy reflects medical practice in the 1960s, 1970s, and 1980s.

Electrocardiographic ST segment and T wave changes are frequently present in patients with FMV/MVP and sudden death or ventricular fibrillation. In a study by Campbell et al.[19] involving 20 patients with MVP without MVR, 14 of the patients were symptomatic. Twenty-four-hour electrocardiographic monitoring was performed in all patients. One patient had syncope secondary to spontaneously terminated ventricular fibrillation and three patients had ventricular tachycardia. Eight of the 20 patients had inferolateral ST and T wave abnormalities on the resting electrocardiogram; ventricular fibrillation or tachycardia occurred in patients with ST and T wave changes.

Winkle et al.[18] reported seven cases with MVP (only two had significant MVR) who have survived one or more episodes of life-threatening ventricular arrhythmias. These arrhythmias included ventricular fibrillation in three patients, cardiac standstill in one patient, and recurrent ventricular tachycardia causing syncope or sustained ventricular tachycardia requiring electrical cardioversion in two patients. Of the seven patients, five had ST and T wave changes in the resting electrocardiogram; all had ventricular arrhythmias on the resting electrocardiogram, during treadmill exercise testing, and during ambulatory electrocardiographic monitoring. At present it is wise to regard these resting electrocardiographic changes with concern, particularly when present in symptomatic individuals, although the lack of data regarding the overall incidence of these electrocardiographic changes in patients with FMV/MVP limits the conclusions that may be drawn.

While prolonged electrical systole corrected for heart rate (QT_c or QTI) and sudden death have been reported in patients with MVP, the overall incidence of QT_c prolongation in patients with FMV/MVP appears to be low.[1,41]

Sudden death in patients with FMV/MVP most often is due to ventricular fibrillation. Among the patients with FMV/MVP–sudden death reported from The Ohio State University Medical Center, ventricular fibrillation was documented in seven patients (Table 4).[15] There is evidence that the incidence of potentially lethal ventricular arrhythmias in patients with MVP is greater than in the general population. Wei et al.[26] found 10 patients with MVP without significant MVR and a similar number of patients without detectable heart disease among 60 consecutive patients referred for the management of refractory complex ventricular arrhythmias. If there is no selection bias and the incidence of FMV/MVP in the general population is 2–4%, then the disproportionately high representation of MVP patients in this series suggests that complex ventricular arrhythmias in patients with MVP may be more frequent than in the general population without heart disease.

Cause of Arrhythmias

The cause of arrhythmias in patients with FMV/MVP is multifactorial (see Chapter 16) and appears to be related to the anatomic substrate and the modulating role of the autonomic nervous system (Table 6).[28] Papillary muscle tension in FMV/MVP may be responsible for ventricular arrhythmias.[42] Membrane depolarization is caused by both gradual and rapid ventricular stretch, but premature ventricular depolarizations are more readily elicited by rapid stretch. Studies have demonstrated the existence of stretch-activated membrane channels in ventricular myocardium; these may contribute to ventricular ectopy under conditions of differential ventricular loading as in FMV/MVP.[28,43] Echocardiographic data demonstrated that in normal subjects the distance between the papillary muscle tips and the mitral annulus during systole remains relatively constant. In contrast, in patients with FMV/MVP, mitral valve leaflet dis-

---

Table 6
Floppy Mitral Valve/Mitral Valve Prolapse: Possible Cause
of Ventricular Arrhythmias

- Likely multifactorial
- Papillary muscle traction/ventricular stretch
- Mechanical stimulation of myocardium by leaflets
- Abnormal innervation of floppy mitral valve
- Endocardial friction lesions
- Autonomic dysfunction ($\uparrow$NE$\rightarrow$ $\downarrow$K+, postural phenomena)
- QT dispersion
- Platelet aggregation–fibrin deposits (emboli of coronary arteries)
- Myocardial fibrosis

Floppy Mitral Valve / Mitral Valve Prolapse

Abnormal Mitral Apparatus

↓

Mitral Leaflet Prolapse

↓

Papillary Muscle Traction
Activation of Stretch Receptors

↓

Papillary Muscle and
Subendocardial Ischemia

↓

Pain
Ventricular Arrhythmias

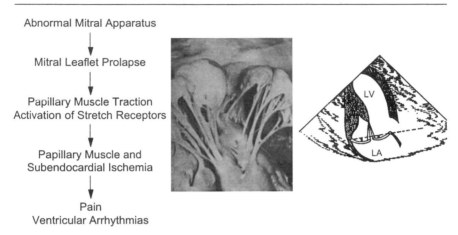

Figure 2. Postulated mechanisms of ventricular arrhythmia and chest pain related to papillary muscle traction and activation of stretch receptors. Floppy mitral valve is shown in the middle. (Used with permission from Edward JE. Circulation 43:606–612, 1971.) Papillary muscle traction during left ventricular (LV) systole is also shown schematically. LA = left atrium.

placement into the left atrium results in papillary muscle displacement that causes traction of the muscle (Fig. 2).[28,42]

Innervation of the mitral valve may also contribute the genesis of cardiac arrhythmias in FMV/MVP.[44] Human cardiac valves have distinct patterns of innervation that comprise both primary sensory and autonomic components. The presence of distinct nerve terminals suggests a neural basis for interactions between the central nervous system and the mitral valve. The subendocardial surface on the atrial aspect at the middle portion of the mitral valve is rich in nerve endings, including afferent nerves; mechanical stimuli from this area caused by abnormal coaptation in MVP may cause abnormal autonomic nerve feedback between the central nervous system and mitral valve nervous system (Fig. 3).[28,44]

Endocardial friction lesions resulting from friction between the chordae and LV myocardium have been reported in patients with FMV/MVP, and it is possible that these lesions may he responsible for, or contribute to, the development of ventricular arrhythmias.[22,23] Platelet aggregation, hemorrhage, and fibrin deposits have been observed in the angle between the LA and the posterior mitral leaflet and microembolism from these deposits may involve the coronary circulation with subsequent myocardial ischemia and ventricular arrhythmias. Chesler et al.[22] reported the clinical pathology in 14 instances of sudden death attributable to arrhythmias associated with FMV/MVP (only two had significant MVR). Endocardial

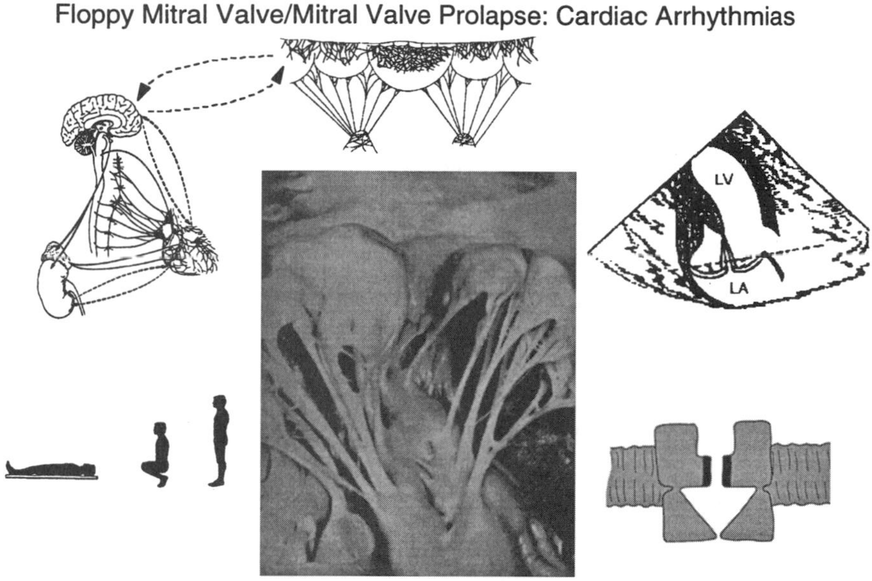

Floppy Mitral Valve/Mitral Valve Prolapse: Cardiac Arrhythmias

Figure 3. The cause of cardiac arrhythmias in floppy mitral valve/mitral valve prolapse is multifactorial. Autonomic dysfunction-neurohormonal abnormalities, papillary muscle traction/ventricular stretch-stretch receptors activation, orthostatic phenomena, innervation of the mitral valve, and mechanical stimulation of myocardium by mitral valve leaflets are contributory factors. Floppy mitral valve is shown in the middle (used with permission from Edward JE. Circulation 43:606–612, 1971); above the mitral valve innervation of the mitral valve is shown schematically; upper right shows papillary muscle traction during ventricular systole; lower right stretch-activated receptor is shown schematically. Left upper part shows schematically interactions between the brain-heart-kidneys and adrenals. Lower left part shows schematically orthostatic phenomena. (Used with permission from Boudoulas H, et al.[28])

friction lesions were present in 11 individuals; five patients had thrombotic lesions containing fibrin and platelets in the angle between the posterior leaflet and the LA wall. Other studies also have suggested that fibromuscular dysplasia was present in the AV node artery in patients with MVP who died suddenly.[45]

Autonomic dysfunction may initiate, precipitate, or contribute to arrhythmias in patients with FMV/MVP syndrome. Increased adrenergic activity, catecholamine regulation abnormality, and adrenergic hyperresponsiveness has been observed in certain patients with FMV/MVP. Altered vagal tone or baroreceptor activity may also play a role in the pathogenesis of cardiac arrhythmias in certain patients.[41,46–52]

Increased adrenergic activity associated with FMV/MVP in some instances may be associated with hypokalemia which, in turn, may contribute to cardiac arrhythmias.[41,46] Autonomic dysfunction and stretch-activated mechanoreceptors may contribute to QT dispersion, which may cause ventricular arrhythmias in some patients with MVP. The incidence of QT dispersion has been reported to be higher in patients with MVP compared to the general population.[28,53,54]

Patients with FMV/MVP often present with postural phenomena such as orthostatic decreases in cardiac output, orthostatic hypotension, tachycardia, and symptoms related to alterations in heart rate, blood pressure, and cardiac output. Orthostatic phenomena are multifactorial in origin. Decreased intravascular volume, an abnormal renin-aldosterone response to volume depletion, a baroreflex modulation abnormality, a hyperadrenergic state, or a parasympathetic abnormality may partially account for these phenomena. Further, inability of patients with FMV/MVP to maintain normal left ventricular diastolic volume in the upright posture will result in greater prolapse and papillary muscle traction.[28,42,55] Greater prolapse in the upright posture and the development of the "third chamber" between the mitral valve annulus and the prolapsed mitral valve leaflets (see Chapter 21) may contribute to orthostatic phenomena. These changes in LV size and mitral valve apparatus may contribute to orthostatic changes in cardiac arrhythmias.

Incidence of Sudden Death

The magnitude of sudden death in patients with FMV/MVP without significant MVR is difficult to quantify. The incidence of sudden death during follow-up of clinically recognized patients with MVP has varied from 0% to 1.3% per year. Data from these studies, however, most likely represent heterogeneous populations that may include some patients with significant MVR who are more likely to be highly symptomatic and have more complex arrhythmias than unselected patients with FMV/MVP.

Nishimura et al.[56] reported six cases of sudden death among 237 patients with MVP (patients had minimal symptoms) followed for an average of 6 years, suggesting an average risk of approximately 0.4% per year, an incidence of sudden death greater than that for the general population without heart disease. All patients in this study who had sudden death had echocardiographic evidence of mitral leaflet redundancy. Mitral leaflet redundancy was found in 41% of the entire MVP population in this study. Complex ventricular arrhythmias were found in three of the six patients who died suddenly.

Davies et al.[57] had four individuals with FMV/MVP without significant MVR, among 13 cases of sudden death with FMV/MVP during a 5-year forensic necropsy study. During the same period, approximately 250 cases of sudden death per year caused by coronary artery disease were reported in the study population. This suggests that on a yearly basis, 0.3 sudden deaths might be expected among patients with FMV/MVP without significant MVR for every 100 coronary artery disease sudden deaths. Bias, however, may be a problem with these estimations. It is more likely that an autopsy will be performed in patients with FMV/MVP and sudden death than in patients with known coronary artery disease and a history of previous myocardial infarction.

Floppy Mitral Valve/Mitral Valve Prolapse Sudden Death: Diagnostic–Therapeutic Approach

Patients with FMV/MVP who fall into the currently, incompletely defined "high-risk," category should have further diagnostic studies. Such studies should be individualized and address the suspected underlying pathology and pathophysiology. Appropriate therapy would depend on the outcome of such testing, subject to the same limitations and potential benefit of individualized antiarrhythmic therapy.[58,59]

Patients with FMV and significant MVR should undergo reconstructive surgery or valve replacement when indicated (see Chapter 18) to prevent irreversible LV damage.

Standard electrocardiography should be used to identify patients who have evidence of preexcitation or other anomalous AV pathways, or prolongation of the rate-corrected QT interval. Since each of these subgroups may be at increased risk of sudden death, such patients should be separated from the general FMV/MVP population for more intensive evaluation. Diuretics should be avoided to prevent hypokalemia and hypomagnesemia that might initiate or precipitate cardiac arrhythmias. Likewise, caffeine, alcohol, ephedrine-like drugs, or other stimulants should be avoided.

Abnormal AV pathways, when present and particularly when associated with supraventricular arrhythmias, warrant electrophysiological studies and, if indicated, ablation therapy.[58–72] There are data suggesting that FMV/MVP patients with complex ventricular arrhythmias in whom ventricular tachycardia-fibrillation is not inducible by programmed electrical stimulation have a benign short-term natural history. Automatic cardioverter-defibrillator implantation may be necessary in selective cases.[28] Although mitral valve reconstruction in patients without significant MVR has been reported to provide the relief of symptoms including complex ventricular arrhythmias, this therapeutic approach remains controversial.

Patients with FMV/MVP who have recovered from cardiopulmonary resuscitation should undergo a thorough noninvasive and invasive cardiac evaluation to define the electrophysiological substrate, the nature of the arrhythmias, as well as to exclude any other coexisting cardiac pathology. Implantation of automatic defibrillator may be indicated in selected patients.

Floppy Mitral Valve/Mitral Valve Prolapse Sudden Death: Perspective

Uncertainty exists regarding the predictive value of suspected risk factors for sudden death in patients with FMV/MVP. Patients with FMV/MVP who experience sudden death usually represent isolated instances; thus, it will be necessary to establish a centralized data registry to gather these isolated reports. Further, it might be necessary to establish a cooperative study in patients with FMV/MVP at "higher risk" for sudden death in order to define the natural course of these patients. Such studies will improve our ability to define prognostic indicators and to define the effect of therapeutic interventions in a small subset of patients with FMV/MVP who are at higher risk for sudden death.

References

1. Boudoulas H, Wooley CF (eds). Mitral Valve Prolapse and the Mitral Valve Prolapse Syndrome. Mount Kisco, NY, Futura Publishing Company, 1988.
2. Boudoulas H, Kolibash AJ, Baker P, King BD, Wooley CF. Mitral valve prolapse and the mitral valve prolapse syndrome: A diagnostic classification and pathogenesis of symptoms. Am Heart J 118:796–818, 1989.
3. Wooley CF, Baker PB, Kolibash AJ, Kilman JW, Sparks EA, Boudoulas H. The floppy myxomatous mitral valve, mitral valve prolapse and mitral regurgitation. Prog Cardiovasc Dis 33:397–433, 1991.
4. Wooley CF, Sparks EA, Boudoulas H. The floppy mitral valve-mitral valve prolapse-mitral valvular regurgitation triad. ACC Current J Rev July/August 1994, pp 25–26.
5. Boudoulas H, Wooley CF. Mitral valve prolapse and the mitral valve prolapse syndrome. In Yu PN, Goodwin JF (eds). Prog Cardiovasc Dis 14:275–309, 1986.
6. Boudoulas H. Valvular Disease. American College of Cardiology Self-Assessment Program (ADDSAP) 2000, in press.
7. Boudoulas H, Kolibash AJ, Wooley CF. Mitral valve prolapse: The high-risk patient. Practical Cardiol 17:15–31, 1991.
8. Duren DR, Becker AE, Dunning AJ. Long-term follow-up of idiopathic mitral valve prolapse in 300 patients: A prospective study. J Am Coll Cardiol 11:42–47, 1988.
9. Kolibash AJ, Kilman JW, Bush CA, et al. Evidence for progression from mild to severe mitral regurgitation in mitral valve prolapse. Am J Cardiol 58:762–767, 1986.
10. Boudoulas H, Kolibash AJ, Wooley CF. Mitral valve prolapse: A heterogeneous disorder. Primary Cardiol 1991;17:29–43.
11. Boudoulas H, Boudoulas D, Sparks EA, Pearson AC, Nagaraja HN, Wooley CF. Left atrial performance indices in chronic mitral valve disease. J Heart Valve Dis 1995;4(Suppl 2);S242–247.
12. Weissler AM, Boudoulas H. Sudden death: Detecting the vulnerable ventricle by noninvasive methods. J Lab Clin Med 98:654–659, 1981.

13. Moss AJ, Schwartz PJ. Sudden death and the idiopathic long QT syndrome. Am J Med 66:6–7, 1979.
14. Boudoulas H, Sohn YH, O'Neill W, Brown R, Weissler AM. The $QT>QS_2$ syndrome: A new mortality risk indicator in coronary artery disease. Am J Cardiol 50:1228–1235, 1982.
15. Boudoulas H, Schaal SF, Stang JM, et al. Mitral valve prolapse: Cardiac arrest with long-term survival. Int J Cardiol 26:37–44, 1990
16. Jeresaty RM. Sudden death in the mitral valve prolapse-click syndrome. Am J Cardiol 37:317–318, 1976.
17. Sorensen HD, Smith RF. Lethal cardiac arrhythmias in the prolapsing valve syndrome. J Tenn Med Assoc Aug: 667–668, 1975.
18. Winkle RA, Lopes MG, Popp RL, Hancock EW. Life-threatening arrhythmias in the mitral valve prolapse syndrome. Am J Med 60:961–967, 1976.
19. Campbell RWF, Godman MG, Fiddler GI, Marquis RM, Julian DG. Ventricular arrhythmias in syndrome of balloon deformity of mitral valve. Definition of possible high risk group. Br Heart J 38:1053–1078, 1976.
20. Mair WJ. Sudden death in young females with floppy mitral valve syndrome. Austr NZ J Med 10:221–223, 1980.
21. Bharati S, Granston As, Liebson PR, Loeb HS, Rosen KM, Lev M. The conduction system in mitral valve prolapse syndrome with sudden death. Am Heart J 101:667–670, 1981.
22. Chesler E, King RA, Edwards JE. The myxomatous mitral valve and sudden death. Circulation 67:632–639, 1983.
23. Chesler E, Edwards JE. Mitral valve prolapse and sudden death. Primary Cardiol Jan: 75–87, 1984.
24. Pocock WA, Bosman CK, Chesler E, Barlow JB, Edwards JE. Sudden death in primary mitral valve prolapse. Am Heart J 107:378–382, 1984.
25. Roberts WC. Sudden cardiac death: Definitions and causes. Am J Cardiol 57:1410–1413, 1986.
26. Wei JY, Bulkeley BH, Schaeffer AH, Greene HG, Reid Pr. Mitral valve prolapse syndrome and recurrent ventricular tachyarrhythmias: A malignant variant refractory to conventional drug therapy. Ann Int Med 89:6–9, 1978.
27. Ritchie JL, Hammermeister KE, Kennedy JW. Refractory ventricular tachycardia and fibrillation in a patient with the prolapsing mitral leaflet syndrome: Successful control with overdrive pacing. Am J Cardiol 37:314–316, 1976.
28. Boudoulas H, Schaal SF, Wooley CF. Floppy mitral valve/mitral valve prolapse: Cardiac arrhythmias. In Vardas PE (ed): Cardiac Arrhythmias, Pacing, and Electrophysiology, Great Britain, Kluwer Academic Publisher, 1998, pp 89–95.
29. Farb A, Tang AL, Atkinson JB, McCarthy WF, Virmani R. Comparison of cardiac findings in patients with mitral valve prolapse who die suddenly to those who have congestive heart failure from mitral regurgitation and to those with fatal noncardiac conditions. Am J Cardiol 70:234–239, 1992.
30. Dollar AL, Roberts WC. Morphologic comparison of patients with mitral valve prolapse who died suddenly with patient who died from severe valvular dysfunction or other conditions. J Am Coll Cardiol 17:921–931, 1991.
31. Brugada R, Roberts R. The Molecular Genetics of Arrhythmias and Sudden Death. Clin Cardiol 21:553–560, 1998.
32. Loire R, Tabib A. Unexpected sudden cardiac death. An evaluation of 1000 autopsies. Arch Mal Coeur Vaiss 89(1):13–18, 1996.
33. Joint Steering Committees of the Unexplained Cardiac Arrest Registry of Europe and the Idiopathic Ventricular Fibrillation Registry of the US. Survivors of

out-of-hospital cardiac arrest with apparently normal heart: Need for definition and standardized clinical evaluation. Circulation 95:265–272, 1997.

34. Vohra J, Sathe S, Warren R, Tatoulis J, Hunt D. Malignant ventricular arrhythmias in patients with mitral valve prolapse and mild mitral regurgitation. PACE 16:387–393, 1993.
35. Babuty D, Cosney P, Breuillac JC, Charniot JC, Delhomme C, Fauchier L, Fauchier JP. Ventricular arrhythmia factors in mitral valve prolapse. PACE 17:1090–1099, 1994.
36. Levy S. Ventricular arrhythmias and mitral valve prolapse. Acta Cardiologica XlV11,2:125–134, 1992.
37. Vecchia LL, Ometto R, Centofante P, Varotto L, Bonanno C, Bozzola L, Bevilacqua P, Vincenzi M. Arrhythmic profile, ventricular function, and histomorphometric findings in patients with idiopathic ventricular tachycardia and mitral valve prolapse: Clinical and prognostic evaluation. Clin Cardiol 21:731–735, 1998.
38. Corrado D, Thiene G, Nava A, Rossi L, Pennelli. Sudden death in young competitive athletes: Clinicopathologic correlations in 22 cases. Am J Med 89:586–596, 1990
39. Corrado D, Basso C, Nava A, Rossi L, Thiene G. Sudden death in young people with apparently isolated mitral valve prolapse. G Ital Cardiol 27(11):1097–1105, 1997.
40. Loire R, Tabib A. Unexpected sudden cardiac death. An evaluation of 1000 autopsies. Arch Mal Coeur Vaiss 89(1):13–18, 1996.
41. Boudoulas H, Reynolds JC, Mazzaferri E, Wooley CF. Metabolic studies in mitral valve prolapse syndrome. Circulation 61:1200–1205, 1980.
42. Sanfilippo AJ, Harrigan P, Popvic AD, et al. Papillary muscle tension in mitral valve prolapse: Quantitation by two-dimensional echocardiography. J Am Coll Cardiol 19:564–571, 1992.
43. Franz MR, Cima R, Wang D, Proffit D, Kuntz R. Electrophysiological effects of myocardial stretch and mechanical determinants of stretch-activated arrhythmias. Circulation 86:968–978, 1992
44. Marron K, Yacoub MH, Polak JM, et al. Innervation of human atrioventricular and arterial valves. Circulation 1996;94:368–375.
45. Burke AP, Farb A, Tang A, Smialek J, Virmani R. Fibromuscular dysplasia of small coronary arteries and fibrosis in the basilar ventricular septum in mitral valve prolapse. Am Heart J 1997;134:282–291.
46. Boudoulas H, Reynolds JC, Mazzaferri E, Wooley CF. Mitral valve prolapse syndrome: The effect of adrenergic stimulation. J Am Coll Cardiol 2:628–444, 1983.
47. Gaffney AF, Karlsson ES, Campbell W, Schutte JE, Nixon JV, Willerson JT, Blomqvist CG. Autonomic dysfunction in women with mitral valve prolapse syndrome. Circulation 59:894–901, 1979.
48. Coghlan HC, Phares P, Cowley M, Copley D, James TN. Dysautonomia in mitral valve prolapse. Am J Med 67:236–244, 1979.
49. Levitt B, Cagin N, Kleid J, Somberg J, Gillis R. Role of the nervous system in the genesis of cardiac rhythm disorders. Am J Cardiol 37:111–113, 1976.
50. Eliot RS, Buell JC. Role of emotions and stress in the genesis of sudden death. J Am Coll Cardiol 5:95–98B, 1985.
51. Boudoulas H, Schaal SF, Leier CV, Lewis RP. The role of the autonomic nervous system in patients with sinoatrial and atrioventricular node dysfunction. Eur J Cardiol 12;311–319, 1981.

52. Davies AO, Mares A, Pool JL, et al. Mitral valve prolapse with symptoms of beta adrenergic hypersensitivity: Beta$_2$ adrenergic receptor supercoupling with desensitization of isoproterenol exposure. Am J Med 82:193–201, 1987.
53. Boudoulas H, Wooley CF. The floppy mitral valve, mitral valve prolapse, mitral valvular regurgitation. In: Moss and Adams' Heart Disease in Infants, Children and Adolescents. Sixth edition, in press.
54. Zdrojewski TR, Purzycki Z, Rynkiewicz A, Kubasik A, Wyrzkowski B, Krupa-Wojciechowska B. QT/QS2 ratio in mitral valve prolapse syndrome, hyperthyroidism and borderline hypertension: Possible indication of dysautonomia. Am J Noninvas Cardiol 1993;7:19–22.
55. Bashore TM, Grines C, Utlak D, Boudoulas H, Wooley CF. Postural exercise abnormalities in symptomatic patients with mitral valve prolapse. J Am Coll Cardiol 11:499–507, 1988.
56. Nishimura RA, McGoon MD, Shuib C, Miller FA Jr, Ilstrup DM, Tajik AJ. Echocardiographically documented mitral valve prolapse. Long-term follow-up in 237 patients. N Engl J Med 313: 1305–1309, 1985.
57. Davies MJ, Moore BP, Brainbridge MV. The floppy mitral valve: Study of incidence, pathology, and complications in surgical, necropsy and forensic material. Br Heart J 40:468–481, 1978.
58. Wooley CF, Boudoulas H. Mitral valve prolapse. Conn's Current Therapy. Rakel RE, ed., W.B. Saunders Co., 1999, pp.289–293.
59. Boudoulas H, Nelson SD, Schaal SF, Lewis RP. Diagnosis and management of syncope. In Alexander RW, Schlant RC, Fuster V, O'Rourke RA, Roberts R, Sonnenblick EH (eds): Hurst's the Heart, 9th ed. New York, McGraw-Hill, 1998, pp 1059–1080.
60. Ware JA, Magro SA, Luck JC, Mann Dem Nielson AP, Rosen KM, Wyndham CRC. Conduction system abnormalities in symptomatic mitral valve prolapse: An electrophysiologic analysis of 60 patients. Am J Cardiol 53:1075–1078, 1984.
61. Dobmeyer DJ, Stine RA, Leier CV, Schaal SF. Electrophysiologic mechanisms of provoked atrial flutter in mitral valve prolapse syndrome. Am J Cardiol 56:602–608, 1985.
62. Camous JP, Guarino L, Varenne A, Sabetier M, Baudouy M, Guiran JB. Serious arrhythmia in a patient suffering from ventricular pre-excitation and a prolapse of the two mitral valves. Ann de cardiologie et d'angeiologie 26:329–333, 1977.
63. Woodley D, Chambers W, Starke H, Dzindzio B, Forker AD. Intermittent complete atrioventricular block masquerading as epilepsy in the mitral valve prolapse syndrome. Chest 72:369–372, 1977.
64. Swartz MH, Teichholz LE, Donoso E. Mitral valve prolapse. A review of associated arrhythmias. Am J Med 62:377–389, 1977.
65. Sorbo MD, Buja GF, Miorelli M, Nistri S, Perrone C, Manca S, Grasso F, Giordano GM, Nava A. The prevalence of the Wolf-Parkinson-White syndrome in a population of 116,542 young males. G Ital Cardiol 25:681–687, 1995.
66. Fomina IG, Tuzikova OF, Reshetnikova AA, Pogrebkova NS. Disorders of cardiac rhythm in combined ventricular pre-excitation syndrome and primary mitral valve prolapse. Ter Arkh 62:38–42, 1990.
67. Picca M, Bisceglia J, Zocca A, Pelosi G. Prevalence and severity of mitral insufficiency and arrhythmia in mitral valve prolapse. Giornale Italiano di Cardiologia 24(11): 1387–1394, 1994.
68. Rechavia E, Mager A, Birnbaum Y, Sclarovsky S. Mitral valve prolapse, sick sinus and Wolff-Parkinson-White syndromes: Interrelationships with respect

to sudden cardiac death. Israel Journal of Medical Sciences 29(10):654–655, 1993.

69. Vukovic I, Smalcelj A, Buljevic B, Petrac D, Miric D. Risk factors for the onset of ventricular tachycardia in patients with mitral valve prolapse. Lijec Vjesn 117(7–8):159–164, Jul-Aug 1995.

70. You-Bing D, Takenaka K, Sakamoto T, et al. Followup in mitral valve prolapse by phonocardiography, M-mode and two-dimensional echocardiography and Doppler echocardiography. Am J Cardiol 65:349–354, 1990.

71. Marks AR, Choong CY, Chir MBB, et al. Identification of high-risk and low-risk subgroups of patients with mitral valve prolapse. N Engl J Med 320:1031–1036, 1989.

72. Nomura M, Nakaya Y, Kishi F, Kondo Y, Yukinaka M, Saito K, Ito S. Signal averaged electrocardiogram after exercise in patients with mitral valve prolapse. J Med 28(1–2):62–74, 1997.

73. Rosenthal ME, Hamer A, Gang ES, Oseran DS, Mandel WJ, Peter T. The yield of programmed ventricular stimulation in mitral valve prolapse patients with ventricular arrhythmias. Am Heart J 110:970–976, 1985.

74. Morady F, Shen E, Bhandari A, Schwartz A, Scheinman MM. Programmed ventricular stimulation in mitral valve prolapse: Analysis of 36 patients. Am J Cardiol 53:135–138, 1984.

Part XI

Floppy Mitral Valve, Mitral Valve Prolapse, Mitral Valvular Regurgitation:
The Surgeons

Introduction

The Floppy Mitral Valve, Mitral Valve Prolapse, Mitral Valvular Regurgitation:
The Surgeons

Charles F. Wooley, MD,
Harisios Boudoulas, MD, PhD

Transition points in the clinical relevance of floppy mitral valve (FMV) morphology, dysfunction, and connective tissue implications came into sharper focus with a number of surgical–pathological correlative studies during the 1960s and 1970s. These included the following: *Symptomatic Valvular Myxomatous Transformation (The Floppy Valve Syndrome)*,[1] a fundamental study by Read et al. in 1965 in the United States; *Reconstructive Surgery for Mitral Valvular Regurgitation*,[2] a surgical landmark by Carpentier et al. in the 1960s in France; and *Clinical and Pathological Findings in Patients With 'Floppy' Valves Treated Surgically*,[3] an insightful study by McKay and Yacoub in 1973 in England.

Raymond C. Read (Fig. 1) used the term floppy valve syndrome in 1965 to describe patients with significant valvular incompetence with "myxomatous transformation" of the aortic and mitral valves at surgery or autopsy in patients who did not fit the clinical criteria for Marfan syndrome. Valvular regurgitation "resulted because of valve prolapse from either structural fatigue, ruptured chordae, loss of substance, interference with coaptation, or supervening endocarditis. Descriptive teminology—"floppy valve" as a term for myxomatous changes and "prolapse" as a term for the mechanism producing mitral or aortic valvular regurgitation—united evolving imaging and pathological perspectives with surgical observations in the beating heart.

This linkage of surgical observations with imaging and pathological

From: Boudoulas H, Wooley CF. *Mitral Valve: Floppy Mitral Valve, Mitral Valve Prolapse, Mitral Valvular Regurgitation*. Second revised edition. ©Futura Publishing Company, Armonk, NY, 2000.

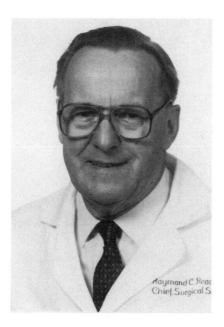

Figure 1. Dr. Raymond C. Read.

correlates enhanced our understanding of the nature of valvular disorders of connective tissue etiology. Evolving concepts about cardiovascular disorders of connective tissue origin, previously based on autopsy studies, were now confirmed during life. Most importantly, the cardiovascular surgeons set the stage for a revolution in the surgical approach to the FMV.

Although surgical repair of the FMV was proposed and performed in the 1960s, FMV replacement with various types of prosthetic valves was the procedure most cardiac surgeons used during the next three decades. The mortality and morbidity of mitral valve replacement and the complexities of postoperative management were such that surgery was usually not recommended until patients were symptomatic with late-stage disease. The clinical indications for surgery included FMV dysfunction with severe mitral valvular regurgitation (MVR), left atrial and ventricular enlargement and dysfunction, atrial fibrillation, and congestive heart failure. The exceptions included patients who experienced acute catastrophic events associated with FMV disruption.

When Lawrence H. Cohn (Fig. 2) discussed surgery for MVR in 1988,[4] he considered the factors that coalesced to stimulate the FMV/MVR repair techniques. These included the limitations of prosthetic heart valves, the positive long-term results of mitral valve reconstructive techniques from several centers, the gathering experimental and clinical data supporting the preservation of the papillary muscle-chordal-annular complex, and the continuing improvements in myocardial preservation. If we fast-forward to the present, Cohn's views of minimally invasive cardiac valve surgery with quality assessed by transesophageal echocardiography incorporate the major developments in the methods and techniques involved in FMV repair.

These surgical developments, better appreciation of the natural history of patients with FMV dysfunction and complications, and the less than optimal surgical results in patients with late-stage disease prompted renewed consideration of the indications and timing of cardiac surgery. The basic premise is that FMV patients with the likelihood of progression and complications should benefit from earlier repair. The challenge lies in the accurate identification of FMV patients at risk for progressive valvular dysfunction and complications.

Traditionally, cardiologists and cardiac surgeons have placed a great deal of reliance on patient symptoms when considering surgical intervention in patients with valvular heart disease. Symptoms also constitute the fundamental components of functional classification schemes used for decision-making and communication purposes.

However, the relations between symptoms in FMV/mitral valve prolapse (MVP)/MVR patients and objective hemodynamic and imaging data are quite different from those in patients with other forms of valvular heart disease such as mitral or aortic stenosis. Quantifying the magnitude and severity of MVR has proven to be a more complex matter than the ritualistic "gold standards" approach based on numbers and dimensions, while awareness by clinicians that FMV/MVP results in a unique form of MVR has been a gradual process. Development of innovative and global approaches to understanding left heart adaptations or accompaniments to FMV complex dysfunction has been a diagnostic and therapeutic challenge. Thus, careful clinical assessment, FMV morphological information, pathophysiological data, and critical evaluation of the evolving imaging technology must be integrated with the ever-changing surgical techniques.[5] Indeed, these steps have been the hallmark of the successful cardiac surgeons in this era.

While extending the indications for FMV repair, and diminishing morbidity and mortality, our surgical colleagues are simultaneously influencing the timing of surgical intervention in FMV patients. As a result, FMV surgical repair has become an integral part of the natural history of the FMV/MVP/MVR triad.

Our respected surgical colleagues from Harvard, Drs. Reul and Dr. Lawrence H. Cohn (Fig. 2), present a current state-of-the-art chapter that

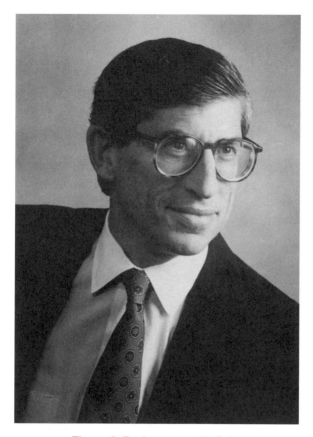

Figure 2. Dr. Lawrence H. Cohn

incorporates their surgical own experience and wisdom, while acknowledging the contributions of the many predecessors and contemporary cardiovascular surgeons around the world.

References

1. Read RC, Thal AP, Wendt VE. Symptomatic valvular myxomatous transformation (the floppy valve syndrome): A possible forme fruste of the Marfan syndrome. Circulation 32:897–910, 1965.
2. Carpentier A, Guerinon J, Deloche A, et al. Pathology of the mitral valve. In Kalmanson D (ed): The Mitral Valve: A Pluridisciplinary Approach. Acton, MA, Mass Publishing Sciences Group, 1976, pp 65–77.
3. McKay R, Yacoub MH. Clinical and pathological finding in patients with "floppy" valves treated surgically. Circulation (Suppl 3);47:63–73, 1973.
4. Cohn LH. Surgery for mitral regurgitation. JAMA 260:2883–2887, 1988.
5. Schlant RC. Timing of surgery for patients with nonischemic severe mitral regurgitation. Circulation 99:338–339, 1999.

18

Surgical Reconstruction of the Complicated Floppy Mitral Valve

Ross M. Reul, MD, Lawrence H. Cohn, MD

Introduction

Mitral valve reconstruction is the treatment of choice for most mitral valve regurgitant lesions requiring surgery. Although most patients with mitral valve prolapse (MVP) generally experience no complications, degenerative mitral valve disease, or the floppy mitral valve syndrome, is now the most common cause of mitral insufficiency in North America.[1] MVP has been reported in 2.5% to 5% of the general population.[2–5] As many as 10% of patients with MVP may develop significant mitral regurgitation.[6] While the incidence of MVP is higher in young females, males over the age of 50 years with MVP are two to three times more likely to require surgery for significant mitral regurgitation than age-matched females with MVP.[7] With advancements in myocardial preservation and surgical valve repair techniques, the morbidity and mortality of surgical treatment for mitral insufficiency continues to decline. Driven by these improvements, the indications for operative intervention are expanding. This has resulted in the ability to offer patients a surgical option with acceptable risks much earlier in the course of this progressive disease, prior to the onset of irreversible left ventricular dysfunction.

From: Boudoulas H, Wooley CF. *Mitral Valve: Floppy Mitral Valve, Mitral Valve Prolapse, Mitral Valvular Regurgitation.* Second revised edition. ©Futura Publishing Company, Armonk, NY, 2000.

History of Mitral Valve Surgery

In 1902, Sir Lauder Brunton, sickened by the devastating prognosis of severe mitral valve disease, suggested using a transventricular valvotomy to correct mitral stenosis.[8] Following years of research,[9–14] Cutler and Levine performed the first successful human valve operation at the Peter Bent Brigham Hospital in 1923.[15] The patient was a 12-year-old girl suffering from end-stage mitral stenosis who underwent a transventricular commissurotomy with a tenotomy knife. Although she recovered well, the next six patients in Cutler's series died and the technique was abandoned. Two years later, Souttar performed a closed finger-dilatation technique for mitral stenosis.[16] In 1948, Harken reported his valvuloplasty technique in a series of patients with mitral stenosis and then expanded this to several thousand closed mitral valvotomy patients.[17] A revolution in cardiac surgery resulted from the introduction of the "heart-lung machine" by Gibbon in 1954.[18] Lillehei used cardiopulmonary bypass to perform the first mitral annuloplasty for mitral insufficiency in 1957.[19] Bailey, Merendino, and McGoon contributed their techniques of chordal shortening, triangular leaflet resection, and exclusion of ruptured chordae tendineae in the late 1950s.[20–22]

Starr implanted the first successful prosthetic mitral valve in 1961 and most surgeons quickly abandoned mitral repair for the relative ease and standardization of the technique of mitral valve replacement (MVR).[23] Carpentier, in 1969, introduced the bioprosthetic valve, which required minimal or no systemic anticoagulation.[24] Wooler, Kay, and Reed continued to advocate and advance the plastic procedures for mitral insufficiency.[25–27] Then, in 1971, Carpentier described his anatomic and physiological approach to repairing the mitral valve. He introduced a rigid prosthetic annuloplasty ring to "remodel the valve on a frame," thus preserving the valve orifice area while preventing further annular dilatation.[28] Five years later, Duran developed the flexible annuloplasty ring to conform to the native mitral annulus throughout the cardiac cycle.[29]

The annuloplasty ring and standardization of mitral valve reparative techniques have greatly enhanced the predictability and the reliability of the procedures. Reports of long-term follow-up following prosthetic MVR showed a significant incidence of thromboembolic, thrombotic, and hemorrhagic complications as well as a high incidence of postoperative left ventricular dysfunction.[30–33] The advantage of low thrombogenicity of bioprosthetic valves was overshadowed by long-term results revealing a vulnerability for structural valve degeneration after 8 to 15 years, especially in young patients and bioprosthetic valves in the mitral position.[34–43] Improvements in myocardial preservation provide longer acceptable cross-clamp times, allowing the surgeon time to assess and attempt to repair most valves. Over the past several years, enthusiasm for mitral valve reconstruction has increased as these results have become available and many centers now will repair the valve whenever technically feasible.[44]

Indications for Surgery

Determining the optimum time to intervene surgically in the asymptomatic or minimally symptomatic patient with mitral regurgitation can present a challenge. The risk:benefit assessment becomes complicated because (1) the variability in the natural history makes it difficult to predict which patients will become severely symptomatic or progress to myocardial dysfunction, (2) the favorable loading conditions of the regurgitant lesions make the prediction of postoperative left ventricular function imprecise, and (3) preoperative evaluation of the etiology and morphologic characteristics of the lesions can be difficult.

Symptomatic patients with 4^+ mitral regurgitation by echocardiography or cardiac catheterization, or patients with any evidence of worsening myocardial function, should undergo mitral valve surgery.[45] Many patients with significant mitral insufficiency do not notice any symptoms of heart failure because of left atrial enlargement and ventricular compensation. In these patients, exercise testing often unmasks severely diminished functional reserve capacity.[46]

The asymptomatic patient with mitral regurgitation and no evidence of left ventricular compromise should be followed closely with serial noninvasive studies every 6 months to evaluate baseline end-systolic dimensions, along with close clinical monitoring. Any evidence of increasing left ventricular dysfunction is an indication for surgical therapy.[45–48] The goal of surgical intervention prior to the onset of irreversible left ventricular dysfunction has prompted many investigators to attempt to predict postoperative left ventricular function from preoperative noninvasive parameters. Many clinicians use the left ventricular ejection fraction (EF) to estimate systolic performance. The loading conditions of mitral regurgitation may result in a falsely elevated estimate of myocardial function. An end-systolic diameter index (ESDI) greater than 2.6 cm/m^2 and an end-systolic volume index (ESVI) greater than 50 or 60 mL/m^2 have been advocated as predictors of postoperative left ventricular dysfunction.[49–51] Others have used wall thickness and left atrial size, myocardial elastance, regurgitant volume, dP/dt, exercise testing, and clinical indicators as preoperative predictors.[46,52–58]

The onset of atrial fibrillation in a patient with mitral regurgitation is an indication for surgery. There is a higher likelihood of conversion to normal sinus rhythm if mitral valve reconstruction is performed within 6 months of the onset of atrial fibrillation.[45,46,59] New-onset atrial fibrillation may be the only clinical evidence of developing left ventricular decompensation. There should be a lower threshold for surgical treatment for patients with coronary artery disease and mitral regurgitation because of the higher risk of ischemic cardiomyopathy.[60–63]

Mitral Valve Reconstruction or Replacement

Most surgeons now attempt to repair rather than replace the mitral valve whenever possible. Although mitral reconstruction is, in general, technically more challenging and may result in longer cross-clamp times when compared to mitral valve replacement, the early and long-term results have been very favorable.[31,44,62,64–70] Prosthetic valves are thrombogenic, requiring systemic anticoagulation. Bioprosthetic valves offer a limited durability due to structural valve degeneration, particularly in the mitral position.

Classic mitral valve replacement involves severing the chordae tendineae and excising the mitral valve leaflets, thus disrupting the connections between the valve and the left ventricle. It is now well established that the mitral valvular–ventricular interactions contribute to left ventricular systolic performance. Rushmer first proposed the importance of the coordinated function of the papillary muscles, chordae tendineae, and mitral valve leaflets in 1956.[71,72] Lillehei corroborated this clinically, reporting improved cardiac output and survival in patients undergoing mitral valve replacement with preservation of the subvalvular apparatus over those undergoing classic mitral valve replacement.[73] Experimental transection of the chordae results in decreased left ventricular contractility that is restored by reattachment.[74–76] Clinically mitral valve replacement with preservation of the subvalvular apparatus results in improved survival, EF, ESD, ESV, end-diastolic pressure (EDP), and exercise capacity when compared to patients undergoing classic mitral valve replacement.[73,77–85]

Mitral valve repair techniques preserve or reconstruct the subvalvular apparatus and as much of the native valve as is feasible. This contributes to the favorable outcomes in terms of postoperative left ventricular function, operative mortality, survival, and thromboembolic complications when mitral repair is compared to mitral valve replacement.

With the development of reproducible plastic techniques for mitral valve reconstruction, most regurgitant lesions of the mitral valve are now amenable to repair. Preoperative assessment of the morphologic characteristics of the diseased mitral valve is not accurate enough to ensure repair will be feasible and the final decision must be made intraoperatively. Therefore, the postoperative risks of mitral valve replacement must be included in discussions with the patient and in the preoperative evaluation.

Unexpected mitral valve replacement is necessary in about 5% of cases in most centers with a large valve surgery experience. Patients with degenerative mitral valve disease are more likely to have lesions that will be amenable to mitral valve repair techniques than other etiologies of mitral insufficiency.

Surgical Exposure

Over the past 75 years, exposure of the heart for cardiac valve operations has been obtained through numerous different thoracic incisions. The median sternotomy, however, has become the most commonly used incision and is versatile for most adult cardiac surgery operations. In mitral valve surgery through a standard median sternotomy, superior and inferior vena caval cannulas are placed, and the arterial cannula is usually placed in the distal ascending aorta. Moderate hypothermia, antegrade and retrograde cardioplegia, and topical cooling are used for myocardial protection.[86–88] Sondergaard's plane is developed and the left atrium is incised near the atrial septum and carried behind the right pulmonary artery and inferior vena cava for mitral valve exposure.[89,90] Alternatively, an anterior right thoracotomy utilizing femoro-femoral bypass is used to avoid median sternotomy in patients with patent substernal bypass grafts, a stented aortic prosthesis, or prior mediastinitis.[91] Axillo-axillary bypass is an alternative in patients with severe lower extremity peripheral vascular disease.[92]

Over the past 15 years, minimally invasive surgical incisions have been popularized in several surgical fields.[93,94] More recently, since 1996, cardiac surgeons have been reporting excellent early results following aortic and mitral valve operations using less invasive techniques.[95–98] In our experience at Brigham and Women's Hospital, a small (6–8 cm) right parasternal incision offers exceptional exposure to perform mitral reconstruction or replacement for most mitral valve lesions. When compared to patients undergoing mitral valve operations through a median sternotomy, the right parasternal group had greater patient satisfaction, required less blood product transfusion, and charges were 20% less. Of 43 patients undergoing mitral valve surgery between July 1996 and April 1997, the operative mortality was 0 (0%). Eighty-six percent of these patients underwent mitral valve repair, all with a Cosgrove annuloplasty ring. Postoperative and intraoperative transesophageal echocardiography showed all repairs had minimal to trace mitral regurgitation postoperatively. There were no postoperative wound infections involving the parasternal wound.[95]

A 6–8 cm right parasternal incision is made, the third and fourth intercostal cartilages are excised, and the pericardium is opened. Femoro-

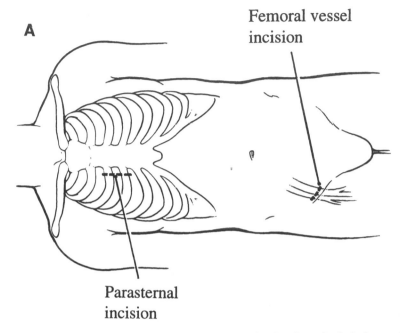

Femoral vessel incision

A

Parasternal incision

Figure 1. Minimally invasive exposure of the mitral valve. **A.** A 6–8 cm right parasternal incision is made over the right 3rd and 4th costal cartilages. *Continued.*

femoral bypass or axillo-axillary bypass is initiated, or the superior and inferior venae cavae and ascending aorta can be cannulated through the parasternal incision. The heart is fibrillated and the aortic cross-clamp is placed followed by antegrade blood cardioplegia and moderate systemic hypothermia. The right atrium is incised, then the septum is opened, exposing the mitral valve (Fig. 1).[95]

Surgical Reconstruction Techniques

Once the mitral valve is adequately exposed, regardless of the approach, the mitral valve apparatus is inspected, including the annulus, leaflets, chordae tendineae, papillary muscles, and the surrounding ventricular myocardium. Carpentier introduced an anatomic classification to accurately describe the location of lesions involving the anterior and posterior mitral valve leaflets and the commissures (Fig. 2).[99] The extent of leaflet prolapse or flail is determined using nerve hooks to place traction on the leaflets and chordae. A rarely prolapsed area on the posterior leaflet in segment P1 is often used as a "reference point" to assess the extent of prolapse of the remaining leaflet.[99,100] The reconstruction technique will

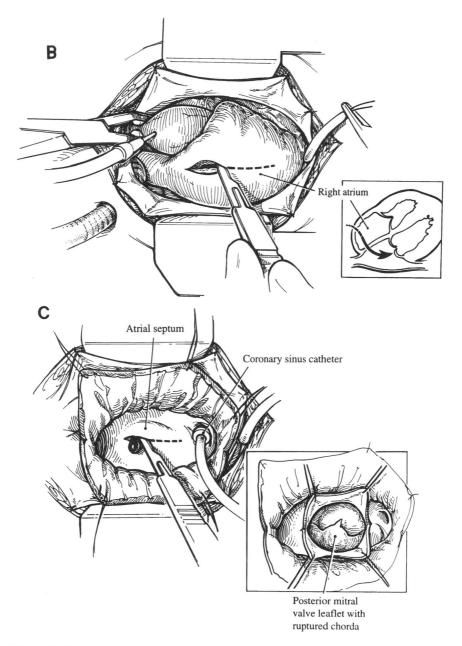

Figure 1. B. Exposure of the right atrium as seen through the right parasternal incision. **C.** The transseptal incision provides excellent exposure of the mitral valve.

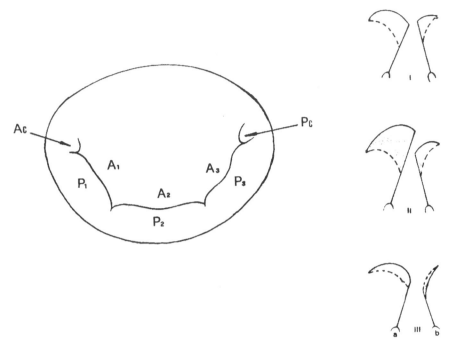

Figure 2. Carpentier's anatomic segments of the mitral valve. Segments A_1, A_2, and A_3 make up the anterior leaflet, P_1, P_2, and P_3 the posterior leaflet, and Ac and Pc represent the anterior and posterior commissures. The anatomic segments are used along with Carpentier's functional classification: (I) normal leaflet motion, (II) leaflet prolapse, and (III) restricted leaflet motion. (Reprinted with permission from the Society of Thoracic Surgeons.[99])

be dictated by the pathoanatomic characteristics of the lesion or lesions causing mitral insufficiency.

Prosthetic Annuloplasty Rings

Most surgeons routinely use an annuloplasty ring to remodel the dilated annulus and prevent further progression of the disease in the years following surgical repair. Carpentier's rigid annuloplasty ring was designed to remodel the dilated annulus resulting in a physiologic 3:4 ratio between the anteroposterior and transverse diameters of the mitral valve (Fig. 3).[101] The normal mitral annular configuration is dynamic throughout the cardiac cycle. It is circular in diastole and elliptical during systole and the normal annular circumference changes throughout each cardiac cycle.[102] Duran introduced the totally flexible annuloplasty ring in 1976

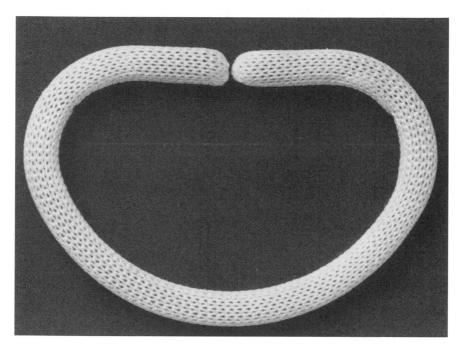

Figure 3. The Carpentier rigid annuloplasty ring. (Courtesy of Baxter Healthcare Corporation.)[101]

(Fig. 4).[29] At Brigham and Women's Hospital, we now routinely use the Cosgrove annuloplasty system (Fig. 5). Similar to Cooley's posterior annular collar prosthesis reported 20 years ago,[103] Cosgrove's incomplete ring provides support to the dilated posterior portion of the annulus while the fibrous, generally stable anterior portion remains uncovered by prosthetic material. The annulus maintains a saddle shape and remains dynamic throughout the cardiac cycle.[104] In a prospective study of 135 consecutive patients undergoing mitral valve repair using the Cosgrove annuloplasty system, with or without concomitant coronary artery bypass or other procedures, there were significant improvements in mitral regurgitation and NYHA functional class. There were two early (systolic anterior motion, valve dehiscence) and three late (two anterior chordal rupture, one progressive anterior leaflet prolapse) valve failures that required MVR. The operative mortality for isolated mitral repair was 0%.[105] Whether a rigid, flexible, or incomplete ring, or no ring at all offers less morbidity is the source of debate.[1,65,101,106–117] It is likely, however, that the most reliable annuloplasty will be the one with which the surgeon is most comfortable and experienced.[1,118]

Often, prosthetic annuloplasty alone will be sufficient to resolve the

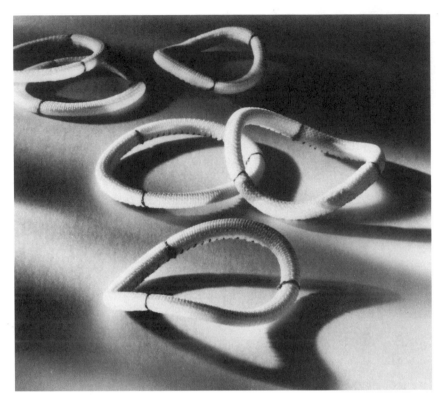

Figure 4. The Duran flexible annuloplasty ring. (Courtesy of Medtronics, Inc.[29])

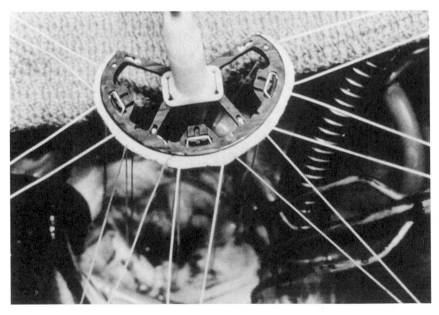

Figure 5. The Cosgrove annuloplasty system.[104]

mitral insufficiency in ischemic mitral regurgitation, but rarely with the prolapsed mitral valve. When other techniques are necessary, they are undertaken prior to tying down the annuloplasty ring. The chordae of the anterior leaflet are placed under tension with a right angle, and the area of the anterior leaflet is approximated with sized obturators. When using a full ring annuloplasty, a series of horizontal mattress sutures are placed around the mitral annulus with equidistant spacing. The sutures placed in the anterior portion of the sewing ring should maintain the same space intervals, whereas the distance between sutures placed in the posterior portion of the annuloplasty ring is decreased to preferentially cinch down the posterior portion of the annulus. For the Cosgrove annuloplasty, the anterior annular sutures are omitted, thus avoiding placing sutures in the vicinity of the atrioventricular node and the aortic valve (Fig. 5) and the posterior portion is performed as described above. The ring is seated on the annulus and the valve is tested for competence prior to tying down the sutures. Competence is evaluated by placing a red rubber catheter through the mitral valve and injecting saline into the left ventricle. Asymmetry along the line of leaflet apposition is an indication of residual leaflet prolapse or restriction.[118-120] We routinely use transesophageal echocardiography in all cases for intraoperative assessment of valve function and intracardiac air.

Infective Endocarditis

The myxomatous degeneration of the fibrosa layer in mitral valve prolapse predisposes the involved leaflets to infectious endocarditis. Small leaflet perforations can be repaired with simple suture plication, or if larger, a patch of glutaraldehyde-treated autologous pericardium can be used.[121,122] If the involved tissue requires extensive debridement, the entire leaflet can be replaced with autologous pericardium.

Posterior Leaflet Prolapse

In mitral valve prolapse complicated by significant regurgitation, intraoperative findings most often include a large, redundant posterior leaflet with elongated or ruptured chordae tendineae. The involved segment and chordae are excised in a quadrangular resection when less than 50% of the posterior leaflet area is flail.[100,123,124] Each edge of the flail segment is incised perpendicular to the annulus and a rectangle of prolapsed tissue excised. The involved portion of the annulus is plicated and the remaining edges of the posterior leaflet are then approximated with a running monofilament suture with the knots tied on the ventricular side to minimize thrombogenicity.[125] When greater than 50% of the annulus is flail, a quadrangular resection will likely excessively reduce the posterior leaflet area and should not be used. In these cases, chordal transfer can be effective. A secondary chorda or chordae can be excised and transferred to the edge of the flail segment.[100]

An excessively dilated leaflet, as seen with Barlow's disease, can result in postoperative systolic anterior motion that may cause left ventricular outflow obstruction.[126,127] In order to minimize the risk of this complication, a sliding leaflet technique may be used with quadrangular resection (Fig. 6). Following the quadrangular resection as described above, the remaining leaflet segments are excised from the annulus toward each commissure for a distance equal to that of the portion excised. The posterior leaflet is then sutured to the annulus, decreasing the height of the remaining posterior leaflet as well as the length of the annulus requiring plication.[101,126,127] The repair is then reinforced with an annuloplasty ring (Fig. 7).

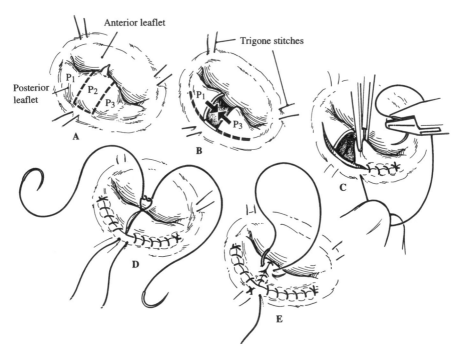

Figure 6. The sliding leaflet technique for posterior leaflet flail. **A.** Prolapsed middle scallop of the posterior mitral leaflet (segment P$_2$). **B.** Quadrangular resection of the flail segment and incision between the leaflet remnants and the annulus toward the commissures for a distance equal to the annular length of the segment resected. The free edges are advanced to the midline and the leaflet remnants reattached to the annulus. **D** and **E.** The free edges are reapproximated.

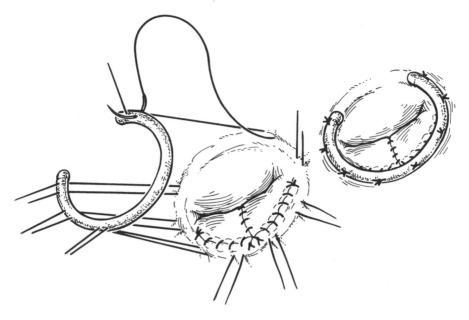

Figure 7. Implantation of the Cosgrove annuloplasty.

Following recent descriptions of techniques to repair the extensively calcified mitral annulus with excellent results, this pathology no longer represents a contraindication to surgical valve repair.[123,128–130] This is usually seen with degenerative valve disease or may be idiopathic, but it is distinct from the calcified leaflet involvement associated with rheumatic valvular disease.[128] Most often, the posterior portion of the annulus is involved with occasional spread anteriorly or into the leaflets and myocardium. When the severely calcified mitral annulus is associated with posterior leaflet prolapse, a quadrangular resection is performed followed by resection of the remaining leaflet from the annulus as described above. The annular calcifications are meticulously debrided using a rongeur, followed by extensive irrigation. The leaflet repair is then completed using the sliding leaflet technique and the annulus reinforced with an annuloplasty ring (Fig. 8).[123]

Anterior Leaflet Prolapse

Anterior leaflet flail may be encountered with or without associated posterior leaflet prolapse. The anterior leaflet triangular resection has been replaced by more reliable techniques with improved postoperative results.[101,119] For mitral insufficiency due to elongated or ruptured anterior

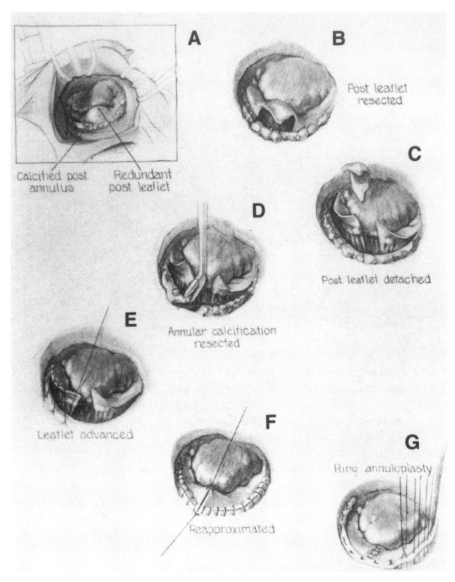

Figure 8. Mitral valve repair with a severely calcified mitral annulus. **A.** Exposure through a left atriotomy. **B.** Quadrangular resection of the prolapsed posterior leaflet. **C.** Free edges of the posterior leaflet are excised from the calcified annulus. **D.** Rongeur debridement of the annular calcifications. **E.** and **F.** Sliding leaflet closure. **G.** Cosgrove ring annuloplasty. (Reprinted with permission by Futura Publishing Co., Inc.[123])

chordae, chordal replacement with expanded polytetrafluoroethylene (ePTFE) suture is now widely utilized with excellent postoperative outcomes (Fig. 9).[124,131–135] A double-armed 5-0 PTFE suture is passed twice through the papillary muscle just below the insertion site of the chordae and tied. The two ends are then passed through the anterior leaflet edge at the site of the elongated or ruptured chordae insertion from the ventricular to the atrial side, then passed through the leaflet again and tied on the ventricular side, using upward traction on a stay suture to ensure the proper length of the neochordae. The chordal replacement sutures have enough tensile strength to withstand the physiologic stress of valve motion throughout the cardiac cycle.[136] Over time, the PTFE sutures become lined with fibrous material.[133,135,137]

Anterior leaflet flail due to ruptured or elongated chordae can also be repaired by chordal transfer, taking healthy secondary or basal chordae from the anterior leaflet (Fig. 10A), or excising a portion of the posterior

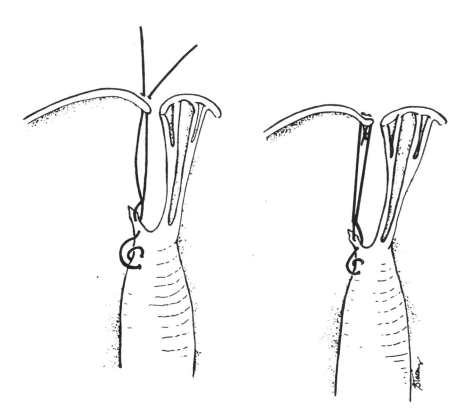

Figure 9. Chordal replacement with ePTFE suture for anterior leaflet flail. (Reprinted with permission by Mosby-Year Book, Inc.[133])

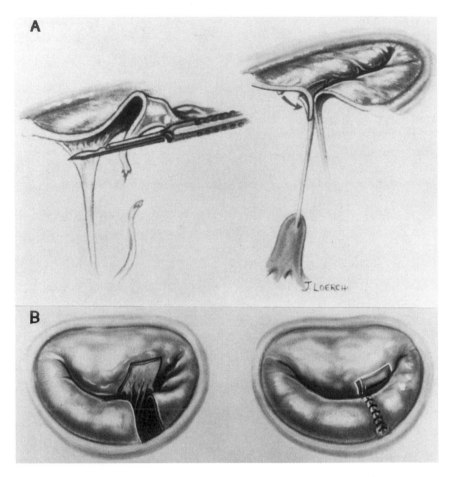

Figure 10. Chordal transfer for anterior leaflet prolapse. **A.** Transfer of a secondary anterior leaflet chorda to the leaflet edge. **B.** Transposition of posterior leaflet chordae to the anterior leaflet flail segment. (Reprinted with permission by Mosby-Year Book, Inc.[138])

leaflet including one or several chordae and suturing this to the edge of the anterior leaflet flail segment (Fig. 10B).[138] Chordal shortening techniques are also used for these etiologies of anterior leaflet flail. A recent report by Smedira and Cosgrove reported superior results from chordal transfer when compared to chordal shortening in patients with anterior leaflet flail.[138] An edge-to-edge technique, advocated by Fucci and others, offers a simple and effective method of repairing the prolapsed anterior mitral leaflet (Fig. 11).[139]

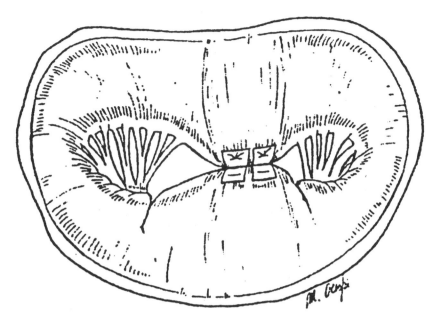

Figure 11. Edge-to-edge repair creating a double orifice mitral valve. (Reprinted with permission by Springer-Verlag.[139])

Surgical Results

Although lacking in prospective, case-matched, randomized clinical trials, several authors have shown favorable long- and short-term outcomes when mitral valve repair is compared with replacement.[31,44,62,64–70] In patients with myxomatous degeneration as the etiology of mitral insufficiency, a high proportion can be repaired and 30-day mortality rates between 0% and 3% are expected following mitral repair.[1,44,106,127] Because the patient population with significant mitral insufficiency from MVP is generally older, coronary artery disease plays a prominent role in evaluating surgical outcomes.[101] While age and requirement for coronary artery bypass grafting (CABG) are not contraindications for mitral valve surgery, they represent high-risk patients. At Brigham and Women's Hospital between March 1984 and October 1997, 1,000 patients underwent mitral valve repair and 501 (50%) of these were for myxomatous mitral regurgitation. The overall operative mortality for myxomatous etiology was 1.8%. The operative mortality was 4.1% and 1.0% in patients that did and did not undergo concomitant CABG, respectively (data not published).

Early and late survival following mitral reconstruction depends on the etiology of the mitral lesion, the preoperative myocardial function, other comorbid patient characteristics, and whether the valve can be repaired or replaced. Actuarial survival following mitral repair for myxomatous valve disease is 90–97% at 1 year, 86–91% at 5 years, 81–88% at 10 years, and 46–71% at 15 years.[1,44,65,101,106,140] There is a slight survival advantage postoperatively in patients with rheumatic valvular disease, likely due to the generally younger patient population.[44] Mitral regurgitation secondary to myocardial ischemia carries a poorer postoperative prognosis when compared to degenerative mitral regurgitation, even when the latter is associated with coronary artery disease.[1,44,120]

Repairing the native mitral valve results in a relatively nonthrombogenic valve, thus eliminating the need for systemic anticoagulation, unless the patient is in atrial fibrillation or has another indication for anticoagulation. In addition, preservation of left ventricular systolic function reduces the risk of thromboemboli. The actuarial freedom from thromboembolic events following mitral valve repair for myxomatous mitral insufficiency is 94–100% at 1 year, 87–99% at 5 years, 82–90% at 10 years, and as high as 90% at 15 years.[1,44,65,106,140]

The excellent long-term freedom from reoperation in most series following mitral repair reflects the durability of the mitral reconstruction techniques. Most reoperations take place within the first year after surgery or several years later. Early residual mitral regurgitation implies a technical error, whereas the later reoperations are more likely due to progression of the patient's underlying disease. As with any complex technical procedure, a learning curve exists early in every surgeon's experience that may influence the outcomes of mitral repair, or the decision regarding repair versus replacement of the valve. In patients with degenerative mitral valve disease, the actuarial freedom from reoperation at 1 year postoperatively is 95–99%, 88–98% at 5 years, 88–98% at 10 years, and 85–90% at 15 years.[1,44,65,101,106,140–143]

The incidence of postoperative infective endocarditis following mitral reconstruction is very low with an actuarial freedom from infective endocarditis of 99–100% through 10 to 15 years of follow-up.[1,44,101,104,106,139,144] Because of the foreign material, prosthetic valve infective endocarditis can be a devastating problem.

The actuarial freedom from all valve-related complications in patients undergoing mitral repair for myxomatous valve disease has been reported between 92% and 95% at 1 year, 74–87% at 5 years, 69–80% at 10 years, and 37–74% at 15 years.[1,44,101,106,140]

Summary

Mitral valve reconstruction is now the procedure of choice for most regurgitant mitral valve lesions. The lesions that complicate MVP are particularly amenable to mitral valve plastic techniques. Improvements in myocardial protection have allowed longer aortic cross-clamp times to safely attempt to repair very complicated lesions. The standardization of surgical techniques and favorable long-term results, along with a more aggressive approach to preserving the native valve, have resulted in an expansion of the indications for surgery for mitral insufficiency to include most lesions and the asymptomatic patient. Minimally invasive mitral valve surgery is being developed with excellent early results. The potential for less expensive, less painful surgical correction of mitral regurgitation may help persuade more patients and physicians to elect surgical intervention prior to the onset of irreversible ventricular dysfunction.

References

1. Cohn LH, Couper GS, Aranki SF, et al. Long-term results of mitral valve reconstruction for regurgitation of the myxomatous mitral valve. J Thorac Cardiovasc Surg 107:143–51, 1994.
2. Marks AR, Choong CY, Sanfilippo AJ, Ferre M, et al. Identification of high-risk and low-risk subgroups of patients with mitral valve prolapse. N Engl J Med 320:1031–1036, 1985.
3. Nishimura RA, McGoon MD, Shub C, et al. Echocardiographically documented mitral valve prolapse: Long-term follow-up of 237 patients. N Engl J Med 313:1305–1309, 1985.
4. Hickey AJ, Wolfers J, Wilcken DEL. Mitral valve prolapse: Prevalence in an Australian population. Med J Aust 1:31–33, 1981.
5. Savage DD, Garrison RJ, Devereux RB, Castelli WP, et al. Mitral valve prolapse in the general population. 1. Epidemiological features: The Framingham study. Am Heart J 105:571–576, 1983.
6. Manteuffel-Szoege L, Nowicki J, Wasniewska M, Sitkowski W, et al. Mitral commissurotomy: Results of 1700 cases. J Cardiovasc Surg 11:350–354, 1970.
7. Wilcken DEL, Hickey AJ. Lifetime risk for patients with mitral valve prolapse if developing severe valve regurgitation requiring surgery. Circulation 78:10–14, 1988.
8. Brunton L. Preliminary note on the possibility of treating mitral stenosis by surgical methods. Lancet 1:352, 1902.
9. MacCallum WG. On the teaching of pathological physiology. Johns Hopkins Hosp Bull 17:251, 1906.
10. Cushing H, Branch JRB. Experimental and clinical notes on chronic valvular lesions in the dog and their possible relation to a future surgery of the cardiac valves. J Med Res 12:471–486, 1907–8.
11. Bernheim BM. Experimental surgery of the mitral valve. Johns Hopkins Hosp Bull 20:107–110, 1909.
12. Schepelmann E. Versuche zur Herz-chirugie. Archiv Klin Chir 97:739–751, 1912.
13. Tuffier T, Carrel A: Patching and section of the pulmonary orifice of the heart. J Exp Med 20:3–8, 1914.
14. Allen DS, Graham EA. Intracardiac surgery: A new method. JAMA 79:1028–1030, 1922.
15. Cutler EC, Levine SA: Cardiotomy and valvotomy for mitral stenosis. Exper-

imental observations and clinical notes concerning an operated case with recovery. Boston Med Surg J 188:1023–1027, 1923.

16. Souttar HS. The surgical diagnosis of mitral stenosis. Br Med J 2:603–607, 1925.

17. Harken DE, Ellis LB, Ware PF, et al. The surgical treatment of mitral stenosis. I. Valvuloplasty. N Engl J Med 239:801–809, 1948.

18. Gibbon JH. Application of a mechanical heart and lung apparatus to cardiac surgery. Minn Med 37:171–185, 1954.

19. Lillehei CW, Gott VL, De Wall RA, Varco RL. Surgical correction of pure mitral insufficiency by annuloplasty under direct vision. Lancet 77:446–449, 1957.

20. Bailey CP, Hirose T. Maximal reconstitution of the stenotic mitral valve by neostrophingic mobilization (rehinging of the septal leaflet). J Thorac Surg 35:559–583, 1958.

21. Merendino KA, Thomas GI, Jesseph JE, et al: The open correction of rheumatic mitral regurgitation and/or stenosis, with special reference to regurgitation treated by posteromedial annuloplasty utilizing a pump-oxygenator. Ann Surg 150:5–22, 1959.

22. McGoon DC. Repair of mitral insufficiency due to ruptured chordae tendineae. J Thorac Cardiovasc Surg 39:357–363, 1960.

23. Starr A, Edwards ML. Mitral replacement: Clinical experience with a ball valve prosthesis. Ann Surg 154:726–740, 1961.

24. Carpentier A, Lemaigre G, Robert L, et al. Biological factors affecting long-term results of valvular heterografts. J Thorac Cardiovasc Surg 58:467–483, 1969.

25. Wooler GH, Nixon PGF, Grimshaw VA, Watson DA: Experiences with the repair of the mitral valve in mitral incompetence. Thorax 17:49–57, 1962.

26. Kay JH, Egerton WS. The repair of mitral insufficiency associated with ruptured chordae tendineae. Ann Surg 157:351–360, 1963.

27. Reed GE, Tice DA, Clauss RH. Asymmetric exagerated mitral annuloplasty: Repair of mitral insufficiency with hemodynamic predictability. J Thorac Cardiovasc Surg 49:752–761, 1965.

28. Carpentier A, Deloche A, Dauptain J, et al. A new reconstructive operation for correction of mitral and tricuspid insufficiency. J Thorac Cardiovasc Surg 61:1–13, 1971.

29. Duran CG, Ubago JLM. Clinical and hemodynamic performance of a totally flexible prosthetic ring for atrioventricular valve reconstruction. Ann Thorac Surg 22:458–463, 1976.

30. Cohn LH, Allred EN, Cohn LA, et al. Early and late risk of mitral valve replacement. J Thorac Cardiovasc Surg 90:872–881, 1985.

31. Angell WW, Oury JH, Shah P. A comparison of replacement and reconstruction in patients with mitral regurgitation. J Thorac Cardiovasc Surg 93:665–674, 1987.

32. Perier P, Deloche A, Chauvaud S, et al: Comparative evaluation of mitral valve repair and replacement with Starr, Bjork and porcine valve prostheses. Circulation 70(Suppl II):II-187–192, 1984.

33. Miller DC, Oyer PE, Stinson EB, et al. Ten to fifteen year reassessment of the performance characteristics of the Starr-Edwards Model 6120 mitral valve prosthesis. J Thorac Cardiovasc Surg 85:1–20, 1983.

34. Reul GJ, Cooley DA, Duncan JM, Frazier OH, et al. Valve failure with the Ionescue-Shiley bovine pericardial bioprosthesis: analysis of 2680 patients. J Vasc Surg 2:192–204, 1985.

35. Cohn LH. Atrioventricular valve replacement with a Hancock porcine xenograft. Ann Thorac Surg 51:683–684, 1991.
36. Glower DD, White WD, Hattent AC, et al. Determinants of reoperation after 960 valve replacements with Carpentier-Edwards prostheses. J Thorac Cardiovasc Surg 107:381–392, 1994.
37. Akins CW, Carrol DL, Buckley MJ, et al. Late results with Carpentier-Edwards porcine bioprostheses. Circulation 82(Suppl IV):IV-65–74, 1990.
38. Pupello DF, Bessone LN, Blank RH, Lopez-Cuenca E, et al: The porcine bioprosthesis: Patient age as a factor in predicting failure. In Bodnar E, Yacoub M (eds): Biological and Bioprosthetic Valves. New York, NY, Yorke Medical Books, 1986, pp 130.
39. Bernal JM, Rabasa JM, Lopez R, Nistal JF, et al. Durability of the Carpentier-Edwards porcine bioprosthesis: Role of age and valve position. Ann Thorac Surg 60:S248–S252, 1995.
40. Geha AS, Laks H, Stansel HC Jr, et al. Late failure of porcine valve heterografts in children. J Thorac Cardiovasc Surg 78:351–364, 1979.
41. Thandroyen FT, Whitton IN, Pirie D, Rogers MA, et al: Severe calcification of glutaraldehyde-preserved porcine xenografts in children. Am J Cardiol 45:690–696, 1980.
42. Jamieson WRE, Rosada LJ, Munro AI, et al. Carpentier-Edwards standard porcine bioprosthesis: Primary tissue failure (structural valve deterioration) by age groups. Ann Thorac Surg 46:155–162, 1988.
43. Jamieson WRE, Tyers GFO, Janusz MT, et al. Age as a determinant for selection of porcine bioprostheses for cardiac valve replacement: Experience with Carpentier-Edwards Standard bioprosthesis. Can J Cardiol 7:181–188, 1991.
44. Reul RM and Cohn LH. Mitral valve repair for mitral insufficiency. Prog Cardiovasc Dis 39:567–599, 1997.
45. Cohn LH. Surgery for mitral regurgitation. JAMA 260:2883–2887, 1988.
46. Mudge GH. Asymptomatic mitral regurgitation: when to operate? J Cardiac Surg 9(Suppl):248–251, 1994.
47. Grossman W. Aortic and mitral regurgitation. JAMA 252:2447–2449, 1984.
48. Gaasch WH, Levine HJ, Zile MR. Chronic aortic and mitral regurgitation: Mechanical consequences of the lesion and the results of surgical correction. In The Ventricle: Basic and Clinical Aspects. Boston, MA, Martinus Nyjhoff, pp 237–258, 1985.
49. Zile MR, Gaasch WH, Carroll JD, Levine HJ. Chronic mitral regurgitation: Predictive value of preoperative echocardiographic indexes of left ventricular function and wall stress. J Am Coll Cardiol 3:235–242, 1984.
50. Crawford MH, Souchek J, Oprian CA, Miller DC, et al: Determinants of survival and left ventricular performance after mitral valve replacement: Department of Veterans Affairs Cooperative Study on Valvular Heart Disease. Circulation 81:1173–1181, 1990.
51. Borow KM, Green LH, Mann T, et al. End-systolic volume as a predictor of postoperative left ventricular performance in volume overload from valvular regurgitation. Am J Med 68:655–663, 1980.
52. Reed D, Abbott RD, Smucker ML, Kaul S. Prediction of outcome after mitral valve replacement in patients with symptomatic chronic mitral regurgitation: the importance of left atrial size. Circulation 84:23–34, 1991.
53. Starling MR, Kirsh MM, Montgomery DG, Gross MD. Impaired left ventricular contractile function in patients with long-term mitral regurgitation and normal ejection fraction. J Am Coll Cardiol 22:239–250, 1993.

54. Levine HJ, Gaasch WH. Ratio of regurgitant volume to end-diastolic volume: A major determinant of ventricular response to surgical correction of chronic volume overload. Am J Cardiol 52:406–410, 1983.
55. Clancy KF, Hakki AH, Iskandrian AS, et al: Forward ejection fraction: A new index of left ventricular function in mitral regurgitation. Am Heart J 110:658–664, 1985.
56. Enriquez-Sarano M, Bailey KR, Seward JB, et al: Quantitative Doppler assessment of valvular regurgitation. Circulation 87:841–848, 1993.
57. Pai RG, Bansal RC, Shah PM. Doppler-derived rate of left ventricular pressure rise: Its correlation with the postoperative left ventricular function in mitral regurgitation. Circulation 82:514–520, 1990.
58. Fleischman KE, Wolff S, Lin CM, et al. Echocardiographic predictors of survival after surgery for mitral regurgitation in the age of valve repair. Am Heart J 131:281–288, 1996.
59. Betrin A, Chaitman BR, Aleazan A, et al. Preoperative determinants of return to sinus rhythm after valve replacement. In Cohn LH, Gallucci V (eds): Cardiac Bioprosthesis. New York, NY, Yorke Medical Books, 1982, pp 184–191.
60. Enriquez-Sarano M, Tajik AJ, Schaff HV, et al. Echocardiographic prediction of left ventricular function after correction of mitral regurgitation: Results and clinical implications. J Am Coll Cardiol 24:1536–1543, 1994.
61. Stewart WJ. Choosing the "golden moment" for mitral valve repair. J Am Coll Cardiol 24:1544–1546, 1994.
62. Hickey MS, Smith LR, Muhlbaier LH, et al. Current prognosis of ischemic mitral regurgitation: Implications for future management. Circulation 78(SupplI):I-51–59, 1988.
63. Dion R. Ischemic mitral regurgitation: When and how should it be corrected? J Heart Valve Disease 2:536–543, 1993.
64. Craver JM, Cohen C, Weintraub WS. Case-matched comparison of mitral valve replacement and repair. Ann Thorac Surg 49:964–969, 1990.
65. Yacoub M, Halim M, Radley-Smith R, et al. Surgical treatment of mitral regurgitation caused by floppy valves: Repair versus replacement. Circulation 64 (Suppl II):II-210–216, 1981.
66. Adebo OA, Ross JK: Surgical treatment of ruptured mitral valve chordae: A comparison between valve replacement and valve repair. Thorac Cardiovasc Surg 32:139–142, 1984.
67. Sand ME, Naftel DC, Blackstone EH, et al. A Comparison of repair and replacement for mitral valve incompetence. J Thorac Cardiovasc Surg 94:208–219, 1987.
68. Akins CW, Hilgenberg AD, Buckley MJ, et al: Mitral valve reconstruction for degenerative and ischemic mitral regurgitation. Ann Thorac Surg 58:668–676, 1994.
69. Dion R, Benetis R, Elias B, et al. Mitral valve procedures in ischemic regurgitation. J Heart Valve Dis 4(Suppl II):S124–S131, 1995.
70. Enriquez-Sarano M, Schaff HV, Orszulak TA, et al. Valve repair improves the outcome of surgery for mitral regurgitation: A multivariate analysis. Circulation 91:1022–1028, 1995.
71. Rushmer RF. Initial phase of ventricular systole: Asynchronous contraction. Am J Physiol 188:187–194, 1956.
72. Rushmer RF, Finlayson BL, Nash AA. Movements of the mitral valve. Circ Res 4:337–342, 1956.
73. Lillehei CW, Levy MJ, Bonnabeau RC. Mitral valve replacement with preser-

vation of papillary muscles and chordae tendineae. J Thorac Cardiovasc Surg 47:532–543, 1964.

74. Hansen DE, Borow KM, Newmann A, et al. Effects of acute lung injury and anesthesia on left ventricular mechanics. Am J Physiol 251:H1195, 1986.

75. Hansen DE, Cahill PD, Derby GC, Miller DC. Relative contributions of the anterior and posterior mitral chordae tendineae to canine global left ventricular systolic performance. J Thorac Cardiovasc Surg 94:45–55, 1987.

76. Sarris GE, Cahill PD, Hansen DE, Miller DC. Restoration of left ventricular systolic performance after reattachment of the mitral chordae tendineae: The importance of valvular-ventricular interaction. J Thorac Cardiovasc Surg 95:968–979, 1988.

77. David TE, Burns RJ, Bacchus CM, et al: Mitral valve replacement for mitral regurgitation with and without preservation of chordae tendineae. J Thorac Cardiovasc Surg 88:718–725, 1984.

78. Rozich JD, Carabello BA, Usher BW, et al. mitral valve replacement with and without chordal preservation in patients with chronic mitral regurgitation: Mechanisms for differences in postoperative ejection performance. Circulation 86:1718–1726, 1992.

79. Hennein HA, Swain JA, McIntosh CL, et al. Comparative assessment of chordal preservation versus chordal resection during mitral valve replacement. J Thorac Cardiovasc Surg 99:828–837, 1990.

80. Hetzer R, Bougioukas G, Franz M, Borst HG. Mitral valve replacement with preservation of papillary muscles and chordae tendineae: Revival of a seemingly forgotten concept. Cardiovasc Surg 31:291–296, 1983.

81. Natsuaki M, Itoh T, Tomita S, et al. Importance of preserving the subvalvular apparatus in mitral valve replacement. Ann Thorac Surg 61:585–590, 1996.

82. Okita Y, Shigehito M, Kusuhara K, Ueda Y, et al: Analysis of left ventricular motion after mitral valve replacement with a technique of preservation of all chordae tendineae: Comparison with conventional mitral valve replacement or mitral valve repair. J Thorac Cardiovasc Surg 104:786–796, 1992.

83. Komeda M, David TE, Rao V, et al. Late hemodynamic effects of the preserved papillary muscles during mitral valve replacement. Circulation 90(Suppl II):II-190–194, 1994.

84. David TE, Ho WC. The effect of preservation of chordae tendineae on mitral valve replacement for postinfarction mitral regurgitation. Circulation 74(Suppl I):I-116–120, 1986.

85. Moon MR, DeAnda A Jr, Daughters GT II, Ingels NB Jr, Miller DC. Experimental evaluation of different chordal preservation methods during mitral valve replacement. Ann Thorac Surg 58:931–944, 1994.

86. Cohn LH, Aranki SF, Rizzo RJ, et al. Decrease in operative risk of reoperative valve surgery. Ann Thorac Surg 56:15–21, 1993.

87. Buckberg GD. Antegrade/retrograde blood cardioplegia to ensure cardioplegic distribution: Operative techniques and objectives. J Cardiac Surg 4:216–238, 1989.

88. Singh AK. Warm retrograde cardioplegia: protection of the right ventricle in mitral valve operations. J Thorac Cardiovasc Surg 106:370–371, 1993.

89. Sondergaard T, Gotzsche M, Ottosen P, Schultz J. Surgical closure of interatrial septal defects by circumclusion. Acta Chir Scand 109:188–196, 1955.

90. Larbalestier RI, Chard RB, Cohn LH. Optimal approach to the mitral valve: Dissection of the interatrial groove. Ann Thorac Surg 54:1186–1188, 1992.

91. Cohn LH, Peigh PS, Sell J, DiSesa VJ. Right thoracotomy, femoro-femoral by-

pass and deep hypothermia for re-replacement of the mitral valve. Ann Thorac Surg 48:69–71, 1989.

92. Bichell DP, Balaguer JM, Aranki SF, Couper GS, Adams DH, Rizzo RJ, Collins JJ Jr, Cohn LH. Axilloaxillary cardiopulmonary bypass: A practical alternative to femorofemoral bypass. Ann Thorac Surg 64:702–705, 1997.
93. Semm K. Die endoskopische Appendektomie. Gynakol Prax 7:131–140, 1983.
94. Muhe E. Laparoscopic cholecystectomy. Z Gastroenterol Verh 26:204, 1991.
95. Cohn LH, Adams DH, Couper GS, Bichell DP, Rosborough DM, Sears SP, Aranki SF. Minimally invasive cardiac valve surgery improves patient satisfaction while reducing costs of cardiac valve replacement and repair. Ann Surg 226:421–428, 1997.
96. Balaguer JM, Cohn LH. Minimally invasive cardiac valve surgery. Adv Cardiovasc Med, in press.
97. Cosgrove DM, Sabik JF. Minimally invasive approach for aortic operations. Ann Thorac Surg 62:596–597, 1996.
98. Falk V, Walther T, Diegler A, et al. Echocardiographic monitoring of minimally invasive mitral valve surgery using an endoaortic clamp. J Heart Valve Dis 5:630–637, 1996.
99. Carpentier A, Lessana A, Relland JYM, et al. The "Physio-Ring": An advanced concept in mitral valve annuloplasty. Ann Thorac Surg 60:1177–1186, 1995.
100. Wells FC. Conservation and surgical repair of the mitral valve. In Wells FC, Shapiro LM (eds.): Mitral Valve Disease. Oxford, UK, Butterworth-Heinemann Ltd, 1996, pp 114–134.
101. Deloche A, Jebra VA, Relland JY, et al. Valve repair with Carpentier techniques: The second decade. J Thorac Cardiovasc Surg 99:990–1002, 1990.
102. Ormiston JA, Shah PM, Tei C, Wong M. Size and motion of the mitral valve annulus in man. I. A two-dimensional echocardiographic method and findings in normal subjects. Circulation 64:113–120, 1981.
103. Cooley DA, Frazier OH, Norman JC. Mitral leaflet prolapse: Surgical treatment using a posterior annular collar prosthesis. Bull Tex Heart Inst 3:438–442, 1976.
104. Cosgrove DM, Arcidi JM, Rodriguez L, et al. Initial experience with the Cosgrove-Edwards annuloplasty system. Ann Thorac Surg 60:499–504, 1995.
105. Cohn LH. Mid-term results for mitral valve repair utilizing the Cosgrove annuloplasty ring. (abstract)
106. David TE, Armstrong S, Zhao S, et al. Late results of mitral valve repair for mitral regurgitation due to degenerative disease. Ann Thorac Surg 56:7–12, 1993.
107. Spence PA, Peniston CM, David TE, et al. Toward a better understanding of the etiology of left ventricular dysfunction after mitral valve replacement: An experimental study with possible clinical implications. Ann Thorac Surg 41:363–371, 1986.
108. van Rijk-Zwiller GL, Mast F, Schipperheyn JJ, et al. Comparison of rigid and flexible rings for annuloplasty of the porcine mitral valve. Circulation 82(Suppl II):II-58–64, 1990.
109. Castro LJ, Moon MR, Rayhill SC, et al. Annuloplasty with flexible or rigid ring does not alter left ventricular systolic performance, energetics, or ventricular-arterial coupling in concious, closed-chest dogs. J Thorac Cardiovasc Surg 105:643–659, 1993.
110. Okada Y, Shomura T, Yamaura Y, Yoshikawa J. Comparison of the Carpentier and Duran prosthetic rings used in mitral reconstruction. Ann Thorac Surg 59:658–663, 1995.
111. David TE, Komeda M, Pollick C, Burns RJ. Mitral valve annuloplasty: The

effect of the type on left ventricular function. Ann Thorac Surg 47:524–528, 1989.

112. Unger-Graeber B, Lee RT, Sutton MSJ, et al. Doppler echocardiographic comparison of the Carpentier and Duran annuloplasty rings versus no ring after mitral valve repair for mitral regurgitation. Am J Cardiol 67:517–519, 1991.

113. Reed GE, Pooley RW, Moggio RA. Durability of measured mitral annuloplasty: Seventeen-year study. J Thorac Cardiovasc Surg 79:321–325, 1980.

114. Czer LSC, Maurer G, Trento A, et al: Comparative efficacy of ring and suture annuloplasty for ischemic mitral regurgitation. Circulation 86(Suppl II):II-46–52, 1992.

115. Cohn LH: Mitral and tricuspid valve repair. Ann Thorac Surg 43:572–573, 1987.

116. Grossi EA, Galloway AC, Parish MA, et al. Experience with twenty-eight cases of systolic anterior motion after mitral valve reconstruction by the Carpentier technique. J Thorac Cardiovasc Surg 103:466–470, 1992.

117. Mihaileanu S, Marino JP, Chauvaud S, et al. Left ventricular outflow obstruction after mitral valve repair (Carpentier's technique): Proposed mechanism of disease. Circulation 78(Suppl I):I-78–84, 1988.

118. Bonchek LI: discussion of (1).

119. Carpentier A. Cardiac valve surgery: the "French correction." J Thorac Cardiovasc Surg 86:323–347, 1983.

120. Cohn LH, Rizzo RJ, Adams DH, et al. The effect of pathophysiology on the surgical treatment of ischemic mitral regurgitation: Operative and late risks of repair versus replacement. Eur J Cardio-thorac Surg 9:568–574, 1995.

121. Cohn LH, Kowalker W, Satinder B, et al. Comparative morbidity of mitral valve repair versus replacement for mitral regurgitation with and without coronary artery disease. Ann Thorac Surg 45:284–290, 1988.

122. Chauvaud S, Jebara V, Chachques JC, et al. Valve extension with glutaraldehyde-preserved autologous pericardium: Results in mitral valve repair. J Thorac Cardiovasc Surg 102:171–177, 1991.

123. Bichell DP, Adams DH, Aranki SF, et al. Repair of mitral regurgitation from myxomatous degeneration in the patient with a severely calcified posterior annulus. J Card Surg 10(4Pt1):281–284, 1995.

124. Cohn LH, Couper GS, Aranki SA, et al. The long-term results of mitral valve reconstruction for the "floppy" valve. J Cardiac Surg 9(Suppl):278–281, 1994.

125. Cohn LH, DiSesa VJ, Couper GS, et al. Mitral valve repair for myxomatous degeneration and prolapse of the mitral valve. J Thorac Cardiovasc Surg 98:987–993, 1989.

126. Jebara VA, Mihaileanu S, Acar C, et al. Left ventricular outflow tract obstruction after mitral valve repair: Results of the sliding leaflet technique. Circulation 88(Suppl II):II-30–34, 1993.

127. Perier P, Clausnizer B, Mistarz K. Carpentier "sliding leaflet" technique for repair of the mitral valve: Early results. Ann Thorac Surg 57:383–386, 1994.

128. Carpentier A, Pellerin M, Fuzellier JF, Relland JYM. Extensive calcification of the mitral valve annulus: Pathology and surgical management. J Thorac Cardiovasc Surg 111:718–730, 1996.

129. Grossi EA, Galloway AC, Steinberg BM, et al. Severe calcification does not affect long-term outcome of mitral valve repair. Ann Thorac Surg 58:685–688, 1994.

130. El Asmar B, Acker M, Couetil JP, et al. Mitral valve repair in the extensively calcified mitral valve annulus. Ann Thorac Surg 52:66–69, 1991.

131. Frater RW, Vetter HO, Zussa C, Dahm M. Chordal replacement in mitral valve repair. Circulation 82(Suppl IV):IV-125–130, 1990.
132. David TE. Replacement of chordae tendineae with expanded polytetrafluoroethylene sutures. J Cardiac Surg 4:286–289, 1989.
133. David TE, Bos J, Rakowski H. Mitral valve repair by replacement of chordae tendineae with polytetrafluoroethylene sutures. J Thorac Cardiovasc Surg 101:495–501, 1991.
134. Zussa C, Polesel E, Da Col U, Galloni M, et al. Seven-year experience with chordal replacement with expanded polytetrafluoroethylene in floppy mitral valve. J Thorac Cardiovasc Surg 108:37–41, 1994.
135. Zussa C, Frater RWM, Polesel E, et al. Artificial mitral valve chordae: Experimental and clinical experience. Ann Thorac Surg 50:367–373, 1990.
136. Frater RWM: Discussion of Zussa et al. (134).
137. Valfre C. Discussion of David et al. (132).
138. Smedira NG, Selman R, Cosgrove DM, et al. Repair of anterior leaflet prolapse: Chordal transfer is superior to chordal shortening. J Thorac Cardiovasc Surg 112:287–292, 1996.
139. Fucci C, Sandrelli L, Pardini A, et al. Improved results with mitral valve repair using new surgical techniques. Eur J Cardiothorac Surg 9:621–627, 1995.
140. Alvarez JM, Deal CW, Loveridge K, et al. Repairing the degenerative mitral valve: Ten- to fifteen-year follow-up. J Thorac Cardiovasc Surg 112:238–247, 1996.
141. Lessana A, Carbane C, Romano M, et al. Mitral Valve repair: results and the decision-making process in reconstruction: Report of 275 cases. J Thorac Cardiovasc Surg 99:622–630, 1990.
142. Galloway AC, Colvin SB, Baumann FG, et al. Long-term results of mitral valve reconstruction with Carpentier techniques in 148 patients with mitral insufficiency. Circulation 78(Suppl I):I-97–105, 1988.
143. Antunes MJ, Magalhaes MP, Colsen PR, et al. Valvuloplasty of rheumatic mitral valve disease: A surgical challenge. J Thorac Cardiovasc Surg 94:44–56, 1987.
144. Bernal JM, Rabasa JM, Vilchez FG, et al. Mitral valve repair in rheumatic disease: The flexible solution. Circulation 88(Suppl I):I-1746–1753, 1993.

19

The Floppy Mitral Valve:

Intraoperative Transesophageal Echocardiography

Michael J. Malkowski, MD

Introduction

Intraoperative transesophageal echocardiography (TEE) has grown in parallel with the impressive results of mitral valve repair for mitral regurgitation due to floppy mitral valve disease. TEE has played a pivotal role in assessing the reparability of the mitral valve, establishing the severity of mitral regurgitation , and determining the success of the repair. Expert knowledge of cardiac anatomy and pathophysiology is essential for successful interaction between the surgeon and echocardiographer. The following section reviews the approach to the preoperative and postoperative assessment of patients undergoing mitral valve surgery for severe mitral regurgitation as a result of floppy mitral valve disease.

Presurgical Transesophageal Echocardiography

The presurgical TEE is used to assess valve anatomy, determine the mechanism of mitral regurgitation , and estimate the severity of regurgitation.

From: Boudoulas H, Wooley CF. *Mitral Valve: Floppy Mitral Valve, Mitral Valve Prolapse, Mitral Valvular Regurgitation.* Second revised edition. ©Futura Publishing Company, Armonk, NY, 2000.

The mitral leaflets, chordae tendineae and mitral annulus may all be abnormal in floppy mitral valve disease.[1] All abnormalities of the mitral apparatus may be identified by TEE. The leaflet thickness is frequently greater than 5 mm due to the increase in spongiosum found histologically. The spectrum of abnormality ranges from mild focal thickening to marked diffuse thickening in floppy valve leaflets. In addition, the leaflets are frequently elongated, accounting for leaflet billowing. The chordae tendineae may also be elongated and have been found to be histolgically abnormal. Chordal elongation also may account for the billowing or prolapse of the leaflets to the left atrial side of the annulus during systole. A torn chordae tendineae may be recognized as a thin hypermobile structure attached to

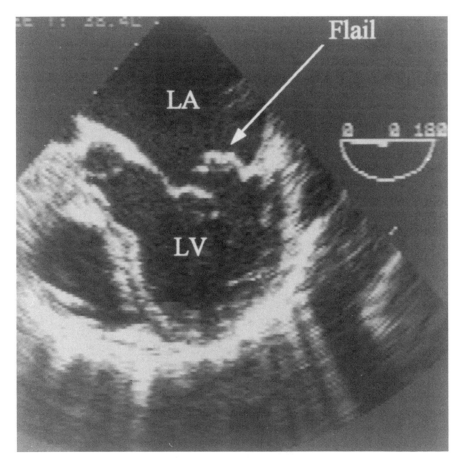

Figure 1. TEE example of a flail posterior leaflet (Flail). Note the leaflet projecting into the left atrium (LA) with the chordae tendineae attached to the leaflet edge. LV = left ventricle.

the valve resulting in a flail portion of the valve.[2] The mitral annulus is frequently dilated in patients with severe mitral regurgitation. The annular structure is abnormal and hypermobile, which may account for the widening of the annulus.[3] In addition, in the case of long-standing mitral regurgitation, the left atrium and left ventricle may dilate and further contribute to annular dilatation. Annular dilatation may contribute to the severity of mitral regurgitation by separating the leaflets and preventing normal coaptation.

The mechanisms of mitral valve regurgitation include flail leaflet, and/or prolapse of one or both leaflets. Flail leaflets are diagnosed with the visualization of the leaflet and/or torn chordae tendineae pointed directly into the left atrium[2,4] (Fig. 1). In addition, the regurgitant jet is very eccentric when there is a flail leaflet and the regurgitant color Doppler jet frequently swirls along the wall of the left atrium opposite from the flail segment.[2] Prolapse of the mitral valve is best described as the leaflets billowing into the left atrium[5] (Fig. 2). Prolapse is due to a combination of elongated chordae tendineae and/or excessive leaflet tissue, which results in malcoaptation of the leaflet margins. Since the mitral annulus is saddle-

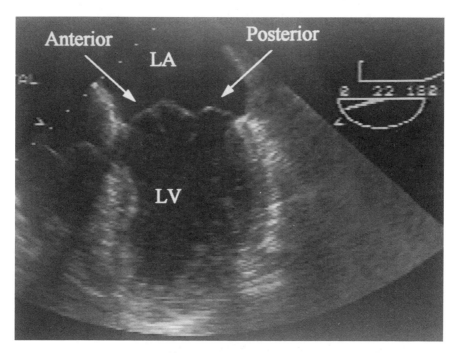

Figure 2. TEE example of marked bileaflet prolapse into the left atrium (LA). At surgery the mitral valve leaflets and chordae were elongated and redundant. LV = left ventricle.

shaped, prolapse of these leaflets should be assessed in the longitudinal view (120°), which would be similar to the parasternal long-axis view on transthoracic echocardiography.[6] When prolapse occurs, leaflet coaptation is incomplete due to the loss of the normal coaptation alignment, allowing regurgitant flow through the valve into the left atrium.

The site of leaflet flail can be accurately determined by TEE.[7,8] Anterior leaflet flail is easily defined by visualization of a free edge of leaflet segment in the left atrium during systole with attached mobile chordae from the transverse (0°) or longitudinal (120°) views (Fig. 3). The anterior leaflet can easily be identified by the close proximity to the aortic valve. Definition of the flail scallop of the posterior leaflet is also possible as previously described by Grewal et al.[8] Flail middle scallop is visualized from the longitudinal (120°) view opposite the longest portion of the anterior leaflet (Fig. 4). Flail lateral scallop is visualized from the transverse four-

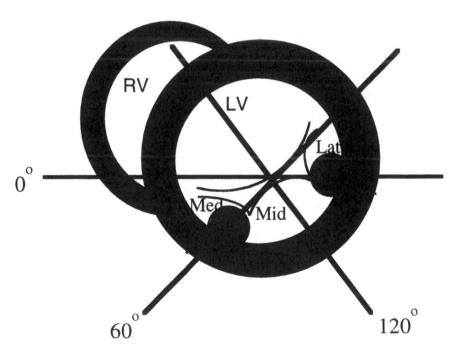

Figure 3. Identification of the flail segment by TEE depends on the position of the imaging angle in relation to the mitral valve anatomy. At 0° the imaging plane transects the anterior leaflet and the posterior leaflet at the junction between the lateral and middle scallop. At 60–90° the imaging plane will transect the anterolateral and posteromedial commisures and the scallops of the posterior leaflet may be identified in relation to those anatomic landmarks. At roughly 120° the imaging plane transects the anterior leaflet and the middle scallop of the posterior leaflet. (Reproduced with permission of the J Am Soc Echocardiogr 11:966–971, 1998.)

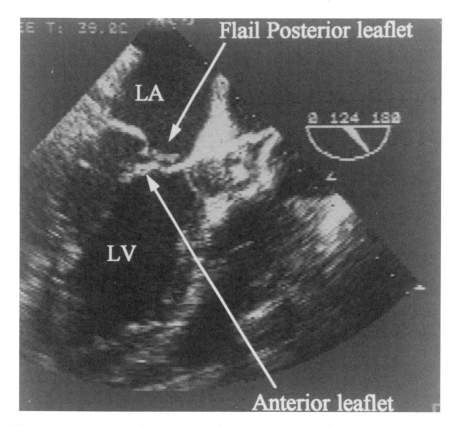

Figure 4. TEE example of a flail middle scallop of the posterior leaflet. This is best visualized with the transducer angle at 120–135°. This is the most common flail scallop in patients with floppy mitral valves. LA = left atrium; LV = left ventricle.

chamber view with the leaflet attached to the lateral aspect of the mitral annulus. This view may also include a portion of a flail middle scallop, and the long-axis view (120°) must be assessed before accurate determination of the flail lateral scallop can be assured. Flail medial scallop is diagnosed when the flail segment is visualized along the posteromedial commisure in the two-chamber (60–90°) view.

Determination of the mechanism of regurgitation is important in determining the surgical approach. In patients with floppy mitral valves, the most common abnormality amenable to surgical repair is a flail posterior leaflet.[9] The most common flail site is the middle scallop of the posterior leaflet. Flail medial or lateral scallops are less common but are also considered reparable lesions. However, there may be some difficulty in assuring valve competence when the commisure is involved. The anterior leaflet flail may be challenging to repair successfully.[9] The anterior leaflet is longer than the posterior leaflet but typically covers only one-third of the annulus. Thus, when resecting a flail portion of the anterior leaflet, there is usually shortening of the leaflet, which may result in poor leaflet coaptation.

Patients with flail leaflets and severe mitral regurgitation have an unstable course resulting in death or requiring mitral valve surgery.[10] Mitral valve repair improves outcome in patients with floppy mitral valves and mitral regurgitation who require mitral valve surgery.[11] Thus, predicting which patients are best suited for valve repair would influence the planning and timing of mitral valve surgery for flail mitral leaflet.

Transesophageal echocardiographic findings predict the potential for mitral valve repair in patients with flail mitral leaflets due to a floppy mitral valve. Specifically, the findings of isolated posterior flail leaflet, anterior leaflet elongation, and marked annular dilatation influence reparative surgery in these patients. Clinical findings favoring repair include a history of mitral valve prolapse and younger age. Mitral annular calcium may also influence the decision to repair a mitral valve. In cases of significant annular calcification, resection of the posterior annular calcium is required for placement of the annuloplasty ring. This procedure is challenging but may be performed successfully.[12]

The severity of regurgitation may be determined by TEE. The methods used include color Doppler for mitral regurgitation jet area, jet width and proximal convergence method, and the pulsed-Doppler techniques assessing transmitral and pulmonary venous flow. Color jet area is the most frequently used parameter but may be the most inaccurate.[13,14] The limitations of color jet area include the influence gain settings and interoperator variability.[14] In addition, the three-dimensional regurgitant jet is being assessed by a two-dimensional technique that may contribute to error. Wall impinging jets undergo spatial distortion and rapidly lose momentum.[15] Thus, jet area in a flail mitral leaflet correlates poorly with regurgitant volume and may significantly underestimate the severity of mitral regurgitation. Jet area is accurate in identifying severe mitral regurgitation when the jet area is greater than 8 cm^2 and mild mitral regurgitation when the maximum jet area of a central free jet is less than 4 cm^2.[13] In determining the spectrum of moderate mitral regurgitation, color Doppler is less precise.

The jet width or vena contracta has gained recent favor as a useful technique to assess mitral regurgitation severity.[16] Recent experimental work has confirmed the utility of measuring the vena contracta.[17] A jet width greater than 0.5 cm has accurately identified severe mitral regurgitation and less than 0.3 has accurately identified mild mitral regurgitation. Again there is a large moderate group with a large spectrum of mitral regurgitation whose clinical significance and natural history is unclear.

Proximal convergence analysis has shown promise as a color Doppler method to determine the regurgitant orifice area but requires offline analysis and has not been gained widespread use.[18]

Pulsed Doppler echocardiography provides additional information regarding the severity of mitral regurgitation. Klein et al. have demonstrated an excellent relationship between pulmonary venous flow reversal and severe mitral regurgitation.[19,20] The right and left pulmonary veins may be identified by TEE and the sample volume placed approximately 2 cm within the pulmonary vein. Systolic flow reversal in the pulmonary veins is very specific for severe mitral regurgitation and correlates strongly with pulmonary wedge pressure v-wave elevation. In floppy mitral valve disease, especially with flail leaflet, eccentric mitral regurgitation is frequently present. Thus, both the right and the left pulmonary veins must be interrogated since reversal may be seen in one or two veins but not the others.

Transmitral Doppler also provides information regarding the severity of regurgitation. With elevation of left atrial pressure, the early filling velocity increases significantly. An increased E velocity and E/A velocity ratio and a shortening of the isovolumic relaxation time or deceleration time on the transmitral flow correlate with an elevated left atrial pressure. The E/A ratio has been shown to increase with the severity of mitral regurgitation.[21] When other factors that may contribute to left atrial pressure elevation are absent (i.e., left ventricular systolic dysfunction), severe mitral regurgitation is frequently the cause of the pressure elevation.

In patients with coronary artery disease requiring coronary artery bypass surgery who have floppy mitral valves, intraoperative TEE may be useful in determining the need for concomitant valve surgery. In cases of flail leaflet, mitral repair or replacement is strongly suggested since progression to symptomatic heart failure is predictable.[10] In addition, recent studies suggest early surgery is preferred to prevent left ventricular dilatation and dysfunction and heart failure.[22] In cases of floppy mitral valve disease and prolapse with regurgitation, the severity of mitral regurgitation may be underestimated due to the effects of general anesthesia.[23] In a recent study of 43 patients comparing the severity of mitral regurgitation during preoperative TEE and intraoperative TEE, the mean jet area, mean jet width, and mean vena contracta all decreased under general anesthesia. Grewal et al. noted that the blood pressure decreased and left ventricular cavity diameter decreased under anesthesia, which resulted in a reduction in mitral regurgitation severity in all groups except those with flail leaflets. There was a significant decrease in jet area, jet width, and pulmonary venous flow.[23] In many cases there was improvement in the severity grade. Thus, general anesthesia alters loading conditions and may reduce the severity of mitral regurgitation except in the presence of a flail leaflet. The effect of loading condition on mitral regurgitation should be considered when planning surgery.

The presurgical TEE serves many purposes in patients with floppy mitral valve disease. It confirms the pathology that was suspected and resulted in the planned surgical intervention. It defines the pathology and helps guide the surgical approach. In cases of surgical intervention (i.e., coronary artery bypass surgery) and uncertainity in the severity of mitral regurgitation, it defines the severity of the mitral abnormality and helps determine the need for mitral valve surgrery.

Anatomic-echo correlates are well defined. Mitral valve repair results in many benefits, including improved left ventricular function and preservation of normal geometry. In additon, repair patients avoid long-term anticoagulation and benefit from a lower endocarditis risk. Thus, the presurgical TEE helps the surgical team determine the feasability of repair and plan the surgical procedure.

Postsurgical Transesophageal Echocardiography

The postoperative TEE is critical in the assessment of the post-repair mitral valve.[24,25] The three findings that must be excluded prior to completion of the operation include residual mitral regurgitation, mitral stenosis, and systolic anterior motion of the anterior mitral leaflet with left ventricular cavity obstruction (Fig. 5). Any of these findings must be brought to the attention of the surgeon immediately, and revision of the repair or mitral valve replacement must be contemplated.

Successful mitral valve repair results in trivial or very mild mitral regurgitation. The most frequent methods of assessing mitral regurgitation involve color Doppler and pulsed-Doppler techniques. The color jet of mitral regurgitation should be very small. The maximal jet area should be less than 3 cm^2 indicative of mild regurgitation. Care must be taken to integrate multiple angles since the repair may result in alteration of the valve geometry and very eccentric jets of regurgitation. In addition, the valve repair must be tested with an adequate blood pressure. Frequently, postoperative hemodynamics are markedly different than awake conditions. In the early postoperative period, most patients are relatively hypotensive. This situation is inadequate for assessing valve competence. The anesthesiologist should titrate medications to provide a blood pressure similar to the preinduction state and the valve should be assessed under these conditions. When valvular dysfunction is detected post bypass, the patient is at risk for major post-operative complications and death.[24] When moderate or severe mitral regurgitation is detected, revision of the repair or mitral valve replacement should be considered. If the flail portion involves the commisure there may be a greater risk of

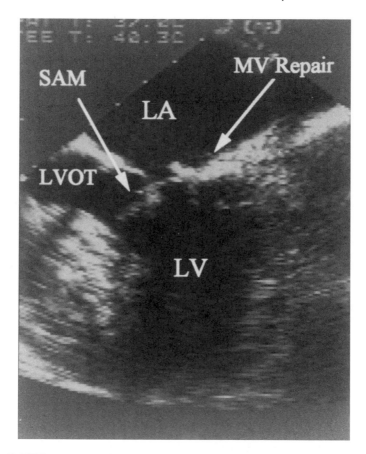

Figure 5. TEE example of systolic anterior motion (SAM) of the anterior mitral leaflet following mitral valve repair with a mitral annuloplasty ring. This finding prompted mitral valve (MV) replacement. LA = left atrium; LV = left ventricle; LVOT = left ventricular outflow tract.

post-repair mitral regurgitation since resection of involved tissue may result in malcoaptation.[26]

As previously described, flail mitral leaflet most commonly involves the middle scallop of the posterior mitral leaflet. Mitral repair is attempted more frequently in the posterior leaflet flail patient than anterior or bileaflet flail patients.[9] However, even when the posterior leaflet is flail and partially resected, the anterior leaflet is frequently elongated and or thickened with abnormal chordal attachments. Thus, following repair specifically when the mitral annular is reduced, the elongated, floppy anterior leaflet is in close proximity to the left ventricular outflow tract. During ventricular systole, the redundant tissue of the anterior leaflet may be pulled by venturi effect forces into the outflow tract below the aortic valve and obstruct flow. The systolic anterior motion of the mitral valve is similar to hypertrophic obstructive cardiomyopathy physiology. Upon making this observation, the surgical team may attempt to alter the postoperative management. Specifically, the left ventricular volume should be increased to alter the orientation of the mitral apparatus and the left ventricle. In addition, withdrawal of inotropic drugs which increase the outflow velocity that pulls the leaflet into the outflow tract should be discontinued. If systolic anterior motion of the anterior leaflet of the mitral valve persists and results in mitral regurgitation and/or outflow tract obstruction, consideration should be given to a revision of the repair or mitral valve replacement.

Mitral stenosis may result from mitral valve repair when the reduction of the annulus results in restriction on leaflet mobility and obstruction to flow. As the annulus size decreases, there is less area to accommodate the enlarged mitral leaflets that define the floppy mitral valve. These enlarged leaflets may obstruct flow even when there is no commissural fusion or rheumatic fibrosis. Doppler echocardiography contributes greatly in the postoperative assessment of the repaired mitral valve. The most helpful aspects of the exam include the assessment of the mean transmitral gradient and the pressure half-time estimate of the mitral valve area.[27] The mean gradient is easily obtainable on most commercially available ultrasound imaging units. The continuous Doppler is directed through the central portion of the valve orifice. The display is then analyzed using software available on the imaging unit. The gradient is dependent on many variables including the stroke volume or flow volume across the valve for each cardiac cycle. Even when there is an adequate effective orifice area, the mean gradient may be elevated when the cardiac output is high or the diastolic filling time is decreased. Thus, in the setting of a normal to high cardiac output, a mean gradient of less than 6 mm Hg is indicative of minimal flow obstruction. When the mean transmitral gradient is elevated, the additional analysis of the pressure half-time may be valuable. This is also performed in the operating room using the software provided. The slope of the early portion of the transmitral envelope is traced and the pressure half-time is calculated. The equation 220/pressure half-time is then used to calculate an estimated valve area. The combination of these methods in the operating room helps identify iatrogenic mitral stenosis and helps prevent a potentially unstable postoperative course.

For anatomic, technical, or clinical reasons, the surgical team may elect to perform a mitral valve replacement. It is widely recognized that preservation of the subvalvular structures is critical to prevent left ventricular dilatation and dysfunction. In preserving these structures, there is a small risk that retained leaflet, especially the anterior leaflet, may partially protrude on the ventricular side of the prosthetic sewing ring. Thus, it is important to assess the subvalvular area for anterior motion of retained vavlular structures off bypass, which may partially obstruct the left ventricular outflow tract.

Chronic mitral regurgitation may result in left ventricular dilatation and dysfunction. In this setting, the left ventricular ejection fraction may remain normal or near-normal despite abnormal myocardial contractility because of altered loading conditions. When mitral regurgitation is present, the left atrium accepts stroke volume at a lower pressure. Thus, the afterload on the left ventricle is diminished. This results in maintenance of the ejection fraction until late in the course of severe mitral regurgitation.[28] There has clearly been a shift toward early valve surgery, especially if the valve appears repairable prior to left ventricular dilatation and dysfunction.[22]

Intracardiac air bubbles are almost always seen as the heart begins to eject and clears air that may collect in the left atrium, left ventricle, and pulmonary vasculature. While a vent is present to prevent systemic distribution of the air bubbles, occasionally these bubbles may embolize down the coronary arteries. In my experience, this occurs in the distribution of the right coronary artery much more frequently than the left. Should a significant amount of air embolize down the right coronary artery, significant right ventricular systolic dysfunction and inferior left ventricular dysfunction may occur. This is an important cause of postoperative hypotension to identify and convey to the anesthesia and surgical team who may delay removing the bypass apparatus until there is return of function.

Summary

Intraoperative TEE has become an important tool in the presurgical and postsurgical assessment of the floppy mitral valve. Presurgical identification of valve pathology and the mechanism of mitral valve regurgitation helps determine the reparability of the floppy mitral valve. In addition, postsurgical assessment following mitral valve repair and replacement assists in the postoperative management by recognizing complications that result from the surgical procedure.

References

1. Malkowski MJ, Guo R, Orsinelli DA, et al. The morphologic characteristics of flail mitral leaflets by transesophageal echocardiography. J Heart Valve Dis 6:54–59, 1997.
2. Pearson AC, St. Vrain J, Mrosek D, Labovitz AJ. Color Doppler echocardiographic evaluation of patients with a flail mitral leaflet. J Am Coll Cardiol 16:232–239, 1990.

3. Hutchins GM, Moore W, Skoog DK. The association of floppy mitral valve with disjunction of the mitral annulus fibrosus. N Engl J Med 314:535–540, 1986.

4. Stewart WJ, Currie PJ, Salcedo EE, Klein AL, Marwick T, Agler DA, Homa D, et al. Evaluation of mitral leaflet motion by echocardiography and jet direction by Doppler color flow mapping to determine the mechanism of mitral regurgitation. J Am Coll Cardiol 20:1353–1361, 1992.

5. Davies MJ, Moore BP, Bainbridge MV. The floppy mitral valve: Study of incidence, pathology, and complications in surgical, necropsy and forensic material. Br Heart J 40:468–481, 1978.

6. Levine RA, Triulzi MO, Harrigan EW, Weyman AE. The relationship of mitral annular shape to the diagnosis of mitral valve prolapse. Circulation 75:756–767, 1987.

7. Stewart WJ, Griffin B, Thomas JD. Multiplane transesophageal echocardiographic evaluation of mitral valve disease. Am J Cardiac Imaging 9:121–128, 1995.

8. Grewal K, Malkowski MJ, Kramer CK, Dianzumba S, Reichek N. Multiplane transesophageal echo identification of the involved scallop in patients with flail mitral leaflet: Intraoperative correlation. J Am Soc Echocardiography 11:966–971, 1998.

9. Cosgrove DM, Stewart WJ. Mitral valvuloplasty. Curr Probl Cardiol 14:359–415, 1989.

10. Ling LH, Enriquez-Sarano M, Seward JB, Tajik AJ, Schaff HV, Bailey KR, Frye RL. Clinical outcome of mitral regurgitation due to flail leaflet. N Engl J Med 335:1417–1423, 1996.

11. Enriquez-Sarano M, Schaff HV, Orszulak TA, Tajik AJ, Bailey KR, Frye RL. Valve repair improves the outcome of surgery for mitral regurgitation. Circulation 91:1022–1028, 1995.

12. Bichell DP, Adams DH, Aranki SF, Rizzo RJ, Cohn LH. Repair of mitral regurgitation from myxomatous degeneration in the patients with a severely calcified posterior annulus. J Cardiac Surg 10:281–284, 1995.

13. Yoshida K, Yoshikawa J, Yamaura Y, Hozumi T, Akasaka T, Fukaya T. Assessment of mitral regurgitation by biplane transesophageal color Doppler flow mapping. Circulation 82:1121–1126, 1990.

14. Sahn DJ. Instrumentation and physical factors related to visualization of stenotic and regurgitant jets by Doppler color flow mapping. J Am Coll Cardiol 12:1354–1365, 1988.

15. Chen C, Thomas JD, Anconina J, et al. Impact of impinging wall jet on color Doppler quantification of mitral regurgitation. Circulation 84:712–720, 1991.

16. Hall SA, Brickner E, Willett DL, Irani WN, Afridi I, Grayburn PA. Assessment of mitral regurgitation severity by Doppler color flow mapping of the vena contracta. Circulation 95:636–642, 1997.

17. Zhou X, Jones M, Shiota T, Yamada I, Teien D, Sahn DJ. Vena contracta imaged by Doppler color flow mapping predicts the severity of eccentric mitral regurgitation better than color jet area: A chronic animal study. J Am Coll Cardiol 30:1393–1398, 1997.

18. Pu M, Vandervoort PM, Griffin BP, Leung DY, Stewart WJ, Cosgrove DM, Thomas JD. Quantification of mitral regrugitation by the proximal convergence method using transesophageal echocardigraphy. Circulation 92:2169–2177, 1995.

19. Klein AL, Stewart WJ, Bartlett J, et al. Effects of mitral regurgitation on pulmonary venous flow and left atrial pressure: An intraoperative transesophageal echocardiographic study. J Am Coll Cardiol 20:1345–1352, 1992.

20. Klein AL, O'Barski TP, Stewart WJ, et al. Transesophageal Doppler echocardiography of the pulmonary vein flow: A new marker of mitral regurgitation severity. J Am Coll Cardiol 18:518–526, 1991.
21. Thomas L, Foster E, Schiller NB. Peak mitral inflow velocity predicts mitral regurgitation severity. J Am Coll Cardiol 31:174–179, 1998.
22. Ling LH, Enriquez-Sarano M, Seward JB, Orszulak TA, Schaff HV, Bailey KR, Tajik AJ, et al. Early surgery in patients with mitral regurgitation due to flail leaflets: A long-term outcome study. Circulation 96:1819–1825, 1997.
23. Grewal KS, Piracha AR, Astbury JC, Reichek N, Malkowski MJ. The effects of general anesthesia on severity of mitral regurgitation by transesophageal echocardiography. J Am Coll Cardiol 31:325A, 1998.
24. Sheikh KH, de Bruijn NP, Rankin JS, Clements FM, Stanley T, Wolfe WG, Kisslo J. The utility of transesophageal echocardiography and Doppler color flow imaging in patients undergoing cardiac valve surgery. J Am Coll Cardiol 15:363–372, 1990.
25. Freeman WK, Schaff HV, Khandheria BK, Oh JK, Orszulak TA, Abel MD, Seward JB, et al. Intraoperative evaluation of mitral valve regurgitation and repair by transesophageal echocardiography: Incidence and significance of systolic anterior motion. J Am Coll Cardiol 20:599–609, 1992.
26. Cormier B, Barabas M, Iung B, Garbarz E, Vahanian A. Commisural prolapse: A marker of severity for mitral valve repair. J Am Coll Cardiol 31(Suppl A):28A, 1998.
27. Nishimura RA, Rihal CS, Tajik AJ, Holmes DR Jr. Accurate measurement of transmitral gradient in patients with mitral stenosis: A simultaneous catheterization and Doppler echocardiographic study. J Am Coll Cardiol 24:152–158, 1994.
28. Enriquez-Sarano M, Tajik AJ, Schaff HV, Orszulak TA, McGoon MD, Bailey KR, Frye RL. Echocardiographic prediction of left ventricular function after correction of mitral regurgitation: Results and clinical implications. J Am Coll Cardiol 24:1536–1543, 1994.

Part XII

Floppy Mitral Valve, Mitral Valve Prolapse

Natural History

Introduction

The Floppy Mitral Valve, Mitral Valve Prolapse, Mitral Valve Regurgitation:
Historical Aspects and Natural History

Charles F. Wooley, MD,
Harisios Boudoulas, MD, PhD

The path to understanding the etiology and pathogenesis of mitral valvular regurgitation (MVR) has been the most tortuous of all the individual valvular lesions. This is related primarily to the complexity and interrelationships of the function of the mitral valve complex within the left atrium and left ventricle. Ignoring or forgetting astute clinical observations by our predecessors also contributed to the process.

Nineteenth century pathologists and clinicians based earlier insights about MVR on clinical assessments correlated with autopsy findings. The correlations of physical diagnosis with autopsy findings reached new levels in 19th century France when Corvisart refined percussion of the thorax and its contents in 1808 and Laennec introduced cardiopulmonary auscultation in 1819. Cardiovascular physical diagnosis developed through the stages of observation, inspection and palpation to the application, and interpretation of the acoustic information inherent in percussion and auscultation. Thus, the presence and interpretation of cardiac murmurs, the detection of cardiac enlargement, and the diagnosis of valvular heart disease became subjects of intense interest to clinicians.

Before clinicians could accurately time cardiac murmurs, it was necessary to understand the timing and origin of the first and second heart sounds. Laennec's belief that the first sound resulted from ventricular contraction and that contraction of the auricles caused the second heart sound led to a period of confusion. Studies during the 1830s by Rouanet, Bouil-

From: Boudoulas H, Wooley CF. *Mitral Valve: Floppy Mitral Valve, Mitral Valve Prolapse, Mitral Valvular Regurgitation.* Second revised edition. ©Futura Publishing Company, Armonk, NY, 2000.

laud, Magendie, Hope, and CJB Williams led to clarification of the heart sound sequence, i.e., that the first heart sound was related to ventricular contraction with closure of mitral and tricuspid valves, and the second heart sound was related to aortic and pulmonic valve closure. Once clinicians could separate systole from diastole, the timing of murmurs and their interpretation became useful clinical currency.

In England, James Hope established the relationship of apical systolic thrills and systolic murmurs with mitral regurgitation as a distinct valvular lesion in the 1830s. Hope incorporated Newtonian principles to the heart's action when he introduced a modern perspective in 1839; he displayed an extraordinary grasp of the hemodynamics of mitral regurgitation:

> When the mitral orifice is permanently patescent [wide open], so that, at each ventricular contraction, blood regurgitates into the auricle, this cavity suffers in a remarkable degree, for it is not only gorged with the blood which it cannot transmit, but, in addition, sustains the pressure of the ventricular contraction. Permanent patescence of the mitral orifice, therefore, constitutes an obstruction on the left side of the heart, and the effect of this, as of contraction of the orifice, may be propagated backwards to the right side. The regurgitation is always considerable when it renders the pulse small and weak.

> When the impediment to the circulation is primitively seated in the lungs, the right ventricle, situated immediately behind them, is the first to experience its influence, and when the cavity is so far overpowered by the distending pressure of the blood as to be incapable of adequately expelling its contents, the obstruction extends to the auricle–the process being exactly the same as that which I have already described, in reference to the left ventricle and auricle.

Hope's contemporary, CJB Williams, provided the pathological correlation for a loud apical systolic murmur heard during life in a patient when the autopsy demonstrated ruptured mitral chordae associated with abnormalities of the mitral valve leaflets.

In the United States in the 1850s, Austin Flint recognized and taught that mitral regurgitation could be long borne without serious inconvenience, with a natural history quite distinct from other forms of valvular disease. This important concept was lost and then resurfaced again later in the 20th century. JP Crozer Griffith, Professor of Clinical Medicine at the University of Pennsylvania, discussed apical mid- and late systolic murmurs of mitral origin as instances of mitral regurgitation at the Association of American Physicians meeting in 1892. JN Hall, in Colorado, encountered late systolic murmurs of mitral insufficiency frequently and considered sudden yielding of the valve unable to withstand left ventricular systolic pressure as the probable mechanism.

Thus, by the beginning of the 20th century, the auscultatory diagnosis of MVR was clearly described, ruptured mitral chordae as a cause of MVR was recognized, and the long natural history of patients with MVR had been defined. So where did clinicians go wrong for the next 100 years?

As is usually the case, the answer involved dogma without data. Information from the cardiovascular physiologists about mitral valve function was just beginning to have an impact in the clinical area. Apical systolic clicks and apical mid- and late-systolic murmurs were regarded as nonorganic or extracardiac in origin by authoritative French auscultators. A coherent approach to the pathophysiology and etiology of mitral regurgitation had not yet surfaced.

British cardiologists, initially Graham Steell and James Mackenzie and later Thomas Lewis and John Parkinson, downplayed the diagnostic significance of apical systolic murmurs. Mackenzie's original intent was to overcome the "tyranny of the stethoscope" and to spare a host of individuals from invalidism and cardiac neurosis. However, during World War I, the concept was expanded on a grand scale so that medical officers could deal specifically with the large numbers of young men with apical systolic murmurs, soldier's heart, and the effort syndrome who presented extraordinary diagnostic, disposition, and pension problems during the war. The doctrine that the apical systolic murmur should be disregarded when not accompanied by other signs of heart disease was developed and implemented under the wartime manpower pressures. The approach became military policy first in Great Britain and then in the United States as the war progressed. Intended to provide medical officers with guidelines about fitness for military service, the net result of setting dogma about individuals with apical systolic murmurs without data was the inhibition of inquiry for several decades.

Thus, as the result of the physical examination of millions of young men in the United States during World War I, several controversial issues regarding physical fitness for military service surfaced. The unexpected frequency of apical systolic murmurs and the interpretation and significance of these murmurs was the primary cardiovascular dilemma. In 1926 in the United States, Richard Cabot attacked the basic concept of mitral regurgitation as a clinical entity in his text, *Facts on the Heart*, when he stated that mitral regurgitation was a lesion almost never verified at postmortem examination. He thought physicians were in error when they diagnosed mitral regurgitation on the basis of the loud apical systolic murmurs and made the outrageous statement that these murmurs were extraordinarily common in all sorts of noncardiac disease as in health. He dated this pernicious habit to the World War I wartime experience noted above:

> . . .Fortunately the mistake was discovered and the rule put into effect that no man should be rejected from military service on account of a systolic murmur no matter how loud it might be.

Cabot expressed doubts that mitral regurgitation could be diagnosed in life but did grant that it might exist as a great rarity. It is not:

> . . .a clinical entity, for it cannot, so far as I can see, be recognized in life. Mackenzie has told us how he gradually came to recognize that no one ever died of mitral regurgitation.

Cabot was widely recognized in the United States for his emphasis on clinical and autopsy correlations and his contributions to medical progress with the case history method of teaching. The Case Records of the Massachusetts General Hospital published in the *New England Journal of Medicine* had their origins in the Clinicopathological Exercises founded by Cabot. Thus, the Mackenzie and Cabot dogma without data had a significant and negative impact on the mitral regurgitation debate that lasted for several decades.

Sir Thomas Lewis continued to teach that "the diagnosis of mitral regurgitation has a very limited importance" in the 1930s. However, clinical cardiologists such as Paul Dudley White and Samuel Levine in Boston realized these positions were incorrect and developed a more reasonable approach to the apical systolic murmur–mitral regurgitation association in the early 1930s.

There were some data developing from experimental studies. Wiggers and Feil[1] described the cardiodynamics of mitral insufficiency in 1922 incorporating and analyzing the earlier German experimental experience. Their state-of-the-art studies involved recording optical pressure curves from the left atrium, the left ventricle, and the aorta, left atrial and left ventricular volumes, and arterial resistance. Mitral regurgitation was related to the events of the cardiac cycle as defined earlier by Wiggers. The time of onset and duration of valvular regurgitation, quantitation of the increased left atrial and left ventricular volumes, and the marked increase in valvular regurgitation associated with increasing arterial resistance were among the results in this classic study.

The Floppy Mitral Valve and Mitral Valvular Regurgitation

The clinical emphasis on inflammatory diseases with scar formation as residual of previous inflammation causing chronic cardiac valvular disorders was appropriate at a time when the life span was short, infections were prevalent, and rheumatic fever and syphilis were rampant. There were exceptions to these categorical classifications based on pathological observations. As early as 1912, Salle described mitral leaflet and chordal abnormalities in a postmortem examination of a patient with Marfan syndrome. Bailey and Hickam (1944) made the association of severe mitral regurgitation with rupture of elongated, thin mitral chordae not related to infectious endocarditis. Mitral cusps were voluminous, showed "fibrosis without stenosis," and ballooned or bulged upward into the left atrium. Dilatation of the mitral annulus was a consistent finding. Valvular connective tissue changes were present without inflammation; a gross anatomic and histological profile led the investigators to exclude a rheumatic etiology. The illustrations in the article establish the paper as a fundamental floppy mitral valve study.

When Brigden and Leatham (1953) described "pure" mitral incompetence in males without a rheumatic history, the clinical features included a long natural history, susceptibility to bacterial endocarditis, and the late onset of rapidly progressive congestive heart failure, forerunners to the floppy mitral valve (FMV) natural history studies later in the century.

A new group of cardiac morphological pathologists described valvular stretch as opposed to valvular scar and contraction as a cause of chronic valvular heart disease. They introduced terms such as mucoid degeneration (Fernex and Fernex, 1958), billowing sail deformity (Oka and Angrist, 1961), or floppy, myxomatous, mucinous, hooded, or balloon mitral valves. The Fernex article, describing cardiomegaly in two patients who had mitral valves with multiple domes, augmentation of the mitral valve surface, and MVR without clinical evidence of Marfan syndrome was a key article emphasizing a connective tissue etiology for floppy mitral valves.

At about the same time an important symposium on MVR in 1958 presented a historical background, clinical and hemodynamic characteristics of MVR, and the important distinctions between mitral valve stenosis and MVR. However, there was no clear-cut consideration of the FMV as an etiologic factor in patients with MVR.

Early 20th century concepts about the incidence, etiology, and pathogenesis of MVR were being revised during the second half of the century by cardiac morphologists and pathologists, clinical cardiologists, cardiac imagers, and cardiovascular surgeons. The sophisticated imaging and surgical approaches to FMV recognition and reconstruction utilizes principles developed by multiple basic and clinical investigators.

The culmination of these basic and clinical developments are best exemplified in the current approaches to the diagnosis of FMV, mitral valve prolapse (MVP), and the documentation of the natural history of the FMV/MVP/MVR triad.

20

Floppy Mitral Valve/Mitral Valve Prolapse/Mitral Valvular Regurgitation:

Natural History

Harisios Boudoulas, MD, PhD,
Albert J. Kolibash, MD,
Charles F. Wooley, MD

Introduction

The long-term natural history of patients with floppy mitral valve (FMV), mitral valve prolapse (MVP), mitral valvular regurgitation (MVR) has been clarified during the past 50 years. It is the purpose of this chapter to review studies that have addressed the clinical course and have described the natural history and potential complications of FMV/MVP/MVR.

Complications Related to FMV/MVP/MVR

Symptoms and serious complications related to mitral valve dysfunction in patients with FMV/MVP include infective endocarditis, thromboembolic phenomena, serious supraventricular or ventricular arrhythmias, atrioventricular conduction defects, progressive MVR, ruptured

From: Boudoulas H, Wooley CF. *Mitral Valve: Floppy Mitral Valve, Mitral Valve Prolapse, Mitral Valvular Regurgitation*. Second revised edition. ©Futura Publishing Company, Armonk, NY, 2000.

The Floppy Mitral Valve - Mitral Valve Prolapse - Mitral Valvular Regurgitation Triad: Natural Progression

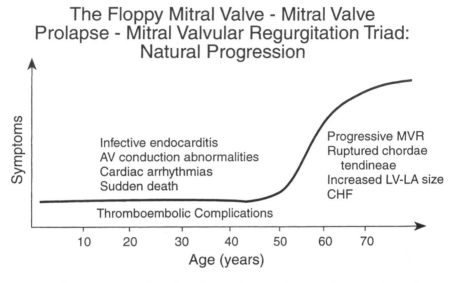

Figure 1. Symptoms are plotted against patient age in years. Increased symptoms occurred after age 50 and are related to progressive mitral valvular regurgitation (MVR), atrial fibrillation, left atrial (LA) and left ventricular (LV) dysfunction, and congestive heart failure (CHF). Thromboembolic complications, infective endocarditis, and cardiac arrhythmias have been reported at a wide range of ages. (Modified with permission from Boudoulas H.[12])

chordae tendineae that require mitral valve surgery, congestive heart failure, and death. As a general rule, complications related to FMV/MVP increase with age (Fig. 1).[1–19]

Natural History in Children and Adolescents

Although FMV/MVP is genetically determined, its clinical manifestations do not usually become evident before adulthood. Children and adolescents with FMV/MVP may have the same symptoms as adults, but the frequency of symptoms appears to be less in children and the overall prognosis is good.[20] Bisset et al.[21] studied 119 children and adolescents for a mean follow-up period of 6 to 9 years. No progress of MVR or deaths have been reported; one patient developed infective endocarditis, one had a cerebrovascular accident, and two required antiarrhythmic therapy for supraventricular arrhythmias. Greenwood[22,23] followed 331 children with isolated MVP for 1 month to 8 years (mean of 2.7 years). Chest pain developed in 12 children; one was treated with propranolol. MVR progressed to heart failure in one patient who developed thyrotoxicosis. Four patients had migraine headaches, and one had a cerebrovascular accident.

Ohara et al.[24] studied the incidence of symptoms in 108 children with MVP. Chest pain was the most common symptom occurring in 11 children (10.2%). The chest pain was nonexertional, located in the left chest, and it was intermittent. Palpitations were present in 7.4%, dyspnea in 3.7%, and syncope in 0.9% of the children.

Kavey et al.[25] performed 24-hour ambulatory monitoring and exercise testing in 103 consecutive children with MVP; a group of 50 normal children served as control subjects. In the MVP group 16% of the patients had exercise-induced premature ventricular beats (PVBs) and 38% had PVBs on ambulatory monitoring. Multiformed PVBs, PVBs in couplets, and ventricular tachycardia were reported in 4% during exercise and in 8% on ambulatory monitoring. No control subject had a single PVB in response to treadmill exercise, and only 8% had rare uniform PVBs on ambulatory monitoring. Physical findings, resting electrocardiogram, and symptoms were not correlated with PVBs in the MVP group. In maximal exercise stress tests, all children reached the predicted maximum or submaximum level of work; exercise time was not different in MVP compared to controls.

Benign arrhythmias on a 24-hour Holter monitor were found in 49.1% of the 108 children with MVP studied by Ohara et al.[24] The evidence of arrhythmia was lower in a group of 70 normal control children (21.4%). PVBs were the most common arrhythmias. The incidence of isolated PVBs was greater in MVP compared to control (27.3% versus 8.5%); the incidence of PVBs increased slightly with age. Isolated atrial premature beats were present in 23.6% of MVP children and 10% in the controls.

Rocchini et al.[26] studied 38 patients ages 1 to 20 years (mean 11.2 years) with recurrent ventricular tachycardia; 17 of the 21 patients with underlying heart disease were symptomatic compared with only six of the 17 patients without heart disease. Of the 21 patients with heart disease, five had MVP. Clinical observations suggest that children with MVP may be at higher risk of arrhythmias during anesthesia and the perioperative period.[20]

The progression of MVR through the spectrum from mild to moderate, and from moderate to severe in patients with FMV/MVP is gradual, and the entire process accelerates after a prolonged asymptomatic interval. Due to the slow gradual progression, significant MVR usually occurs after the fourth or fifth decades and, therefore, is usually not seen in the pediatric population.

Natural History in Adults

In adult patients with FMV, complications increase with age.[1,2] Allen et al.[27] followed 62 patients from 9 to 22 years, mean 13.8 years, seven of whom had serious complications related to FMV/MVP. These included two deaths, five bacterial endocarditis, one ruptured chordae tendineae, one mitral valve replacement, and one progressively severe MVR. Ten additional patients showed a lesser form of deterioration. Only 41 of 62 patients had no significant cardiac event during the follow-up period.

Mills et al.[28] followed 53 patients from 10 to 22 years, mean 13.7 years, 8 of whom (15%) had complications including two cardiac deaths, one ventricular fibrillation, three bacterial endocarditis, and five severe MVR. Koch et al.[29] followed 40 patients with MVP for an average of 10 years and noted serious complications in seven; five sudden deaths and two congestive heart failure.

Belardi et al.[30] followed 137 patients from 1 to 11 years, mean 4.2 years, 22 of whom (16%) developed significant complications: 11 required mitral valve replacement, five died (two sudden death and three severe congestive heart failure), three had bacterial endocarditis, and three required pacemakers for complete AV block. Beton et al.[31] reported 182 patients, mean age 48, who had multiple complications including 24 with supraventricular tachycardia, 22 with atrial fibrillation, 12 with severe MVR, five with mitral valve replacement, 27 with congestive heart failure, eight with bacterial endocarditis, and three with symptoms of cerebral ischemia. Follow-up time was not reported in this study. Devereux et al.[32] reported that the odds ratios in patients with MVP to develop endocarditis and to have chordae tendineae rupture was much greater compared to the general population.

Duren et al.[33] from Amsterdam, Netherlands, reported the results of a long-term prospective follow-up study in 300 patients with MVP diagnosed by clinical, cineangiographic, and echocardiographic criteria. All patients had auscultatory findings consistent with MVP. The ages ranged from 10 to 87 years (mean 42.2 years). The study included all patients with MVP irrespective of clinical condition at the onset, with an average follow-up period of 6.1 years. The clinical condition remained stable in 153 patients. Twenty-seven of the 153 patients developed supraventricular tachycardia that was controlled with medications; 20 patients developed signs of MVR but remained clinically asymptomatic. Serious complications developed in 100 patients. Sudden death occurred in three, ventricular fibrillation in two, ventricular tachycardia in 56, and infective endocarditis in 18. Twenty-eight patients had mitral valve surgery because of progressive MVR; an additional eight patients with severe MVR were considered surgical candidates. Eleven patients had cerebrovascular accidents. Although the study population may not be representative for the entire FMV/MVP population, the results strongly support the concept that FMV/MVP may be associated with significant morbidity and mortality.

Nishimura et al.[34] from the Mayo Clinic, Rochester, Minnesota, determined prognosis in a prospective (mean 6.2 years) follow-up study in 237 minimally symptomatic or asymptomatic patients with MVP documented by echocardiography. The average age was 44 years (range 10 to 69 years). Sudden death occurred in six patients. In multivariable analysis of echocardiographic factors, the presence or absence of redundant mitral valve leaflet, (i.e., FMV) present in 97 patients, emerged as the only variable associated with sudden death. Ten patients sustained a cerebral embolic event; one had a left ventricular (LV) aneurysm with apical thrombus, one had infective endocarditis, six were in atrial fibrillation with left atrial (LA) enlargement, and two were in sinus rhythm. Infective endocarditis occurred in three patients. Progressive MVR prompted valve replacement in 17 patients. A LV end-diastolic diameter exceeding 60 mm was the best echocardiographic predictor of the subsequent need for mitral valve surgery. Twenty patients had no clinical auscultatory findings of a systolic click or murmur; none of these patients had any complications during follow-up. The authors concluded that although most patients with echocardiographic evidence of MVP have a benign course, subsets of patients can be identified by echocardiography (i.e., patients with FMV) that are at high risk for the development of progressive MVR, sudden death, cerebral embolic events, infective endocarditis.

Marks et al.[35] from Massachusetts General Hospital, Boston, Massachusetts, confirmed Nishimura's data in a retrospective study. Clinical and two-dimensional echocardiographic data from 456 patients with MVP were analyzed. Two groups of patients were compared: those with thickening of mitral valve leaflet and redundancy (i.e., FMV) and those without leaflet thickening. Complications, or a history of complications (i.e., infective endocarditis, MVR, and the need for mitral valve replacement), were more prevalent in those with leaflet thickening and redundancy (i.e., patients with FMV) compared to those without leaflet thickening. The incidence of stroke, however, was similar in the two groups.

The Ohio State University Medical Center Experience

Kolibash et al.[17] reported the natural history in 86 patients with ages 26 to 82 years (mean age, 60) who presented with symptoms at The Ohio State University Medical Center. These patients included 53 men and 23 women. Thirteen patients (15%) had a remote history of documented infective endocarditis. All 86 patients had apical systolic murmurs. Atrial fibrillation was present in 48 of 86 patients (56%) and congestive heart failure in 73 (85%).

MVP was seen in 57 of 75 patients (75%) with adequate echocardiograms and in 61 of 84 patients (73%) who underwent contrast left ventriculography. Seventy-five patients had mitral valve replacement of whom 39 (51%) had ruptured chordae tendineae. All had FMV with extensive myxomatous changes, collagen degeneration in the valve leaflets and chordae tendineae on histological examination.

Eighty patients had a known heart murmur before their admission. Figure 2 shows the chronological relationship between the ages at which a murmur was first detected and the ages at which symptoms first developed. The average age at which a murmur was first detected was 34 years and the average age at which symptoms first developed was 59; thus, patients had an asymptomatic period on average of 24 years (Fig. 3). Sixty-two patients (72%) had a known murmur before the age of 50. Only 11 patients (13%) had symptoms before age of 50 whereas 75 (87%) developed

Relationship Between Detection of Murmur and Onset of Symptoms

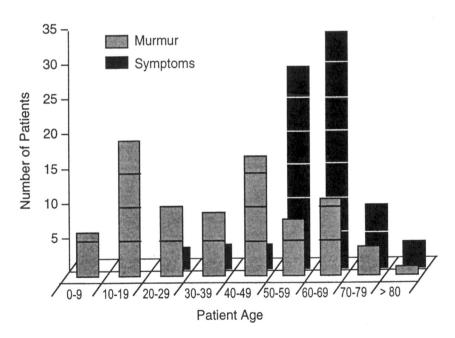

Figure 2. The decades of life when a heart murmur was first detected (cross-hatched bars) and when symptoms first developed (black bars) are shown. Note that 62 patients (72%) were under 50 years when first informed of having a murmur and 75 patients (87%) were over 50 when they first became symptomatic. (Used with permission from Kolibash, et al.[17])

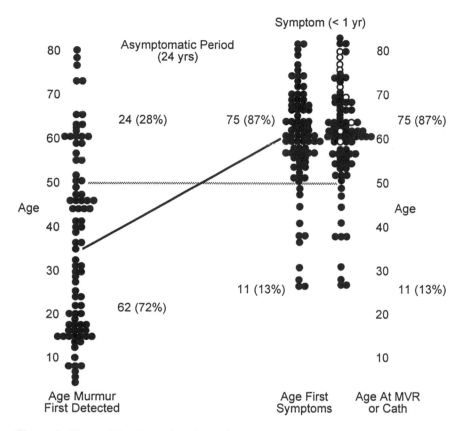

Figure 3. These data show the chronological relationships between the ages at which a murmur was first detected (left column), the ages at which symptoms first developed (middle column), and the ages at which mitral valve surgery was considered (right column). Each dot in each column represents a patient. The open dots in the right column signify those patients who did not have surgery. The horizontal broken line separates patients over and under 50 years of age and the solid line connects the mean ages between the two columns. The average age at which a murmur was first heard was 34 years with 62 patients (72%) less than 50 years. The average age at symptom onset was 59 with 75 patients (87%) above 50 years. The average age when mitral valve surgery was considered was 60 years with 75 patients (87%) over 50 years. Note the prolonged period of 24 years (ages 34–59) of an asymptomatic heart murmur and the short period of 1 year (ages 59–60) between symptom onset and surgical consideration. MVR = mitral valve replacement. (Used with permission from Kolibash, et al.[17].)

symptoms after age 50. Importantly, after the onset of symptoms, mitral valve surgery was usually required within 1 year.

Twenty-eight patients had one or more serial studies including auscultatory examinations, chest X-rays, M-mode echocardiograms, and cardiac catheterization, including contrast left ventriculography. Figure 4

Type of murmur	(# Pts.)	Age First Described	Age MVR	Murmur at MVR	(# Pts.)
Mid to Late Systolic	(5)	50	57	HSM	(5)
Late Systolic	(4)	46	58	HSM	(3)
				LSM	(1)
LSM-MSC	(5)	51	57	HSM	(4)
				LSM	(1)
Holosystolic	(12)	51	56	HSM	(12)

Figure 4. Descriptions of heart murmurs in 26 patients (Pts) examined on two occasions an average of 7 years apart. Note that initially nine patients had late systolic murmurs, five of whom had mid-systolic clicks. At the time of the most recent examination, 24 patients had holosystolic murmurs. HSM = holosystolic murmur; LSM = late systolic murmur; MSC = mid-systolic click; MVR = mitral valve replacement.

shows auscultatory changes in 26 patients examined on two occasions on an average of 7 years time interval. All but two patients had holosystolic murmur at the time of mitral valve surgery whereas only 12 had holosystolic murmur at the time of the first examination. Significantly, nine patients initially had late systolic murmurs, five of whom also had mid-systolic clicks.

Twenty-five patients had at least two chest x-rays taken at an average interval of 6 years. Initially, 14 patients had a normal chest x-ray, eight patients had LV enlargement, and three patients had LA enlargement only. Eleven of the 14 with normal chest x-rays showed LV enlargement and two of the 14 showed LA enlargement 6 years later. All eight patients with initial LV enlargement showed at least a 2-cm progressive increase in the cardiac silhouette several years later. The three patients with LA enlargement subsequently developed LV enlargement as well. Figure 5 shows three chest x-rays that demonstrate progressive cardiomegaly over a 31-month period in a patient who developed congestive heart failure and a loud holosystolic murmur.

Figure 6 shows echocardiographic changes in LA size in 11 patients over a 2-year period. LA size increased from 4.4 ± 7 to 5.0 ± 8 cm (p<0.02).

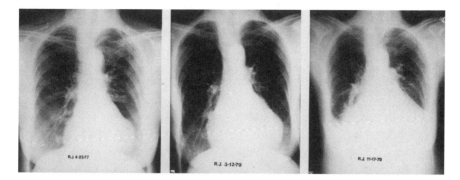

Figure 5. Progressively enlarging cardiac silhouette over a 31-month period in an individual who developed severe congestive heart failure and a loud holosystolic murmur.

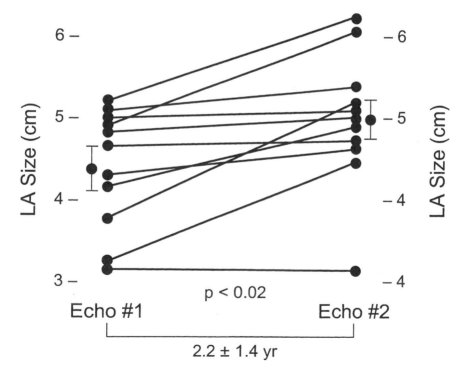

Figure 6. Echocardiographic changes in left atrial (LA) size in 11 patients over a 2-year period (4.4 ± 7 cm to 5.01 ± 8 cm). Mitral valve prolapse was identified on the initial echocardiogram in 9 of 11 patients.

Although LV end-diastolic and end-systolic volumes increased as well, the changes were not significant. These studies suggest that LA size may be affected prior to increase of LV size. Of additional importance is that nine of the 11 patients had MVP on the initial echocardiograms.

At least two cardiac catheterizations were performed in 15 patients at an average interval of 7 years. Findings included a slight increase in LV end-diastolic and systolic volumes between the two studies. The average LV ejection fractions were normal at each study. However, the mean pulmonary capillary wedge pressure increased from 10 to 18 mm Hg ($p<0.02$) and the average V wave amplitude increased from 18 to 25 mm Hg ($p<0.1$).

Obvious worsening in the degree of angiographic MVR occurred between the two studies as shown in Figure 7. Of 15 patients, 14 showed angiographic evidence of progressive MVR. Significantly, 11 of these 15 patients had MVP at the time of each study.

The results of this study strongly suggest that FMV/MVP with mild MVR is a progressive disease in certain patients who develop symptoms of congestive heart failure and require mitral valve surgery late in life. The presence of an asymptomatic heart murmur in 80 patients (93%) suggests that an abnormality of the mitral valve had been present many years before their presentation. During this period of an asymptomatic murmur, patients were able to live productive, comfortable lives. However, once symptoms related to MVR developed, deterioration was usually rapid and mitral valve surgery was often required within 1 year. The rapid deterioration may, in part, be contributed to the onset of atrial fibrillation or ruptured chordae tendineae, both of which occurred with a high incidence in the study.

Although the incidence of documented endocarditis was high (13 patients, 15%), the average time between the acute infection and surgery was 5.6 years. No patient had evidence of active endocarditis at the time of surgery. Thus, active endocarditis was not a major factor contributing to the acute clinical deterioration of these patients.

The observations noted in the 28 patients with serial clinical studies are particularly important since each of these patients had objective evidence of progressive MVR that occurred in the presence of FMV/MVP by initial auscultatory, echocardiographic, and angiographic criteria. Thus, patients with FMV/MVP documented earlier in life by currently accepted clinical criteria had evidence of progressive MVR by one or more similar studies performed later in life.

These long-term follow-up studies in patients with FMV/MVP permit several conclusions: (1) serious complications do occur in patients with FMV/MVP/MVR, (2) FMV/MVP patients constitute a nonhomoge-

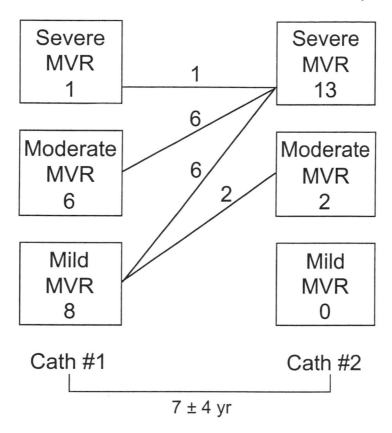

Figure 7. Qualitative changes in the severity of angiographic mitral valvular regurgitation (MVR) in 15 patients having two left ventriculograms at average intervals of 7 years. The degree of MVR had worsened in 14 of the 15 patients at the time of the second study. Eleven patients had angiographic mitral valve prolapse at the time of each angiogram.

neous population, (3) complications are directly related to the specific subset of FMV/MVP patients included in the study, (4) complications in patients with FMV/MVP appear to occur primarily in patients with diagnostic auscultatory findings, and (5) redundant mitral valve leaflets and increased LV/LA size in patients with FMV/MVP are associated with a high frequency of serious complications (Table 1, Fig. 8). The possibility that a patient with FMV/MVP will require mitral valve surgery increases with age. Male FMV/MVP patients required mitral valve surgery more often than female patients with FMV/MVP (Fig. 9).

Table 1
Floppy Mitral Valve/Mitral Valve Prolapse: The High Risk Patient

---

Men, age >50
Mitral systolic murmur
Thick redundant mitral valve leaflets
Left ventricular–left atrial enlargement
Combinations of the above

FMV/MVP/MVR: The High-Risk Patient

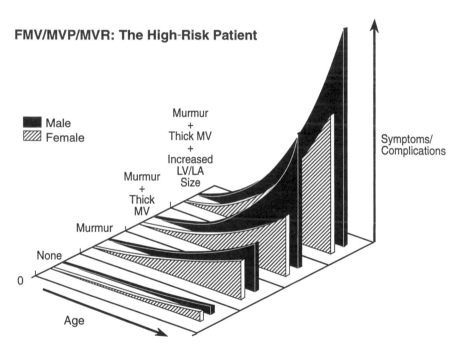

Figure 8. Patients with floppy mitral valve (FMV), mitral valve prolapse (MVP), and systolic murmur, thick, redundant mitral valve (MV) leaflets, and men over age 50 are at higher risk of developing complications. Left ventricular (LV) enlargement in patients with FMV/MVP predicts the need for mitral valve surgery. Presence of two or more of the above abnormalities markedly increases the likelihood of complications. Absence of all three of these features identifies patients with FMV/MVP at extremely low risk. LA = left atrium. (Used with permission from Boudoulas H, et al.[18])

A
FMV/MVP/MVR: Surgery

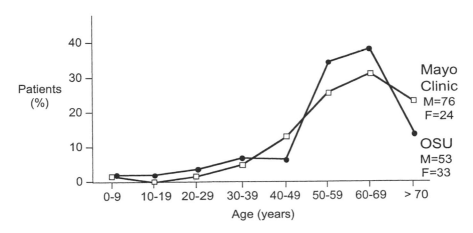

B
FMV/MVP/MVR: Estimated Lifetime Risk of Mitral Valve Surgery

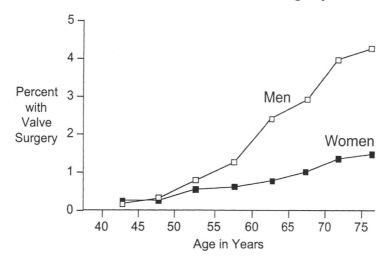

Figure 9. A. mitral valve surgery for mitral valvular regurgitation (MVR) secondary to floppy mitral valve (FMV), mitral valve prolapse (MVP) in relation to age. Data from The Ohio State University (OSU) and Mayo Clinic. (Constructed with permission from Wooley C, et al.[7] and Freed LA, et al.[15]) **B.** Estimated lifetime risk of mitral valve surgery by age and sex among cohorts diagnosed as having MVP. Age-specific events were calculated from the State of New South Wales, Australia. (Used with permission from Wilcken DEL, et al.[42]) M = male; F = female.

Pathophysiology of Chronic Mitral Valve Regurgitation

In certain patients with FMV/MVP/MVR, the mitral valve abnormalities progress with time and mild MVR may become severe. Clinical progression in patients with chronic MVR is usually gradual, permitting adaptive compensatory mechanisms (Fig. 10).[36] During LV systole, part of LV volume is ejected into the low-pressure left atrium. The left atrium dilates gradually and accommodates this extra volume load; as a result there is only minimal or moderate increase in LA pressure during LV systole. The LV diastolic volume also increases gradually, since in addition to the blood flow from the pulmonary veins, blood ejected into the left atrium during LV systole returns into the left ventricle during diastole. As a result of this gradual dilatation, the left ventricle ejects two or more times its nor-

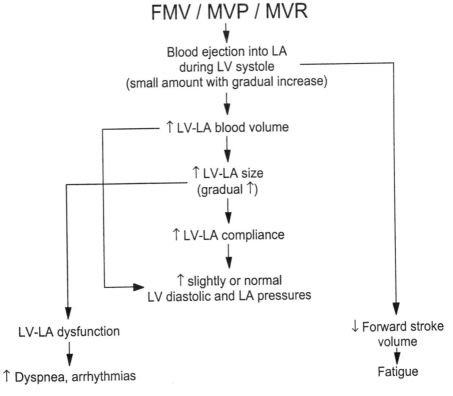

Figure 10. Floppy mitral valve (FMV), mitral valve prolapse (MVP), mitral valvular regurgitation (MVR). Pathophysiologic mechanisms. Schematic presentation. LA = left atrium; LV = left ventricle; ↑ = increase; ↓ = decrease.

mal stroke volume, a portion of which goes into the left atrium (regurgitant volume). As a general rule, MVR progresses gradually. Factors that accelerate the natural course of MVR include infective endocarditis, the development of atrial fibrillation, chordae tendineae rupture, and LA and LV dysfunction (Fig. 11).[36]

Timing for Surgery

Patients with FMV/MVP, mitral valvular dysfunction, and/or MVR may require mitral valve surgery (see Chapter 18). In most instances, patients may live long productive lives after mitral valve surgery. Thus, we consider mitral valve surgery as part of the natural history of FMV/MVP/MVR.

The timing of surgery for patients with FMV/MVP/MVR, particularly in the asymptomatic or mildly symptomatic patient, may be a difficult decision. Preservation of LA and LV function are important considerations. If LV dysfunction is mild and contractile reserve still exists, patients will generally experience symptoms or limitations with only a mild fall in LV ejection performance. If LV dysfunction has become severe, surgery may be associated with a severe fall in LV ejection performance, persistence of symptoms, and even death from congestive heart failure. Thus, the ideal timing for mitral valve surgery is at the onset of LV dysfunction, when good surgical results should be expected.[37-48]

Thus, proper timing of mitral valve surgery requires recognition of LV dysfunction before it has become severe. Unfortunately, the clinical evaluation of LV function has been difficult in MVR because the lesion causes significant alterations in loading conditions. Indeed, in MVR, increased preload with decreased afterload results in an augmentation of the ejection performance with a supernormal ejection fraction. Good postoperative results have been reported when % shortening of the LV internal diameter (%ΔD) is greater than 32%. Once %ΔD or ejection fraction has fallen into the low normal range, a severe postoperative fall in ejection performance may occur. Thus, preoperative ejection fraction may not be a good predictor of postoperative ejection fraction, but when the ejection fraction is frankly subnormal, survival is greatly reduced. Values of LV ejection fraction and end-systolic indexes, which may define patients with poor outlook for benefit from surgery, are: LV ejection fraction <55%; end-systolic diameter index >2.5 cm/m²; end-systolic volume index >60 mg/m²; and end-systolic stress/end-systolic volume index <2.4 (Table 2). These are only guidelines and no single value can be used exclusively in deciding when to perform mitral valve surgery. This decision must be made with comprehensive knowledge of the individual patient's natural

FMV/MVP/MVR:
Dynamic Spectrum & Natural Progression

A

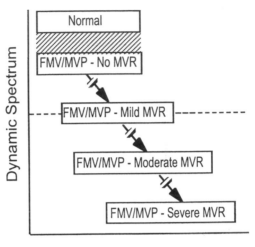

Time (years)

FMV/MVP/MVR:
Natural History - Precipitating Factors

B

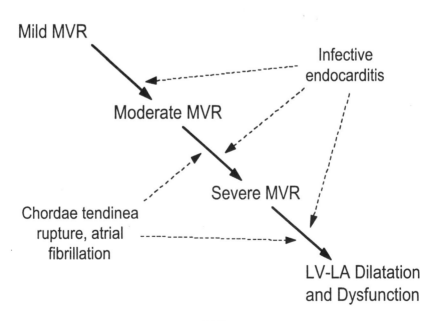

Table 2
Predictors for Suboptimal Response to Mitral Valve Replacement in Patients with Floppy Mitral Valve, Mitral Valve Prolapse, and Mitral Valvular Regurgitation

LV end-diastolic diameter index	>40 cm/m^2
LV end-systolic diameter index	>2.6 cm/m^2
LV end-diastolic volume index cm^2/m^2	>220
LV end-systolic volume index	>60 cm^2/m^2
LV ejection fraction	<55%
%ΔD	<32%
End-systolic stress/end-systolic volume index	<2.4

LV = left ventricular; %ΔD = % fractional shortening of the LV internal diameter.

history, individual indicators of LV function, and the evolving state of mitral valve surgery for MVR.[36,37]

Development of symptoms in chronic MVR usually coincides with onset of LV dysfunction. As such, even mild symptoms are probably significant. If symptoms are present and ventricular function has begun to decline, surgery should be considered. A question often asked is how should I manage the asymptomatic patient who is beginning to show signs of LV dysfunction by physical or echocardiographic examination? It is difficult to recommend surgery for a truly asymptomatic patient. The guidelines for operative intervention, based in part on signs of developing LV dysfunction, are not perfect predictors of outcome. Thus, a poor outcome could occur despite favorable preoperative indexes. Some patients who claim to be asymptomatic have in fact limited their activities to avoid symptoms. In most instances, an exercise tolerance test will help delineate normal or reduced exercise tolerance. The patient who is truly asymptomatic, who has normal exercise tolerance in an objective evaluation, and who is beginning to show signs of LV dysfunction by echocardiography requires very close follow-up. If LV function continues to worsen or response to medical therapy is limited, mitral valve surgery should be considered (Fig. 12).[36]

Figure 11. A. The dynamic spectrum, time in years, and the progression of floppy mitral valve (FMV), mitral valve prolapse (MVP) are shown. A subtle gradation (cross-hatched area) exists between the normal mitral valve and the valves with mild FMV/MVP, without mitral valvular regurgitation (No MVR). Progression from one to another level may or may not occur. **B.** Natural history and precipitating factors in chronic MVR. Schematic presentation. LV = left ventricle; LA = left atrium.

Chronic Mitral Regurgitation (MVR): Timing for Surgery

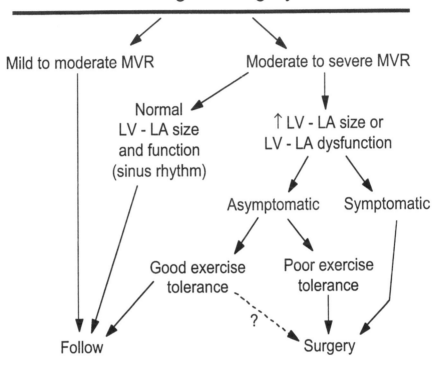

Figure 12. Timing for surgery in patients with floppy mitral valve, mitral valve prolapse, mitral valvular regurgitation (MVR), based on left ventricular (LV) and left atrial (LA) size and function and exercise tolerance.

Mitral Valve Replacement Versus Reconstructive Surgery

Papillary muscle integrity plays a major role in normal ventricular contraction. Removal of the chordae tendineae affects the role of the papillary muscle and decreases overall ventricular performance. Recent studies demonstrate that mitral valve repair or replacement with chordae tendineae left intact helps preserve postoperative LV function. Mitral valve repair has the advantage of leaving the patient with a native mitral valve instead of a prosthesis, eliminating certain complications associated with prosthetic valve.[38,39]

The optimal timing for mitral valve surgery has been changing with the evolution of reparative mitral valve surgery with preservation of the papillary muscle complex. The clinician may be inclined to proceed with surgery earlier to preserve LV function when there is a high probability of a mitral reparative procedure rather than a replacement procedure. Experience with mitral valve repair suggests that localized valve pathology without extensive calcification lends itself to mitral valve repair. Mitral valve replacement, with preservation of at least the posterior papillary muscle, should be performed in those patients with a greatly dilated annulus or severe valve dysfunction, particularly those with extreme calcification. Recent techniques, however, allow reconstructive surgery even in patients with massive mitral annular dilatation. Mitral valve reconstruction in experienced hands appears to be widely applicable with potential for fewer complications. Thus, mitral valve repair should be the goal of both cardiologists and surgeons.

A second factor in the timing of mitral valve surgery is information about the prognostic implications of chronic atrial fibrillation. Atrial fibrillation was thought to be a relatively benign rhythm that could be controlled by digoxin therapy. Several studies, however, have shown that this rhythm is not benign and is associated with increased long-term morbidity and mortality. Studies from the insurance industry have shown that even in the absence of structural heart disease, individuals with chronic atrial fibrillation do not live as long as those with sinus rhythm. Likewise, the Framingham study has shown that patients with chronic atrial fibrillation experience more cardiovascular events and do not live as long as those who have normal sinus rhythm. Patients with atrial fibrillation of less than 12 months' duration have a high probability of conversion to normal sinus rhythm, but after a year, the patient with chronic atrial fibrillation is unlikely to revert to normal sinus rhythm. Thus, the appearance of atrial arrhythmias in a patient with MVR suggests LA dysfunction; in those patients further diagnostic studies and the possibility of mitral valve surgery should be considered.[36,37,49]

Rarely, mitral valve surgery has been performed in patients with FMV/MVP without severe MVR, for life-threatening arrhythmias, pain, or dyspnea. Analyses of the combined results indicate that the symptoms may improve in some patients but success is not consistent (see case in FMV/MVPS chapter). Because of the small sample size, short follow-up, and incomplete postoperative evaluation, inadequate data are available to formulate conclusions regarding the appropriateness of surgery for these indications, and at present surgery for these indications in patients with FMV/MVP without significant MVR must be considered investigational.[36]

Case Presentation

A 64-year-old white male with FMV/MVP/MVR had mitral valve reconstructive surgery in May 1989. A graphic presentation of the patient's history is shown in Figure 13. His cardiac history began in 1975 when he had an abnormal stress electrocardiogram as a part of a routine evaluation for employment.[36] A cardiac catheterization was performed that was reported normal at that time. He remained asymptomatic.

In 1977 a new murmur was noted on a routine physical examination and was attributed to FMV/MVP. He developed chest pain in 1985 and presented for the first time to The Ohio State University Medical Center (OSUMC) for further evaluation. Cardiac catheterization was performed that revealed normal coronary artery anatomy, increased LV and LA size, normal LV systolic function, and FMV/MVP with severe MVR. Cardiac catheterization data are shown in Table 3. A radionuclide exercise test demonstrated good exercise tolerance, a resting ejection fraction of 58%, which increased to 72% with exercise.

In November 1986 the patient developed flu-like symptoms (chills, dry cough, myalgias, anorexia). He was treated elsewhere in December 1986 with oral erythromycin without improvement. In January 1987 he re-

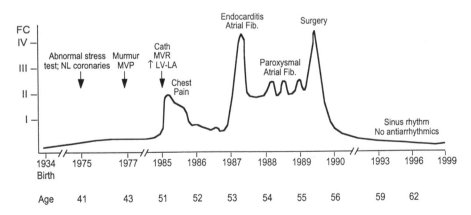

Figure 13. Natural history of a patient with floppy mitral valve (FMV), mitral valve prolapse (MVP), and mitral valvular regurgitation (MVR). Note the long natural history. NL = normal; cath = cardiac catheterization; LV = left ventricle; LA = left atrium; Fib = fibrillation.

Table 3
Floppy Mitral Valve, Mitral Valve Prolapse, Mitral Valvular Regurgitation: Hemodynamic Data

	1985	1989
RA pressure (mm Hg)		
Mean	5	10
A	5	9
V	9	14
Pulmonary artery pressure (mm Hg)		
Systolic	45	36
Diastolic	20	17
PW pressure (mm Hg)		
Mean	18	14
A	18	10
V	35	20
LV pressure (mm Hg)		
Systolic	110	124
Diastolic	16	10
Aortic pressure (mm Hg)		
Systolic	110	124
Diastolic	65	76
CI (liter per min/BSA, green dye)	4.10	4.39
LV-EDVI (cm^3/BSA)	182	220
LV-ESVI (cm^{3}BSA)	70	75
LV ejection fraction (%)	62	66
CI (liter per min/BSA, angiographic)	7.84	011.01
Regurgitant fraction (%)	48	60
LV end-systolic stress (kdynes/cm^2)	140	165
End-systolic stress/LV-ESVI	2.0	2.2

RA = right atrium; PW = pulmonary capillary wedge; LV = left ventricular; CI = cardiac index; EDVI = end-diastolic volume index; ESVI = end-systolic volume index; BSA = body surface area.

ported having nightly fever up to 102°, nightly sweats, and palpitations. He denied dyspnea, orthopnea, paroxysmal nocturnal dyspnea, or edema. Dental procedures had been performed in October 1986 with oral antibiotic prophylaxis prior to the dental work.

He returned to the OSUMC for further evaluation and therapy. The diagnosis of infective endocarditis was confirmed when blood cultures were positive for *Streptococcus sanguis*, and he received a 6-week course of intravenous antibiotics. At the time of admission his rhythm was atrial fibrillation with rapid ventricular response. Digitalis therapy was associated with conversion to sinus rhythm. An echocardiogram demonstrated a re-

dundant mitral valve with vegetations on the atrial surface of the posterior
mitral valve leaflet. He was maintained on digitalis therapy and dis-
charged. He returned to full-time work as an executive vice president of a
regional company. Between January 1987 and February 1989, he had two
episodes of atrial fibrillation for which he came to the emergency department at the OSUMC. The first episode converted spontaneously without
additional therapy. After the second episode of atrial fibrillation, therapy
with quinidine and digitalis was initiated.

In April 1989 the patient had another episode of atrial fibrillation
that was associated with mild shortness of breath and he was admitted
to the hospital for 2 days. The physical examination during this admission revealed a pleasant 55-year-old man in no distress. His height and
arm span were 72", with an upper segment to lower segment ratio of
0.92". His blood pressure was 120/80 in both arms, and his heart rate
was 84 beats/min and irregular. The jugular venous pressure was nor-

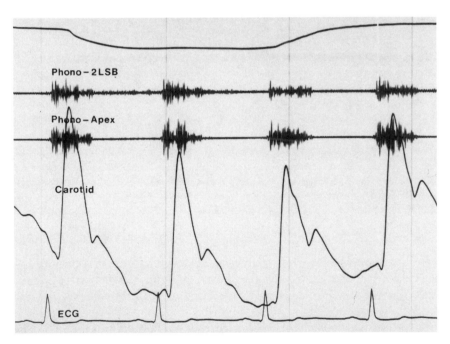

Figure 14. Phonocardiogram (phono) obtained from the second intercostal space
left sternal border (2LSB) and from the cardiac (apex), carotid arterial pulse
(carotid), and electrocardiogram (ECG). Note the holosystolic murmur and the
rapid carotid upstroke.

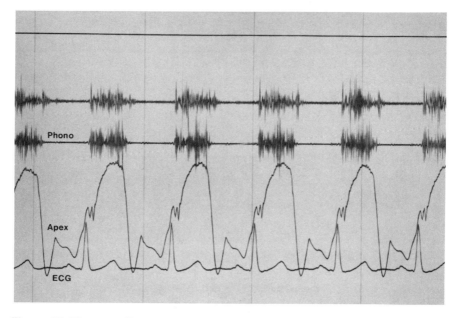

Figure 15. Phonocardiogram recorded at cardiac apex (phono), apex cardiogram (apex), and electrocardiogram (ECG). The apex impulse is sustained with an exaggerated rapid filling wave. An S_3 gallop which coincides with the rapid filling wave was also recorded on the phono.

mal with slightly increased V wave. The carotid pulse was brisk (Fig. 14). The cardiac apex was in the 6th intercostal space at the mid-clavicular line; it was sustained and diffusely enlarged (Fig. 15). A loud grade IV–V/VI apical systolic murmur masked the first heart sound and radiated to the left axilla and left sternal border. An S_3 gallop was present. A soft murmur of tricuspid regurgitation was heard at the lower left sternal border and was increased in intensity with inspiration. The lungs were clear, and there was no peripheral edema or hepatosplenomegaly. The electrocardiogram on admission showed atrial fibrillation, increased precordial voltage, and ST and T wave changes to which digitalis and quinidine may add (Fig. 16). At the time of discharge the electrocardiogram showed sinus rhythm (Fig. 16). The chest x-ray showed slightly increased cardiac size with clear lung fields.

The echocardiogram demonstrated increased LV and LA size, FMV/MVP, and voluminous and redundant mitral valve. Doppler and color Doppler echocardiography demonstrated severe MVR. Because of

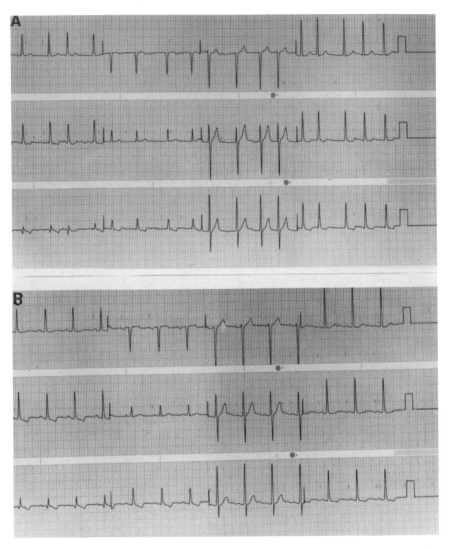

Figure 16. A. Atrial fibrillation with ST and T wave changes especially in the inferolateral leads. **B.** Sinus rhythm with ST and T wave changes in the inferolateral leads.

the frequency of episodes of paroxysmal atrial fibrillation and progressive LV and LA enlargement, mitral valve surgery was recommended.

Cardiac catheterization performed prior to surgery demonstrated large LV and LA size, floppy mitral valve, and severe MVR (Fig. 17). The coronary arteries were normal. A patent foramen ovale with a small left-

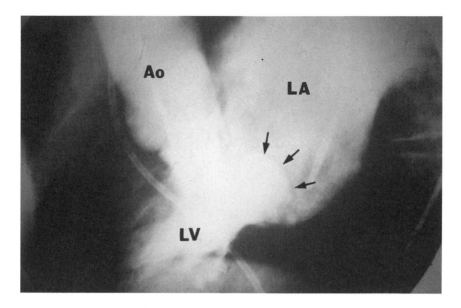

Figure 17. Left ventriculogram in a patient with floppy mitral valve, mitral valve prolapse, and severe mitral valvular regurgitation. Note the large left atrial size. The mitral valve leaflets are thick and prolapsing into the left atrium.

to-right shunt was also demonstrated. The hemodynamic findings are summarized in Table 3. Reconstructive mitral valve surgery and closure of the atrial septal defect were performed. The mitral valve reconstruction included chordal repair and use of annuloplasty ring. Doppler and color Doppler echocardiography were used during the operation to assess surgical results. Postoperative atrial arrhythmias were treated medically. After surgery, the patient returned to work and remained physically active without any limitations. A few years after surgery, antiarrhythmic therapy was discontinued and the patient remained in normal sinus rhythm.

Ten years after the operation (January 1999), the patient continued to be asymptomatic. Physical examination included normal jugular venous pressure, clear lungs, and no peripheral edema. The first heart sound was decreased in intensity with normal splitting of the second heart sound and no murmurs in any body position (Fig. 18). The echocardiogram demonstrated normal LV and mild increase of LA size, and thickened mitral valve; there was no MVP. Doppler echocardiogram demonstrated no MVR and trivial to mild tricuspid regurgitation. Serial echocardiographic measurements are shown in Table 4.

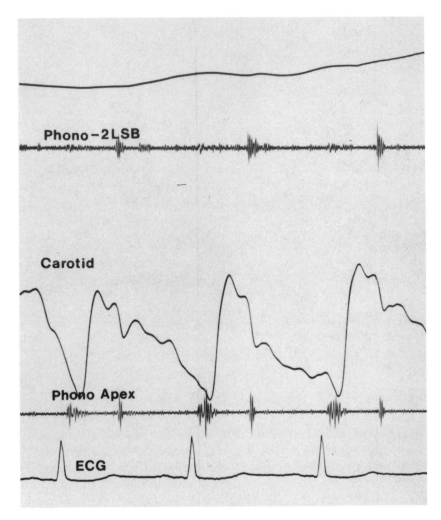

Figure 18. Phonocardiogram obtained from the second intercostal space (phono-2LSB) and from the cardiac apex (phono apex) simultaneously with electrocardiogram (ECG) 6 months after surgery. Note the absence of heart murmur. (Compare with the phono before surgery in Figs. 14 and 15.)

Floppy Mitral Valve/Mitral Valve Prolapse/Acute Mitral Valvular Regurgitation

The most common causes of acute MVR are chordae tendineae rupture, papillary muscle rupture, and infective endocarditis.[50,51] Distinguishing the three most common types of acute mitral regurgitation clinically is reasonably straightforward. Rupture of the chordae

Table 4
Chronic Mitral Regurgitation: Serial Echocardiographic Measurements

	1985	1986	1987	1988	1989	MV Surg. ↓ 1989	1999
LV end-diastolic diameter	5.7	5.7	6.1	6.0	6.8	5.7	5.7
LV end-diastolic diameter index	2.6	2.6	2.7	2.67	3.0	2.6	2.6
LV end-systolic diameter	3.6	3.9	4.0	4.3	4.3	3.6	3.6
LV end-diastolic diameter index	1.6	1.8	1.8	1.9	1.9	1.6	1.6
%ΔD	37	32	34	28	37	37	37
LA diameter	4.7	4.7	4.6	5.5	6.0	5.1	4.3

LV = left ventricular; %ΔD = % fractional shortening of the LV internal diameter; LA = left atrial.

tendineae is the most common cause of acute MVR in an otherwise healthy person.

Pathophysiology of Acute Mitral Valvular Rregurgitation

Patients with acute MVR have entirely different clinical presentation than patients with chronic MVR. This reflects the unique pathophysiology of acute MVR.[36] The immediate direct effects of regurgitant blood flow into the LA in patients with acute MVR are obvious because there is no time for LA adaptation. In severe acute MVR, a large regurgitant volume is ejected into the LA during LV systole. Since there is not time for the LA and LV to dilate, the large LA volume and consequently the large LV diastolic volume will result in striking elevation of LA and LV diastolic pressures. Left atrial V wave pressures of 60 mm Hg or greater are common. The marked increase in pulmonary venous pressure results in pulmonary congestion and pulmonary edema. The patient complains of severe dyspnea. Since the LV is of normal size and a large amount of blood goes into the LA during LV systole, the forward LV stroke volume is markedly diminished. The net result in addition to pulmonary congestion is tissue hypoperfusion, low cardiac output, hypotension and shock (Fig. 19).

Physical Findings

The physical findings in a patient with severe acute MVR usually include an LV S_4 gallop; an S_3 gallop may also be present. However, since

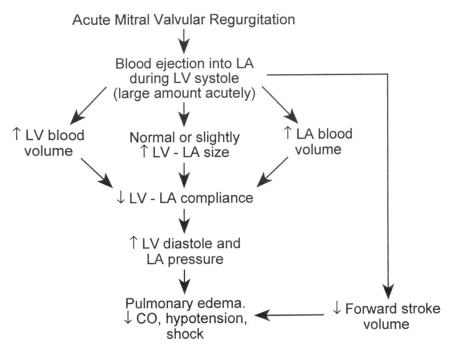

Figure 19. Pathophysiological mechanisms in acute mitral regurgitation. Schematic presentation. LV = left ventricular; LA = left atrium; CO = cardiac output; ↑= increase; ↓= decrease.

acute MVR is associated with sinus tachycardia, a summation gallop is commonly heard. The systolic murmur has several characteristics that distinguish it from the holosystolic murmur of chronic MVR. The murmur may peak in mid-systole and diminish in intensity before the second heart sound (Fig. 20). If the mitral regurgitant jet is directed toward the intra-atrial septum and impinges on the aortic root, the murmur may radiate toward the base of the heart and appear loudest in the second and third left intercostal space at the left sternal border. The result is a crescendo-decrescendo systolic murmur that seems to disappear before the second heart sound and may be heard best at the base of the heart. Although these findings may suggest valvular aortic stenosis, the carotid pulse rises rapidly and is short in duration, and the murmur does not usually radiate into the neck (Fig. 20). The wide splitting of the second heart sound due to early aortic closure is also inconsistent with LV outflow tract obstruction. In the case of anterior chordae tendineae rupture, the murmur may radiate posteriorly to the spine.

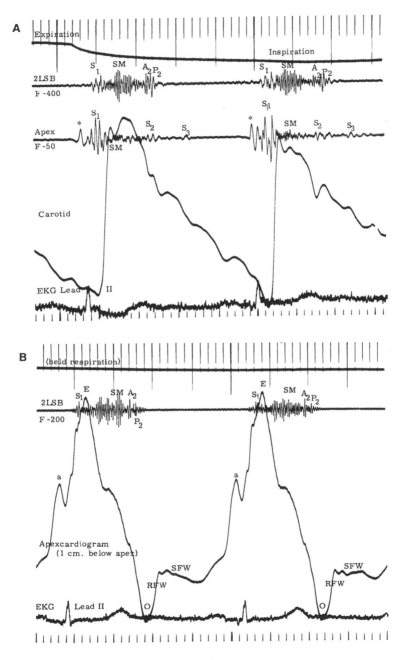

Figure 20. A. Phonocardiogram second intercostal space, left sternal border (2LSB) and apex. S_1 = first heart sound, SM = systolic murmur, A_2 P_2 = aortic and pulmonic components of the second heart sound, S_3 = S_3 gallop, EKG = electrocardiogram. Note the rapid upstroke of the carotid arterial pulse. **B.** Phonocardiogram and apex cardiogram. Note the prominent a (a) and rapid filling waves (RFW); SFW = slow filling wave; F = frequency.

Laboratory Findings

The electrocardiogram usually shows nonspecific findings.

Chest x-ray shows normal or slightly increased heart size with pulmonary congestion or pulmonary edema.

The echocardiogram usually shows normal or slightly increased LV and LA size with normal LV systolic function. Chordae tendineae rupture or flail mitral leaflet may be seen, especially in the transesophageal echocardiogram. Echo Doppler and color Doppler echocardiography shows severe MVR; the direction of the regurgitant flow can also be evaluated.

Cardiac catheterization with left ventriculography shows severe MVR into a slightly enlarged LA chamber. LA pressure is elevated and a large V wave is present in the LA pressure recording. LV diastolic pressure is high. The LV size may be normal or only slightly increased.

Diagnosis

The sudden appearance of a new systolic murmur accompanied by shortness of breath in the middle-aged patient should raise the strong suspicion of acute severe MVR. In certain cases, a patient with known murmur may present with acute deterioration of symptoms (mostly dyspnea and/or fatigue). Infective endocarditis or myocardial infarction can usually be identified on the basis of the clinical history and the physical examination. It should be emphasized that chordae tendineae rupture may occur in a patient with FMV who developed infective endocarditis. The so-called "spontaneous" rupture most often occurs in the presence of chordal structural abnormalities in patients with FMV/MVP or Marfan syndrome.

Physicians who are not familiar with the syndrome of acute MVR may be confused by the presence of acute interstitial pulmonary congestion in a patient with relatively normal LV and LA size. To the inexperienced ear, the murmur—which decreases in intensity before the second heart sound and radiates to the base of the heart—may seem to suggest ventricular outflow obstruction. Awareness of the fine points of the differential diagnosis of MVR may be critical, since time is of the essence.

Natural History

In cases of severe acute MVR, the patient's clinical status deteriorates rapidly despite "good" medical management and leads to death without surgical intervention. The natural history of acute MVR depends on the etiology, the degree of mitral valve dysfunction, the severity of the MVR, and the functional status of the left ventricle and left atrium. Patients with less severe MVR may progress less rapidly, respond to medical therapy, and may not require emergency surgical intervention.[36]

Two patients with chordae tendineae rupture, one who required mitral valve replacement immediately after the event and another in whom surgery was performed several months after chordae tendineae rupture, are presented.

Case #1

EM was a 50-year-old man who developed acute dyspnea and collapsed during strenuous physical activity. He transferred to the OSUMC in December 1966. On physical examination, the intensity of the first heart sound was diminished, a wide splitting of the second heart sound and an S₃ gallop were present. The systolic murmur was louder in the second intercostal space at the left sternal border and was terminated well before the second heart sound (Fig. 20). The apex was sustained, with large a wave and prominent rapid filling wave (Fig. 20). Cardiac catheterization demonstrated normal LV systolic function and severe MVR. Mitral valve replacement was performed after cardiac catheterization. The mitral valve was redundant; the posterolateral chordae tendineae were ruptured, resulting in severe acute MVR.

Case #2

The other patient is an 80-year-old woman with known heart murmur for many years. She developed chronic atrial fibrillation approximately 2 years prior to mitral valve replacement. Despite the atrial fibrillation, she remained relatively asymptomatic until approximately 7 months prior to mitral valve surgery when she started to complain of dyspnea with mild exertion. Symptoms improved significantly with mild diuresis and she continued to do well without major limitations of her physical activities. On physical examination she had a holosystolic murmur at the apex radiating to the left sternal border. There were no gallops. An echocardiogram at the time of deterioration of her symptoms demonstrated severe MVR, FMV/MVP, normal LV systolic function, marked LA enlargement, and flail posterior mitral valve leaflet. The patient elected not to have surgery. She continued to have mild symptoms, mostly related to exertion. Natural history of the disease with and without surgery were discussed in detail on several occasions with the patient and her family. After several months, the patient decided to go ahead with surgery. Transesophageal echocardiogram prior to surgery demonstrated flail posterior mitral valve leaflet, severe MVR, FMV/MVP, large LA, normal LV systolic function, and

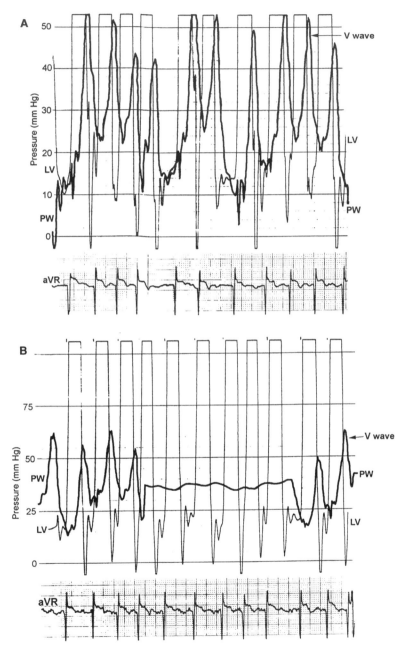

Figure 21. Left ventricular (LV) and pulmonary capillary wedge (PW) pressures. Note the prominent V wave.

heavy mitral annular calcification. Cardiac catheterization demonstrated pulmonary hypertension and large V waves in the pulmonary capillary wedge pressure tracing (Fig. 21). Coronary arteries were free of significant stenosis. The patient had mitral valve replacement with a porcine valve. Reconstructive surgery was not performed because of severe mitral annular calcification. FMV, severe MVP and rupture of the posterior chordae tendineae were found during surgery. The postoperative course was uneventful but the patient remained in atrial fibrillation.

Timing for Surgery

Patients with acute severe MVR, pulmonary congestion, and hypotension require emergency surgical intervention. Any delay will result in irreversible clinical deterioration. Mitral valve reconstructive surgery is preferable when feasible, but mitral valve replacement may be necessary in certain circumstances. Patients with less severe acute MVR without pulmonary congestion or tissue hypoperfusion may be managed medically without emergency surgical intervention. Data, however, suggest that most of the patients will benefit with early surgical intervention.[36,37,47] Decisions about surgical therapy should be based on the patient's symptoms, clinical status, the presence of atrial fibrillation, LV and LA size, and function as discussed above in the section dealing with patients with chronic MVR.

Comments

Chronic MVR due to FMV/MVP, as a general rule, is characterized by a long natural history. A heart murmur is present for many years before the patient becomes symptomatic. There is a progressive enlargement of LV and LA size with gradual alterations of LV filling and LA pressures. Progressive LA and LV chamber enlargement due to volume overload may lead to progressive LV and LA dysfunction without surgical intervention.

Infective endocarditis, chordae tendineae rupture, and onset of atrial fibrillation accelerate the natural progress of the disease, increase the degree of MVR, and may initiate or precipitate symptoms. The development of symptoms, atrial fibrillation, progressive LV and LA dilatation, early signs of LV dysfunction, and increased LV end-systolic stress should prompt surgical intervention. It should be emphasized that LV dysfunction in patients with significant MVR may be masked because of increased preload and decreased afterload. For these reasons, exercise stress testing should be performed in asymptomatic patients with MVR and early signs of LV dysfunction in order to subjectively evaluate exercise tolerance and ventricular function. If exercise tolerance is good, the patient should be followed closely and surgery should be considered if symptoms progress or deterioration of LV performance occurs. The increasing use of mitral valve repair coupled with the realization that chronic atrial fibrillation leads to decreased long-term survival has and will continue to influence the timing and type of surgery. The intraoperative use of echo Doppler and color Doppler has enhanced surgical results.

Sudden disruption of mitral valve integrity results in acute, massive MVR in the presence of relatively normal LV and LA size. This results in a marked increase in LA and pulmonary capillary wedge pressure with the development of pulmonary edema. Because of the relatively normal LV size in the presence of significant MVR, the forward stroke volume is decreased significantly; this will result in a significant decrease in tissue perfusion, hypotension, and shock. For these reasons, emergency cardiovascular evaluation followed by emergency surgical intervention is indicated in patients with severe acute MVR. Patients with less severe acute MVR without pulmonary congestion and tissue hypoperfusion may be managed medically without emergency surgery. Experience, however, suggests that these patients will require surgical intervention.

References

1. Boudoulas H, Kolibash AJ Jr, Baker P, King BD, Wooley CF. Mitral valve prolapse and the mitral valve prolapse syndrome: A diagnostic classification and pathogenesis of symptoms. Am Heart J 118:796–818, 1989.
2. Wooley CF, Baker P, Kolibash AJ, Kilman JW, Sparks EA, Boudoulas H. The floppy myxomatous mitral valve, mitral valve prolapse and mitral regurgitation. Prog Cardiovasc Dis 33:397–433, 1991.
3. Wooley CF, Sparks EA, Boudoulas H. The floppy mitral valve-mitral valve prolapse-mitral valvular regurgitation triad. ACC Current Journal Review July/August 1994, pp 25–26.
4. Boudoulas H. Mitral valve prolapse: Serious or not? Hospital Med 43–62, Sept 1992.
5. Boudoulas H, Wooley CF. Mitral valve prolapse and the mitral valve prolapse syndrome. In Yu PN, Goodwin JF (eds): Prog Cardiovasc Dis 14:275–309, 1986.
6. Davies MJ, Moore BP, Brainbridge MV. The floppy mitral valve: Study of incidence, pathology, and complications in surgical, necropsy and forensic material. Br Heart J 40:468–481, 1978.
7. Wooley CF, Boudoulas H. Mitral valve prolapse. Conn's Current Therapy. In Rakel RE (ed): Philadelphia, W.B. Saunders Co., 1999, pp 289–293.
8. Boudoulas H. Valvular Disease. American College of Cardiology Self-Assessment Program (ACCSAP) 2000, in press.
9. You-Bing D, Takenaka K, Sakamonto T, et al. Follow-up in mitral valve prolapse by phonocardiography, M-mode and two-dimensional echocardiography and Doppler echocardiography. Am J Cardiol 65:349–354, 1990.

10. Baker PB, Bansal G, Boudoulas H, Kolibash AJ, Kilman J, Wooley CF. Floppy mitral valve chordae tendineae: Histopathologic Alterations. Human Pathology 19:507–512, 1988.
11. Boudoulas H, Kolibash AJ, Wooley CF. Mitral valve prolapse: The high-risk patient. Practical Cardiol 17:15–31, 1991.
12. Boudoulas H. Mitral valve prolapse and the mitral valve prolapse syndrome. In Toutouzas P, Boudoulas H (eds): Cardiac Diseases, Parissianos Medical and Scientific Editions, Athens, 2:135–156, 789–793, 1991.
13. Boudoulas H, Schaal SF, Wooley CF. Floppy mitral valve/mitral valve prolapse: Cardiac arrhythmias. In Vardas PE (ed): Cardiac Arrhythmias, Pacing, and Electrophysiology. Great Britain, Kluwer Academic Publisher, 1998, pp 89–95.
14. Malkowski MT, Boudoulas H, Wooley CF, Guo R, Pearson AC. The spectrum of structural abnormalities in the floppy mitral valve: Echocardiographic evaluation. Am Heart J 132:145–151, 1999.
15. Freed LA, Levy D, Levine RA, Larson MG, Evans JC, Fuller DL, Lehman B, et al. Prevalence and clinical outcome of mitral valve prolapse. N Engl J Med 341:1–17, 1999.
16. Barlow JB, Bosman CK, Pocock WA, Marchand P. Late systolic murmurs and nonejection (mid-late) systolic clicks: An analysis of 90 patients. Br Heart J 30:203–218, 1968.
17. Kolibash AJ, Kilman JW, Bush CA, Ryan JM, Fontana ME, Wooley CF. Evidence for progression from mild to severe mitral regurgitation in mitral valve prolapse. Am J Cardiol 58:762–767, 1986.
18. Boudoulas H, Kolibash AH, Wooley CF. Mitral valve prolapse: A heterogeneous disorder. Primary Cardiol 17:29–43, 1991.
19. Barnett HJM, Jones MW, Boughner DR, et al. Cerebral ischemic events associated with prolapsing mitral valve. Arch Neurol 33:777–782, 1976.
20. Boudoulas H, Wooley CF. The floppy mitral valve, mitral valve prolapse, and mitral valvular regurgitation. In Moss and Adams: Heart Disease in Infants, Children, and Adolescents. Sixth edition, in press.
21. Bisset GS III, Schwartz DC, Meyer RA, et al. Clinical spectrum and long-term follow-up of isolated mitral valve prolapse in 119 children. Circulation 62:423–429, 1980.
22. Greenwood RD. Mitral valve prolapse: Incidence and clinical course in a pediatric population. Clin Pediatr 23:318–320, 1984.
23. Greenwood RD. Mitral valve prolapse in childhood. Hosp Pract 41–42, Aug 1986.
24. Ohara N, Mikajima T, Takagi J, Kato H. Mitral valve prolapse in childhood: The incidence and clinical presentation in different age groups. Acta Paediatr Jpn 4:467–475, 1991.
25. Kavey REW, Blackman MS, Sondheimer HM, Byrum CJ. Ventricular arrhythmias and mitral valve prolapse in childhood. J Pediatr 105:885–890, 1984.
26. Rocchini AP, Chun PO, Dick M. Ventricular tachycardia in children. Am J Cardiol 47:1091–1097, 1981.
27. Allen H, Harris A, Leatham A. Significance and prognosis of an isolated late systolic murmur: A 9 to 22 year follow-up. Br Heart J 36:525–532, 1974.
28. Mills P, Rose J, Hollingsworth J, Amara I, Craige E. Long-term prognosis of mitral valve prolapse. N Engl J Med 297:13–18, 1977.
29. Koch FH, Hancock EW. Ten year follow up of forty patients with the midsystolic click/late systolic murmur syndrome. Am J Cardiol 37:149, 1976.
30. Belardi J, Lardani H, Manubens S, Sheldon WC, Moreyra A. Idiopathic pro-

lapse of the mitral valve: A follow-up study in 137 patients studied by angiography. Am J Cardiol 37:120, 1976.

31. Beton DC, Brear SG, Edwards JD, Leonard JC. Mitral valve prolapse: An assessment of clinical features, associated conditions and prognosis. Quart J Med 52:150–164, 1983.

32. Devereux RB, Hawkins I, Kramer-Fox R, Lutas EM, Hammond IW, Spitzer MC, Hochreiter C, et al. Complications of mitral valve prolapse. Disproportionate occurrence in men and older patients. Am J Med 81:751–758, 1986.

33. Duren DR, Becker AE, Dunning AJ. Long-term follow-up of idiopathic mitral valve prolapse in 300 patients: A prospective study. J Am Coll Cardiol 11:42–47, 1988.

34. Nishimura RA, McGoon MD, Shub C, Miller FA, Ilstrup DM, Tajik AJ. Echocardiographically documented mitral valve prolapse: Long-term follow up of 237 patients. N Engl J Med 313:1305–1309, 1985.

35. Marks AR, Choong CY, Chir MBB, et al. Identification of high-risk and low-risk subgroups of patients with mitral valve prolapse. N Engl J Med 320:1031–1036, 1989.

36. Boudoulas H, Wooley CF. Mitral regurgitation: Chronic versus acute. Implications for timing of surgery. In Bowen JM, Mazzaferri EL (eds): Contemporary Internal Medicine, Vol 3, New York and London, Plenum Medical Book Co, 1991, pp 1–35.

37. Cohn LH, Couper GS, Aranki SF, Rizzo RJ, Kinchla NM, Collins JJ Jr. Long-term results of mitral valve reconstruction for regurgitation of the myxomatous mitral valve. J Thorac Cardiovasc Surg 107:143–150, 1994.

38. Skoularigis J, Sinovich V, Joubert G, Sareli P. Evaluation of the long-term results of mitral valve repair in 254 young patients with rheumatic mitral regurgitation. Circulation 90:II167–174, 1994.

39. Enriquez-Sarano M, Tajik AJ. Natural history of mitral regurgitation due to flail leaflets. Eur Heart J 18:705–707, 1997.

40. Ling LH, Enriquez-Sarano M, Seward JB, Orszulak TA, Schaff HV, Bailey KR, Tajik AJ, et al. Early surgery in patients with mitral regurgitation due to flail leaflets: A long-term outcome study. Circulation 96:1819–1825, 1997.

41. Enriquez-Sarano M, Schaff HV, Frye RL. Early surgery for mitral regurgitation: The advantages of youth. Circulation 96:4121–4123, 1997.

42. Wilcken DEL, Hickey AJ. Lifetime risk for patients with mitral valve prolapse of developing severe valve regurgitation requiring surgery. Circulation 78:10–14, 1988.

43. Hickey AJ, Wilcken DEL, Wright JS, Warren BA. Primary (spontaneous) chordal rupture: Relation to myxomatous valve disease and mitral valve prolapse. J Am Coll Cardiol 5:1341–1346, 1985.

44. Salomon NW, Stinson EB, Griepp RB, Shumway NE. Surgical treatment of degenerative mitral regurgitation. Am J Cardiol 38:463–468, 1976.

45. McKay R, Yacoub MH. Clinical and pathological findings in patients with floppy valves treated surgically. Circulation 47(Suppl 3):63–73, 1973.

46. Tribouilloy CM, Enriquez-Sarano M, Schaff HV, Orszulak TA, Bailey KR, Tajik AJ, Frey RL. Impact of preoperative symptoms on survival after surgical correction of organic mitral regurgitation: Rationale for optimizing surgical indications. Circulation 99:400–405, 1999.

47. Schlant RC. Timing of surgery for patients with nonischemic severe mitral regurgitation. Circulation 99:338–339, 1999.

48. Lee EM, Shapiro LM, Wells FC. Superiority of mitral valve repair in surgery for degenerative mitral regurgitation. Eur Heart J 18:655–663, 1999.
49. Boudoulas H, Boudoulas D, Sparks EA, Pearson AC, Nagaraja HN, Wooley CF. Left atrial performance indices in chronic mitral valve disease. J Heart Valve Dis 4(Suppl 2):S242–247, 1995.
50. Boudoulas H, Vavuranakis M, Wooley CF. Valvular heart disease: The influence of changing etiology on nosology. J Heart Valve Dis 3:516–526, 1994.
51. Lucas RV, Edwards JE. The Floppy Mitral Valve. Chicago, Year Book Medical Publishers, 1982.

Part XIII

The Floppy Mitral Valve, Mitral Valve Prolapse, Mitral Valvular Regurgitation:

Effects on the Circulation

Introduction

The Floppy Mitral Valve, Mitral Valve Prolapse, Mitral Valvular Regurgitation:

Effects on the Circulation

Charles F. Wooley, MD,
Harisios Boudoulas, MD, PhD

Our clinical and physiological cardiovascular predecessors were concerned with the state of the "Circulation," always spelled with a capital "C." Their initial cardiac catheterization studies in humans at mid-20th century were intended to provide the requisite information and data about the intact circulation and the interrelations of circulatory phenomena. However, during the past few decades, cardiac diagnostic evaluations have become more fragmented or compartmentalized, and less attention is directed to the study and analysis of the intact circulation.

Chapter 21 presents our consideration of the floppy mitral valve (FMV), mitral valve prolapse (MVP), mitral valvular regurgitation (MVR) triad within the intact circulation, calling attention to the global cardiovascular implications and effects of FMV dysfunction.

The concept that the exuberant FMV prolapses into the left atrium in such a dynamic manner that the prolapsing FMV becomes a space-occupying lesion within the left atrium is fundamental to these considerations. Another significant result of the prolapsing FMV into the left atrium is the development of a "third chamber" within the left atrium during ventricular systole, between the left ventricle, the mitral annulus, and the remaining left atrial chamber (Fig. 1).

The FMV/MVP dynamics also alter left ventricular papillary muscle traction, altering the patterns of left ventricular contraction and relaxation, activating papillary muscle and left ventricular stretch receptors, and con-

From: Boudoulas H, Wooley CF. *Mitral Valve: Floppy Mitral Valve, Mitral Valve Prolapse, Mitral Valvular Regurgitation.* Second revised edition. ©Futura Publishing Company, Armonk, NY, 2000.

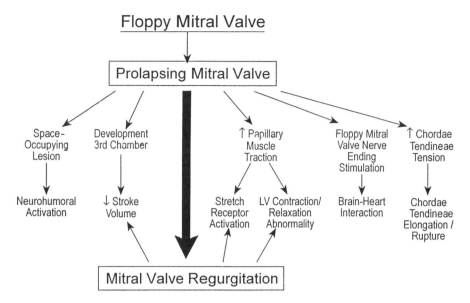

Figure 1. Results of the prolapsing FMV into the left atrium.

tributing to the production of cardiac arrhythmias. FMV innervation patterns with distinct nerve terminals suggest a neural basis for other brain-heart interactions, augmented by mechanical stimuli from the prolapsing FMV.

The histopathology of FMV chordae is abnormal in a nonuniform fashion as described in Chapter 5. The dynamic changes in the FMV complex during MVP increase FMV chordal tension. This increase in tension on abnormal FMV chordae may result in elongation of affected chordae, and under certain circumstances, rupture of the affected FMV chordae tendineae.

The dynamic changes within the left heart chambers with the development of the third chamber may have significant effects on cardiac output, since the blood in the third chamber does not contribute to forward stroke volume. Similarly, the development and progression of MVR further affects forward stroke volume.

Left atrial performance is important in patients with the FMV/MVP/MVR triad. With the onset of MVR, and gradual progression of the MVR from mild to moderate to severe, multiple left atrial performance indices change with increases in left atrial chamber size and alterations in left atrial dimensions. The development of left atrial myopathy further reduces left atrial efficiency, results in left atrial failure, with the histopathologic and electrophysiological changes conducive to the development of atrial fibrillation.

Aortic function is extremely important within the entire cardiovascular system, however, it is not currently evaluated in clinical practice on a routine basis. As a connective tissue disorder, FMV/MVP may be associated with abnormal structural and elastic properties of the aorta, with resultant changes in aortic function. Progression of MVR and the aging process per se also affect aortic function indices in an adverse manner (Fig. 2).

The phenomena associated with FMV dysfunction, with prolapse of the mitral valve into the left atrium (MVP), and the unique, resultant forms of MVR, are dynamic in nature. As the long-term natural history of these interrelated phenomena is being clarified, it is apparent that the FMV/MVP/MVR triad influences the circulation in a global fashion.

Floppy Mitral Valve – Mitral Valve Prolapse – Elastic Properties of the Aorta

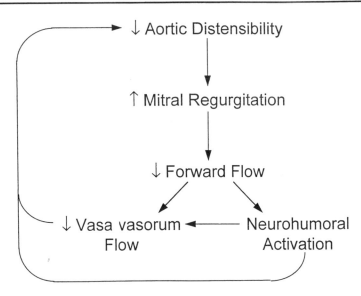

Figure 2. FMV/MVP: elastic properties of the aorta.

21

Floppy Mitral Valve/Mitral Valve Prolapse/Mitral Valvular Regurgitation:

Effects on the Circulation

Harisios Boudoulas, MD, PhD,
Charles F. Wooley, MD

Introduction

Floppy mitral valve (FMV) function is a reflection of the broad FMV pathologic spectrum and the changes that occur in the FMV complex with time. The expressions of FMV dysfunction are dynamic and are expressed over time through the morphogenic changes in FMV.[1-8] The phenomena associated with FMV dysfunction, mitral valve prolapse (MVP), mitral valvular regurgitation (MVR), affect left atrial (LA) and left ventricular (LV) function. In time, these cumulative effects influence the circulation in a global fashion.

Prolapse of the FMV is a unique situation in which the redundant FMV prolapses into the left atrium during LV systole. As a result, a number of dynamic events are set in motion. The prolapsing FMV becomes a space-occupying section of the LA chamber; this results in the development of a third chamber within the border of the mitral valve annulus and the prolapsing mitral valve leaflet(s) (Figs. 1 and 2).[1,2,5,9] Physiologically,

From: Boudoulas H, Wooley CF. *Mitral Valve: Floppy Mitral Valve, Mitral Valve Prolapse, Mitral Valvular Regurgitation*. Second revised edition. ©Futura Publishing Company, Armonk, NY, 2000.

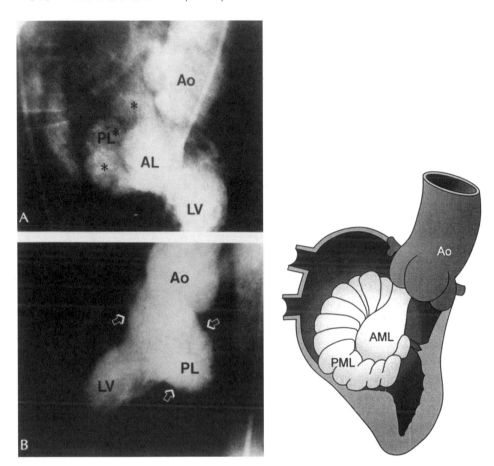

Figure 1. Left. Left ventriculography in right and left oblique projections. **A.** Right oblique projection shows prolapsing anterior (AL) and posterior (PL) mitral valve leaflets. The asterisks indicate individual redundant scallops of posterior leaflet. **B.** Left oblique projection shows the halo or saturn ring appearance of the myxomatous, prolapsing mitral valve associated with increased valve surface area. LV = left ventricle; Ao = aorta. Note that the redundant floppy, prolapsing mitral valve occupies a large part of the left atrium. There is no mitral valvular regurgitation. Right. Prolapsing anterior and posterior mitral valve leaflets (AML), (PML) are shown schematically. Note the redundancy of mitral valve leaflets.

the third chamber acts like an LV aneurysm since blood within this space does not contribute to the effective stroke volume. Thus, during LV systole, the left heart consists of three chambers: the left ventricle, the left atrium, and the third chamber between mitral annulus and the prolapsing leaflet(s).

The prolapsing mitral valve also affects papillary muscle traction

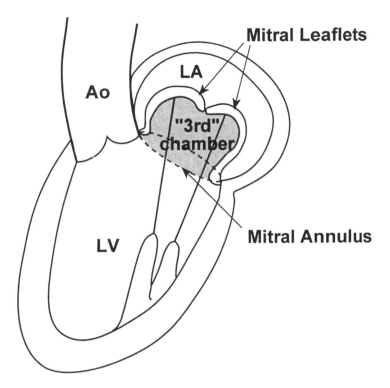

Figure 2. The third space between the mitral valve anulus and the prolapsing mitral valve leaflets are shown schematically. LV = left ventricle; LA = left atrium; Ao = aorta.

with the activation of stretch receptors. Altered papillary muscle traction may result in LV contraction and relaxation abnormalities, while activation of stretch receptors may provide a stimulus for cardiac arrhythmias. [10–13]

The physiological/pathophysiological consequences of the third chamber effect, altered papillary muscle traction, and the resultant LV contraction abnormalities are not well understood, but probably play important roles in the clinical presentation of FMV/MVP/MVR triad and the FMV/MVP syndrome. The extent of these changes may determine the natural history of the disease.

When patients with FMV/MVP develop MVR on an intermittent or chronic basis, changes in LV, LA, and aortic function occur. While LV structural and functional changes have been extensively studied in MVR, much less attention has been given to LA and aortic changes in chronic MVR. All of these factors will be discussed in this chapter.

Prolapse of Floppy Mitral Valve: A Space-Occupying Lesion–Development of Third Chamber

FMV, when prolapsing into the left atrium, occupies part of the LA cavity, the degree of which depends on the severity of mitral leaflet prolapse and the size of mitral valve leaflets (Figs. 1 and 2).[1,2,5,9] This space-occupying lesion may provide stimulus for neurohumoral activation and alter atrial hemodynamics.

Because of the prolapse of the mitral valve leaflet(s), a new chamber develops between the mitral annulus and the prolapsing mitral valve leaflet(s) during LV systole. Thus, during LV systole, in cases of FMV/MVP, even without MVR, a certain amount of blood occupies the space between the mitral annulus and the mitral valve leaflets (the third space), as a result of FMV prolapse into the left atrium. In severe prolapse, the amount of blood may represent a large amount of the total potential stroke volume, resulting in a significant decrease of the effective stroke volume. The degree of MVP increases in the upright posture. This may contribute to a further decrease in effective stroke volume and forward cardiac output. Decreased cardiac output may contribute to fatigue and exercise intolerance in certain patients with FMV/MVP syndrome. Indeed, studies from our laboratory have shown the inability of patients with FMV/MVP to maintain normal LV diastolic volume in the upright exercise; it also was noted that the cardiac output was decreased during upright exercise.[14]

Floppy Mitral Valve/Mitral Valve Prolapse: Papillary Muscle Traction, Left Ventricular Contraction and Relaxation

In normal subjects, the distance between the papillary muscle tips and the mitral annulus during LV systole remains relatively constant. In contrast, in patients with FMV/MVP, mitral valve leaflet displacement into the left atrium results in papillary muscle displacement that increases traction on the papillary muscles (Fig. 3).[10,12] Since normal LV contractile function and symmetry are dependent on the integrity of papillary muscle and chordae tendineae function, alterations in papillary muscle traction and stress result in disorders of contractile patterns of LV contraction.[15–24]

Scambardonis et al.[15] analyzed LV contraction patterns in 87 patients with FMV/MVP. Sixty-nine percent had no or mild MVR and 42% of the patients had pronounced leaflet prolapse (3+ to 4+) of the posterior, or both posterior and anterior mitral valve leaflets. Distinctly abnormal patterns of LV contraction were present in 82% of the patients (Fig. 4).

Floppy Mitral Valve / Mitral Valve Prolapse

Abnormal Mitral Apparatus

↓

Mitral Leaflet Prolapse

↓

Papillary Muscle Traction
Activation of Stretch Receptors

↓

Papillary Muscle and
Subendocardial Ischemia

↓

Pain
Ventricular Arrhythmias

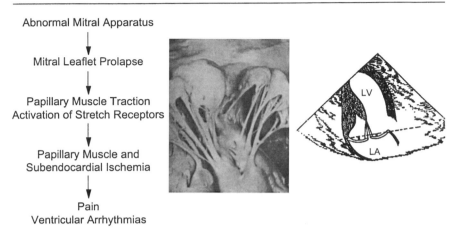

Figure 3. Floppy mitral valve is shown in the middle. (Used with permission from Edwards JE. Circulation 43:606–612, 1971). Papillary muscle traction during left ventricular (LV) systole is shown schematically. LA = left atrium.

Type I: Ballerina Foot Pattern

This pattern was the most frequently seen, was present in 27 patients (38%), and was characterized by early vigorous contraction of the posteromedial portion of the left ventricle with anterior convexity, giving rise to the configuration resembling ballerina foot at end-systole. An anterior bulge in early diastole often accompanied this contraction pattern.

Type 2: Hour-Glass Pattern

A vigorous ring-like contraction involving the middle portions of both anterior and posterior LV walls, usually beginning from the posterior LV wall, was demonstrated in 22 patients (27%).

Type 3: Inadequate Long-Axis Shortening

The contraction pattern was otherwise normal with symmetrical shortening of all other axes. There were 12 cases (15%) in this group.

Type 4: Posterior Akinesis

Eight cases (10%) exhibited vigorous anterior wall contractions with posterior wall akinesis. Ejection fractions were normal.

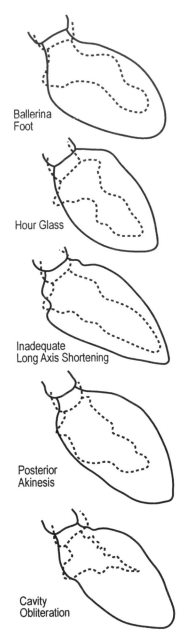

Figure 4. Left ventricular contraction patterns in patients with floppy mitral valve, mitral valve prolapse. (Used with permission from Scabardonis et al.[15]).

Type 5: Cavity Obliteration

In two cases (3%), hyperdynamic LV contraction resulted in an almost complete approximation of anterior and inferior LV walls. This was seen at the apical and middle portions of the left ventricle and was reminiscent of the cavity obliteration pattern seen in hypertrophic myocardiopathy.

Diastolic Phase

In addition to abnormal contraction patterns, abnormalities in the mode of LV relaxation were also noted in 48 cases (55%), of which 44 were associated with abnormal systolic contraction patterns.[15,25] The most frequently observed abnormality was an early bulge of the anterior and/or apical portions of the left ventricle, presumably a result of the normal relaxation in these portions and sustained contraction in other portions of the myocardium.

Floppy Mitral Valve/Mitral Valve Prolapse Papillary Muscle Stretch: Stretch Receptors and Cardiac Arrhythmias

Papillary muscle traction in FMV/MVP may be a contributing factor in the production of arrhythmias.[12] Activation of stretch receptors results in membrane depolarization; membrane depolarization is caused by both gradual and rapid ventricular stretch, but premature ventricular depolarizations are more readily elicited by rapid stretch. Recent studies have demonstrated the existence of stretch-activated membrane channels in ventricular myocardium; these may contribute to ventricular ectopy under conditions of differential ventricular loading as in FMV/MVP (Fig. 5).[11,12]

Floppy Mitral Valve/Mitral Valve Prolapse: Mitral Valve Innervation/Mitral Valve–Brain Interactions

Human cardiac valves have distinct patterns of innervation that comprise both primary sensory and autonomic components.[12,26] The presence of these distinct nerve terminals suggests a neural basis for interactions between the central nervous system and the mitral valve. The subendocardial surface on the atrial aspect at the middle portion of the mitral valve is rich in nerve endings, including afferent nerves; mechanical stimuli from this area caused by abnormal coaptation in FMV/MVP may cause an abnormal autonomic nerve feedback between the central nervous system and mitral valve nervous system (Fig. 5).[12]

Floppy Mitral Valve/Mitral Valve Prolapse: Cardiac Arrhythmias

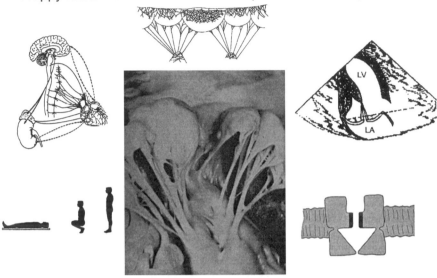

Figure 5. Floppy mitral valve is shown in the middle (used with permission from Edwards JE. Circulation 43:606–612, 1971); above the mitral valve, innervation of the mitral valve is shown schematically; upper right shows papillary muscle tension during ventricular systole; lower right stretch-activated receptor is shown schematically. Left upper part shows schematically interactions between the brain-heart-kidneys and adrenals. Lower left part shows schematically orthostatic phenomena.

Left Atrial Performance: Multidimensional Left Atrial Performance Indices

In contrast to LV emptying, which is monophasic, LA emptying is biphasic. LA emptying from the beginning of the mitral valve opening to the onset of atrial systole is related primarily to LV structure and hemodynamics and less to LA function, while LA emptying from the onset of LA systole to the mitral valve closure is directly related to LA systolic function (Fig. 6).[27]

Evaluation of LA function in most clinical studies evolved from estimation of LA diameter, LA pressure recordings, A-wave velocity with Doppler echocardiography, and measurements of LA volume based on echocardiographic, cineangiocardiographic, and magnetic resonance imaging techniques. LA function, however, is complex and multidimensional. Similar to LV contraction, LA contraction due to atrial myocardial fiber shortening results in a decreased LA volume, a generation of force, and ejection of blood into the left ventricle. Further, the velocity and ac-

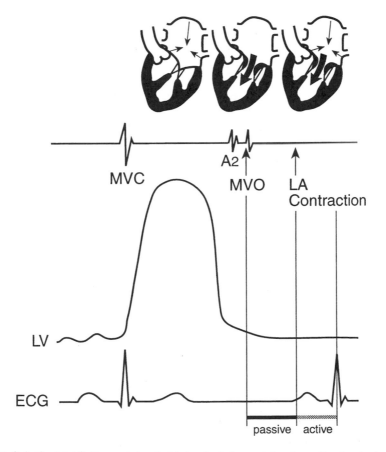

Figure 6. Left atrial (LA) emptying is biphasic. LA emptying from the beginning of mitral valve opening to the onset of atrial contraction is related primarily to left ventricular (LV) structure and dynamics, while LA emptying from the beginning of atrial systole to mitral valve closure is directly related to LA systolic function. MVC = mitral valve closure; MVO = mitral valve opening; A_2 = aortic component of the second heart sound; ECG = electrocardiogram.

celeration of blood ejected into the left ventricle, and the duration of LA contraction may be altered in patients with LA dysfunction.

Comprehensive evaluation of LA function requires analysis of multiple indices of LA performance (Fig. 7). These include LA ejection fraction to estimate the degree of atrial myocardial fiber shortening; LA stroke volume to estimate the amount of blood ejected into the left ventricle; A-wave velocity and A-wave acceleration time to estimate the velocity and acceleration of blood ejected into the left ventricle, and left atrial kinetic energy (LAKE) to estimate LA work. LA dysfunction may result in abnormality(ies) in one or several of the above parameters.[27]

Left Atrial Performance Indices

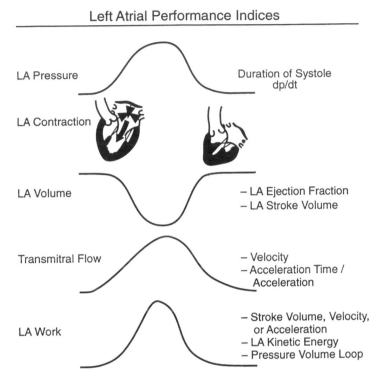

LA Pressure	Duration of Systole dp/dt
LA Contraction	
LA Volume	– LA Ejection Fraction – LA Stroke Volume
Transmitral Flow	– Velocity – Acceleration Time / Acceleration
LA Work	– Stroke Volume, Velocity, or Acceleration – LA Kinetic Energy – Pressure Volume Loop

Figure 7. Left atrial (LA) function is complex and multidimensional (see text for details). (Used with permission from Boudoulas H, et al.[27])

Left Atrial Performance in Chronic Mitral Valvular Regurgitation

During LV systole, part of the LV stroke volume in chronic MVR is ejected into the low-pressure left atrium. The left atrium dilates gradually and accommodates this extra load. Chronic LA dilatation results in an increase in LA compliance with a relatively normal LA pressure despite the large LA volume (Fig. 8).[27] Thus, in chronic MVR, significant LA dilatation and dysfunction may occur. In fact, the left atrium may be affected more than the left ventricle, similar to the way the left ventricle is affected in patients with aortic regurgitation. To better understand the natural history of MVR, the effect of mitral regurgitation on LA structure and function is critical. Thus, LA performance indices in MVR may provide important information defining the optimal timing for surgical intervention in such patients.

Atrial dysfunction in chronic mitral valve disease is related both to the effects of progressive LA hypertension with increased LA volumes and to LA fibrosis. In a study of patients with FMV/MVP and mild to se-

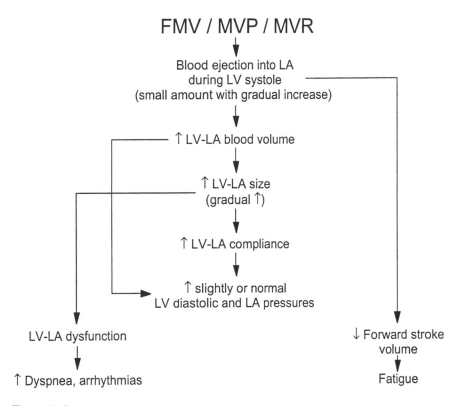

Figure 8. Pathophysiology of chronic mitral valvular regurgitation (MVR). LV = left ventricle; LA = left atrium; ↑= increase; ↓= decrease; FMV = floppy mitral valve; MVP = mitral valve prolapse.

vere MVR, LA maximal volumes ranged from normal to markedly enlarged. The wide range of LA maximal volume was related to the severity of MVR. As the LA maximal volume was increased, the LA stroke volume was also increased. While the LA maximal volume and LA stroke volume were increased, the LA ejection fraction remained relatively unchanged (Fig. 9).[27] In contrast to LA volumes, which were markedly increased, the A-wave velocity and the A-wave acceleration time remained within normal range, the LAKE, an index of LA work, was increased significantly in MVR, compared to normal subjects. Since LAKE is the product of LA stroke volume and A-wave velocity, the increased LAKE in MVR was mostly related to large LA stroke volume (Fig. 10). The increase in LAKE in normal subjects is increased with age while in chronic MVR, LAKE is related to the severity of mitral regurgitation and not to the age (Fig. 11).

Longstanding LA volume overload and increased LA work in chronic

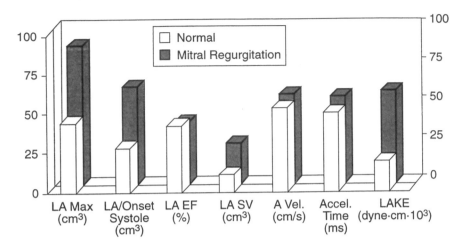

Figure 9. Left atrial maximal volume (LA max), volume at onset of atrial systole, LA ejection fraction (EF), LA stroke volume (SV), A-wave velocity (Vel), A-wave acceleration (Accel) time, and left atrial kinetic energy (LAKE) in mitral valve regurgitation and normal subjects. LA dysfunction may result in abnormality(ies) in one or several of these parameters. Evaluation of LA function, therefore, should be based on multiple indices of LA performance. (Modified with permission from Boudoulas H, et al.[27]).

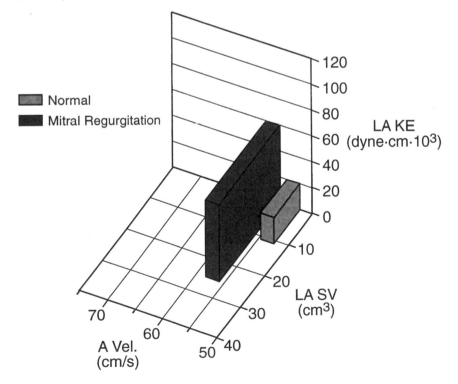

Figure 10. Left atrial kinetic energy (LAKE) was greater in mitral regurgitation compared to normal subjects (p<0.001). A vel = A-wave velocity; LA SV = left atrial stroke volume.

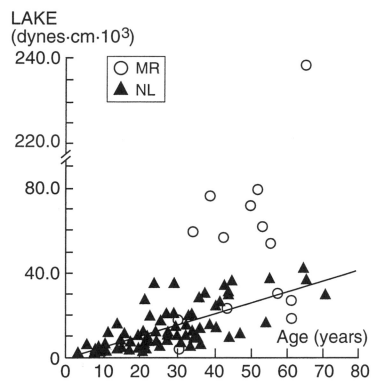

Figure 11. Relationship between left atrial kinetic energy (LAKE) and age in patient with chronic mitral valvular regurgitation (MR) and normal subjects (NL).

MVR results in LA fatigue and failure. Thus, LA status is an important determinant of the natural history in patients with chronic MVR.

Aortic Function

Beyond serving a conduit function, the aorta plays important roles maintaining LV performance, myocardial perfusion, and arterial function throughout the entire cardiovascular system. Stiffening of the aorta may provide resistance to LV ejection and facilitate mitral regurgitation.[28–30] Thus, stiffening of the aorta with aging may play an important role in the deterioration of MVR in patients with FMV/MVP which usually occurs after the age of 50 to 60 years.

The aorta expands during LV systole and recoils during diastole. Under normal conditions, a large proportion of the LV stroke volume is stored in the aorta during LV systole, while during diastole, the stored blood flows into the periphery. This function of the aorta is important for maintaining blood flow and pressure throughout the cardiac cycle.

The ejection of blood from the LV during systole generates pressure and pulse waves that are perceived in peripheral vessels as arterial pressure and arterial pulse, respectively. The pulse wave velocity (PWV), defined as the speed at which the pulse wave travels in the aorta, is directly related to the elastic properties of the aortic wall. A decrease in the elastic properties of the aorta increases the PWV. When the pulse waves reach the periphery, they then return to the ascending aorta as reflected waves. Normally, the reflected waves reach the ascending aorta early in diastole, causing formation of the diastolic wave (Fig. 12). Reflected waves that reach the aortic valve early in diastole facilitate coronary blood flow. When the elastic properties of the aorta are diminished and the PWV increases, the reflected waves from the periphery return earlier into the ascending aorta, fuse with the systolic part of the pulse, with an increase in systolic pressure and disappearance of the diastolic wave. Thus, decreased compliance of the aorta will result in increased aortic systolic pressure, decreased aortic diastolic pressure, and increased pulse pressure.

LV–vascular coupling is an important determinant of LV performance. In patients with LV dysfunction without appropriate adaptation of the vasculature, overall circulatory performance may not improve and in fact may be diminished despite positive inotropic interventions. In addition, stiffening of the aorta may produce impaired relaxation and decreased early diastolic filling, necessitating an increase in LA contribution in order to maintain LV stroke volume. Further, aortic function is an important determinant of myocardial perfusion. Indeed, experimental studies have indicated that decreased aortic distensibility has a detrimental ef-

---

Figure 12. Upper panel. During left ventricular systole, the aorta expands and a large proportion of stroke volume is stored in the aorta. During diastole, aortic pressure is falling, the aorta recoils and the stored blood flows into periphery. The long black arrow shows schematically the velocity of the pulse wave. When the pulse wave reaches the periphery, it returns back to the ascending aorta. Normally, the reflected waves reach the ascending aorta early in diastole; this results in the formation of the diastolic wave (DW). Lower panel. The storage capacity of the aorta is related to its elastic properties; large proportion of storage capacity is lost in disease states and in elderly individuals. The reflected waves (helicoid arrows) are also shown. When the elastic properties of the aorta are diminished and the pulse wave velocity increases, the reflected waves from the periphery return earlier into the ascending aorta, fuse with the systolic part of the pulse, and result in an increase in pulse pressure, a late systolic peak in the pulse, and the disappearance of the DW. Note that the velocity of reflected waves in the stiff aorta is faster (lower panel). The shapes of the arterial pulse in elastic (upper panel) and stiff aorta (lower panel) are also shown. (Used with permission from Boudoulas H, et al.[28]).

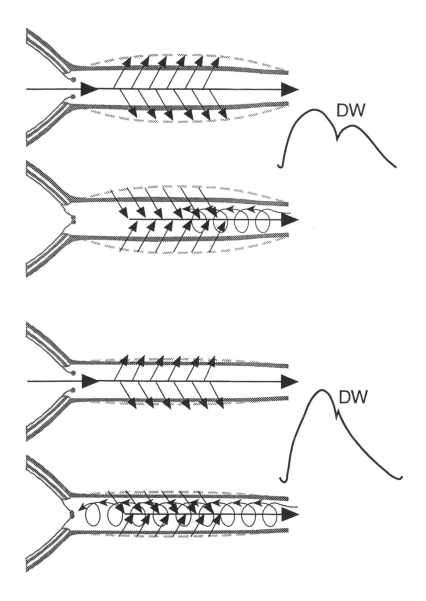

fect on the dynamics of coronary flow and has an aggravating effect on myocardial ischemia in the presence of coronary artery stenosis.[28]

Decreased aortic distensibility may precipitate LV dilatation and dysfunction in patients with chronic aortic or mitral valvular regurgitation. Patients with aortic regurgitation who require valve replacement have lower aortic distensibility when compared with patients who do not require valve replacement.

Effect of Age on Aortic Function and Mitral Valvular Regurgitation

Aortic stiffening and LAKE increase with age, even in normal subjects at a time when parameters related to LV structure and systolic function are relatively unaffected. Several factors may contribute to stiffening of the aorta with age. Any change of structure of the arterial wall may result in abnormal aortic function. In experimental animals, changes of the arterial wall structure during the progression and regression of atherosclerosis paralleled indices of aortic elastic properties. Similar findings have been reported during the development and treatment of arterial hypertension.[29]

Abnormal aortic function, however, may be present in cases where structural abnormalities of the aortic wall cannot be precisely defined with contemporary technology. For example, acute changes of blood supply to the aortic wall due to a decrease in vasa vasorum flow may result in aortic dysfunction. Endothelium-derived relaxant factor (nitric oxide), endothelin, atrial natriuretic peptides, catecholamines, and prostaglandins may alter the elastic properties of the aorta directly through their effects on smooth muscle of the aortic wall and indirectly by their effects on vasa vasorum flow. In addition, the autonomic nervous system may play a significant role in the determination of aortic wall function through a direct effect on smooth muscle, vasa vasorum flow, or neurohormonal activation. All of these factors mentioned, to a certain degree, alter with age. In addition, collagen content of the aortic wall may increase while elastin content may decrease with age. Further, studies have suggested that vasa vasorum flow is decreased with age.[29]

Recent data from our laboratory suggested that patients with FMV/MVP have abnormal aortic distensibility.[30] Decreased aortic distensibility may provide resistance to LV ejection, which will increase the degree of MVR. The decrease in aortic distensibility with age may provide a partial explanation as to why MVR in patients with MVP/FMV is accentuated after the age of 50 to 60 years. Whether pharmacological agents that improve the elastic properties of the aorta will slow the progression of mitral valvular regurgitation in patients with MVP/FMV remains to be determined.

Conclusions

The pathophysiological consequences of mitral valve apparatus function and dysfunction in FMV/MVP are incompletely understood at present. Certainly, prolapsing mitral valve leaflet(s) resulting in occupation of LA space, increased papillary muscle traction, activation of stretch receptors, and development of a third chamber or neutral space between the mitral annulus and the prolapsing mitral valve leaflet contribute significantly to the clinical picture of FMV/MVP and FMV/MVP syndrome while influencing the natural history of the disease. Future research will help to better define the incompletely understood complex phenomena related to function or dysfunction of the FMV complex.

LA function is an important determinant of the natural history in patients with chronic MVR. LA dilatation and dysfunction often occur prior to LV structural and functional changes. Monitoring of LA performance indexes therefore provides important information for the understanding of the natural history of the disease.

Aortic function is an important determinant of LV performance and myocardial perfusion. Elastic properties of the aorta decrease with age. In addition, patients with FMV/MVP/MVR have decreased aortic distensibility compared to normal subjects. Stiffening of the aorta may increase the degree of MVR and precipitate the natural history in patients with FMV/MVP. Determination of the elastic properties of the aorta in clinical practice may help us to better understand and define the natural history of the disease with the potential for new forms of therapeutic intervention.

Thus, prolapsing FMV into the left atrium results in the development of a third chamber and decreased cardiac output, papillary muscle traction, and stretch receptor stimulation, which may result in myocardial ischemia and cardiac arrhythmias, stimulation of the mitral valve apparatus nerve endings, and interaction of mitral valve innervation with the central nervous system. Further, alterations in papillary muscle traction may lead to LV contraction and relaxation abnormalities, while FMV/MVP/MVR may lead to LA dilatation and dysfunction. Moreover, elastic properties of the aorta may be abnormal in patients with FMV/MVP. Thus, FMV/MVP/MVR has a global effect on the cardiovascular system.

References

1. Boudoulas H, Kolibash AJ, Baker P, King BD, Wooley DF. Mitral valve prolapse and the mitral valve prolapse syndrome: A diagnostic classification and pathogenesis of symptoms. Am Heart J 118:796–818, 1989.
2. Wooley CF, Baker PB, Kolibash AJ, Kioman JW, Sparks EA, Boudoulas H. The floppy myxomatous mitral valve, mitral valve prolapse and mitral regurgitation. Prog Cardiovasc Dis 33:397–433, 1991

3. Wooley CF, Sparks EA, Boudoulas H. The floppy mitral valve-mitral valve prolapse-mitral valvular regurgitation triad. ACC Current J Rev July/August 1994, pp 25–26.
4. Barlow JB, Pocock WA. Mitral leaflet billowing and prolapse. In Barlow JB (ed): Perspectives on the Mitral Valve. Philadelphia, FA Davis Company, 1987, pp 45–112.
5. Boudoulas H, Wooley CF. Mitral valve prolapse and the mitral valve prolpase syndrome. In Yu PN, Goodwin JF (eds): Progress in Cardiovasc Dis 14:275–309, 1986.
6. Wooley CF, Boudoulas H. Mitral valve prolapse. In Raken RE (ed): Con's Current Therapy. Philadelphia, W.B. Saunders Co., 1999, pp 289–293.
7. Boudoulas H. Valvular Disease: American College of Cardiology Self-Assessment Program (ACCSAP) 2000, in press.
8. Boudoulas H, Kolibash AJ, Wooley CF. Mitral valve prolapse: A heterogeneous disorder. Primary Cardiol 17:29–43, 1991.
9. Fontana ME, Wooley CF, Leighton RF, et al. Postural changes in left ventricular and mitral valvular dynamics in the systolic click- late systolic murmur syndrome. Circulation 51:165–173, 1975.
10. Sanfilippo AJ, Harrigan P, Popvic AD, et al. Papillary muscle tension in mitral valve prolapse: Quantitation by two-dimensional echocardiography. J Am Coll Cardiol 19:564–571, 1992.
11. Franz MR, Cima R, Wang D, Proffit D, Kuntz R. Electorphysiological effects of myocardial stretch and mechanical determinants of stretch-activated arrhythmias. Circulation 86:968–978, 1992.
12. Boudoulas H, Schaal SF, Wooley CF. Floppy mitral valve/mitral valve prolapse: Cardiac arrhythmias. In Vardas PE (ed): Cardiac Arrhythmias, Pacing, and Electrophysiology. Great Britain, Kluwer Academic Publisher, 1998, pp 89–95.
13. Tavi P, Han C, Weckstrom M. Mechanisms of stretch-induced changes in Ca^{2+} in rat atrial myocytes. Role of increase troponin C affinity and stretch-activated ion channels. Circulation Res 83:1165–1177, 1998.
14. Bashore TM, Grines C, Utlak D, Boudoulas H, Wooley CF. Postural exercise abnormalities in symptomatic patients with mitral valve prolapse. J Am coll Cardiol 11:499–507, 1988.
15. Scampardonis G, Yang SS, Maranhao V, Golberg H, Gooch A. Left ventricular abnormalities in prolapsed mitral leaflet syndrome. Circulation 48:287–297, 1973.
16. Cobbs WB Jr, King SB. Ventricular buckling: A factor in the abnormal ventriculogram and peculiar hemodynamics associated with mitral valve prolapse. Am Heart J 93:741–758, 1977
17. Colle JP, LeGoff G, Ohayon J, Bonnett J, Bricaud H, Besse P. Quantitative frame by frame analysis of regional contraction and lengthening on left ventricular cineangiograms: Application to the study of normal left ventricles and left ventricles with mitral valve prolapse. Clin Cardiol 9:43–51, 1986.
18. Liedtke JA, Gault JH, Leaman DM, Blumenthal MS. Geometry of left ventricular contraction in the systolic click syndrome. Circulation 48:27–35, 1973.
19. Grossman H, Fleming RJ, Engle MA, Levin AH, Ehlers KH. Left ventricular abnormality, mitral insufficiency, late systolic murmur, and inversion of T waves. In Grossman H, et al (eds): Angiocardiography in the Apical Systolic Click Syndrome. Radiology 91:898–904, 1968.
20. Reece IJ, Cooley DA, Painvin GA, Okereke OUJ, Powers PL, Pechacek LW, Fra-

zier OH. Surgical treatment of mitral systolic click syndrome: Results in 37 patients. Ann Thoracic Surg 29:155–158, 1985.

21. Mathey DG, Decoodt PR, Allen HN, Swan HJ. Abnormal left ventricular contraction pattern in the systolic click-late systolic murmur syndrome. Circulation 56:311–315, 1977.

22. Pastenac A, Abbou B, Gervais AR. Abnormalities of left ventricular contraction in the mitral valve prolapse syndrome. Arch Mal Coeur Vaiss 72:248–257, 1979.

23. Delhomme C, Casset-Senon D, Babuty D, Charniot JC, Fauchier L, Fauchier JP, Philippe L, Cosnay P. A study of 36 cases of mitral valve prolapse by isotopic ventricular tomography. Arch Mal Coeur Vaiss 89:1127–1135, 1996.

24. Tebbe U, Schicha H, Neumann P, Voth E, Emrich D, Neuhaus KL, Kreuzer H. Mitral valve prolapse in the ventriculogram: Scintigraphic, electrocardiographic, and hemodynamic abnormalities. Clin Cardiol 8:341–347, 1985.

25. Corrao S, Scaglione R, Arnone S, Licata G. Left ventricular diastolic filling alterations in subjects with mitral valve prolapse: A Doppler echocardiographic study. Eur Heart J 14:369–372, 1993.

26. Marron K, Yacoub MH, Plak JM, et al. Innervation of human atrioventricular and arterial valves. Circulation 94:368–375, 1996.

27. Boudoulas H, Boudoulas D, Sparks EA, Pearson AC, Nagaraja HN, Wooley CF. Left atrial performance indices in chronic mitral valve disease. J Heart Valve Dis 4 (Suppl 2):S242–247, 1995.

28. Boudoulas H, Toutouzas PK, Wooley CF (eds). Functional Abnormalities of the Aorta. Armonk, NY, Futura Publishing Company, Inc., 1996.

29. Breithaupt-Grogler K, Ling M, Boudoulas H, Belz GG. Protective effect of chronic garlic intake on elastic properties of the aorta in the elderly. Circulation 96:2649–2655, 1997.

30. Malkowski MT, Boudoulas H, Wooley CF, Guo R, Pearson AC. Abnormal elastic properties of the aorta in mitral valve prolapse. Circulation 92(Suppl I):357, 1995.

Part XIV

Floppy Mitral Valve, Mitral Valve Prolapse, Mitral Valvular Regurgitation:

The Japanese Experience

Introduction

The Floppy Mitral Valve, Mitral Valve Prolapse, Mitral Valvular Regurgitation:
The View from Japan

Charles F. Wooley, MD,
Harisios Boudoulas, MD, PhD

The intensity, energetics, and excellence of the Japanese cardiovascular investigators must be experienced first hand to be fully comprehended. The editors had the benefit of personal visits with Dr. Sakamoto (Fig. 1)

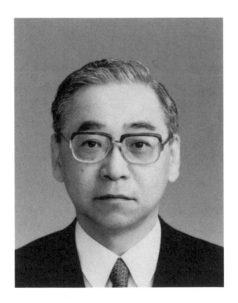

Figure 1. Dr. Tsuguya Sakamoto.

From: Boudoulas H, Wooley CF. *Mitral Valve: Floppy Mitral Valve, Mitral Valve Prolapse, Mitral Valve Regurgitation.* Second revised edition. ©Futura Publishing Company, Armonk, NY, 2000.

and his Japanese colleagues, participating in dynamic and collegial conferences in Japan, and can attest to these qualities.

The series of Conferences on Mitral Valve Prolapse and on Valve and Valvular Diseases referenced in the following chapter began in 1986, continued into the 1990s, and were published in the *Journal of Cardiology*. These conferences and proceedings represent the comprehensive nature of the work by Japanese cardiologists integrating their work with global developments. Guests from around the world were invited to participate in these individual conferences, and contributed to the exchanges about the clinical entities.

Dr. Tsuguya Sakamoto provides us with the essence of these carefully performed, imaginative studies published in the *Journal of Cardiology* of the Japanese College of Cardiology. He shares the wealth of the Japanese experience with us along with his personal and perceptive insights into the floppy mitral valve/mitral valve prolapse/mitral valvular regurgitation triad as seen and investigated in Japan.

22

Mitral Valve Prolapse:

Contributions of Japanese Investigators *

Tsuguya Sakamoto, MD

Introduction

As in the occidental countries, mitral valve prolapse (MVP) has been extensively debated in our country for more than 20 years. This chapter is a short summary of clinical as well as experimental work done in Japan. Particular emphasis is placed on describing pioneering work, opinions that are partially or totally different from the occidental contributions, and our activity in the study of this puzzling entity.

Historical Background

A phonocardiographic study of the mid-systolic click in Japan was first done by Hinohara in 1941 and published in the *American Heart Journal*.[1] As in the earlier reports, he did not mention the connection of this auscultatory sign with MVP, and there was confusion about distinguishing it from the ejection and other systolic sounds. After World War II,

* Supported in part by a Grant-in-Aid for Scientific Research from the Ministry of Education, Science, and Culture of Japan (#58480235) and a Grant-in-Aid for the mitral valve prolapse project from the Ministry of Health and Welfare of Japan.
From: Boudoulas H, Wooley CF. *Mitral Valve: Floppy Mitral Valve, Mitral Valve Prolapse, Mitral Valvular Regurgitation*. Second revised edition. ©Futura Publishing Company, Armonk, NY, 2000.

phonocardiographic research in Japan rapidly developed. Yamakawa, an inventor of intracardiac phonocardiography (1953), described in his book[2] the phonocardiographic features of mid-systolic click. Among the Japanese textbooks on auscultation and phonocardiography, we[3] first devoted one chapter (of 12 pages) to describing various facets of mid- and late systolic clicks including the effects of respiration and posture and the evanescent characteristics of the clicks. However, the theory of innocent or extracardiac origin advocated by several authorities heavily influenced our description.

In 1966, when the Third Meeting of Laennec Society met in New York, NY, to celebrate the 150th anniversary of the invention of the stethoscope, we presented the pharmacodynamic phonocardiography to emphasize the capability of this test to provoke many silent states, including valvular regurgitation.[4] The provocation of late systolic murmur in cases of mid-systolic click and also in many cases of hyperthyroidism was documented.[5] It was particularly the methoxamine-induced late or pansystolic murmur in cases with mid-systolic click that led to suspicion of the intracardiac origin of this sound, and we had a great interest in the works published by the South African group[6–8] and others.[9–12]

Following the establishment of the Japanese Society of Cardiovascular Sound, 1970, several reports of mid-systolic click or late systolic murmur were published, including a surgical report describing an abnormal valve movement in systole during surgery. In 1974, 161 consecutive cases from 5,963 phonocardiographic records (2.7%) were retrospectively reported from our laboratory, including 70 cases of apical mid-systolic click, 53 cases of late systolic apical murmur with or without mid-systolic click, 26 cases of basal mid-systolic click and/or late systolic murmur, and 12 cases of provoked apical systolic click and/or late systolic murmur.[13] By analyzing these cases, results were ascertained as in the previous reports, except for the important difference in pharmacodynamic phonocardiography. A two-dimensional echocardiogram was illustrated to show the late systolic prolapse of the anterior leaflet into the left atrium, and this is probably the first report in the world of a two-dimensional echocardiogram showing MVP. The next year Tanaka et al.[14] reported the detailed M-mode and two-dimensional echocardiographic findings in seven cases with MVP, including nearly all of the features reported by the succeeding investigators.

Though we had a session about MVP at the VIII World Congress of Cardiology (Tokyo, 1978), which Dr. J.B. Barlow and I presided over, the first symposium of Japanese doctors was held the next year and 12 presentations were discussed extensively.[15] In 1981, controversies in diagnosing MVP by echocardiography and angiography were debated in a panel and several new criteria were proposed.[16] These criteria were discussed at a symposium on valvular heart disease.[17] In 1985, mitral valve prolapse was a theme of a fireside conference of the Japanese Circulation Society,[18] and from that year on, a 2-day conference on MVP was to be an annual meeting, inviting outstanding authorities as guests (Table 1).

Finally, in 1986 the Department of Health and Welfare in Japan organized the National Study Group on MVP syndrome, and the first meeting was held in Osaka in October 1986. The Conference on "Mitral Valve Prolapse" sponsored by the Japanese College of Cardiology lasted 5 years and developed into the Conference on "Valve and Valvular Diseases" in 1990,

---

Table 1

Guest Speakers and Titles of their Presentations at the Conferences on Mitral Valve Prolapse (1986–1990) and Valve and Valvular Diseases (1991–present)

1986   Harisios Boudoulas (The Ohio State University, Columbus, OH)
Mitral Valve Prolapse Syndrome: Evidence of Autonomic Dysfunction

1987   Robert M. Jeresaty (University of Connecticut School of Medicine, Hartford, CT)
Mitral Valve Prolapse: An Overview

1988   Tsung O. Cheng (The George Washington University School of Medicine, Washington DC)
Mitral Valve Prolapse: An Overview

1989   Pravin M. Shah (Loma Linda University Medical Center, Loma Linda, CA)
Mitral Valve Prolapse vs. Mitral Valve Prolapse Syndrome: What is the Difference?

1990   John B. Barlow (University of the Witwatersrand, Johannesburg, South Africa)
Aspects of Mitral and Tricuspid Regurgitation

1991   F. I. Caird (Southern General Hospital, Glasgow, U.K.)
Valvular Disease of the Heart in the Elderly

1992   John Michael Criley (UCLA School of Medicine, Torrance, CA)
Valve Function During Cough Cardiopulmonary Resuscitation (Cough-CPR)

1993   Robert A. Levine (Massachusetts General Hospital, Boston, MA)
1) Mitral Valve Prolapse: Clinical Impact of New Diagnostic Criteria and Insight from Three-Dimensional Echocardiography
2) Unifying Concepts of Mitral Valve Function and Disease: SAM, Prolapse and Ischemic Mitral Regurgitation

1994   Morris N. Kotler (Temple University School of Medicine, Philadelphia, PA)
Mitral Regurgitation: A New Look at an Old Entity

1995   Ryozo Okada (Juntendo University School of medicine, Tokyo)
Clinicopathological Analysis of Rheumatic Heart Disease

1996   Kohei Kawazoe (Iwate Medical University School of Medicine, Morioka)
Adherence to Valve Repair Surgery: From the Mitral to Aortic Valve

1997   Yashuharu Nimura (National Cardiovascular Center, Osaka)
Echocardiographic Information of the Cardiac Valves

Table 2
Activities of Japanese Investigators in Research on
Mitral Valve Prolapse

1941	Phonocardiographic report
1956	Description of phonocardiographic features
1963	Overview of midsystolic click and late systolic murmur
1966	Provocation of midsystolic click and late systolic murmur
1974	Clinical study of 161 cases with mitral vavle prolapse
1975	Diagnostic criteria with two-dimensional echocardiography
1978	Session on mitral valve prolapse (VIII World Congress of Cardiology, Tokyo)
1979	Symposium on mitral valve prolapse (Japanese Society of Cardio-vascular Sound)
1981	Panel discussion: Controversies about diagnostic criteria (ibid.)
1981	Symposium on valvular heart disease (Japanese Circulation Society)
1985	Fireside conference (ibid.)
1985	Conference on mitral valve prolapse (annual meeting)
1986	Grant-in-aid for the study of mitral valve prolapse from the Ministry of Health and Welfare in Japan
1991	Conference on Valve and Valvular Diseases (annual meeting)

dealing with a wider spectrum of the valve problem. The proceedings have been published yearly as a supplement issue of *Journal of Cardiology*. The above-mentioned history is summarized in Table 2.

Individual Studies

Auscultation and Phonocardiography (Including Mechanocardiography)

As it has been emphasized, "the essential aim of auscultation is to clinch the diagnosis."[19] In cases of mitral valve prolapse, the key auscultatory signs should be phonocardiographically proved;[20] otherwise a tiny click is often overlooked and the exact timing of the murmur is apt to be misjudged.

Phonocardiographic Screening

In the Kita ward of Tokyo, phonocardiographic screening for cardiac disease was started in 1976. School children in the fourth grade of elementary school (9 year olds) and school boys and girls in the second grade of middle school (13 year olds) were examined phonocardiographically by well-trained technicians. All cases with abnormal records were reinvestigated by both auscultation and phonocardiography, and then at the non-invasive laboratory of the University of Tokyo. This was a good source for our study of mitral valve prolapse[21-24] (Fig. 1).

The prevalence of the mid-systolic (rarely early systolic) click in these age groups was nearly 1%, and it was higher in females than in males

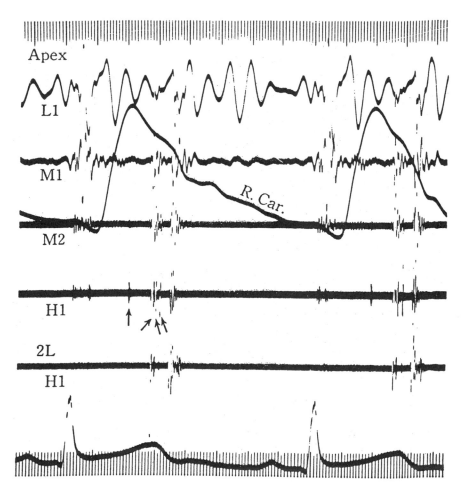

Figure 1. Phonocardiogram in an elementary schoolboy with mid-systolic click and mitral valve prolapse. Mid-systolic click is multiple (arrows). This case had mid-systolic buckling of the mitral valve echo and the two-dimensional echocardiogram showed the prolapse of the anterior mitral leaflet. Methoxamine provoked late systolic murmur, but the boy had no complaints and no abnormality except auscultatory signs. Apex = apical phonocardiograms; 2L = second left intercostal space along the sternal margin. L1, M1, M2 and H1 indicate filters used (almost flat, 100 Hz/12 dB, 200/24, and 400/24, respectively). Paper speed: 100 mm/sec. Time lines: 0.01 and 0.1 sec.

Table 3
Prevalence of Phonocardiographic Signs of Mitral Valve Prolapse in School Children in Kita Ward, Tokyo (1975–1986)

Elementary School (4th grade: 9 year olds)		Middle School (2nd grade: 13 year olds)		Total
Males	Females	Males	Females	
183/33,863	309/31,460	290/26,967	405/25,503	1,187/117,793
(0.540%)	(0.982%)	(1.075%)	(1.588%)	(1.008%)
492/65,323		695/52,470		
(0.753%)		(1.325%)		

Prevalence in males: 0.778%; in females: 1.253%.
Denominator means cases examined by using phonocardiography and auscultation, and numerator means cases with mid-systolic click with or without late systolic murmur or whoops. From 1979 about one-half of middle school students were being rechecked because they had the same examination in elementary school.

(Table 3). Middle school pupils showed definitely higher prevalence than elementary school children, and this tendency has recently been verified by the screening of high school students (in whom the incidence was approximately 2%). Thus, the auscultatory signs of MVP increased in frequency with age even within the first and second decades. This study disclosed, however, that the late systolic murmur or occasionally pansystolic murmur related to MVP was seldom observed in elementary school children and it developed only occasionally in middle school pupils[24] and more frequently in high school students. In addition to the previous report,[13] these prospective studies indicated a sizable number of cases with MVP in our country, contrary to a report suggesting the rarity of this anomaly in the Orient.[25]

Problem of Silent Mitral Valve Prolapse

Since a mid-systolic click or sometimes a late systolic murmur is evanescent in some cases, silent prolapse, in which the auscultatory signs are absent, may be present in any study population. The daily practice of using pharmacodynamic phonocardiography revealed such cases in as high as 12% of cases of MVP[13] in a clinical context.

Pharmacodynamic Studies

Phonocardiography using vasoactive drugs was extensively performed in our laboratory. The effects of amyl nitrite and methoxamine (or phenylephrine) were of particular interest (Fig. 2). In our earlier study,[13] methoxamine provoked a late systolic murmur in 6 of 29 cases with mid-systolic click, definitely intensified a late systolic murmur in 17 of 20 cases, and provoked a new systolic click in 5 of the latter. In 12 cases without systolic click or late systolic murmur, the former developed in 3 and the latter in 11. In cases with basal late systolic murmur along the lower left sternal border, the murmur was also intensified occasionally (2 of 9 cases). On the other hand, amyl nitrite had a reverse effect with rare exceptional cases in which a late systolic murmur was provoked in cases with mid-systolic click (2 of 40 cases) or in a case of a normal phonocardiogram (1 of 8 cases).

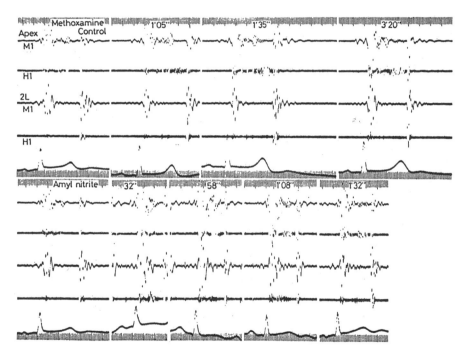

Figure 2. Pharmacodynamic phonocardiography using methoxamine and amyl nitrite in a middle school girl with early to mid-systolic clicks and mitral valve prolapse. **Top:** Following injection of methoxamine (0.08 mg/kg/25 sec), a late systolic crescendo-decrescendo high-pitched murmur was newly developed and lasted several minutes. The systolic clicks did not move toward the second heart sound, probably because of development of significant mitral regurgitation. A reversed splitting of the second heart sound is seen at the timing of 1′35″. **Bottom:** Amyl nitrite inhalation in this case also caused a late systolic murmur, and it lasted about 3 minutes. It is rather exceptional to observe similar changes caused by amyl nitrite. An ejection systolic murmur developed at the base (second intercostal space 2L), but it differs in timing and time course from the apical systolic murmur.

These results combined with those obtained by echocardiographic observation are not compatible with the concept that decreased left ventricular volume has a primary importance in the occurrence of prolapse. Ventricular pressure pulse and the level of the ventricular pressure reached are probably much more important to the changes in the auscultatory signs, as evidenced by the echocardiographic studies discussed below.

An increase of the systolic murmur after inhalation of amyl nitrite may be due to the transmission of a basal ejection systolic murmur, which is extremely common during this procedure. We always use a multifilter system and record two to three areas simultaneously to avoid such an erroneous interpretation.

An Atypical Apical Systolic Murmur

A phonocardiographic study using vasoactive drugs combined with M-mode and two-dimensional echocardiography with the Doppler method revealed that in approximately one-half of the cases, an apical systolic murmur during early or mid-systole actually denotes mitral regurgitation related to MVP. Although such cases are not common, it seemed important to recognize the presence of MVP not having a late systolic or pansystolic regurgitation murmur.[26]

Thyrotoxicosis and Mitral Valve Prolapse

The frequent occurrence of a late systolic crescendo murmur following methoxamine injection in hyperthyroidism was reported earlier.[4] A cumulative study disclosed that a mitral regurgitant murmur, mainly late systolic in timing and occasionally accompanied by a faint early to mid-systolic murmur, was provoked in 19 of 52 cases examined. This prevalence was definitely higher than that in normal subjects; a simultaneously recorded echocardiogram disclosed a concomitant MVP in 3 of 8 cases examined.[27]

Mid-Systolic Click and the Apex Cardiogram

In MVP the mid-systolic click may accompany a mid-systolic notch or cleft in the apex cardiogram. The coincidence in their timing has been interpreted as meaning that they are derived from the same physiological phenomenon. However, there are exceptions.[28] In cases with echocardiographically proven MVP and a mobile click, the apex cardiogram recorded during held expiration did not change shape significantly while the click was moving. This resulted in a discordant time relation between the two signs: the notch or cleft in the apex cardiogram and the mid-systolic click in the phonocardiogram. Usually, the notch or cleft did not change in timing, so that we have to be very careful when considering their relationship (Fig. 3).

Mid-systolic click has been regarded as an important auscultatory and phonocardiographic sign in MVP, but we do not know the exact relationship to the echocardiogram. Correlative study with phonocardiography and two-dimensional echocardiography showed that click(s) appeared in only 30% of cases and that there was a tendency to have a louder click in cases with echocardiographically distinct prolapse.[29]

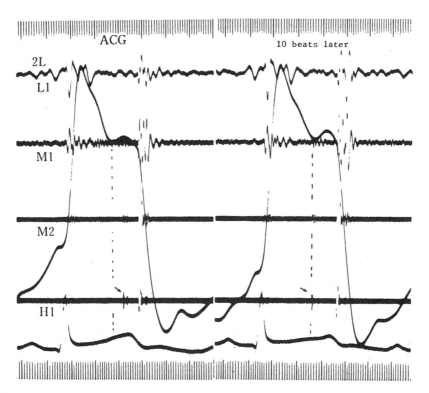

Figure 3. Phonocardiograms and apex cardiograms in a case with mitral valve prolapse showing a discrepant timing of mid-systolic click and the notch in the apex cardiogram. This is the same case shown in Figure 1, but the tracings were taken separately. The two tracings shown in this figure were taken from the continuous tracing and 10 beats apart. The configuration of the apex cardiograms was essentially the same and the timing of the mid-systolic notch remains constant. However, the mid-to late systolic click is mobile (a sliding click), and the time coincidence between the two phenomena was lost frequently.

Systolic Time Intervals

Left ventricular function, as assessed by systolic time intervals and other methods in cases with MVP, may be impaired,[20,30] but our data suggested that there were no abnormal values in the systolic time intervals. The only exception was the secondary prolapse caused by Marfan's syndrome, although in those cases exercise tolerance was not impaired.[31]

Echocardiography

Echocardiographic study of MVP started relatively early in Japan, and the controversies concerning the diagnostic criteria are reviewed every year as mentioned above.

Diagnostic Criteria

Several diagnostic criteria were proposed in our country.[14,32–35] The most important echocardiographic sign of MVP was regarded as the mid- to late systolic buckling of the mitral valve echo on the M-mode echocardiogram. Pansystolic bowing (or hammocking) had been criticized from the start, and the angle of the ultrasonic beam induced by a malpositioned transducer in the upper sternal border was recognized as early as 1975,[36] well before the report of Markiewicz et al.[37] This is likely to occur in subjects with a thin chest and straight back.

As for two-dimensional echocardiography, the worldwide criterion of Gilbert et al.[38] has also been adopted by many Japanese investigators. However, it has a shortcoming in overlooking mild prolapse and thus was modified by Yoshikawa et al.[39,40] They proved the presence of an immobile portion at the base of the anterior mitral leaflet, and proposed a new line of the mitral valve ring in the parasternal long-axis view of the left heart that avoids the immobile portion as shown in Figure 4. Mild prolapse was thus diagnosed echocardiographically.

A rather unique approach to the echocardiographic diagnosis of MVP was proposed by Nagata et al.[33,34] They ignored the setting of the mitral valve ring and defined prolapse by the systolic dislocation of the coaptation zone of the mitral leaflets (Fig. 5). They were able to diagnose echocardiographically even the mildest case with no valve overshooting beyond the mitral valve ring and to correlate these cases with the data from invasive and other noninvasive investigations.

Prevalence of Mitral Valve Prolapse

The prevalence of MVP shown by two-dimensional echocardiography varies. In Japan also, we have two extremes.[41,42] Both reports dealt with

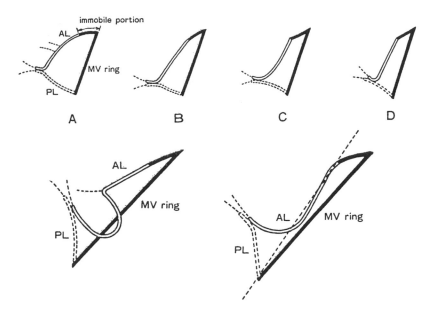

Figure 4. Diagrams showing normal and pathological mitral echo patterns. **Top:** Diagrams showing various normal mitral valve echo patterns. The anterior leaflet is convex to the left ventricle (A), straight (B), slightly concave (C), and the coaptation point of the anterior leaflet deviated toward the mitral valve ring, (D). D is often observed in subjects with a straight back. Note the immobile portion of the anterior leaflet. Whenever the line of the valve ring is depicted, we have to omit this portion to prevent the underestimation of prolapse. AL = anterior leaflet; PL = posterior leaflet; MV ring = mitral valve ring. **Bottom:** Correction of Gilbert's criterion. When the prolapse is marked (left figure), mitral valve ring depicted according to Gilbert et al. does not overlook prolapse, but it may be missed in cases of mild prolapse as shown in the figure at right. When the immobile portion is ignored, it is possible to diagnose prolapse (straight broken line). (From Yoshikawa et al.,[39] used with permission.)

university students, but the prevalence was 11% in one (29 of 265 students)[41] and only 0.92% in the other (42 of 4,517 students).[42] In addition, the striking difference between these reports was that almost all cases (28 of 29) had no phonocardiographic abnormality in the former report,[41] whereas in the latter many cases of prolapse had phonocardiographic abnormalities (systolic murmur: 76%, systolic click: 33%). It is evident that, even though the age and sex are nearly matched, something unknown is different between these two studies. Later on, well-performed two-dimensional echocardiographic studies in 2,016 apparently healthy university freshmen (18–20 year-olds) disclosed grade I prolapse (slight slip of tip of the anterior leaflet) in 17%, grade II (considerable discrepancy keeping a normal convex shape in the body of the anterior leaflet) in 7%, and grade III (sig-

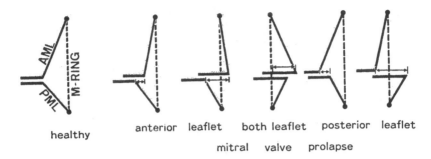

healthy

anterior leaflet both leaflet posterior leaflet

mitral valve prolapse

Figure 5. Diagrams showing a new approach to the diagnosis of mitral valve prolapse using systolic dislocation of the coaptation zone of the mitral leaflets. Irrespective of the setting of the mitral valve ring, prolapse is defined by the dislocated coaptation zone, and thus even prolapse of the mildest degree is easily diagnosed. (From Nagata et al.,[33] used with permission.)

moid configuration of the displaced anterior leaflet) in 1.7%.[43] We are performing a similar study at the University of Tokyo, and the result in 1989 was the same (1.7%: 56 out of 3,379 students; males 1.5%, females 2.7%). Interestingly enough, this percentage raised 14.6% if the subjects were confined to 383 pupils with cardiovascular complaints or some abnormalities compatible with MVP syndrome. However, our impression is that the percentage largely depends on the echocardiographic interpretation, and university students are no longer representative of their contemporaries.

Pharmacodynamic Studies

As previously mentioned, pharmacodynamic tests using vasoactive drugs were performed concomitantly with phonocardiographic studies.[44] Contrary to the widely accepted results, amyl nitrite gave a decrease of murmur, and an increased murmur or provoked murmur in cases with systolic click was not a rule (only 14 out of 91 tested). However, the murmur of prolapse was often provoked in cases of echocardiographically proved silent prolapse by amyl nitrite inhalation (7 out of 8 cases) (Table 4). On the other hand, methoxamine provoked the same murmur in 9 of 21, and in all 14 cases, the regurgitant murmur was intensified by methoxamine. A simultaneous observation of the echocardiograms disclosed an increased prolapse in 8 of 15 cases tested, an unchanged or increased prolapse in 5, and a slightly decreased prolapse in 2 (Table 5). The intensity of an apical regurgitant murmur is not necessarily related to the severity of prolapse; the above-mentioned results may indicate that the arterial pressure level is more important than ventricular volume in permitting the leaflet to billow into the left atrium.[45,46]

Table 4
Results of Pharmacodynamic Phonocardiography in Cases with
Echocardiographically Proved Mitral Valve Prolapse

PCG Finding Before Test	Regurgitant Systolic Murmur	Amyl Nitrite	Methoxamine
Mid-systolic click	Provoked Not provoked	14 77 }/92	9 12 }/21
Regurgitant systolic murmur	Intensified Decreased or unchanged	5 20 }/25	14 0 }/14
No signs (silent prolapse)	Provoked Not provoked	7 1 }/8	2 0 }/2

PCG = phonocardiographic; Provoked = the murmur of mitral valve prolapse was provoked by a drug (late systolic or, occasionally, pansystolic murmur of pansystolic murmur with late systolic accentuation).

It was said that an increase of the systolic murmur after inhalation of amyl nitrite has been attributed to a more marked prolapse due to the diminished left ventricular volume, leading aggravated mitral regurgitation. Doppler study denied this assumption, because the intensified systolic murmur by amyl nitrite was not associated with newly developed

Table 5
Effects of Methoxamine on Echocardiographic and Phonocardiographic
Signs of Mitral Valve Prolapse (Simultaneous Observations)

Degree of MVP on Echocardiogram	Phonocardiographic Changes	Number of Cases Observed
Increased	LSM: intensified	3
Increased	PSM: intensified	3
Increased	MSM: changed to PSM	1
Increased	SC only	1
Increased or unchanged	LSM: intensified	1
Increased or unchanged	SC: SC with LSM	2
Increased or unchanged	SC: changed to LSM	1
Unchanged	LSM: intensified	1
Decreased	LSM: intensified	1
Decreased	SC only	1
		15

LSM = late systolic murmur; PSM = pansystolic murmur; MSM = mid-systolic murmur; SC = mid-systolic click.

regurgitant signals during and after the test.[47] Because of some difficulties to obtain echocardiograms of good quality, we tried the same maneuver in 23 patients with MVP by using transesophageal echocardiography, by which a stable image was obtained during the acute course of amyl nitrite inhalation.[48] Left ventricular end-diastolic dimension decreased significantly (40 ± 6→37 ± 5 mm) according to the increased heart rate (84 ± 20→104 ± 25 beats/min). Prolapse of both the anterior and the posterior leaflets increased significantly, but mitral regurgitant signal area measured by color-coded Doppler flow imaging significantly decreased (1.10 ± 1.25→0.65 ± 1.23 cm^2). These results indicate that the left ventricular volume reduction enhances prolapse, but left ventricular pressure drop eliminates the regurgitation. More recently, we disclosed that, using phonocardiography and various ultrasound techniques, mitral systolic murmur greatly increased by dobutamine, but regurgitation estimated by color Doppler diminished (regurgitant flow area from 618 to 364 mm^2). Important determinants of the intensification of the murmur were the regurgitant blood velocity (from 4.4 to 5.1 m/sec) and decrease in the mitral valve ring size. This rule can be applied to any kind of mitral regurgitation.[49] Thus, we obtained the conclusion as to the relationships among the grade of valve prolapse, regurgitant volume, regurgitant murmur, and regurgitant velocity.

It is apparent that MVP has some relation to autonomic dysfunction.[50] Various mental tests (calculation, unpleasant memories, etc.) may cause increases in prolapse and the A/R ratio in continuous wave Doppler (A: atrial inflow; R: rapid inflow).[51] These changes were not observed in normal persons, and are probably caused by the excessive secretion of catecholamine in patients with prolapse.

Doppler Echocardiography

It has been stated that Doppler echocardiography depicts mitral regurgitant jet in most cases of mitral regurgitation. For example, in a large series, the sensitivity was 92%, the specificity 96%, and the predictive accuracy 93% by two-dimensional Doppler echocardiography when left ventriculography was used as the gold standard.[52] However, in MVP, the regurgitant jets are likely to be directed at unusual sites. In general, the jet directs backward in cases with anterior prolapse. In cases in which the posterior leaflets prolapse, the jet directs anteriorly in prolapse of the middle scallop, laterally in medial scallop, and inward in lateral scallop.[53] However, it takes a long time to obtain such direction by the usual Doppler technique, so that the effort was not practical.

Recently developed color flow-mapping (real-time two-dimensional Doppler echocardiography[54] or simply color Doppler) enables us to perform a prompt scan of the whole heart. We can visualize not only the presence but the instantaneous changes in the magnitude and direction of the abnormal flow, providing an estimation of the severity of the concomitant mitral regurgitation. In reality, a regurgitant echo signal was often detected even in cases with simple mid-systolic click.[55]

Today, transesophageal Doppler echocardiography is extensively used clinically in Japan, and there are many articles concerning MVP. Some insist that it is possible to localize the site of prolapse (medial, middle, and lateral scallops of the posterior leaflet) by the transthoracic approach, but it seems difficult because of the limited direction of the echo section. Much more information was obtained by transesophageal technique about the structural abnormalities, such as rupture of the chordae tendineae.[56] Equivocal case by transthoracic method is easily diagnosed by transesophageal route. However, we have had another difficulty with color Doppler in its extreme sensitivity in detecting regurgitant signals. Studies from two laboratories revealed nearly the same results, in which presumably normal valves were incompetent in a large number of subjects, except for the aortic valve.[57,58] Such regurgitant signals increased in the elderly.[59] Esophageal color Doppler further disclosed *pansystolic* regurgitant signals from the mitral valve in *all* cases examined.[60] With increased experience and a very rapid improvement in technology, we have moved inevitably to a Copernican change in our physiological concept of valve mechanics.

In this situation, we have faced certain difficulties. First, when we detect mitral regurgitant signals in the left atrium by color Doppler in cases with MVP, we may not connect these two phenomena if we ignore the reasonable connection between them. Second, when we cannot obtain any clinical data concerning regurgitation, what is the meaning of the regurgitant signals detected only by color Doppler? Are they pathological? If not, how does one differentiate between physiological and pathological regurgitation? Further extensive studies are required to solve these problems.

Diagnostic Criteria

In 1986, Perloff et al.[61] proposed major and minor criteria for the clinical diagnosis of MVP. My criteria[62] are similar to theirs with minor differences (Table 6). An important problem is how to decide whether to use the mitral valve ring or the mitral annular plane to evaluate prolapse.

At present, we have new criteria in the era of color Doppler echocardiography[63]: (1) phonocardiographic or auscultatory evidence indicative of mitral regurgitation or abnormalities of the mitral complex, (2) a systolic bulging or an apparent systolic ballooning of the mitral valve by two-dimensional echocardiography, and (3) mitral regurgitant signals with an

Table 6
Diagnostic Criteria for Mitral Valve Prolapse[62]

Auscultation and phonocardiography (at the apex)
  Mid-systolic (or late systolic) click, particularly sliding click
  Mid-systolic click with late systolic murmur
  Mid-systolic click provoked by amyl nitrite or methoxamine
    Late sytolic murmur with or without mid-systolic click provoked by amyl
    nitrite or methoxamine
M-mode echocardiography
  Mid-systolic buckling
  Pansystolic bowing (hammocking) of 3 mm or more recorded from lower
    intercostal space
Two-dimensional echocardiography
  Systolic protrusion of mitral valve leaflets beyond the mitral valve ring
    determined by the line connecting the junction between the anterior leaflet
    and the valve ring and the top of posterior wall echo of the left ventricle[39]
Combinations of these

acceleration flow at the site of prolapse by Doppler color flow mapping. In a strict sense, new criteria exclude an echocardiography-induced prolapse and stress in the clinical state of the patients. If a presumably healthy person has one or two of the criteria, we had better follow such a case, but not as a patient.

Very recently, three-dimensional display of MVP was attempted using biplane transesophageal echocardiography.[64] This is attractive and it is important to reestablish MVP as a disease with concomitant abnormalities and clinical complications of the pathological process.[65] At the present time, this methodology is not real-time, but the works by Roelandt and Pandian are now in process.[66] We have an expectancy for the three-dimensional diagnostic approach.

Clinical Problems

As previously described, the clinical signs and symptoms of MVP largely depend on the age of the study group. In younger people, the clinical significance of MVP may be trivial, but in the older age group, arrhythmias, mitral regurgitation, and other clinical manifestations cannot be neglected. Of these, I have to mention follow-up studies, sudden death, and changing concepts of surgical therapy.

Follow-Up Studies

Using criteria advocated by the National Cardiovascular Center,[33] echocardiographic progression of MVP was not evident in all 27 follow-up cases (mean 7.1 years). Left atrial dimension increased with an advance of age, particularly in cases with atrial fibrillation or ruptured chordae tendineae.[67] Our data also confirmed the similar results.[68] Phonocardiographically and echocardiographically proved MVP was followed 1 to 14 (mean 4.3) years in 116 patients (48 men and 68 women, mean age 27 years). Echocardiographic prolapse (no phono signs: silent prolapse) remained unchanged in 10 of 18 patients, but mid- or late systolic click appeared in 7. Of 57 patients with such clicks it remained unchanged in many cases (35 of 57), but significant systolic click appeared in 7 from 18 cases of silent state, while clicks disappeared in 15. Systolic murmurs are unchanged in most cases and the echocardiogram did not show the advanced degree of prolapse during the follow-up periods.

A great interest is the natural course of school children with a phonocardiographic sign of MVP. With increase in age, the prevalence of systolic click becomes higher,[24] but the course of an individual case is rather unknown. Our more than one thousand school children were annually followed, but fortunately no cardiac event happened so far. Limited echo study in only 24 cases 20 years later showed no change and these were anterior leaflet prolapse in all. Prolapse of the posterior leaflet or both the anterior and posterior leaflets are rare in school children (only 1 out of 1,187 cases). One girl had a tendency to develop a late systolic murmur, but the follow-up was not performed after graduation from high school. Predisposing factors to progressive deterioration are aging, male gender, posterior leaflet prolapse, increased thickness of the leaflet, and holosystolic murmur at the initial examination.[69] Isolated click, if otherwise it is within normal limits and has no change by provocation, has practically no prognostic value.

Sudden Death

Sudden death, probably the most serious aspect of MVP, is very rare in Japan. So far, a few cases of sudden death connected with MVP have been reported, but nearly all were resuscitated.[70] For one example, I have checked about 270,000 school children during the past 11 years and encountered three cases of sudden death. Mitral valve prolapse was not noted either on clinical grounds or by autopsy. During this period about 1,000 cases of MVP were followed, but no death was encountered. Sustained ventricular tachycardia was observed in two cases without prolapse, but not in cases with prolapse. Up to the present time, we do not know the reason for the difference between the Japanese and the occidental patients. We have an impression that the serious symptoms are likely to occur in patients with *mild* prolapse. Although right ventricular endomyocardial biopsy showed endocardial thickening, interstitial myocardial fibrosis, myocardial hypertrophy, myocardial degeneration, or myocardial disarray, these changes are always mild[71] and their relation to clinical findings has not been confirmed yet.

Surgical Therapy

Since 1987, surgery for mitral valvular regurgitation due to MVP has changed from prosthesis to repair.[72,73] The enthusiasm for repair is now a new trend in some institutions,[74] and intraoperative transesophageal echocardiography is regarded as an excellent tool in monitoring the surgical procedure.[75]

An Experimental Study

An experimental model of MVP was not attempted until Imataka et al. produced a similar state in rabbits by vagal manipulations.[76,77] After clipping or crushing the cervical vagi, papillary muscle lesions and mitral valve injuries were found in 46.8% and 47.7%, respectively. These include deposits of colloidal carbon previously injected after operation, swelling, increased stiffness, degeneration of myocardial cells, and interstitial fibrosis.[78] In nearly one-half of cases, the phonocardiograms disclosed a systolic murmur with or without a mid-systolic click. This study is now in progress,[79–82] and it was speculated that ventricular premature contractions frequently occurred during vagal manipulation closely related to the development of initial mitral valve bleeding followed by swelling and then fibrosis of the papillary muscles.

Innervation of the mitral valve was studied in four autopsied hearts not having heart disease and it was disclosed that acetylcholine-esterase-positive nerve fibers that are identical with vagal nerve were present in the mitral valve and the distribution, density, and structure were different in various areas, suggesting that the vagal innervation could play an important role for mitral valve function.[83] On the other hand, immunohistochemical study showed that S-100 protein and sympathetic nerve distributed in the coaptation zone, which may give stimuli to the nerve ending and mechanically cause autonomic nerve dysfunction.[84]

Myocardial distribution of the ^{123}I-metaiodobenzylguanidine (MIBG) washout was observed in cases with MVP (increased washout at the apical area and posterobasal interventricular septum), suggesting the abnormality of local myocardial sympathetic nerve function.[85]

Aside from the conventional pathological findings of MVP, a large number of autopsies (about 4,000 cases) disclosed some specific pathological conditions related to MVP. These include the objection to the association of floppy mitral valve with dysfunction[86] of the mitral valve fibrosis advocated by Hutchins,[87] partial absence of commissural chordal insertion,[88] and congenital absence of the commissural chordae tendineae[89] (12/4,800 autopsy cases). Other abnormalities were described, but we do not know if these are congenital or acquired.

Conclusion

In proportion to the worldwide flood of information, many reports covering nearly all the aspects of MVP have been presented in Japan also. I have introduced some of them in this chapter. We know that MVP is not infrequent among the oriental peoples, and all the features are the same as in the occidental peoples, though they are generally mild in Japan. Our investigations include research now in progress to elucidate the puzzle of this peculiar disease.

References

1. Hinohara S. Systolic gallop rhythm. Am Heart J 22:726, 1941.
2. Yamakawa K. Auscultation of the Heart, 2nd ed. Tokyo, Igaku-Shoin, 1956.
3. Ueda H, Kaito G, Sakamoto T. Clinical Phonocardiography. Tokyo, Nanzando, 1963, Ch 16, pp 219–30.
4. Ueda H, Sakamoto T. Detection of silent valve disease by functional phonocardiography using vasoactive drugs. Presented at the Third Meeting of Laennec Society, New York, October 20, 1966.
5. Ueda H, Sakamoto T, Uozumi Z, Inoue K, Kawai N, Yamada T. The use of methoxamine as a diagnostic aid in clinical phonocardiography. Jpn Heart J 7:204, 1966.
6. Reid JVO. Mid-systolic clicks. S Afr Med J 35:353, 1961.
7. Barlow JB, Peacock WA, Marchand P, Denny M. The significance of late systolic murmurs. Am Heart J 66:443, 1963.
8. Barlow JB, Bosman CK. Aneurysmal protrusion of the posterior leaflet of the mitral valve: Auscultatory-electrocardiographic syndrome. Am Heart J 71:166, 1966.
9. Segal BL, Likoff W. Late systolic murmur of mitral regurgitation. Am Heart J 67:1757, 1964.
10. Ronan JA, Perloff JK, Harvey WP. Systolic clicks and the late systolic murmur: Intracardiac phonocardiographic evidence of their mitral valve origin. Am Heart J 70:319, 1965.
11. Leon DF, Leonard JJ, Kroetz FW, Page WL, Shaver JA, Lancaster JF. Late systolic murmurs, clicks, and whoops arising from the mitral valve. Am Heart J 72:325, 1966.
12. Criley JM, Lewis KB, Humphries JO, Ross RS. Prolapse of the mitral valve: Clinical and cineangiocardiographic findings. Br Heart J 28:488, 1966.
13. Sakamoto T, Ichiyasu H, Hayashi T, Matsuhisa M. Clinical, electro-, phono-, mechano-, and echocardiographic observations of "click syndrome." Cardiovasc Sound Bull 4:507, 1974.
14. Tanaka M, Kosaka S, Terasawa Y, Kashiwagi M, Hikichi H, Meguro T, Watanabe S, et al. A significance of the mitral valve movement to the genesis of the late systolic murmur in mitral insufficiency. Cardiovasc Sound Bull 5:679, 1975.

15. Symposium on Mitral Valve Prolapse (T Sakamoto, Y Komatsu, eds.). J Cardiogr 10:1–121, 1980.
16. Panel Discussion on Diagnostic Considerations Concerned with Mitral Valve Prolapse (T Sakamoto, ed.). J Cardiogr 12:761–801, 1982.
17. Symposium on Current Problems in Valvular Heart Disease (T Sakamoto, H Manabe, eds.). Jpn Circ J 46:335–441, 1982.
18. Mitral Valve Prolapse. Fireside Conference (presided over by T Sakamoto, J Yoshikawa). Jpn Circ Soc, March 29, 1985.
19. Barlow JB. Perspectives on the Mitral Valve. Philadelphia, F.A. Davis, 1987, p 43.
20. Jeresaty RM. Mitral Valve Prolapse. New York, Raven Press, 1979.
21. Sakamoto T, Amano K, Hada Y, Yamaguchi T, Ishimitsu T, Hayashi T, Ichiyasu H, et al. Prevalence of click syndrome in school children. J Cardiogr 10:59, 1980.
22. Sakamoto T. Prospective phonocardiographic study of mitral valve prolapse: Prevalence of the nonejection click in school children. In Diethrich EB (ed): Noninvasive Assessment of the Cardiovascular System, Bristol, John Wright, PSG, 1982, pp 153–157.
23. Sakamoto T. Phonocardiographic assessment of the prevalence of mitral valve prolapse in the prospective survey of heart disease in school children: A seven-year cumulative study. Acta Cardiol 38:261, 1983.
24. Sakamoto T, Hada Y, Amano K, Yamaguchi T, Takenaka K. Population study of mitral valve prolapse: Eight years experience. Circulation 70:II–162, 1984.
25. Iqbal MZ, Eybel CE, Messer JV. Mitral valve prolapse associated with bicuspid aortic valve. Cardiovasc Rev Rep 1:465, 1980.
26. Amano K, Sakamoto T, Hada Y, Takenaka K, Hasegawa I, Takahashi T, Suzuki J, et al. Clinical significance of early or mid-systolic apical murmurs: Analysis by phonocardiography, two-dimensional echocardiography and pulsed Doppler echocardiography. J Cardiogr 16:433, 1986.
27. Sakamoto T, Yamaguchi T, Ichiyasu H, Hayashi T, Amano K, Hada Y, Tei C. Valvular disease in thyroid dysfunction: The use of pharmacodynamic phonocardiography. J Cardiogr 10:859, 1980.
28. Sakamoto T. Sliding systolic click(s). Int Med 44:671, 1979.
29. Fukuda N, Oki T, Kawano K, Okumoto T, Emi S, Uchida T, Kawano T, et al. Systolic clicks in mitral valve prolapse: Their pathophysiological relationship to the grade and causes of prolapse. J Cardiol 18(Suppl 18):45, 1988.
30. Yazaki N, Niwayama H, Onishi M, Sunami Y, Nishimoto Y, Masuda Y, Inagaki Y. Systolic time intervals in mitral valve prolapse syndrome. J Cardiol 19(Suppl 21):75, 1989.
31. Sakamoto T, Ishimitsu T, Hada Y, Amano K, Yamaguchi T, Takenaka K. Systolic time intervals in mitral valve prolapse. Acta Cardiol 32:325, 1981.
32. Inoh T, Maeda K, Oda K. Diagnosis and classification of the mitral valve prolapse by the ultrasoundcardiotomography and the evaluation of the M-mode technique. Jpn Circ J 43:405, 1979.
33. Nagata S, Sakakibara H, Beppu S, Hayashi T, Matsuhisa M, Kimura E, Masuda Y, et al. New echocardiographic criterion in the diagnosis of mitral valve prolapse. J Cardiogr 12:779, 1982.
34. Nagata S, Sakakibara H, Mikami T, Beppu S, Park YD, Matsuhisa M, Nimura Y. Idiopathic mitral valve prolapse: Analysis by real-time two-dimensional echocardiography. Jpn Circ J 46:369, 1982.
35. Yoshikawa J, Owaki T, Yanagihara K, Kato H, Okumachi F, Takagi Y, Yamaoka S. Diagnostic problems of M-mode and cross-sectional echocardiography in mitral valve prolapse. J Cardiogr 10:101, 1980.

36. Tanaka K, Yoshikawa J, Owaki T, Kato H, Okumanchi F, Takagi Y, Ishihara K, et al. Echocardiographic problem in diagnosing prolapsed mitral valve. Proc Jpn Soc Ultras Med 27:225, 1975.
37. Markiewicz W, London E, Popp RL. Effect of transducer placement on echocardiographic mitral valve motion. Am Heart J 96:555, 1978.
38. Gilbert BW, Schatz RA, VonRamm OT, Behar VS, Kisslo JA. Mitral valve prolapse: Two-dimensional echocardiographic and angiographic correlation. Circulation 54:716, 1976.
39. Yoshikawa J, Kato H, Yanagihara K, Okumachi F, Takagi Y, Yoshida K, Asaka T, et al. Criteria for the diagnosis of prolapsed mitral valve using phonocardiography and echocardiography. J Cardiogr 12:773, 1982.
40. Yoshikawa J, Karo H, Yanagihara K, Okumachi F, Shiratori K, Koizumi K, Yoshida K, et al. Echocardiographic diagnosis of mitral valve prolapse. Cardioangiol 15:680, 1984.
41. Sasaki H, Ogawa S, Handa S, Nakamura Y, Yamada R. Two-dimensional echocardiographic diagnosis of mitral valve prolapse syndrome in presumably healthy young students. J Cardiogr 12:23, 1982.
42. Kumaki T, Yokota Y, Kaku K, Toh S, Takarada A, Seo T, Kobo M, et al. Study on the mitral valve prolapse. I. Incidence in Kobe University students. II. Follow-up study. Jpn Circ J 49:1307, 1985.
43. Fujii K, Ishida Y, Tanouchi J, Ishihara K, Matsuyama T, Nishioka H, Uematsu M, et al. Mitral valve prolapse: Two-dimensional echocardiographic screening in apparently healthy students. J Cardiol 18(Suppl 18):9, 1988.
44. Sakamoto T, Takenaka K, Amano K, Hasegawa I, Suzuki J, Shiota T, Takahashi H, et al. Pharmacodynamic echocardiography. Echocardiography 6:131, 1989.
45. Sakamoto T. Pharmacodynamics of mitral valve prolapse. International Symposium on Auscultation and Phonocardiography. Srinagar, August 16–18, 1983.
46. Sakamoto T. Syndrome of mitral valve prolapse. Jpn J Int Med 72:714, 1983.
47. Suzuki J, Sakamoto T, Hada Y, Amano K, Takenaka K, Hasegawa I. Pharmacodynamic tests in patients with mitral valve prolapse. J Cardiol 17(Suppl 14):149, 1987.
48. Takenaka K, Sakamoto T, Amano W, Shiota S, Igarashi T, Suzuki J, Sugimoto T. Effect of amyl nitrite on mitral valve prolapse and mitral regurgitation: A transesophageal echocardiographic study. Am J Noninvas Cardiol 5:257, 1991.
49. Sonoda M, Takenaka K, Suzuki J, Amano W, Igarashi T, Watanabe F, Aoki T, et al. Effects of augmented left ventricular function on mitral regurgitation. J Cardiol 23(Suppl 34):77, 1993.
50. Boudoulas H, Wooley CF. Mitral valve prolapse syndrome: Evidence of autonomic dysfunction. J Cardiol 17(Suppl 14):3, 1987.
51. Tei C, Park JC, Horikiri Y, Tanaka N, Mizukami N, Toyama Y. Mental stress echocardiography for patients with mitral valve prolapse. J Cardiol 20(Suppl 23):61, 1990.
52. Ohwa M, Sakakibara H, Miyatake K, Okamoto M, Kinoshita N, Ueda E, Funabashi T, et al. Mitral regurgitation: Detection and quantitative evaluation by two-dimensional Doppler echocardiography. J Cardiogr 15:807, 1985.
53. Kitabatake A, Matsuo H, Asao M, Tanouchi J, Mishima M, Hayashi T, Abe H. Intra-atrial distribution of mitral regurgitation in mitral valve prolapse visualized by pulsed Doppler technique combined with electronic beam sector scanning echocardiography. J Cardiogr 10:111, 1980.
54. Omoto R. Real-Time Two-Dimensional Doppler Echocardiography [color atlas]. Tokyo, Shindan-to-Chiryo-sha, 1983.

55. Sakamoto T. Real-time two-dimensional color-coded Doppler echocardiography in detecting valvular regurgitation: Comparison with phonocardiographic evaluation. First International Congress on Cardiac Doppler. Pisa, October 16, 1985.
56. Joh Y, Yoshikawa J, Yoshida K, Akasaka T, Shakudo M, Hozumi T, Kato H. Transesophageal echocardiographic findings of mitral valve prolapse. J Cardiol 19(Suppl 21):85, 1989.
57. Yoshikawa J. Valvular regurgitation. Second Meeting of Laennec Club Japan, Kumamoto, November 1, 1986.
58. Miyatake K. Valvular regurgitation. Second Meeting of Laennec Club Japan, Kumamoto, November 1, 1986.
59. Akasaka T, Yoshikawa J, Yoshida K, Shiratori K, Okumachi F, Kato H. Age-related valvular regurgitation: A study by pulsed Doppler echocardiography. Circulation 72:III-99, 1985.
60. Roelandt J, Rijsterborgh H, van der Borden B. Variability of Doppler velocities: Potential risk for diagnostic errors. Second International Congress on Cardiac Doppler, Kyoto, November 29, 1986.
61. Perloff JK, Child JS, Edwards JE. New guidelines for the clinical diagnosis of mitral valve prolapse. Am J Cardiol 57:1124, 1986.
62. Sakamoto T. Diagnostic criteria for mitral valve prolapse. Int Med 55:1201, 1985.
63. Jyo Y, Yoshikawa J, Yoshida K, Kato H, Shakudo M. A new diagnostic criteria of mitral valve prolapse syndrome. J Cardiol 18(Suppl 18):29, 1988.
64. Mikami T, Teranishi J, Miyamoto N, Takatsuji H, Fukuda H, Kitabatake A, Sakamoto S, et al. Reconstruction of dynamic three-dimensional image of the mitral valve from transesophageal longitudinal echocardiography: Depiction of mitral valve prolapse. J Cardiol 23(Suppl 34):95, 1993.
65. Levine RA. Mitral valve prolapse: Clinical impact of new diagnostic criteria and insights from three-dimensional echocardiography. J Cardiol 24(Suppl 38):3, 1994.
66. Roelandt JRTC, Pandian NG. Multiplane Transesophageal Echocardiography. Churchill Livingstone Inc., New York, 1996.
67. Okano Y, Nagata S, Ishikura F, Asaoka N, Beppu S, Ohmori F, Tamai J, Miyatake K. Progression of idiopathic mitral valve prolapse estimated by echocardiography. J Cardiol 20(Suppl 23):73, 1990.
68. Deng Y-B, Takenaka K, Sakamoto T, Hada Y, Suzuki J, Shiota T, Amano W, et. al. Follow-up in mitral valve prolapse by phonocardiography, M-mode and two-dimensional echocardiography and Doppler echocardiography. Am J Cardiol 65:349, 1990.
69. Fukuda N, Oki T, Iuchi A, Tabata T, Manabe K, Kageji Y, Hama M, et al. Predisposing factors of severe mitral regurgitation in idiopathic mitral valve prolapse. J Cardiol 26(Suppl 1):17, 1995.
70. Iwase M, Kimura M, Matsuyama H, Wang J, Ando T, Kurokawa H, Nomura M, et al. Prolapse and thickening of the anterior mitral valve leaflet in a 17-year-old high school boy temporarily resuscitated from sudden cardiac death. J Cardiol 26(Suppl 1):85, 1995.
71. Yokota Y, Kumaki T, Miki T, Fukuzaki S. Right ventricular endomyocardial biopsy findings in idiopathic mitral valve prolapse: Comparison with clinical findings. J Cardiogr 16(Suppl XI):117, 1986.
72. Okada Y, Shomura T, Yoshida K, Yoshikawa J. Valve reconstruction for mitral regurgitation secondary to mitral valve prolapse. J Cardiol 20(Suppl 23):95, 1990.

73. Okada Y, Nasu M, Shomura T, Yoshida K, Yoshikawa J. Mitral valve repair for mitral valve prolapse. J Cardiol 23(Suppl 34):117, 1993.
74. Kawazoe K. Adherence to valve repair surgery: From the mitral to aortic valve. J Cardiol 29(Suppl 2):3, 1997.
75. Takeda M, Morizuki O, Obuchi T, Sekiguchi A, Yagyu K, Matsunaga H, Furuse A. Intraoperative evaluation of mitral valve repair: Comparison of transesophageal Doppler echocardiography with ventricular filling test. J Cardiol 23(Suppl 34):125, 1993.
76. Imataka K, Seki A, Tomono S, Fujii J. Experimental production of papillary muscle and mitral valve lesions by cervical vagal nerve clipping in the rabbit. Igaku-no-Ayumi 110:215, 1979.
77. Fujii J, Imataka K. Neurogenic cardiomyopathy. Igaku-no-Ayumi 116:985, 1981.
78. Imataka K, Takahashi N, Seki A, Fujii J. Experimental production of papillary muscle and mitral valve lesions. Jpn Circ J 45:362, 1982.
79. Imataka K, Yamaoki K, Seki A, Takayama Y, Fujii J. Peculiar mitral valve and papillary muscle lesions induced by vagus manipulations in rabbits: An experimental model for nonrheumatic mitral regurgitation. Jpn Heart J 27:377, 1986.
80. Imataka K, Sakamoto H, Okamato E, Ieki K, Fujii J. Effects of administration of three kinds of catecholamine on mitral complex. J Cardiol 22(Suppl 28):47, 1992.
81. Ashida T, Sakurai S, Takahashi N, Fujii J. Experimental production of mitral valve and papillary muscle lesions by premature ventricular contractions in rabbits: Effects of premature ventricular contractions induced by left ventricular pacing. J Cardiol 26(Suppl 1):77, 1995.
82. Ashida T, Kiraku J, Sakurai S, Takahashi N, Fujii J. Experimental production of tricuspid valve and papillary muscle lesions by premature ventricular contractions due to ventricular stimulation in rabbits. J Cardiol 27(Suppl 2):15, 1996.
83. Kawano H, Kawai S, Okada R. Vagal innervation in the human atrioventricular valves. J Cardiol 22(Suppl 28):17, 1992.
84. Kawano T, Oki T, Uchida T, Iuchi A, Ogawa S, Hayashi M, Fukuda N, et al. Innervation of the mitral valve in normal and prolapsed mitral valves. J Cardiol 19(Suppl 21):43, 1989.
85. Kishi F, Nomura M, Yukinaka M, Saito K, Tabata T, Iuchi A, Fukuda N, et al. Evaluation of myocardial sympathetic nerve function in patients with mitral valve prolapse using iodine- 123-metaidobenzylguanidine myocardial scintigraphy. J Cardiol 27(Suppl 2):21, 1996.
86. Sugiura M, Ohkawa S, Watanabe C, Toku A, Imai T, Kuboki K, Shimada H. Morphological observation of the mitral annulus fibrosus in patients with mitral valve prolapse. J Cardiol 20(Suppl 23):21, 1990.
87. Hutchins GM. The association of floppy mitral valve with disjunction of the mitral annulus fibrosus. N Engl J Med 314:535, 1986.
88. Fujimoto T, Oki T, Kiyoshige K, Iuchi A, Tabata T, Manabe K, Tanimoto M, et al. Mitral valve prolapse associated with partial absence of commissural chordal insertion: Report of two cases. J Cardiol 22(Suppl 28):27, 1992.
89. Ohkawa S, Sugawara T, Imai T, Kuboki K, Chida K, Sakai M, Watanabe C, et al. Mitral regurgitation induced by congenital "absence of the commissural chordae tendineae." J Cardiol 24(Suppl 38):29, 1994.

Part XV

Floppy Mitral Valve, Mitral Valve Prolapse Syndrome

The Superior Physician
He is skeptial toward the data of his own profession, welcomes discoveries which upset his previous hypothesis, and is still animated by human sympathy and understanding.
> —Alfred North Whitehead
> Dialogues (Lucien Price)
> 1954

Introduction

From Irritable Heart in the U.S. Civil War and Soldier's Heart in World War I to the Floppy Mitral Valve

Charles F. Wooley, MD,
Harisios Boudoulas, MD, PhD

The rich historic heritage of the floppy mitral valve, mitral valve prolapse, and mitral valvular regurgitation parallels developments in the anatomic and pathologic era of the 18th century and the rise of cardiac physical diagnosis. At the same time, clinicians were dealing with the distinctions between organic heart disease, i.e., cardiac disorders with demonstrable physical findings in life and cardiac pathology at autopsy, and functional heart disease, i.e., patients with disabling cardiovascular symptoms and minimal changes on physical examination. Thus, individuals with the symptom complex of chest pain, palpitations, dyspnea, fatigue, syncope, and the inability to perform sustained physical activities were placed into the category of functional cardiac disorders. These distinctions reached new levels of significance in the United States and Great Britain during the U.S. Civil War and in World War I.

The U.S. Civil War 1861–1865

Cardiac causes of disability in the young Union troops at the time of the Peninsula Campaign in Virginia in 1862 were topics of great concern. The intensive study of these young men in a section at the Turner's Lane Hospital in Philadelphia marks the beginnings of clinical cardiovascular research in the United States.

Jacob Mendez DaCosta described these men in his classic studies "On Irritable Heart," the profile of a peculiar form of functional cardiac disease

From: Boudoulas H, Wooley CF. *Mitral Valve: Floppy Mitral Valve, Mitral Valve Prolapse, Mitral Valve Regurgitation*. Second revised edition. ©Futura Publishing Company, Armonk, NY, 2000.

causing disability among the young troops in this campaign. DaCosta, a Jefferson Medical College graduate with European training, brought contemporary physical diagnostic skills and the perspective of a physician trained in internal medicine to the task. His studies received national and international recognition.

Between the Wars

Similar dilemmas faced British Army medical officers during the 1860–1970 decade when disabled young British soldiers with cardiac symptoms were invalided back to England from the far reaches of the British Empire, particularly from service in great heat. Chest pain, palpitations, breathlessness, fatigue, syncope, and the inability to perform sustained physical activity caused disability similar to that seen and described by DaCosta. "Irritable heart" was widely recognized as a significant cause of disability in the British Army, and was the subject of medical inquiry and government commissions.

World War I: The British Experience

"Irritable heart" resurfaced during World War I and identity with DaCosta's syndrome was postulated. The disorder was renamed "soldier's heart," and the term was applied to the symptomatic and disabled young troops, many from the Western Front. The increasing numbers of men disabled with "soldier's heart" led to the establishment of the Military Heart Hospital, a government-sponsored specialty hospital in England.

At the time, manpower pressures were extreme, and the initiation of conscription was a source of controversy. Both the military hierarchy and the military physicians were dealing with the consequences associated with the army's intake of large numbers of physically unfit or poorly prepared men.

Social, economic, and other medical factors were operative as well. Social activism in England in the early 1900s brought about legislative enactment of the National Insurance Acts, forerunners of legislation that later established the National Health Service. As a result, the Military Heart Hospital research was funded by mechanisms involving the government-insurance-military interactions. The economic aspects involved the mounting concerns in World War I England about the large numbers of young soldiers with soldier's heart, their prolonged hospital stays, the subsequent disability evaluations, and the economic consequences of awarding pensions to young men.

The other medical factors were more subtle and related to the growth and development of the specialties of neurology, psychiatry, and cardiology, which inserted new, incompletely formed, or totally erroneous, concepts about neurasthenia, anxiety states, shell shock, and functional heart disease into the controversies surrounding the soldier's heart debates.

World War I: The U.S. Experience

The U.S. Army Surgeon General's decision to send U.S. Army Medical Officers to the Military Heart Hospital in England in 1917–1918 was based on the premise that the unsatisfactory British experience could be avoided. Careful studies of the disorder, accompanied by revision of physical examination standards, so as to exclude unfit recruits, were major considerations. When the U.S. Army Medical Officers submitted their report to the United States Surgeon General, they renamed soldier's heart as neurocirculatory asthenia.

At the beginnings of U.S. involvement in World War I during 1917–1918, U.S. Army physical examination criteria retained Civil War doctrine and required revisions on multiple occasions. The nationwide examination of 4 million young men required large numbers of qualified examiners and appropriate facilities. In order to resolve many of the problems associated with cardiac disorders in the young soldiers, the first cardiovascular center in the U.S. was established at the U.S. Army Hospital No. 9, Lakewood, New Jersey. The training of selected physicians to be cardiac examiners and supervisors of the national physical examination process was one of the goals of the center.

Graded physical activity, introduced as part of the management of symptomatic soldiers in place of traditional bed rest, followed the earlier British model. Cardiac rehabilitation had its origins, first with the British experiences with soldier's heart, and then in the United States, at Lakewood, New Jersey. Reduction of the length of hospital stay and fewer inappropriate disability pensions were the desired goals.

Soldier's Heart: The Impact

The strides in the detection, description, classification, and management of cardiac disorders in young soldiers in the U.S. Civil War and in World War I were balanced or offset by errors due to medical ignorance, the overriding military manpower pressures, and military medical arrogance. The accomplishments and the failures are best understood within the military medical continuum that began in the U.S. Civil War and extended through World War I.

The World War I soldier's heart studies involved contemporary and future leadership figures in British and American medicine and cardiology, and the many interactions resulted in long-term friendships and collegial activities. Many of the lasting effects of these activities on military and civilian medicine may be traced through developments in cardiology and psychiatry throughout the 20th century.

The "irritable heart," "soldier's heart," and "neurocirculatory asthenia" studies during the two wars provoked a rethinking of traditional concepts about the genesis and classification of heart disease, and the distinctions between organic heart disease and functional cardiac disorders in young men. In particular, the unexpected frequency of young men with apical systolic murmurs detected in the physical examination of millions of potential recruits was a source of great concern and debate about the incidence and etiology of mild mitral valvular regurgitation in young individuals.

Government-sponsored cardiovascular research in specialty hospitals, the appearance of cardiovascular clinical investigators, and the introduction of cardiac rehabilitation into British and American medicine were among the important results. In fact, the organized activities on both sides of the Atlantic during the two wars may be viewed as the coming of age of anglo-American cardiology.

This introduction to Chapter 23 serves as background to the genesis of medical thought about the origins of the floppy mitral valve/mitral valve prolapse syndrome.

The diagnostic and therapeutic considerations in Chapter 24 constitute a work in progress, reflecting the limitations of our understanding of autonomic nervous function and brain–heart interactions.

23

From Irritable Heart to the Floppy Mitral Valve and the Mitral Valve Prolapse Syndrome

Charles F. Wooley, MD,
Harisios Boudoulas, MD, PhD

Introduction

Palpitation, a word denoting the sensation of rapid or irregular heartbeat, was recognized in the medicine of antiquity, but our discussion begins with the work of William Harvey and the Oxford scientists (Fig. 1), with *De Motu Cordis* in 1628 and culminating with Richard Lower's *De Corde* in 1669.[1]

De Motu Cordis

William Harvey's dedication of *De Motu Cordis*[2] refers to his opinion concerning the motion and use of the heart and circulation of the blood . . .confirmed by ocular demonstration for 9 years and more. . . . This little book, really a tract, *Concerning the Movement of the Heart and of the Blood in Animals*, has been referred to as the most important medical text ever writ-

From: Boudoulas H, Wooley CF. *Mitral Valve: Floppy Mitral Valve, Mitral Valve Prolapse, Mitral Valvular Regurgitation.* Second revised edition. ©Futura Publishing Company, Armonk, NY, 2000.

Palpitations, Nervous Heart, Anxiety, and Cardiovascular Syndromes:
A Cardiologist's Historical Perspective

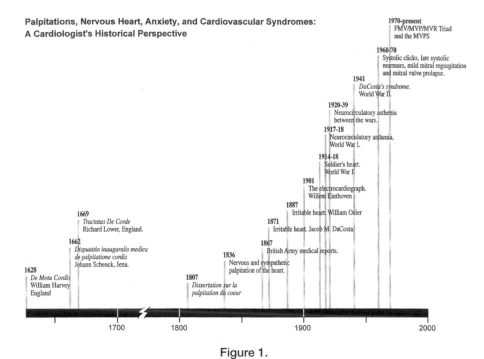

Figure 1.

ten. Published in 1628 in Frankfurt-on-the-Main in a poorly printed volume of only 72 pages with two plates, *De Motu Cordis* generated a storm of protest in the world of philosophy and medicine.

Origin and Conduction of the Heartbeat: The Auricular–Ventricular Rhythm

In his lectures on the *History of Physiology During the Sixteenth, Seventeenth and Eighteenth Centuries*, Foster emphasizes Harvey's clear conception of the work of the auricles and the ventricles: ventricular filling during diastole, both ventricles emptying during systole, the blood moving in a circle ("which motion we may be allowed to call circular") from the left side of the heart, through the arteries, the tissues, and the veins to the right side of the heart, and hence through the lungs to the left side of the heart.[3]

In the words of Harvey, "Two sets of movement occur together, one of the auricles, another of the ventricles. These are not simultaneous, but that of auricles precedes that of the rest of the heart. The movement seems to start in the auricles and to spread to the ventricles." The translator

Leake comments that this was the first clear statement on the problem of the origin and conduction of the heartbeat.

Harvey continues: "These two motions, one of the auricles, the other of the ventricles, are consecutive with a rhythm between them like the mechanism in firearms, where touching the trigger brings down the flint, lights a spark, which falls in the powder and explodes it, firing the ball, which reaches the mark. All of these events because of their quickness seem to occur simultaneously in the twinkling of an eye."[4]

Tractatus De Corde

Richard Lower was one of Oxford's great doctors. Translating his *De Corde*,[5] Franklin noted that "through Harvey's discovery he [Lower] escaped, to an extent that even Harvey did not, from the dominance of older writers."[6] According to Franklin, Lower had as good a knowledge of the nervous system as any of his contemporaries, an outgrowth of his anatomic studies with Thomas Willis. His contributions to the understanding of the nervous system, the circulation, and respiration were multiple and substantial.

Lower's chapter, "The Movement of the Heart," in his *De Corde*[5] displays a remarkable appreciation of fundamental cardiac physiology. Like Harvey, he differentiated auricular systole from ventricular systole and diastole, observing that the auricles were the first to move and not only provided the first impulses for the heart's motion but were "the spark which sets off the whole." Lower used the term *palpitation* to describe a symptom complex in a physiological setting, referring to the "perversion" of the orderly movement of the heart that occurred in emotional states such as anger, joy, and sudden fright.

Palpitation: A Disorder of the Orderly Movement of the Heart

Thus, the term palpitation and its meaning evolved along with the insights into the physiology of the circulation that resulted from Harvey's studies. Harvey's exposition of the sequence of the orderly movement of the heart, the origin and conduction of the heartbeat, and the consecutive motions of the auricles and the ventricles, the auricular–ventricular rhythm, was the essential observation. Lower then extended Harvey's exposition of the sequence of the orderly movement of the heart, incorporating the concepts of the innervation of the heart as substrate, and the interactive role of the brain–heart connections, into his description of palpitation as a symptom complex with a physiological basis arising from a disorder of the orderly movement of the heart.[1]

Palpitation and the Nervous Heart

Evan Bedford traced the early medical literature about palpitation and nervous heart to the thesis by Johann Schenck in Jena in 1662 ("palpitation of the heart. . .a popular subject at Jena at this time") and the dissertation by Laurent Banizette at Montpellier, France, in 1807.

John Calthrop Williams of Nottingham, England, participated in the cardiac diagnosis revolution that accompanied the dissemination of the techniques of percussion and auscultation from the European continent. Williams incorporated the cardiac and neurological physiology of the day in his 1836 text when he attempted to separate nervous or sympathetic palpitations from palpitations associated with organic forms. He associated palpitation with nervous disturbances, precordial pain, vasovagal attacks with syncope, used the term disordered action of the heart, and drew attention to the brain–heart connection:

> Patient. . .suffering for considerable length of time under palpitation. . .and we are unable to discover signs of organic disease . . .may be certain that disordered action of the heart is of functional nature. . .mental emotions a very frequent cause of sympathetic disturbance of heart. . .influence directly from brain to the heart. Palpitation. . .frequent indication that functional derangement is established in the heart. Not many diseases which excite in the mind of the patient so much alarm.[8]

Williams's text provides a window on the cardiovascular and neurophysiology of the day, the origins of the functional heart disorders and the causes that excite them, the early association of "inorganic" murmurs and palpitations with nervous affections of the heart, and the very important concept that functional derangement may terminate in organic disease.

1860–1870: Disability in Young Soldiers

Disability in young soldiers as a result of fatigue, palpitation, dyspnea, and chest pain, the inability to perform demanding or sustained physical tasks under duress or stress, was described as a specific entity in military medical reports from both sides of the Atlantic during the 1860s.

British Army Medical Reports on Irritable Heart

W.C. MacLean, Professor of Military Medicine at the Army Medical School, lectured to men training to be military surgeons at the Royal Victoria Hospital at Netley.[9] Young men invalided with heart disease from foreign and home stations passed through the Medical Division for evaluation and were entered on the lists as cases of valvular disease, but frequently had none of the signs of valvular disease. MacLean described these men under the heading of "irritable heart,"that "rapid, often tumultuous action so common among soldiers," which once established is never gotten rid of so long as a man remains in the army and wears the dress and accoutrements of infantry soldiers. Irritable heart, widely recognized in the British Army, was an important cause of medical disability. The clinical syndrome was frequently classified under the category of valvular heart disease for administrative purposes. Tight accoutrements, constricting uniforms, heavy packs, overexertion, and drill techniques were considered as possible causes. The magnitude of the problem was such that governmental inquiry and commissions mandated widespread changes in uniform, pack, and drill, but the irritable heart remained.

DaCosta's Syndrome

The hidden war that took place in the hospital wards during the Civil War has been obscured by the haze and pall of the battlefields—the casualties, the carnage, the trauma, the amputations, and their sequelae. In reality, medical disorders and infections caused greater morbidity and mortality than wounds.

The physical fitness of the enlistees in the North was not subjected to careful scrutiny until 1863 with enlistments expiring, manpower pressures intense, and conscription coming into effect. Reform of the selection process included the establishment of uniform physical examination standards, which are essentially unchanged since the War of 1812. The large numbers of the physically unfit, the malingerers intent on leaving or avoiding service, and the bounty seekers attempting to hide disabilities complicated matters.

Cardiac causes of disability in the young troops at the time of the Peninsula Campaign was a topic of great concern. The intensive study of these young men at the Turner's Lane Hospital in Philadelphia marks the beginnings of clinical cardiovascular research in the United States. Jacob Mendez DaCosta described these men in his classic studies *On Irritable Heart*, the profile of a peculiar form of functional cardiac disease causing disability among the young troops in this campaign. DaCosta, a Jefferson Medical College graduate with European training, brought contemporary physical diagnostic skills and the perspective of a physician well trained in internal medicine to the task. His studies received national and international recognition.[10]

DaCosta published his initial, preliminary reports in 1862 and 1864 about "irritable heart" based on studies at the U.S. Army Hospital for Injuries and Diseases of the Nervous System, Turners Lane, Philadelphia, during the War. His definitive, classic paper on "irritable heart" was published in 1871,[11] received wide attention, and the disease is still referred to as DaCosta's syndrome. DaCosta thought it was similar to one described earlier among British troops in India and the Crimea.

During the Civil War, the U.S. Army developed the specialty hospital approach. A large, heterogeneous group of soldiers with functional heart disease was sent to the Turner's Lane Hospital, where they were evaluated by DaCosta. His careful clinical description of irritable heart was accompanied by follow-up studies. DaCosta realized that the outcome varied: some men returned to normal function, others experienced persistent disability, whereas a third group had worsening of the clinical situation with progression to cardiac hypertrophy. Although the group at Turner's Lane Hospital was heterogeneous, DaCosta was dealing primarily with young men with disabling symptoms.

William Osler: The Irritable Heart in Civil Life

William Osler was in Philadelphia from 1884 until 1889 as Professor of Clinical Medicine at the University of Pennsylvania, and he had contact with DaCosta during that time. Osler presented a paper in 1887 on *Irritable Heart in Civil Life*, a condition comparable to the irritable heart mentioned by DaCosta as occurring in military life. Osler acknowledged the DaCosta lineage, but emphasized the occurrence of irritable heart in civil life, i.e., this was not specifically a disorder of soldiers, as indeed DaCosta had done earlier. Osler noted the more frequent association of the symptom complex (palpitations, chest pain, and exertional dyspnea) with neurasthenia in women. Osler carried the message with him to Baltimore, and presented the subject in his textbook under Functional Affections of the Heart in a discussion of palpitation, where among other things he described striking palpitation in neurasthenic women, postural tachycardia, and polyuria after attacks of tachycardia.

19th Century Auscultatory Concepts: Systolic Clicks and Apical Systolic Murmurs

Tracing the irritable heart–mitral valve prolapse lineage requires an awareness of nineteenth century auscultatory dogma as well as an understanding of what clinicians meant by functional heart disease.[13]

Systolic Clicks

The association of systolic clicks with functional heart disorders occurred early in the descriptive auscultatory era. Laennec used the term "cliquement metallique," or metallic tinnitus; Austin Flint considered this finding a sign of excited action of the organ. James Hope related the metallic ringing sound to a smart blow of the apex striking the fifth rib, while William Stokes thought its principle cause to be the energy of muscular contraction with or without a great degree of tension of the auriculo-ventricular waves ("common in the hysteric excitement of the heart"). DaCosta described split heart sounds, systolic clicks, and apical systolic murmurs in the young troops with irritable heart described above. Later in the 19th century Potain ascribed sharp systolic clicking sounds to the tensing of pericardial adhesions, and influenced medical thought for the next 60 years.

Apical Systolic Murmurs

Potain was an authoritative source of French auscultatory wisdom, and also held that "circumscribed" systolic murmurs, those occurring in early, mid- or late systole, were nonorganic as compared with the holosystolic murmur of mitral regurgitation. By the end of the century, Griffith and Hall, working independently in the United States, described mid- and late apical systolic murmurs of mitral insufficiency. In particular, Hall presented advanced insights into potential mechanisms for mid- and late "yielding" of the mitral valve as a basis for the timing of these murmurs. Authoritative dogma prevailed, however, and for the next half century systolic clicks remained extracardiac in origin, and mid- and late systolic murmurs were regarded as nonorganic.[13]

The association of systolic clicks and apical mid- and late systolic murmurs with functional heart disease during the early auscultatory era led to rigid clinical thinking that has persisted until the present.

1901–1905: The Electrocardiograph and the Phonocardiograph

August Waller used a capillary electrometer with a mirror galvanometer in studies of electrical currents in the heart (1887). Willem Einthoven's description of the string galvonometer in 1901 and his continued research led to the development of the electrocardiograph, which "marked a change in the nature of the instrumentation of medical diagnosis."[14] The far-reaching results of this scientific medical invention, used in hospitals throughout the world, included a role in the development of those physicians who would become the cardiologists of later decades. Moreover, the palpitations described by Schenck in 1662, Lower in 1669, John Calthrop Williams in 1836, and Jacob DaCosta in 1871 became the electrocardiographic cardiac rhythms and arrhythmias of the 20th century.

1914–1918: Soldier's Heart and the Effort Syndrome

"Irritable heart" resurfaced during World War I and identity with Da-Costa's syndrome was established. The disorder was renamed "Soldier's Heart," and the term was applied to the symptomatic and disabled young troops from the Western Front. Manpower pressures were extreme, the initiation of conscription was controversial, and the large numbers of physically unfit or poorly prepared men were operative factors. The large numbers of men disabled with "soldier's heart" led to the establishment of the British Military Heart Hospital, a government-sponsored specialty hospital in England.

The British World War I Military Heart Hospital idea was proposed by James MacKenzie[15] in order to investigate the causes of soldier's heart, a problem of increasing magnitude as the war progressed. Clifford All-butt,[16] Regius Professor of Medicine at Cambridge, and William Osler, now Regius Professor of Medicine at Oxford, supported Mackenzie "and after a considerable amount of discussion, it was granted to us." The idea became reality at Hampstead and later at Colchester. While the distinguished trio functioned as Advisory Committee and consultant physicians, the younger men, Thomas Lewis as director, with John Parkinson, Jonathan Meakins, Thomas Cotton, et al. as associates, grasped the opportunity and initiated a scientific inquiry into the basic mechanisms of symptoms. Clinical evaluations were augmented by the chest x-ray, electrocardiogram, and exercise testing. These studies were reported in the 1917–1918 Medical Research Committee Report, the 1918 text *The Soldier's Heart and Effort Syndrome* by Lewis,[17] a series of articles in the journal *Heart* 1915–1917, and the *British Medical Journal*.

The British "soldier's heart" experience has been analyzed by Howell.[18] The concepts that emerged from these experiences were greater precision in cardiac diagnosis, improved recruit selection methods, early approaches to cardiac rehabilitation, rational criteria for disability and pensions, the centralized aggregation of patients resulting in shorter hospital stays, and the specialty-oriented clinical research center approach. However, apical systolic murmurs without other signs of heart disease were deliberately ignored, and the diagnosis and differentiation of mitral regurgitation from irritable heart continued to pose diagnostic and classification problems.

1917–1918: The U.S. Experience with Neurocirculatory Asthenia

Sir William Osler advocated recruiting American physicians to participate in British civil and military hospital activities before U.S. involvement in World War I. During the early months of U.S. involvement in the war, a group of U.S. medical officers attached to the British Medical Corps working at the British Military Heart Hospital included B.S. Oppenheimer, S.A. Levine, R.A. Morison, M.A. Rothschild, W. St. Lawrence, and F.N. Wilson. These close contacts with Lewis set the stage for continued Anglo-American collaborations and exchanges. When the U.S. medical officers presented their report to the U.S. Surgeon General they renamed irritable heart, soldier's heart, effort syndrome, and disorderly action of the heart (DAH) as neurocirculatory asthenia (NCA), which became official U.S. military terminology.[19]

The mass mobilization in the United States led to the physical examination of 4 million young men. Although the British experience and the U.S. medical officers' report formed the basis for certain of the cardiovascular standards for military fitness, the debate about the diagnosis of irritable heart, NCA, and mitral insufficiency continued. U.S. Army General Hospital #9 was established at Lakewood, New Jersey as a center for cardiovascular diseases. Frances Peabody was placed in charge of studies and established a research group that included a psychiatrist. These efforts were cut short by the armistice.

Physical Fitness, Military Duty, and Heart Disease in Young Men, from the U.S. Civil War Through World War I

The incidence of truly physically fit young men in any society at any given time reflects the public health, nutrition, hygiene, and levels of well-being in the population, and has genetic, socioeconomic, and geopolitical overtones. Such incidence figures were published by individual European countries during the 1800s. When used in the United States during the Civil War as a measure or index of military aptitude, i.e., as an expression of the number of men found fit for service, these figures were based on the U.S. census of 1860, which listed a population of 31.4 million. This figure was then corrected for the numbers of men lost to the Union by secession. Five million men 18–45 years old comprised the potential population available for military service, of whom 3.8 million were considered fit for service. During the 4 years of war, 50% of the entire population of the 18–45-year-old men served.

Most of the young men entered the U.S. military service in 1861 after minimal, cursory, or limited physical examinations. The existing military physical examination standards were residual of the War of 1812, and were modified according to the reformed U.S. Army physical examination standards in 1863. Where possible, the physical functions that could be measured or tested with the available limited technology were quantitated. The cardiovascular examination relied on a superficial medical history, measurement of the heart rate, the "state" of the arteries and veins, and the cardiac examination using cardiac palpation, percussion, and auscultation.

The evolution of the changes in the U.S. Army physical examination standards were analyzed after the Civil War, and these data formed the template for the U.S. Army World War I experience when 4 million young men were examined in the recruitment and conscription activities of 1917–1918. The template was revised on multiple occasions as the examination, selection, terminology, and classification processes were modified. New technology such as the measurement of blood pressure was introduced, and cardiac specialists were designated or trained to deal with the questions about cardiac murmurs, tachyarrhythmias, and cardiovascular fitness.

Physical examination standards, the interpretation of individual variations in physical examination phenomena, and the criteria for establishing fitness for military service were moving targets during both wars. The manpower pressures of 1863 were driving forces that brought about conscription and the payment of enlistment bounties in the United States. Similar manpower pressures on the Western Front in 1914–1916 eventually brought conscription to Great Britain although the decision was controversial. These manpower pressures brought about reconsideration and revisions of the criteria that defined physical fitness and fitness for duty. In the final analysis, these physical fitness and examination standards were the major factors in determining the body of men at risk for disability when exposed to the rigors of the military experience.

During the latter part of the 20th century cardiologists became increasingly aware of a broad spectrum of cardiac diseases in young men that were as yet undefined and undescribed during 1861–1918. Changes in heart size or dimensions associated with athletic conditioning, the so-called athlete's heart, now measured with the echocardiogram, meant that cardiologists could differentiate this condition from a variety of cardiovascular diseases associated with cardiovascular symptoms, collapse, or sudden death in competition or in training.

For the most part these cardiovascular disorders were simply not known to the physicians of 1861–1918 when contemporary emphasis was placed on chronic rheumatic valvular heart disease, syphilitic heart disease with aortic valvular regurgitation, and acute and chronic myocarditis. Soldiers with most of these now well-defined clinical entities would have been classified having as irritable heart or soldier's heart.

The World War I apical systolic murmur controversies were primarily British creations. Dogmatic assertions, originally by James Mackenzie and then by Thomas Lewis, carrying the weight of authority, led to the downgrading of cardiac auscultation. Ignoring the apical systolic murmur unless other cardiac abnormalities were present was intended to separate the more esoteric matter of cardiac diagnosis from the practicalities of cardiac function, the latter being the end point when considering a man's fitness for military service. This meant that young men with apical systolic murmurs associated with hypertrophic cardiomyopathy, or floppy mitral valves producing mitral valve prolapse and mitral valvular regurgitation, were judged fit for military service unless significant hypertrophy was present. This dogma was a sticking point for a number of the U.S. medical officers; however, in the short term the British view prevailed. DaCosta's postulate about the unusual forms of mitral regurgitation being responsible for the apical systolic murmurs, and Allbutt's wise observations about the natural, life-long and progressive history of individuals with apical systolic murmurs and mitral valvular regurgitation were largely ignored until the second half of the 20th century.

"Functional" cardiac disease remained a diagnosis of exclusion throughout the Civil War–World War I period, meaning that the then known "organic" diseases of the period were excluded primarily by the absence of cardiac enlargement or significant cardiac murmurs. However, the separation process was evolving in a subtle manner as revised physical examination criteria were introduced (Fig. 2). When designated cardiology examiners reinforced the standard medical examiners in World War I, they set new standards for cardiovascular competence among the examiners.

When blood pressure determination was introduced into the physical examination, the impact was limited. However, epidemiologic information about the range of blood pressure in large numbers of young American men began to appear during this time, and for the first time we find incidence figures of arterial hypertension in a defined population. While the early use of blood pressure recording in the examination of large numbers was of some value in the determination of physical fitness during the war, the true significance of blood pressure determination in large populations came later in the 20th century. In terms of the irritable heart–soldier's heart experience, the introduction of the blood pressure movement to the physical examination meant that large numbers of young men with hypertension were separated from the functional cardiovascular disease category.

The use of the chest x-ray and the electrocardiograph during World War I added another objective dimension to cardiopulmonary diagnosis. Although the direct impact of these new techniques on the physical examination of large numbers of recruits was limited, two powerful diagnostic methods were now available in the ongoing process of separating "functional" and "organic" cardiovascular and cardiopulmonary disorders. When the chest x-ray was used in studies of symptomatic men at the Military Heart Hospital in England, the men with soldier's heart had small

Palpitations, Nervous Heart, Anxiety, and Cardiovascular Syndromes: A Cardiologist's Historical Perspective

1628	*De Motu Cordis.* The orderly movement of the heart. William Harvey, England
1662	*Disputatio inauguralis medica de palpitatione cordis.* Johann Schenck, Jena
1669	*Tractatus De Corde.* Palpitation—a disorder of the orderly movement of the heart. Richard Lower, England
1807	*Dissertation sur la palpitation du coeur.* Laurent Banizette, Montpellier Ecole De Medecine
1836	Practical observations on nervous and sympathetic palpitation of the heart. John Calthrop Williams, Nottingham, England
1867	British Army medical reports on irritable heart. W.C. MacLean, Royal Victoria Hospital, Netley, England
1871	Irritable heart. U.S. Civil War experience. Jacob M. DaCosta, Turners Lane Hospital, Philadelphia, Pa. United States
1887	Irritable heart in civil life. William Osler, Philadelphia and Baltimore, United States
1901	The electrocardiograph. The phonocardiograph. Willem Einthoven, Utrech, The Netherlands
1914-18	Soldier's heart. The effort syndrome. World War I. The British experience. James Mackenzie and Thomas Lewis, Military Heart Hospital, Hampstead and Colchester, England
1917-18	Neurocirculatory asthenia. World War I. The U.S. experience. Frank Wilson, Samuel Levine, et al. Military Heart Hospital, England and U.S. Army Hospital No. 9, Lakewood, NJ, United States
1920-39	Neurocirculatory asthenia between the wars. Paul Dudley White and Mandel Cohen, Boston, Mass., United States
1941	Mill Hill Center, England (World War II) DaCosta's syndrome—Paul Wood; Psychiatric aspects—Aubrey Lewis
1960-70	Systolic clicks, late systolic murmurs, mild mitral regurgitation and mitral valve prolapse. John Barlow, South Africa; J. Michael Criley, United States
1970-80	Floppy mitral valve, mitral valve prolapse, mitral valve regurgitation—universal phenomena
1980	Mitral valve prolapse syndrome—neuroendocrine and autonomic nervous system mechanisms

Figure 2.

volume hearts. This was an important observation, since individuals with small hearts have smaller circulating blood volumes than their robust colleagues, and are more susceptible to volume depletion, blood loss, and neuroendocrine stimuli. The introduction of the chest x-ray in cardiac diagnosis provided an objective technique to classify patients with cardiac disorders into two major groups: those with large volume hearts contrasted with individuals with small volume hearts. The distinction, although important, was not completely appreciated at the time.

The use of the electrocardiograph was quite limited. However, the symptoms of palpitation could now be translated into a specific diagnosis of cardiac arrhythmia, patients with electrocardiographic changes associated with myocarditis could be identified, and an appreciation of certain electrocardiographic conduction defects with myocardial disease was developing. It is important to emphasize that during the 1861–1918 interval, young men with disorders of cardiac conduction (Wolff-Parkinson-White syndrome, certain forms of heart block, bundle branch block), and most of the cardiac arrhythmias (supraventricular tachycardia, paroxysmal atrial tachycardia, ventricular arrhythmias), were classified as functional disorders. It was not until much later in the 20th century when the electrocardiograph came into widespread use and ambulatory monitoring of cardiac rhythm was feasible that clarification of the role of cardiac arrhythmias in the symptom complexes associated with irritable heart and soldier's heart was possible.

Lessons Learned from U.S. Army Physical Examinations

Lewis Atterbury Conner, one of the founding group of the American Heart Association in 1924 and its first president in 1924–1925, was an influential figure in U.S. cardiology.[20]

Conner was chief of the Army Medical Corps Division of Internal Medicine, with the rank of major in 1917. He was involved in the selection and training of cardiovascular specialists whose responsibilities involved the interpretation and clarification of cardiovascular signs and symptoms, reconciling cardiovascular physical findings with the military criteria for fitness for duty. Later in the war, Conner represented the Surgeon General's office in the implementation of the first Cardiovascular Medicine Center at U.S. Army Hospital #9 at Lakewood, NJ.

Conner took "stock of what has been accomplished by all this elaborate effort" in the United States when he presented "Cardiac Diagnosis in the Light of Experiences With Army Physical Examinations" at the Association of American Physicians meeting in Atlantic City in June 1919. Clarification of the vague, preexisting cardiovascular physical examination standards and terminology was a major concern. His translation of the wartime lessons learned about cardiac diagnosis, the pathogenesis of cardiac disorders, functional disorders of the heart, and valvular heart disease, in particular mitral regurgitation, was directed to the problems physicians faced in civil life. Many of his observations and conclusions surfaced in his later publications and in his discussions of papers presented at the American Heart Association meetings.

During the U.S. experience in World War I, approximately 4 million young men were examined, when the incidence of cardiovascular defects was appreciable. Mitral valvular regurgitation (MVR) was the most frequent valve lesion and far exceeded all other valve lesions, individual or combined. The repetitive theme, that MVR is a common phenomenon, extends from World War I to the 1980s and has gained new clinical importance as we learn more about the natural history of the FMV, MVP, and MVR.

When we reviewed these data, we concluded that the prevalence of apical systolic murmurs and the diagnosis of MVR in young Americans during World War I parallels the prevalence of apical systolic murmurs and MVP among young men documented in the 1980s.[21]

1920–1939: Neurocirculatory Asthenia Between the Wars

During the two decades following World War I, earlier military experiences were summarized, after histories of symptomatic men from the military were developed, and NCA was identified and studied in the civilian population. Attention was directed away from the heart, and the idea of cardiac neurosis was widely presented and accepted. Paul Dudley White, a cardiologist with World War I military experience who also had worked with Thomas Lewis, and Mandel Cohen, a psychiatrist, began their remarkable NCA collaborative studies, which extended over several decades and involved classification, exercise testing, psychiatric evaluation, and follow-up studies.[22]

1941: World War II–DaCosta's Syndrome Revisited

The Mill Hill Center in England was the World War II successor to the World War I British Military Heart Hospital. The experience was notable for the collaboration of two eminent physicians, Paul Wood, a cardiologist, and Aubrey Lewis, a psychiatrist. Following an intense historical review, Wood performed an equally intense, year-long clinical analysis of 300 patients and resurrected the DaCosta's syndrome terminology. Wood concluded that the problem was really a psychosomatic pattern and not a distinct clinical entity, while Aubrey Lewis emphasized the psychiatric aspects of the effort syndrome.[23] Wood, an influential figure in postwar

British cardiology, relegated the matter in his widely read textbook to cardiovascular disturbances associated with psychiatric states.

1960–1970: Systolic Clicks, Late Systolic Murmurs and Mild Mitral Regurgitation

The mid-20th century, a period of incredible activity in cardiovascular diseases, was marked by sweeping changes in the clinical and basic areas as a result of the cardiovascular diagnostic and surgical era. Basic concepts in auscultation were challenged by diagnostic techniques that included external and intracardiac phonocardiography, cardiac catheterization, angiographic, and echocardiographic techniques. Precepts arising from the descriptive auscultation-pathologic correlate era were blended with newer methods of timing and correlating heart sounds and murmurs with multiple physiological or pathophysiological events.

During this time, mild mitral valvular regurgitation was established as the cause of apical mid- and late systolic murmurs, apical systolic clicks were recognized as nonejection clicks arising from the mitral valve apparatus, and these auscultatory findings were associated with billowing or prolapsing mitral leaflets. John Barlow of South Africa was a central figure during this and the next three decades. Certain of the historical events that preceded and succeeded these observations are outlined and discussed in Chapter 6.

1970–1980: The Floppy Mitral Valve, Mitral Valve Prolapse, and Mitral Valvular Regurgitation

There was a tremendous outpouring of information during the 1970s, extending into the 1980s. Although there were nosological differences, the MVP concept and terminology received wide usage and acceptance; during the 1970s, MVP became a universal phenomenon.

1980: Mitral Valve Prolapse Syndrome–Neuroendocrine and Autonomic Nervous System Mechanisms

From this point forward, the literature generally follows two pathways or themes: one segment deals with the FMV/MVP/MVR triad, while the other deals with the MVP syndrome, much the way we have outlined them in the classification chapter.

The concept of a syndrome comes from the Greek, "a set of symptoms which occur together; the sum of signs of any morbid state; a symptom complex. In genetics a combination of phenotypic manifestations."[24] The following chapter reviews the rationale for considering the MVP syndrome as a clinical entity.

The current interest in and controversy about the mitral valve prolapse syndrome results from the influences of recent brain–heart research on contemporary cardiology and neuropsychiatry, in particular the extensive research into cardiovascular neuroendocrinology and autonomic nervous system function and dysfunction, which is just beginning to have an impact on clinical cardiology.

References

1. Wooley CF. Palpitation: Brain, heart, and 'spirits' in the seventeenth century. J R Soc Med 91:157–160, 1998.
2. Willis R. The Works of William Harvey, MD. Translated from the Latin. London, Sydenham Society, 1843.
3. Foster M. Lectures on the History of Physiology During the Sixteenth, Seventeenth and Eighteenth Centuries. London, Cambridge University Press, 1907, pp 41–45.
4. Harvey W. Exercitatio anatomica De Motu Cordis et sanguinis in animalibus. Translated by Leake CD. Illinois, Charles C. Thomas, 1970, pp 39–48.
5. Lower R. Tractatus de Corde, Chap 2. London, 1669. (Translated by KJ Franklin) Alabama, Classics of Medicine Library, 1969.
6. Franklin KJ. Some notes on Richard Lower (1631–1692), and his De Corde, London 1669. Ann Med Hist 3:599–602, 1931.
7. The Evan Bedford Library of Cardiology: Catalogue of Books, Pamphlets and Journals. London, Royal College of Physicians, 1977, p 196.
8. Williams JC. Practical observations on nervous and sympathetic palpitation of the heart, particularly as distinguished from palpitations as the result of organic disease. London, Logman, Rees, Orme, Browne, 1836.
9. Wooley CF. From irritable heart to mitral valve prolapse: British army medical reports. Am J Cardiol 44:1107–1109, 1985.
10. Wooley CF. Jacob Mendez DaCosta - medical teacher, clinician and clinical investigator. Am J Cardiol 50:1145–1148, 1982.
11. DaCosta JM. On irritable heart. Am J Med Sci 61:17–52, 1871.
12. Wooley CF. From irritable heart to mitral valve prolapse: The Osler connection. Am J Cardiol 53:870–874, 1984.
13. Wooley CF. From irritable heart to mitral valve prolapse: Systolic clicks, apical murmurs and the auscultatory connection in the 19th century. Am Heart J 113:413–419, 1987.
14. Burnett J. The origins of the electrocardiograph as a clinical instrument. In Bynum WF, Lawrence C, Nutton V (eds): The Emergence of Modern Cardiology. Med History (Suppl 5):53–76 1985.
15. Wooley CF. From irritable heart to mitral valve prolapse: World War I, the British experience and James Mackenzie. Am J Cardiol 57:463–466, 1986.
16. Wooley CF. From irritable heart to mitral valve prolapse: World War I, the British experience and Clifford Allbutt. Am J Cardiol 59:353–357, 1987.
17. Lewis T. The Soldier's Heart and Effort Syndrome. London, Shaw, 1918.
18. Howell JD. Soldier's heart: The redefinition of heart disease and specialty formation in early twentieth-century Great Britain. In Bynum WF, Lawrence C, Nutton V (eds): The Emergence of Modern Cardiology. Med History (Suppl 5):34–52, 1985.

19. Wooley CF. From irritable heart to mitral valve prolapse: World War I, the U.S.
20. experience and the origin of neurocirculatory asthenia. Am J Cardiol 59:1183–1186, 1987.
21. Wooley CF, Schneider D, Lerner AA. Lewis Atterbury Conner. Appreciation and bibliography. Circulation 9:1449–1455, 1998.
22. Wooley CF, Boudoulas H. From irritable heart to mitral valve prolapse: World War I, the U.S. experience and the prevalence of apical systolic murmurs and mitral regurgitation in drafted men compared with present day mitral valve prolapse studies. Am J Cardiol 61:895–899, 1988.
23. Cohen ME, White PD. Neurocirculatory asthenia. Concept Mil Med 137:142, 1972.
24. Wood P. Diseases of the Heart and Circulation. Philadelphia, J.B. Lippincott, 1968, pp 1074–1084.
25. Dorland's Illustrated Medical Dictionary. Philadelphia, W.B. Saunders, 1965.

The Floppy Mitral Valve, Mitral Valve Prolapse and the Mitral Valve Prolapse Syndrome

Harisios Boudoulas, MD, PhD, Charles F. Wooley, MD

Introduction

Certain patients with the floppy mitral valve (FMV) and mitral valve prolapse (MVP) have symptoms that cannot be explained on the basis of valvular dysfunction alone.[1-14] Neuroendocrine-cardiovascular or autonomic nervous system function abnormalities have been postulated to explain the symptoms in this group of patients. At present, we classify these patients as FMV/MVP syndrome.

Whether there is a FMV/MVP syndrome, or whether a cardiac process (FMV/MVP) coexists with neuroendocrine abnormalities, autonomic dysfunction, or states of anxiety is controversial.[15-18] Our opinion, based on clinical experience, is that symptomatic patients with FMV/MVP without significant mitral valvular regurgitation (MVR) may manifest a constitutional, neuroendocrine-cardiovascular process resulting from a close, possibly genetic, relationship between FMV/MVP and centrally or peripherally mediated states of autonomic or neuroendocrine dysfunction or imbalance.

From: Boudoulas H, Wooley CF. *Mitral Valve: Floppy Mitral Valve, Mitral Valve Prolapse, Mitral Valvular Regurgitation.* Second revised edition. ©Futura Publishing Company, Armonk, NY, 2000.

Clinical Presentation

Symptoms in patients with FMV/MVP syndrome frequently occur against a background of acute or gradual increases in the physical or emotional stresses of life, quite often with a precipitating event such as trauma, an operation, an illness, marital separation or divorce, a demanding or stressful job, working two jobs, or an impending job change or loss. When the excessive use of caffeine, cigarettes, alcohol, chemical substances, or over-the-counter or prescription drugs is added to the above stresses, the sum contributes to symptoms in susceptible individuals.[1,2]

The true incidence of symptoms in patients with FMV/MVP syndrome is not known; the incidence of symptoms may be exaggerated because most of the studies have been performed in academic institutions and thus may reflect a selection bias.

When Savage and associates used echocardiographic criteria as evidence of MVP in an analysis of the Framingham Heart Study population,[15,16] they found that the incidence of chest pain, syncope, and atrial or ventricular arrhythmias in MVP was similar to those of the general population. However, there are major problems with interpretation of these studies. First, an extremely low proportion of patients with echocardiographic findings of the MVP had diagnostic ausculatory findings (approximately 10%). Second, a high proportion of the non-MVP control subjects had cardiac arrhythmias (17% supraventricular tachycardia and 40% complex ventricular arrhythmias). Thus, when compared with other MVP studies, the MVP group was different because of the very low evidence of auscultatory findings (i.e., patients probably did not have FMV), and the incidence of arrhythmias in the control group was much higher than that reported in a "normal" population.

Devereux et al.[17] also addressed this issue by studying all first-degree relatives of symptomatic MVP patients. Undiagnosed MVP was identified by echocardiography and physical examination in one-third of the relatives. The referred MVP patients had a higher incidence of symptoms than the undiagnosed MVP patients, and the entire MVP cohort had a significantly greater frequency of palpitations, documented arrhythmias, and chest pain than did non-MVP relatives. Bias in the data analysis, however, also constitutes a problem with this study. When symptomatic patients seeking medical care are excluded, the incidence of symptoms in the remainder of the patient population not seeking medical care will not be representative of the entire population with the disease.

The most common symptoms patients with FMV/MVP syndrome present are summarized in Table 1 and Figure 1. Patients with FMV/MVP syndrome may become symptomatic at any age, but in our experience the

Table 1
Floppy Mitral Valve/Mitral Valve Prolapse Syndrome:
Clinical Presentation

Chest pain	Postural phenomena
Palpitations	Orthostatic hypotension
Fatigue–exercise intolerance	Orthostatic tachycardia
Dyspnea	Orthostatic arrhythmias
Syncope–presyncope	Neuropsychiatric symptoms

greatest proportion of the patients became symptomatic in the second or third decades. As a general rule, female patients presented with more symptoms than males (Fig. 2).[1,9]

Chest Pain

As an initial complaint, chest pain occurred in approximately 50% of the men and in 35% of the women. Overall, chest pain was present in approximately 60% of the men and women. Several types of chest pain have been described (Table 2). The pain may be frequent and incapacitating. Patients may report precordial, brief, sharp, sticking sensations or intermittent recurrent pain without a consistent relationship to effort. This has led to characterizing the pain as "atypical" for myocardial ischemia. Some patients experience persistent substernal pressure or heaviness following moderate, brief and intense, or unusual physical exertion; this may persist for hours without rest-related relief. Some patients are able to continue their activities despite the pain; it may also disappear completely for months without treatment. In some patients with FMV/MVP syndrome, chest pain is often relieved in the supine posture.[1,2,19–25]

Initial or recurrent attacks of chest pain may result from emotional stress, trauma, or a surgical procedure. The cycle may begin without obvious reason, but it seems to occur more often in fatigue states. Certain patients describe pain similar to that of angina pectoris, and in some FMV/MVP patients, obstructive or vasoreactive coronary artery disease may be the basis for chest pain. The various types of chest pain, and the interrelationships between chest pain, fatigue, anxiety, arrhythmias, and stress are such that multiple observations and a variety of diagnostic tests may be necessary in individual situations in order to identify the patterns of pain or the settings in which pain occurs.

The cause of chest pain is multifactorial in patients with FMV/MVP syndrome (Table 3). It is well understood how fixed coronary artery steno-

Floppy Mitral Valve / Mitral Valve Prolapse Syndrome:
Initial Symptoms

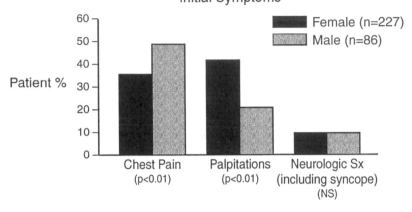

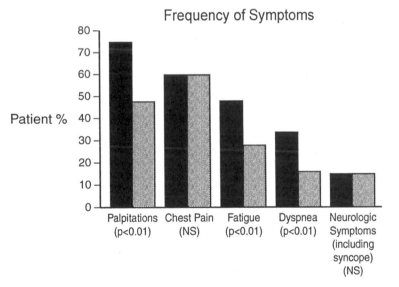

Figure 1. Initial symptoms and frequency of symptoms in patients with FMV/MVP syndrome. P values indicate differences between male and female; Sx = symptoms; NS = nonsignificant. (Used with permission from Boudoulas H, et al.[1])

Figure 2. Mean age of onset of symptoms and number of symptoms in patients with FMV/MVP syndrome. The number of symptoms was greater in female than in male patients. NS = nonsignificant. (Used with permission from Boudoulas H, et al.[1])

Table 2
Floppy Mitral Valve/Mitral Valve Prolapse Syndrome:
Characteristics of Chest Pain

Relationship to Effort–Precipitating Factors:
    Occurs more often in fatigue states
    Initial or recurrent attacks may result from emotional stress, trauma, or
        surgery
    No consistent relationship to effort
    Patient may continue activities despite the pain
    May be relieved in the supine position
    May disappear for months without treatment
Types of Chest Pain:
    Brief duration
    Recurrent
    Frequent–incapacitating
    May persists for hours
    Sharp
    Sticking sensations
    Precordial
    Substernal pressure or heaviness

Floppy Mitral Valve / Mitral Valve Prolapse Syndrome:
Mean Age of Onset of Symptoms.

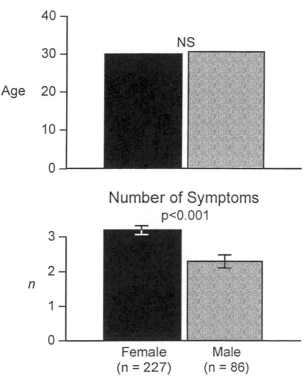

Table 3
Floppy Mitral Valve/Mitral Valve Prolapse Syndrome: Potential Mechanisms of Chest Pain

Valve and Support Apparatus
> Excessive chordae stretching–increased papillary muscle tension
> Inappropriate postural or stress-related tachycardia

Metabolic Causes
> Increased adrenergic tone
> Hyperresponse to adrenergic stimulation
> Excessive lactate production

Coronary Artery Vasoregulation
> Dynamic reduction of the coronary artery caliber
> Inadequate coronary vascular reserve
> Small coronary artery constriction
> Abnormal vasodilatory response

Aortic Pain

Noncardiovascular Origin
> Chest wall
> Esophageal dismotility
> Hyperventilation

Combination of the Above Factors

sis and thrombotic lesions can produce myocardial ischemia and chest pain. The dynamic reduction of the caliber of the coronary arteries or a decreased coronary vasodilatory reserve capacity under certain conditions may also result in myocardial ischemia and chest pain. This dynamic reduction of coronary artery caliber or an inadequate coronary vascular reserve flow capacity may be related to altered coronary arterial responsiveness or regulation. Thus, myocardial ischemia may be brought about by conditions that limit the potential for an increase in coronary flow.[1,2,26–30]

Excessive stretching of the chordae tendineae has been suggested as a possible mechanism for chest pain.[31] Increased tension of the chordae tendineae presumably causes forceful traction on the papillary muscles and the adjacent left ventricular (LV) wall, which may produce variations in papillary muscle and subendocardial blood flow and oxygen demand with resultant papillary muscle ischemia and chest pain (Fig. 3; see also Chapter 21).

Chest pain may be of aortic origin. Decreased aortic distensibility has been reported in certain patients with FMV/MVP. Abnormal elastic properties of the aorta may decrease coronary blood flow, while abnormal function of the aorta may result in chest pain due to aortic stretch (see Chapter 21).[27,28,32,33]

Subendocardial blood flow may be estimated from the diastolic pres-

Floppy Mitral Valve / Mitral Valve Prolapse

Abnormal Mitral Apparatus

↓

Mitral Leaflet Prolapse

↓

Papillary Muscle Traction
Activation of Stretch Receptors

↓

Papillary Muscle and
Subendocardial Ischemia

↓

Pain
Ventricular Arrhythmias

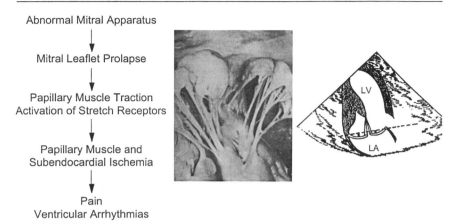

Figure 3. Postulated mechanisms for chest pain and ventricular arrhythmias related to papillary muscle traction and activation of stretch receptors. Floppy mitral valve is shown in the middle (From Edwards JE. Circulation 43:606–612, 1971). Papillary muscle traction during left ventricular (LV) systole is shown schematically. LA = left atrium.

sure time index (DPTI) and myocardial oxygen demand from the tension time index (TTI).[34] Ischemic response to sudden strenuous exercise has been reported in healthy persons when the DPTI:TTI ratio falls below 0.44. It is possible that FMV/MVP syndrome patients may have papillary muscle or subendocardial ischemia with even greater values of this ratio when tension on the papillary muscle and adjacent ventricular wall increases with the degree of prolapse.

Subendocardial blood flow is totally diastolic and thus depends on the duration of diastole (Fig. 4).[35] Inappropriate sinus tachycardia with excessive postural changes, physical and emotional stresses may occur in patients with FMV/MVP syndrome (Fig. 5). Sudden heart rate increases will produce disproportionately greater decreases in the diastolic time necessary for subendocardial flow than in systolic time because of a nonlinear relationship between heart rate and diastolic time (Fig. 6).[36] An increase in adrenergic tone may coexist in patients with FMV/MVP syndrome, which further increases myocardial oxygen consumption. A decrease in plasma volume associated with orthostatic hypotension may also play a role.[36–51]

Myocardial or subendocardial ischemia may occur because of combinations of these factors and may represent a final common pathway. This hypothesis would explain pain with tachycardia. Indeed, studies using rapid atrial pacing have shown myocardial lactate production with chest

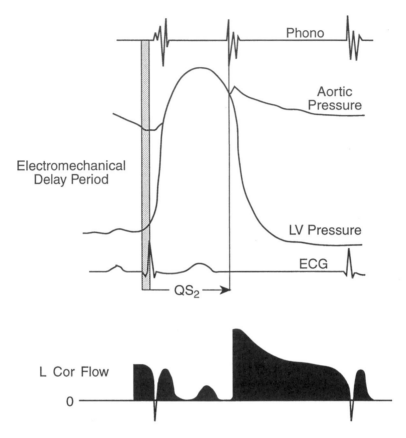

Figure 4. Schematic presentation of left coronary flow (L Cor Flow) in relationship to the cardiac cycle. The greatest proportion of coronary flow occurs in diastole. The cross-hatching represents the electromechanical delay. Phono = phonocardiogram; QS_2 = electromechanical systole; ECG = electrocardiogram. (Used with permission from Boudoulas H, et al.[35])

pain and ischemic electrocardiographic changes in certain patients with FMV/MVP syndrome and normal coronary arteries.[52] Isoproterenol infusions in patients with FMV/MVP syndrome induced chest pain in seven of the 16 patients studied.[38]

Coronary artery spasm has been suggested in a few patients with FMV/MVP syndrome. "Corkscrew" coronary arteries have been observed angiographically and are casually dismissed by angiographers;[53] however, these phenomena have not been intensively studied and their significance is yet uncertain. The coronary anatomy using intravascular ultrasound in patients with FMV/MVP syndrome has not been evaluated. At least one study suggested that congenital abnormalities of the coronary

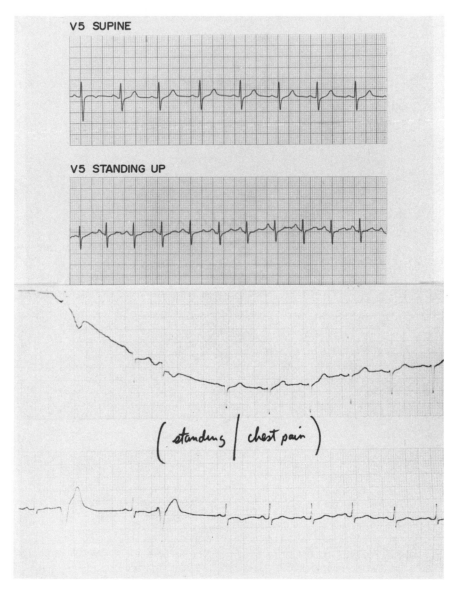

Figure 5. Upper panel. Electrocardiographic lead V_5 in a patient with floppy mitral valve/mitral valve prolapse syndrome (FMV/MVPS). Note the sinus tachycardia in the upright posture. Lower panel. Sinus tachycardia and premature ventricular beats in the upright posture in a patient with FMV/MVPS, at that time patient reported chest pain. (Used with permission from Boudoulas H, et al.[1])

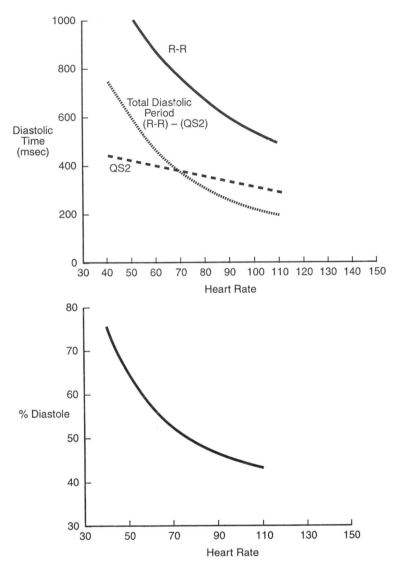

Figure 6. Relationship between heart rate, systolic time (QS$_2$), diastolic time, cardiac cycle (R-R) and % diastole. (Used with permission from Boudoulas H, et al.[36])

arteries in patients with MVP may be more frequent compared to general population.[30]

Excessive lactate production during daily physical activities or an increased adrenergic tone and hyperresponse to adrenergic stimulation may also contribute to the pathogenesis of chest pain. Finally, chest pain may be of extracardiac origin.[54,55]

Palpitations

As an initial symptom, palpitations occurred in approximately 40% of the women and in 20% of the men (Fig. 1), palpitations may be related to cardiac arrhythmias (Fig. 7; see also Chapter 16).[1,2] Arrhythmias may start with postural changes, decrease during exercise, and become more frequent after exercise (Fig. 8).[1,2] Ambulatory monitoring in these patients, however, often demonstrates a discordance between rhythm abnormalities and symptoms. Patients frequently record "palpitations" while in sinus tachycardia, and often fail to record symptoms when atrial or ventricular ectopy are present. The cause of palpitations in patients with FMV/MVP syndrome while in sinus rhythm is not completely understood. Abrupt, posturally induced changes in heart rate make the patients aware of their "heartbeat" and probably contribute to the pathogenesis of palpitations.

Fatigue

Overall, fatigue is present in approximately 50% of the women and in 30% of the men (Fig. 1).[1,2] Fatigue may be increased by exercise, but it is

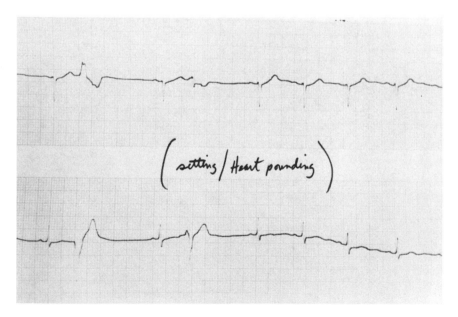

Figure 7. Sinus tachycardia and premature ventricular beats in a patient with floppy mitral valve/mitral valve prolapse syndrome. Patient reported "palpitations" and "heart pounding."" (Used with permission from Boudoulas H, et al.[1])

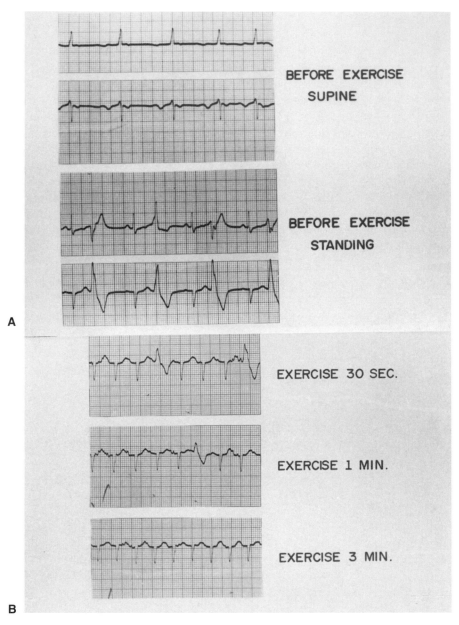

Figure 8. Electrocardiogram before (**A**), during (**B**) and after (**C**) exercise treadmill stress testing on a 35-year-old woman with floppy mitral valve/mitral valve prolapse syndrome. Note the frequent premature beats (PVBs) before and particularly immediately after exercise. PVBs were not present during exercise. (Used with permission from Boudoulas H, et al.[20]) Continued.

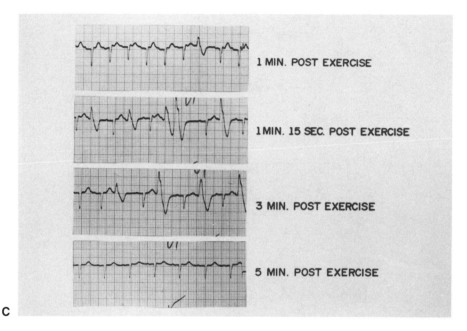

1 MIN. POST EXERCISE

1 MIN. 15 SEC. POST EXERCISE

3 MIN. POST EXERCISE

5 MIN. POST EXERCISE

C

Figure 8C. *(Continued)*

usually described as present to some degree at all times. The complaint is usually of "always feeling tired." Frequently a pattern develops in which fatigue results in a progressive decrease in activity and, thus, fatigue brings more fatigue. Exertional fatigue and asthenia are poorly understood. In postural exercise studies from our laboratory, control subjects exercised longer and achieved a greater workload in both supine and upright positions than the FMV/MVP syndrome patients. FMV/MVP syndrome patients consistently exhibited a smaller LV end-diastolic volume and cardiac output in the upright position when compared to the supine, and this difference was maintained throughout the exercise period (Fig. 9; see Chapter 21).[41] In contrast, the control subjects exhibited a fall in the LV end-diastolic volumes upright, but by the time peak exercise was achieved, the upright volumes were quite similar to the supine values. Other studies also suggested that MVP patients without MVR at rest may develop significant MVR with exercise.[56] These data provided an objective basis for the exercise intolerance in certain FMV/MVP syndrome patients, demonstrated that this intolerance may be accentuated in the upright position, and further suggested that the FMV/MVP syndrome patients' LV end-diastolic volumes remained inappropriately low during upright exercise.

Fatigue also is a common and nonspecific symptom of an underlying

Left ventricular end-diastolic volume index (LVEDVI) in the supine and upright posture, at rest and during exercise

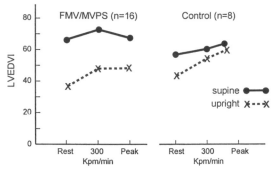

Cardiac index (CI) in the supine and upright posture, at rest and during exercise

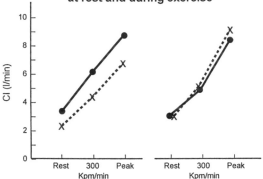

Ejection Fraction in the supine and upright posture, at rest and during exercise

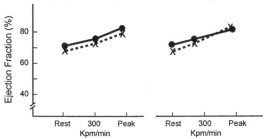

Figure 9. In normal subjects at rest, the left ventricular end-diastolic volume index (LVEDVI) in the upright posture was less compared to the supine position, but at peak exercise LVEDVI was similar in the supine and upright positions; in contrast, in patients with floppy mitral valve/mitral valve prolapse syndrome (FMV/MVPS), LVEDVI in the upright posture remained significantly less compared with the supine position throughout the exercise. Cardiac index in patients with FMV/MVPS was less in the upright posture compared with the supine position; in normal subjects cardiac index was similar in the supine and upright positions. Ejection fraction was similar in the supine and upright positions, in both control subjects and patients with FMV/MVPS.

630

physical or emotional disorder and can be conceptualized as one of two neurobiological emergency systems used by most higher organisms for self-preservation: the fight–flight response mediated through the sympathetic neuroendocrine system and the conservation–withdrawal response, characterized by a general dampening of metabolic and physical activity.[1,2,57] Common precipitating factors include physical or emotional crisis, physical exhaustion, diminished sleep, and disease. Thus, fatigue is more than a state of mind and may be associated with physiological alterations.

Dyspnea

Overall, dyspnea was noted in approximately 35% of women and in 15% of men (Fig. 1).[1,2] Patients often described the need to take an extraordinarily deep breath as dyspnea. Sighing respiration and frank hyperventilation may be observed during the examination of these patients. Dyspnea cannot be explained on the basis of overt cardiac or pulmonary abnormalities. Pulmonary function abnormalities have been described in patients with FMV/MVP syndrome but are not severe enough to explain the dyspnea.[58] Further, pulmonary function abnormalities were not demonstrated in patients with FMV/MVP syndrome and dyspnea. LV function and central hemodynamics are usually normal in FMV/MVP syndrome patients with dyspnea. The respiratory awareness and symptoms in patients with the FMV/MVP syndrome may represent alterations in centrally modulated breathing cycle control. These are areas for further investigation.

Syncope and Presyncope

Syncope or presyncope is a relatively common symptom in patients with FMV/MVP syndrome. The cause in certain patients with FMV/MVP syndrome is multifactorial (Table 4).[1,2] Arrhythmias may play some role in certain patients (Fig. 10), while orthostatic hypotension may also be responsible in certain patients with FMV/MVP syndrome.[59–84] Other factors such as dehydration, medications that impair circulatory responses, postural changes, and the metabolic abnormalities may also play a role. Increased adrenergic activity with decreased intravascular volume may also precipitate neurocardiogenic syncope. Syncope or presyncope, like palpitations, often correlates poorly with cardiac arrhythmias. A given arrhythmia, however, may not always produce the same symptoms, depending on the setting in which it occurs (e.g., supine versus upright position). Further, the occurrence of syncope related to activity may depend not only on the kind of activity but also on its level of intensity. Failing to consider these important factors is one of the major reasons for failure to establish cause–effect relationships in patients with syncope.

Table 4
Floppy Mitral Valve/Mitral Valve Prolapse Syndrome:
Potential Mechanisms of Syncope and Presyncope

Neurocardiogenic
Decreased intravascular volume
Postural phenomena
    Orthostatic tachycardia
    Orthostatic hypotension
    Orthostatic arrhythmias
    Orthostatic low ventricular volume
    Orthostatic increased mitral valve prolapse
    Prolapsing mitral valve may stimulate neurohormonal activation
    Development of "third" chamber
Arrhythmia
Sympathetic abnormality
Parasympathetic abnormality
Baroreflex modulation abnormality

Postural Phenomena

Patients with FMV/MVP syndrome often present with postural phenomena such as an orthostatic decrease in cardiac output, orthostatic hypotension, tachycardia, arrhythmias, and symptoms related to alterations in heart rate, blood pressure, and cardiac output.[41,48,63,65] Studies from our

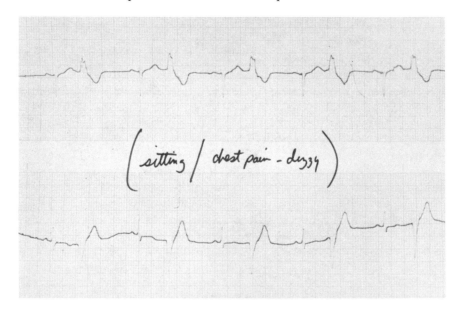

Figure 10. Ventricular bigeminy in a patient with floppy mitral valve/mitral valve prolapse syndrome. Patient reported dizziness and chest pain.

laboratory have shown that orthostatic changes in cardiac output, heart rate, and blood pressure in patients with FMV/MVP syndrome were greater than in controls.[41,47,73,85] The orthostatic changes in heart rate and blood pressure were exaggerated with intravascular volume depletion produced with furosemide administration (Fig. 11). Orthostatic phenomena may be multifactorial in origin (Table 5). A decreased intravascular volume, an abnormal renin–aldosterone response to volume depletion, a baroreflex modulation abnormality, a hyperadrenergic state, or a

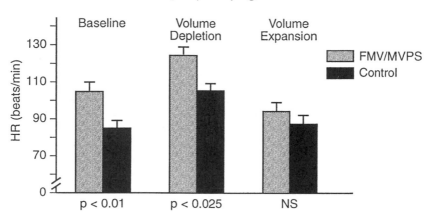

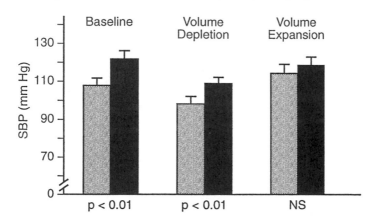

Figure 11. Heart rate (upper panel) and blood pressure (lower panel) in the upright position in patients with floppy mitral valve/mitral valve prolapse syndrome (FMV/MVPS). Note that orthostatic changes are exaggerated after volume depletion and are blunted after volume expansion. NS = nonsignificant.

Table 5
Floppy Mitral Valve/Mitral Valve Prolapse Syndrome:
Potential Mechanisms of Postural Phenomena

Decreased intravascular volume
Decreased left ventricular diastolic volume in the upright posture
Increased mitral valve prolapse in the upright posture
Prolapsing mitral valve may stimulate neurohormonal activation
Development of "third" chamber
Renin-aldosterone regulation abnormality
Hyperadrenergic state
Parasympathetic abnormality
Baroreflex modulation abnormality
Orthostatic hypotension, tachycardia, and cardiac arrhythmias

parasympathetic response abnormality may partially account for these phenomena. Further, the development of the third chamber between mitral valve annulus and the prolapsing mitral valve leaflet(s), especially in the upright position, the inability of patients with FMV/MVP syndrome to maintain normal LV diastolic volume in the upright position are also important factors and may contribute to orthostatic changes (see also Chapter 21).

Neuropsychiatric Symptoms

A consistent finding in many clinical studies of patients with FMV/MVP syndrome has been the high incidence of anxiety, panic attacks, and other complaints that are considered to be neuropsychiatric symptoms.[1,2] Further, the incidence of FMV/MVP is greater in patients with conditions associated with autonomic dysfunction (Table 6).[86–101] Thus, FMV/MVP syndrome was present in 38% of a group of patients with panic disorders, in 40% with agoraphobia, in 35% with mixed disorders presenting with anxiety attacks, in many patients with migraine

Table 6
Floppy Mitral Valve/Mitral Valve Prolapse Syndrome:
High Incidence in Conditions Associated with Autonomic Dysfunction

Panic disorders	Migraine headache
Agoraphobia	Primary sleep disorders
Anxiety	Anorexia nervosa

headache, and in 20% to 50% with primary disorders of sleep. The relationship between FMV/MVP and anxiety disorders remains something of an enigma, however; other studies have showed no association of FMV/MVP in patients with anxiety disorders, questioned the basis for the diagnosis of MVP in the earlier studies, and concluded that MVP and neurosis are independent conditions.[102–104] In some patients with FMV/MVP syndrome, neuropsychiatric symptoms may be related to increased plasma lactate levels or to a hyperadrenergic state.

Metabolic–Neuroendocrine Abnormalities/Pathogenesis of Symptoms in Floppy Mitral Valve/Mitral Valve Prolapse Syndrome

Metabolic–Neuroendocrine Abnormalities

From the symptoms described above, it is obvious that certain patients with FMV/MVP syndrome present with a symptom complex that suggests a hyperadrenergic state, autonomic dysfunction, metabolic disturbances, or a combination thereof. Metabolic and neuroendocrine abnormalities in patients with FMV/MVP syndrome have been reported from our institution and other laboratories and are summarized in Table 7.[1,2]

FMV/MVP syndrome patients studied in the Clinical Research Center in our institution had normal thyroid function tests, normal plasma cortisol, normal diurnal variation of cortisol, normal excretion of 24-hour urinary 17-ketosteroids and 17-hydroxycorticosteroids, and normal response to oral glucose although the glucose and insulin levels were higher than those of control patients (Fig. 12).[37]

Table 7
Floppy Mitral Valve/Mitral Valve Prolapse Syndrome: Metabolic-Neuroendocrine Abnormalities

High catecholamines
Catecholamine regulation abnormality
Hyperresponse to adrenergic stimulation
Parasympathetic abnormality
Baroreflex modulation abnormality
Renin-aldosterone regulation abnormality
Decreased intravascular volume
Decreased left ventricular diastolic volume in the upright posture
Atrial natriuretic factor secretion abnormality

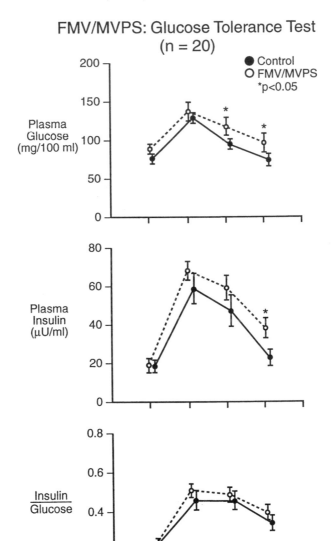

Figure 12. Patients with floppy mitral valve/mitral valve prolapse syndrome (FMV/MVPS) had a normal response to oral glucose administration, but higher glucose and insulin levels than those of controls. (Used with permission from Boudoulas H, et al.[37])

These FMV/MVP syndrome patients also had higher 24-hour urinary epinephrine (E) and norepinephrine (NE) excretion compared with normal controls (Fig. 13).[37] In addition, the frequency of premature ventricular beats (PVBs) detected by ambulatory monitoring paralleled urinary catecholamine excretion; both PVBs and urinary E and NE decreased significantly during the night. When 24-hour urine E and NE were measured for 3 consecutive days, there was no day-to-day variability in these values.[37]

Plasma E and NE at rest were also higher in patients with FMV/MVP syndrome compared with controls. Plasma E and NE increased after exercise in FMV/MVP syndrome patients and in controls, but plasma levels after exercise were not different in FMV/MVP syndrome compared with controls (Fig. 14). However, plasma E plus NE increase was greater in patients whose number of PVBs with exercise increased more than 10 per minute compared with patients in whom the frequency of PVBs remained relatively unchanged.[37]

Pasternac et al. also demonstrated that MVP syndrome patients had higher total plasma catecholamine levels and NE levels when compared with normal subjects, both in the supine and upright positions. When plasma catecholamines were measured in the same patients 6 years later, the catecholamine levels were similar in both measurements.[105]

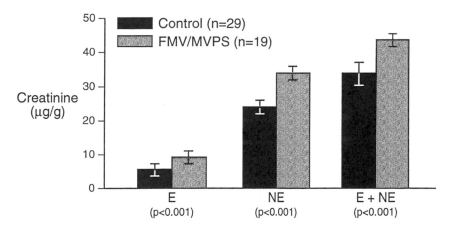

FMV/MVPS: 24 Hour Urinary Epinephrine (E) and Norepinephrine (NE) Excretion

Figure 13. Twenty-four-hour urinary epinephrine (E) and norepinephrine (NE) excretion. Patients with floppy mitral valve/mitral valve prolapse syndrome (FMV/MVPS) had higher levels than normal controls. (Used with permission from Boudoulas H, et al.[37])

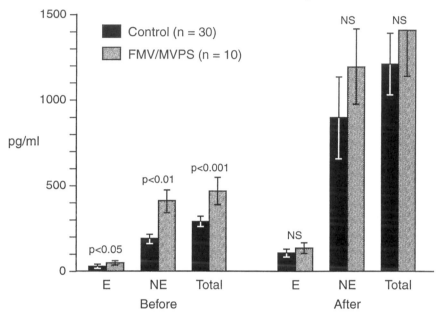

Plasma Epinephrine (E), Norepinephrine (NE) and Total Plasma Catecholamines Before and Immediately After Exercise

Figure 14. Plasma epinephrine (E), norepinephrine (NE), and total plasma catecholamines (total) before exercise were significantly higher in patients with floppy mitral valve/mitral valve prolapse syndrome (FMV/MVPS) than in control subjects but were not statistically different immediately after exercise. NS = nonsignificant. (Used with permission from Boudoulas H, et al.[38])

Studies in patients with coronary artery disease demonstrated that increased urinary catecholamine excretion was associated with a shorter total electromechanical systole corrected for heart rate (QS_2I), while isoproterenol infusion in normal subjects produced an abbreviation of the QS_2I. Patients with FMV/MVP syndrome had a shorter QS_2I compared with normals; this provided further evidence of increased adrenergic activity.[49]

Young women with FMV/MVP syndrome who were subjected to changes in intravascular volume were then studied in the recumbent and upright positions, and demonstrated that volume expansion with normal saline failed to suppress plasma catecholamines in FMV/MVP syndrome patients when compared with controls in both the supine and upright positions, suggesting a disorder of catecholamine regulation (Fig. 15).[47]

Increased adrenergic tone in patients with FMV/MVP/MVP syndrome prompted a study of adrenergic stimulation response. During isoproterenol infusion, none of the control subjects developed symptoms, ex-

Plasma Epinephrine (E) and Norepinephrine (NE) in Patients with FMV/MVPS
and in Control Subjects Before and After Volume Expansion

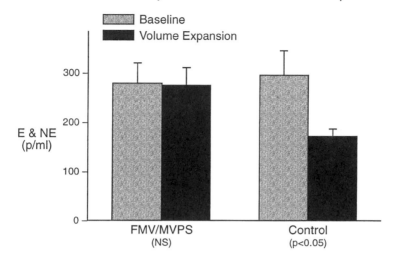

Figure 15. Plasma E + NE decreased significantly in control subjects after volume expansion. In contrast, plasma E + NE remained unchanged after volume expansion in patients with floppy mitral valve/mitral valve prolapse syndrome (FMV/MVPS). NS = nonsignificant.

cluding palpitations. Conversely, isoproterenol infusion reproduced symptoms in patients with FMV/MVP syndrome on a dose-related basis. During isoproterenol infusion 3 of 16 patients developed symptoms with 0.5 μg/min of isoproterenol infusion, 5 of 13 patients developed symptoms with 1.0 μg/min of isoproterenol infusion, and 9 of 11 patients developed symptoms with 2.0 μg/min of isoproterenol infusion. The symptoms related to isoproterenol infusion included chest pain in 7 patients, extreme postinfusion fatigue in 6 patients, dyspnea in 6 patients, dizziness in 4 patients, and panic attacks in 2 patients. Four patients had cool hands during isoproterenol infusion.[38]

The increase in heart rate during isoproterenol infusion was significantly greater in patients with FMV/MVP syndrome compared with controls and was dose related, whereas the baseline heart rate was not significantly different between FMV/MVP syndrome patients and control subjects (Figs. 16 and 17). Changes in pulse pressure were also dose related but similar in both FMV/MVP syndrome patients and in controls.[38]

Diastolic time per beat and per minute decreased significantly in both groups (FMV/MVP syndrome and control subjects) during isoproterenol infusion.[38] Diastolic time has a nonlinear relationship with heart rate. Thus, small changes in heart rate will result in significant changes in dias-

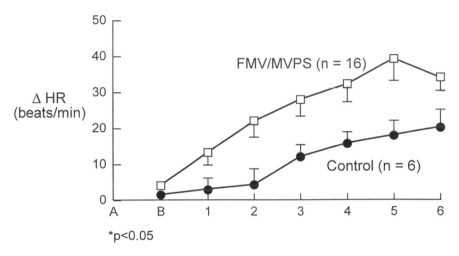

Figure 16. Changes in heart rate during isoproterenol infusions in patients with floppy mitral valve (FMV), mitral valve prolapse syndrome (MVPS), and normal subjects. Note that at any particular time during the infusion, heart rate was faster in FMV/MVP syndrome patients compared to control subjects.

tolic time (Fig. 6).[36] However, the decrease in diastolic time with isoproterenol infusion was significantly greater in FMV/MVP syndrome patients than the decrease in controls (Fig. 18) because of a greater increase in heart rate. Under certain circumstances these changes in diastolic time may be of clinical significance because the greater proportion of coronary blood flow occurs in diastole and subendocardial flow is almost totally diastolic. Spontaneous, inappropriate sinus or ectopic tachycardia in patients with FMV/MVP syndrome results in a significant decrease in diastolic time, which under certain conditions may produce subendocardial ischemia.

The duration of electrical systole (QT) in normal subjects is shorter and parallels the duration of electromechanical systole (QS_2) throughout the normal range of resting heart rate (Fig. 19).[106,107] The QT–QS_2 interval represents a basic cardiac electrical mechanical relation; synchrony or parallel behavior appears to be a normal phenomenon while asynchrony is abnormal. Changes in QT–QS_2 relationship during isoproterenol infusions were dose related both in FMV/MVP syndrome patients and in control subjects. Isoproterenol infusion resulted in a QT prolongation relative to QS_2 ($QT > QS_2$) in FMV/MVP syndrome and in controls, but the relative QT prolongation in relation to QS_2 (QT minus QS_2 interval) was

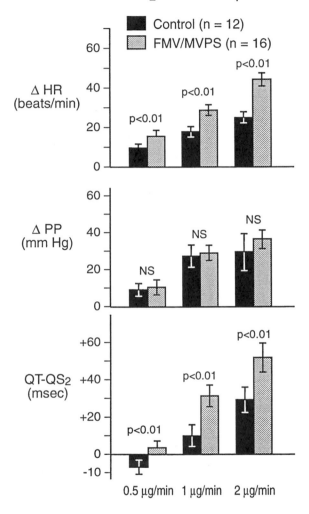

Figure 17. Effect of isoproterenol infusions on heart rate (HR), pulse pressure (PP), and in the relation between electrical (QT) and electromechanical systole (QS$_2$). Changes (Δ) in HR and QT minus QS$_2$ (QT-QS$_2$) with each isoproterenol infusions were significantly greater in patients with floppy mitral valve/mitral valve prolapse (FMV/MVPS) than in control subjects; changes in PP were not different in patients with FMV/MVPS compared with control subjects. NS = nonsignificant. (Used with permission from Boudoulas H, et al.[38])

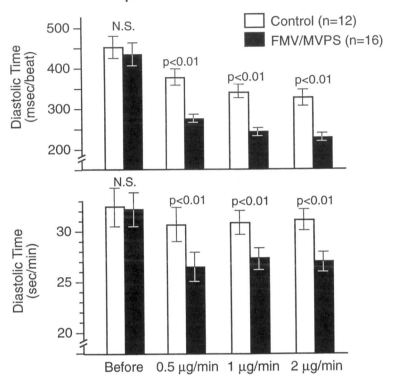

Figure 18. Effect of isoproterenol infusions on diastolic time per beat (upper panel) and per minute (lower panel). The decrease in diastolic time with each isoproterenol infusion was significantly greater in patients with floppy mitral valve/mitral valve prolapse syndrome (FMV/MVPS) than in normal controls. (Used with permission from Boudoulas H, et al.[38])

significantly greater in FMV/MVP syndrome compared with controls (Figs. 17 and 20).[38] This is an interesting observation because this electrical–mechanical asynchrony may be related to the production or occurrence of arrhythmias. Spontaneous transient appropriate or inappropriate increases of catecholamines during daily activities in patients with FMV/MVP syndrome may produce transient $QT > QS_2$. Hyperresponse to adrenergic stimulation has been attributed to altered β-adrenergic receptor coupling to adenylate cyclase. Studies have shown that at rest, the proportion of receptors binding to agonist with high affinity was greater in the MVP subjects compared to controls, even though receptor number was similar in the two groups. The increase in high-affinity receptors in

Relationship Between Electrical Systole (QT) Electromechanical Systole (QS2) and Heart Rate

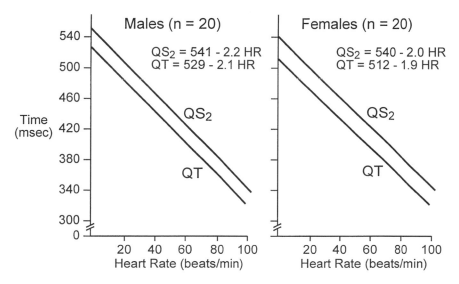

Figure 19. Regression lines of electrical systole (QT) and electromechanical systole (QS$_2$) in 20 males and 20 females. (Used with permission from Boudoulas H, et al.[106])

MVP was associated with greater cyclic AMP production due to isoproterenol stimulation compared to controls. During exercise, however, the β-adrenergic receptor function was similar in the two groups. Thus, MVP subjects are not at increased risk for hyperadrenergic symptoms during exercise.[39,44–46]

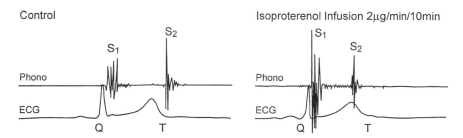

Figure 20. Electrical systole (QT) and electromechanical systole (QS$_2$) before (left) and during isoproterenol infusion (right). Phono = phonocardiogram; ECG = electrocardiogram; S$_1$ = first heart sound; S$_2$ = second heart sound. (Used with permission from Boudoulas H, et al.[51])

Coghlan et al.[42] studied heart rate and blood pressure response to a standardized Valsalva maneuver and postural test in MVP syndrome patients. The directional change of blood pressure and heart rate were similar in MVP syndrome patients and in controls during the Valsalva maneuver and postural test. However, MVP syndrome patients had exaggerated and prolonged bradycardia during the recovery phase of the Valsalva maneuver and following their return to recumbency in the posture test when compared with controls. This bradycardia persisted for 30 to 90 seconds after blood pressure returned to control values. In addition, patients with MVP syndrome had a greater heart rate increase and a widely oscillating heart rate during upright posture compared to controls. From these findings, it was postulated that an abnormal central modulation of baroreflexes was present in MVP syndrome patients. Reflex baroreceptor abnormality in patients with MVP syndrome was also reported from our laboratory (Fig. 21).[73]

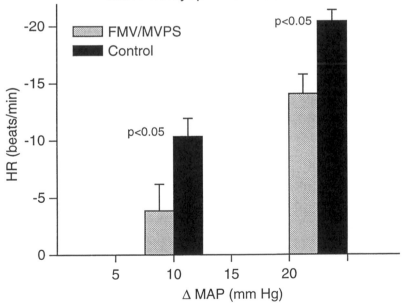

Changes in Heart Rate (HR) and Mean Arterial Pressure (MAP) in Patients with FMV/MVPS and in Control Subjects with Phenlyephrine Infusion.

Figure 21. Changes (decrease) in heart rate were significantly greater in patients with floppy mitral valve/mitral valve prolapse syndrome (FMV/MVPS) than in normal controls, while changes in mean arterial pressure in response to phenlyephrine infusions were similar in both groups.

Gaffney et al.,[40,43] found that heart rate responses to the diving reflex and to phenylephrine infusion were diminished in patients with MVP compared with controls. During lower body negative pressure, patients with MVP had significantly less venous pooling of blood in the legs but greater arterial vasoconstriction compared with normals. They concluded that the autonomic dysfunction in patients with MVP syndrome involves both the sympathetic and the parasympathetic nervous system. These autonomic abnormalities may be a result of defective sensing, inadequate central processing and output, or altered end-organ responsiveness, with or without underlying structural abnormalities of the nervous system.

Pasternac et al.[105] studied patients with MVP syndrome and demonstrated a lower heart rate compared with normal controls in the supine position but the heart rate returned to normal in the upright position. The same patients had higher resting catecholamine levels compared with controls. It was their conclusion that patients with MVP syndrome have increased resting sympathetic tone, and that the associated supine bradycardia suggested that increased vagal tone might also be present at rest.

Other studies from this and other laboratories in FMV/MVP syndrome patients have shown decreased intravascular volume. In addition, patients with FMV/MVP syndrome consistently exhibited a smaller LV end-diastolic volume and cardiac output in the upright position when compared with the supine, and this difference was maintained throughout the exercise period (Fig. 9). There was no difference in the ejection fraction in the upright when compared with the supine position both in FMV/MVP syndrome patients and in controls at rest and during exercise.[41,48]

Plasma renin activity in patients with FMV/MVP syndrome was inappropriately low for the decreased intravascular volume. Further decreases in intravascular volume with furosemide administration produced subnormal renin and aldosterone responses in FMV/MVP syndrome patients compared with controls (Fig. 22).[83,85,108]

Twenty-four-hour urinary sodium excretion was lower in patients with FMV/MVP syndrome compared with controls. There was an inverse correlation between urinary NE and urinary sodium excretion for patients with FMV/MVP syndrome but not for controls (Fig. 23).[38] An inverse relation between sodium intake and urinary catecholamines has been reported previously. The 24-hour sodium excretion was not significantly different in the study patients from day to day during the hospitalization. Serum sodium in patients with FMV/MVP syndrome was within normal limits; serum potassium, however, in most instances was in the low-normal range (Fig. 24).[38] This low serum potassium may be related to high catecholamines.

Plasma Aldosterone (Aldo) After Volume Depletion

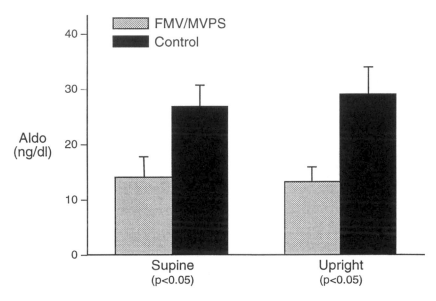

Figure 22. Plasma aldosterone after volume depletion was significantly lower in patients with floppy mitral valve/mitral valve prolapse syndrome (FMV/MVPS) than in control subjects in the supine and upright positions.

Relationship Between Urinary Norepinephrine (NE) and Sodium Excretion

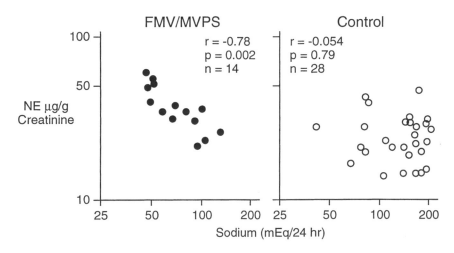

Figure 23. An inverse relation was present between 24-hour urinary NE and sodium excretion in patients with floppy mitral valve/mitral valve prolapse syndrome (FMV/MVPS) but not in control subjects. (Used with permission from Boudoulas H, et al.[38])

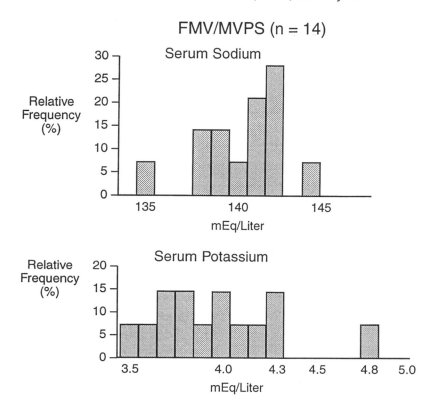

Figure 24. Upper panel: Serum sodium in patients with floppy mitral valve/mitral valve prolapse syndrome (FMV/MVPS) was within normal limits. Lower panel: Serum potassium in patients with FMV/MVPS was in the lower normal limits. (Used with permission from Boudoulas H, et al.[1])

Pathogenesis of Symptoms

The pathogenesis of symptoms in patients with FMV/MVP syndrome is not completely understood, but it appears to be multifactorial, possibly related to autonomic dysfunction, altered cardiac reactivity, and increased papillary muscle tension.[31,109] Increased papillary muscle stretch in patients with FMV/MVP may also play a role in the development of certain arrhythmias and in the pathogenesis of chest pain (see also Chapter 21).

The increased adrenergic activity, catecholamine regulation abnormality, and adrenergic hyperresponsiveness observed in certain patients with FMV/MVP syndrome suggest that some symptoms may be catecholamine related or mediated. Altered vagal tone, adrenergic receptor activity, or baroreceptor activity may also play a role in the pathogenesis of symptoms in certain patients with FMV/MVP syndrome. These mechanisms may result from primary autonomic nervous system disorders, while the heart and the cardiovascular system may be considered as target organs (Fig. 25).[1]

The observations that patients with FMV/MVP syndrome have low intravascular volume and a subnormal increase in renin and aldosterone with volume depletion may explain why certain patients with FMV/MVP syndrome may be more susceptible to volume depletion in clinical settings such as acute illness, the use of diuretics, dehydration from vigorous physical activity, and operative or trauma blood loss. The further contraction of plasma volume under these circumstances may be poorly tolerated because of the already decreased plasma volumes observed in the baseline state. The cyclical volume changes that occur in menstruating females and the protracted volume changes present in pregnant females may produce modifications in the sense of well-being or in symptoms that are related to these mechanisms.

There are several possible explanations for the observed intravascular volume, catecholamine, renin, and aldosterone abnormalities. Increased NE appears to be an appropriate response to low intravascular volume. However, the inability to suppress plasma NE after volume expansion in certain patients with FMV/MVP syndrome suggests an abnormal regulation of intravascular volume. Further, a subnormal renin and aldosterone increase after volume depletion despite a normal increase of plasma norepinephrine suggests a defective recognition of intravascular volume or a renin-receptor abnormality. It also seems reasonable to hypothesize that in certain patients with FMV/MVP syndrome, an inappropriate secretion of atrial natriuretic factors may contribute to the pathogenesis of symptoms.[1,110]

Papillary muscle traction in FMV/MVP may also be responsible for cardiac arrhythmias. Membrane depolarization is caused by both gradual and rapid ventricular stretch, but premature ventricular depolarizations are more readily elicited by rapid stretch. Recent studies have demonstrated the existence of stretch-activated membrane channels in ventricular myocardium; these may contribute to ventricular ectopy under conditions of differential ventricular loading as in FMV/MVP.[31,64,109]

FMV, when prolapsing into the left atrium, occupies part of the left atrial (LA) cavity, the degree of which depends on the severity of mitral leaflet prolapse and the size of mitral valve leaflets (Fig. 26). Because of the prolapse of the mitral valve leaflet(s), a new cavity develops between the mitral annulus and the prolapsing mitral valve leaflet(s) during LV systole.[111] Thus, in cases of MVP, even without MVR, during LV systole, a certain amount of blood occupies the space between the mitral annulus and the mitral valve leaflets (the third chamber), prolapsing into the left

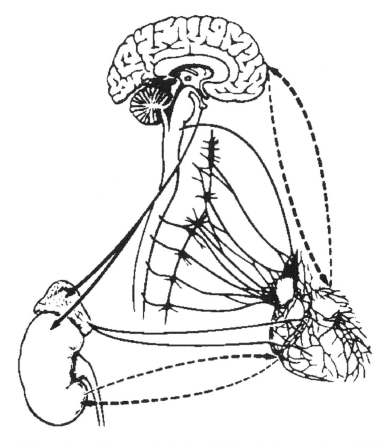

Figure 25. Symptoms in floppy mitral valve (FMV), mitral valve prolapse (MVP syndrome cannot be explained on the basis of valvular abnormalities alone and result from various forms of neuroendocrine or autonomic dysfunction present in certain patients with FMV/MVP. (Used with permission from Boudoulas H, et al.[1])

atrium. In severe prolapse, the amount of blood may represent a large amount of the total stroke volume, resulting in a significant decrease of the effective stroke volume. The degree of prolapse increases in the upright posture. This may result in a greater decrease in effective stroke volume and forward cardiac output. Decreased cardiac output may explain fatigue and exercise intolerance in certain patients with FMV/MVP syndrome.

Human cardiac valves have distinct patterns of innervation that comprise both primary sensory and autonomic components.[64,112,113] The presence of distinct nerve terminals suggests a neural basis for interactions between the central nervous system and the mitral valve. The subendocardial surface on the atrial aspect at the middle portion of the mi-

Floppy Mitral Valve/Mitral Valve Prolapse: Cardiac Arrhythmias

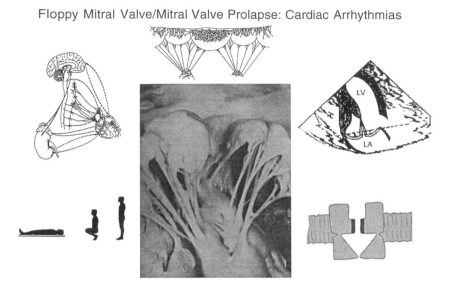

Figure 26. Left: The prolapsing mitral valve becomes a space-occupying lesion of the left atrial chamber and may stimulate neurohormonal activation. Floppy mitral valve is shown in the middle (from Edwards JE. 43:606–612, 1971); above the mitral valve innervation of the mitral valve is shown schematically; upper right shows papillary muscle traction during left ventricular (LV) systole; lower right stretch-activated receptor is shown schematically. Left upper panel shows schematically interactions between the brain-heart-kidneys and adrenals. Lower left shows schematically orthostatic phenomena (from Boudoulas H, et al.[64]).

tral valve is rich in nerve endings, including afferent nerves; mechanical stimuli from this area caused by abnormal coaptation in FMV/MVP may cause an abnormal autonomic nerve feedback between the central nervous system and mitral valve nervous system (see also Chapter 21).

The pathophysiological consequences of mitral valve apparatus function and dysfunction in FMV/MVP are not completely understood at present. Certainly, prolapsing mitral valve leaflet(s) resulting in occupation of LA space, papillary muscle traction, activation of stretch receptors and development of a third chamber between the mitral annulus and prolapsing mitral valve leaflet(s), contribute significantly to the clinical picture of FMV/MVP and FMV/MVP syndrome and also influence the natural history of the disease. Future research will help to better define these incompletely understood complex phenomena related to function or dysfunction of mitral valve apparatus.

Lactate infusion in patients with anxiety has produced symptoms similar to those associated with the FMV/MVP syndrome.[54] This occurred when serum lactate was raised to levels approximating those associated with exercise or other physiological stress. In other studies, plasma lactate elevations were found to be excessive in patients with "neurocirculatory asthenia."[1,54] The symptoms induced with lactate infusion persist for several hours. Thus, it is possible that some of the symptoms in patients with FMV/MVP syndrome may be related to excess plasma lactate production during daily activities.

The relationship between FMV/MVP and the constellation of symptoms that we currently refer to as the FMV/MVP syndrome requires further definition. It appears that FMV/MVP represents a spectrum of manifestations that range from the asymptomatic normal variant mitral valve to significant valvular abnormalities with progression to severe MVR.

Diagnostic Evaluation

The diagnosis of FMV/MVP syndrome is based on the presence of FMV/MVP plus the associated symptom complex. It is apparent that the diagnostic evaluation of patients with FMV/MVP syndrome will lead clinicians into areas of neuroendocrinology, neuropsychiatry, neurocirculatory control, cardiovascular metabolic determinants, and autonomic nervous system function, which in turn will require the development of new methods and approaches to traditional problem solving. Suffice it to say, our own approach has been to believe the patient's descriptions of symptoms and events, to investigate the underlying mechanisms as far as possible with current technology and traditional problem-solving methods, and to avoid the ritualistic reassurance that physicians frequently invoke when faced with puzzling clinical phenomena and armed with minimal data.

Chest Pain

Evaluating chest pain in FMV/MVP syndrome patients requires clinical judgment and common sense. The patient's age, sex, and family history require proper consideration, as do other possible contributing factors. Atypical chest pain in the young patient with FMV/MVP is an enigma. Currently, our diagnostic armamentarium is limited by a poor understanding of its pathophysiology and an inability to ask the correct questions. Typical anginal chest pain in a FMV/MVP patient usually requires further evaluation.

Since the therapy and prognosis of the patient with FMV/MVP-associated chest pain may be quite different from those in patients whose chest pain is related to obstructive coronary artery disease or other forms of myocardial or valvular disease, the recognition, differentiation, definition, or

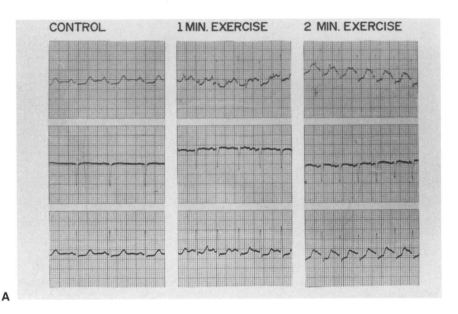

CONTROL   1 MIN. EXERCISE   2 MIN. EXERCISE

A

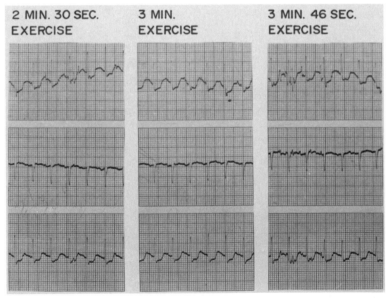

2 MIN. 30 SEC. EXERCISE   3 MIN. EXERCISE   3 MIN. 46 SEC. EXERCISE

B

Figure 27. Electrocardiogram before, during, and after exercise treadmill testing on a 48-year-old woman with floppy mitral valve/mitral valve prolapse syndrome. Note the ST segment depression during and after exercise. Patient had normal coronary arteries. (Used with permission from Boudoulas H, et al.[20]) Continued.

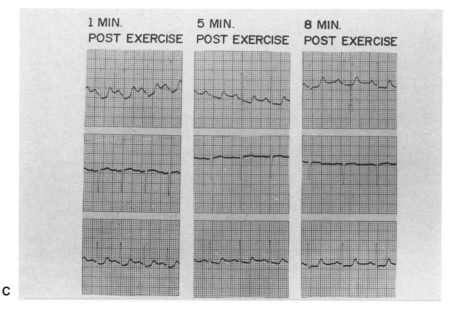

Figure 27C. *(Continued)*

coexistence of these entities is critical. The resting electrocardiogram (ECG) and the results of exercise testing are not specific discriminators; resting or posture-related ECG abnormalities are common in FMV/MVP syndrome patients. The spectrum of ECG changes may be similar to those observed in coronary artery or myocardial disease, including nonspecific ST and T wave changes, inverted T waves in inferior leads, or diffuse T wave inversion. Spontaneous ECG changes may be noted, particularly with postural intervention. ST segment wave changes during exercise have been reported that are not always associated with the presence of chest pain. A high incidence of "false positives" ECG exercise stress tests with ST segment depressions greater than 2 mm have been reported in patients with FMV/MVP syndrome (Fig. 27).[20] Thus, ECG exercise responses must be interpreted with care. Although propranolol administration has been reported to normalize exercise-induced ECG changes in FMV/MVP syndrome patients with normal coronary arteries, similar effects have also been reported in patients with coronary artery disease.[114–118]

Thallium-201 myocardial imaging and exercise radionuclide angiography are frequently normal in patients with FMV/MVP syndrome and normal coronary arteries; however, exceptions have been reported. Thus, within the limits of the tests, a normal exercise myocardial imaging or exercise radionuclide study may be considered as evidence against the coexistence of coronary artery disease in the presence of FMV/MVP syndrome.[119] Stress echocardiography may also provide important information. Data, however, in patients with FMV/MVP are not available. It must be emphasized that in certain situations where the diagnosis is uncertain, coronary arteriography may be necessary to diagnose or exclude coronary artery disease.

Palpitations

The differential diagnosis of palpitations involves arrhythmia detection and definition. The diagnostic evaluation of arrhythmias is presented in Chapter 16.

Dyspnea

When patients with FMV/MVP syndrome present with dyspnea, cardiac or pulmonary causes of this symptom should be excluded.

Fatigue

Fatigue is a nonspecific symptom and its presence is often a cause of concern for both patients and physicians. The first step for the evaluation of fatigue is to separate organic from psychological causes. This is accomplished best by carefully defining the chief complaint. For example, fever, cough, or weight loss should suggest specific diagnoses. A careful exploration of hematopoietic, endocrine, renal disorders, or chronic infection may reveal important clues to the diagnosis. For the patient who is simply fatigued without other complaints, a thorough social history will be very useful. Conscientious, compulsive, or driven individuals who are engaged in multiple activities or quests beyond their capabilities frequently require and benefit from mature counseling and advice about life activities. Certain clinical descriptions of fatigue, such as fatigue that is greatest in the morning and decreases in the afternoon, favors psychological causes. Certain drugs and physical and emotional stress may produce fatigue. The laboratory evaluation should be guided by positive findings in the history and physical examination.

Syncope and Presyncope

These are among the most difficult symptoms to evaluate.[60,72] While syncope is not associated with severe circulatory disease or a poor prognosis in many patients, in others it may be a harbinger of sudden death. As an initial approach to the diagnosis, it is essential to investigate and identify the basic mechanisms: neurocardiogenic, cardiac, and unknown. Clearly the evaluation of syncope utilizing these basic clinical steps must be rooted in a thorough knowledge of the various causes of syncope. Based on these findings, further evaluation is predicated on one's estimation of mortality and morbidity risk. In patients considered at high risk (cardiac arrhythmias), the diagnosis should be pursued via appropriate noninvasive and invasive testing. While cost effectiveness should be practiced in diagnosis, this should not minimize the need for an assiduous search when lethal and life-threatening arrhythmia is suspected.

Postural Phenomena

Physical examination (auscultation, blood pressure, and heart rate measurements) in general and in patients with FMV/MVP syndrome should be performed in the supine and upright postures. Orthostatic changes in blood pressure, heart rate, and arrhythmias, therefore, should be easily detected in a routine physical examination.

Neuropsychiatric Symptoms

Patients who present with anxiety or nervousness require a detailed history and complete physical examination. Consideration of diagnostic studies requires an element of clinical wisdom. Psychiatric consultation may be important in circumstances where precision in psychiatric diagnosis influences appropriate therapy.

Therapeutic Considerations

General Approach

Although individuals with FMV/MVP syndrome may recall chest pain, palpitations, or exercise intolerance dating from childhood or adolescence, most of the symptomatic patients who come to us seeking medical care are young adults, in their 20s and 30s (Fig. 28).[1,13] The age at presentation to the physician is important, since any therapeutic decision involving long-term drug therapy must anticipate and answer the inevitable question: How long will I have to take this medicine? The basic principles of managing patients with FMV/MVP syndrome are shown in Table 8.[1,120] A concerned approach by the physician is important because patient uncertainty, fear, and inability to understand alterations of body

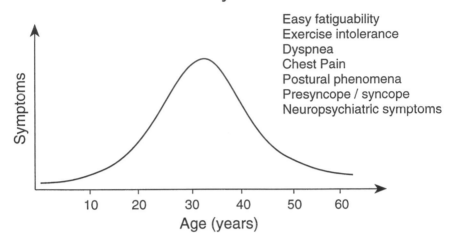

FMV / MVP - syndrome

Easy fatiguability
Exercise intolerance
Dyspnea
Chest Pain
Postural phenomena
Presyncope / syncope
Neuropsychiatric symptoms

Figure 28. Floppy mitral valve/mitral valve prolapse syndrome symptoms are plotted against patient age in years. The greatest proportion of patients become symptomatic during the second or third decades. (Used with permission from Boudoulas H.[13])

function are the usual motivating factors for seeking medical help. In our opinion, the single most important noninvasive test and therapeutic step is a carefully taken medical history and properly performed physical examination.

Symptoms frequently occur against a background of acute or gradual increases in the physical or emotional stresses of life, quite often with a precipitating event such as trauma, an operation, an illness, marital separation or divorce, a demanding or stressful job, working two jobs, or an impending job change or loss. A common sense approach to stress modi-

---

Table 8
Floppy Mitral Valve/Mitral Valve Prolapse Syndrome:
General Principles of Management

Explain and reassure
Avoid volume depletion and the use of diuretics
Avoid catecholamines or other cycle-AMP stimulants
Avoid drugs that may increase adrenergic receptor sensitivity (e.g., caffeine, thyroxine)
Avoid long-term drug therapy
Exercise program

fications, where possible and feasible, may seem too fundamental to the physician to even mention; however, such an approach may never have occurred to the patient who is wrapped up in attempts to meet demands well beyond his or her capabilities. The reestablishment of order in a patient's chaotic life may be an enormous contribution by the physician, and may require assistance from family members, clergy, or a counselor. Undue anxieties, phobias, or panic attacks may form the basis for consultation with an informed psychiatrist.

Nonspecific electrocardiographic changes, stress test or echocardiographic changes, and borderline laboratory results, which in turn may lead to inappropriate, poorly conceived programs of long-term drug therapy, often without clear-cut goals regarding duration of therapy. A careful explanation of the physician's findings, an explanation of what is known about the mechanism of symptoms and the best possible answers to the anxious patient's list of questions constitute the cornerstone of long-term management.[1,120]

FMV/MVP syndrome patients appear to be quite sensitive to volume depletion; women may note an exaggeration of symptoms at the time of menstrual periods. We have found it advisable to avoid or discontinue chronic diuretic therapy in this group of patients, particularly since a diuretic-induced hypokalemia may also contribute to the production or exaggeration of cardiac arrhythmias, setting up a vicious cycle.

The removal of catecholamine and cyclic AMP stimulation by abstinence from caffeine, cigarettes, alcohol, and prescribed or over-the-counter drugs containing epinephrine or ephedrine is an important step.[120,121] Agents, such as thyroxine, that may increase the sensitivity to catecholamines by modifying the function of β-adrenergic receptors should be avoided.

We attempt to avoid long-term drug therapy in patients, given the young age of the patients, the frequency with which they experience undesirable effects from drugs, and the limitations of what frequently amounts to symptomatic therapy.[120]

Questions about physical activities, physical fitness, and exercise programs should be addressed. Fatigue and previous exercise intolerance may have resulted in the avoidance of exercise or in very limited exercise attempts. If there are no serious exercise-induced abnormalities or arrhythmias, enrollment in a cardiac rehabilitation program for gradual aerobic conditioning may be accompanied by gratifying physical, physiological, and psychological benefits.[122] Although the precise mechanism of the beneficial effect of exercise is not known, it is suggested that the beneficial effect of exercise may be mediated through the catecholamine-receptor system, since exercise may alter catecholamine levels or adrenergic receptor activity, or both.[123]

The Management of Specific Symptoms

Chest Pain

The basic principles of the management of chest pain in patients with FMV/MVP/MVP syndrome are shown in Table 9. The management of patients with FMV/MVP syndrome with severe or incapacitating chest pain may be a source of frustration for patient and physician alike as long as our understanding of its pathogenesis remains limited.[1,21] Certainly some individuals with chest pain may have pain associated with coronary artery disease, tachyarrhythmias, or myocardial abnormalities with alterations in myocardial perfusion or diastolic function; identifying this subset of individuals obviously leads to more specific therapy with β-blockers, nitrates, or calcium antagonists. It is important to educate the patient about the nature of the disorder and its symptoms and, especially, to emphasize the positive aspects of the long-term outlook. It is also essential to educate the patient about the factors that may initiate or precipitate symptoms.

In more severe cases, medical management may be indicated. β-Blocking agents may be effective in treating chest pain associated with FMV/MVP syndrome. Although the mechanism of action is not clear, β-blocking agents are known to produce an increase in LV volume, a decrease in LV contractility, and consequently a reduction of papillary muscle tension, a decrease in the degree of prolapse and the size of the "third chamber" (see Chapter 21), and an increase in diastolic time and in diastolic pressure time index. It should be emphasized that rigorous controlled studies dealing with the therapy of pain with β-blocking drugs in FMV/MVP syndrome are lacking.

The effect of α-blocking agents, calcium channel blocking agents, and vasodilators on chest pain in patients with FMV/MVP syndrome also has not yet been subjected to critical study. Theoretically these agents should

---

Table 9
Chest Pain in Floppy Mitral Valve/Mitral Valve Prolapse Syndrome: Basic Principles of Management

Rule out obstructive coronary artery disease or other forms of myocardial or valvular disease.
Educate patient about the nature of the disorder and what may trigger chest pain.
Emphasize positive aspects of the long-term outlook.
Stress management; a regular supervised exercise program may be of value.
Avoid sympathomimetic substances and drugs.
β-Blockers may be beneficial in certain cases.
Amitriptyline may be beneficial in some patients.

be effective in patients with chest pain secondary to coronary artery vasoregulatory abnormalities; however, these agents might increase the degree of mitral valve leaflet prolapse because of their effect on LV volume. The effect of other centrally acting sympathetic blocking drugs such as clonidine on chest pain in patients with FMV/MVP syndrome has not been subjected to critical evaluation. Studies have suggested that low doses of imipramine may improve chest pain in patients with chest pain and normal coronary arteries.[124,125] The effect of this drug, however, specifically in patients with FMV/MVP syndrome has not been studied.

Palpitations

If palpitations are demonstrated to be related to specific cardiac arrhythmias, the management of cardiac arrhythmias should proceed, as is discussed in Chapter 16. If palpitations are related to inappropriate sinus tachycardia during routine daily activities, small amounts of β-blocking drugs may be beneficial.

Fatigue

If there are no contraindications, enrollment in a cardiac rehabilitation program may be beneficial. Aerobic conditioning may help some patients who present with easy fatigability.

Dyspnea

There is no specific therapy for patients who present with dyspnea. Again, an exercise program and an explanation to the patient about the nature of the symptom and the positive long-term outlook may be beneficial in certain patients.

Syncope–Presyncope

Considering the wide variety of disorders that can result in syncope or presyncope, it is clear that effective treatment demands accurate diagnosis. Therapy for the patient with syncope varies from simple maneuvers, such as avoiding precipitating factors, to more direct forms of therapy including potent antiarrhythmic drugs, cardiac pacemakers, or defibrillators. For the patient with neurocardiogenic syncope, avoiding the precipitating factors may be sufficient. For the patient with arrhythmic syncope, control of cardiac arrhythmias with antiarrhythmic drugs, a cardiac pacemaker, ablation, or surgery may be necessary. For the patient with syncope related to orthostatic hypotension, increased sodium and fluid intake should be advised; in certain patients, therapy with florinef may improve symptoms. Therapy with clonidine has been reported to improve some of the orthostatic symptoms. In patients with syncope of "unknown origin," attempts to define the underlying cause should be continued. In patients with combined causes of syncope, the underlying pathophysiological mechanisms should be corrected.[60,72]

Postural Phenomena

Patients with FMV/MVP syndrome appear to be quite sensitive to volume depletion. Postural phenomena may be related to decreased intravascular volume, an abnormal renin and aldosterone response to volume depletion, a hyperadrenergic state, parasympathetic abnormality, or baroreflex receptor abnormality. Diuretic therapy should be avoided in these patients. Increased sodium and fluid intake in certain patients may be beneficial. Therapy with florinef may improve symptoms in more severe cases. Clonidine in low doses (0.3–0.4 mg daily) may improve symptoms related to postural phenomena. Clonidine also may reduce standing plasma NE levels, total peripheral resistance, diastolic blood pressure, and increased plasma volume. The precise mechanisms for the beneficial effect of clonidine remain to be defined. The improvement of sympathetic, parasympathetic, and baroreflex abnormalities may partially account for these beneficial effects.[126]

Neuropsychiatric Symptoms

An explanation to the anxious patient of what is known about the mechanism of symptoms constitutes the best approach. In certain patients, therapy with psychotropic drugs or psychiatric evaluation may be necessary.

Natural History

The natural history of patients with FMV/MVP syndrome is not well defined. Some patients may become asymptomatic, while others continue to have symptoms. Almost all patients with FMV/MVP syndrome benefit from careful evaluation, thoughtful explanations, physician time, and continued follow-up. Our long-term experience supports the wisdom of individual patient analysis, implementation of the many practical recommendations noted above, and the role of experienced clinicians and nurse clinicians as individual sounding boards for these concerned patients. A small proportion of patients with FMV/MVP syndrome may develop symptoms directly related to mitral valve abnormalities and complications (Fig. 29).

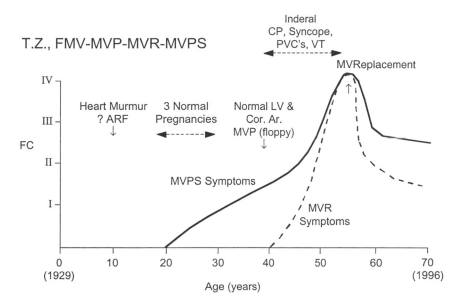

Figure 29. Symptoms and complications in a patient with floppy mitral valve (FMV), mitral valve prolapse syndrome (MVPS). At a younger age, the patient had symptoms related to autonomic dysfunction (MVPS). Later developed symptoms related to severe mitral valvular regurgitation (MVR). After mitral valve replacement, patient continued to have symptoms related to autonomic dysfunction. ARF = acute rheumatic fever; LV = left ventricle; Cor Ar = coronary arteriography; CP = chest pain; PVCs = premature ventricular beats; VT = ventricular tachycardia.

Case Presentation

July 1994, 38-year-old female.

I was diagnosed with mitral valve prolapse syndrome approximately 13 years ago, was treated with various β-blockers, some calcium channel blockers, had my symptoms wax and wane, but overall, 'learned to live with it,' remaining fairly active.

About 3 years prior to the valve repair surgery, I began to notice what I eventually realized to be significant changes in the cardiac symptoms, then having them become increasingly debilitating. To be myself that I could no longer continue to take β-blockers because of consistently low blood pressure, at times falling dangerously low. My internist, who I found to be well-versed in problems associated with MVP syndrome, suggested, upon my obviously worsening condition that I seek further cardiac consultation. Thus, I began a 'journey.' While some certainly helpful, much of the advice/determinations from the cardiologists I consulted I found confusing, discouraging, and patronizing. I recall being misdiagnosed, had noticeably conflicting echo reports, and an overall attitude of not being taken seriously.

The patient was complaining of fatigue, exercise intolerance, palpitations, orthostatic phenomena, dizzy spells. An echocardiogram obtained on September 22, 1992, demonstrated normal LV size and function (LV diastolic diameter 5.2 cm, systolic diameter 3.4 cm, LA diameter 3.2 cm, LV ejection fraction 65%). The mitral valve was redundant with severe MVP and mild to moderate late systolic MVR; there was trivial tricuspid regurgitation. Because of symptoms, the patient had mitral valve repair and tricuspid valve repair performed at another medical center in January 1993. Surgery was complicated with high-grade atrioventricular block requiring a temporary pacemaker, pleural effusions, and a pericardial effusion that required pericardial window. After this stormy postoperative period, the patient recovered, but in October 1995 three sternal wires had to be removed because of the development of an "inflammatory process."

The patient continued to experience the same symptoms she experienced prior to surgery. In December 1993, she started an exercise program in a rehabilitation center which she continued until May 1994 with some improvement in her symptoms. The patient came to see us for the first time in August 1994, still complaining of the same symptoms (palpitations, fatigue, exercise intolerance, orthostatic tachycardia).

On physical examination she was a pleasant woman in no acute distress. Her weight was 114 pounds and she was 56 1/2" tall. Her heart rate in the supine, sitting, and upright positions were 85, 95, and 103 beats/minute, respectively. Blood pressures in the supine, sitting, and standing positions were 118/74, 106/82, and 120/82, respectively. The respiration was 16/min. The joints in distal phalanges were flexible; there was a high arch palate. The jugular venous pressure was normal, the lungs were clear; there was no peripheral edema or hepatosplenomegaly. The carotid upstroke was good, there were no bruits; the peripheral pulses were good and equal. The heart sounds were unremarkable; there were no murmurs, gallops, or clicks. An ECG was within normal limits. On echocardiogram, the LV size was within normal limits and the ejection fraction was estimated at 54%. Both leaflets of the mitral valve were thickened. The LA volumes, maximal, onset of atrial systole and minimal were 51 cm^3, 36 cm^3, and 22 cm^3, respectively. The LA stroke volume was 14 cm^3, the LA ejection fraction was 39%, and the LA kinetic energy was 43025 dyne.cm.

The clinical experience presented here is typical of patients with FMV/MVP syndrome, with mild mitral regurgitation, normal LV size and function, and normal LA size. The patient's symptoms most likely were related to autonomic dysfunction, and persist after valve surgery. In this case, misinterpretation of symptoms influenced the decision and timing of cardiac surgery. Careful analysis of the mechanisms of symptoms in patients with FMV/MVP syndrome is required for informed management of these patients.

Concluding Remarks

Symptoms in patients with FMV/MVP may be directly related to mitral valve dysfunction and progressive MVR. However, in certain patients with FMV/MVP, symptoms cannot be explained on the basis of mitral valve abnormality alone. An activation of the neuroendocrine or autonomic nervous system is required for the explanation of symptoms in this group of patients presently classified under the term FMV/MVP syndrome (Table 10, Fig. 30).[1,2] The clinical utility of this classification is ap-

---

Table 10
Classification of Floppy Mitral Valve–Mitral Valve Prolapse*

Floppy Mitral Valve (FMV), Mitral Valve Prolapse (MVP), Mitral Valvular Regurgitation (MVR)	Floppy Mitral Valve/Mitral Valve Prolapse Syndrome
• Common mitral valve abnormality with a spectrum of structural and functional changes, mild to severe The basis for:	• Patients with FMV/mitral valve prolapse
• Systolic click; mid-late systolic murmur	• Symptom complex: palpitations, fatigue, exercise intolerance, dyspnea, chest pain, postural phenomena, syncope-presyncope, neuropsychiatric symptoms.
• Mild or progressive mitral valve dysfunction	• Neuroendocrine or autonomic dysfunction (high catecholamines, catecholamine regulation abnormality, β-adrenergic receptor abnormality, hyperresponsive to adrenergic stimulation, parasympathetic abnormality, baroreflex modulation abnormality, renin-aldosterone regulation abnormality, decreased intravascular volume, decreased left ventricular volume with upright posture, atrial natriuretic factor secretion abnormality) may provide explanation for symptoms.
• Progressive mitral valvular regurgitation, atrial fibrillation, congestive heart failure	
• Infective endocarditis	
• Embolic phenomena	
• Characterized by long natural history	
• May be heritable, or associated with heritable disorder of connective tissue	
• Conduction system involvement possibly leading to arrhythmias and conduction defects	• Floppy mitral valve/mitral valve prolapse - a possible marker for autonomic dysfunction
• FMV/MVP/MVR postsurgical intervention	

* From Ref. 1

FMV/MVP/MVR:
Dynamic Spectrum & Natural Progression

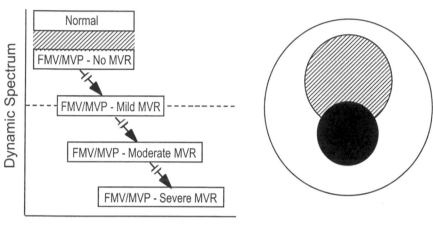

Figure 30. Left panel: The dynamic spectrum, time in years, and the progression of floppy mitral valve (FMV), mitral valve prolapse (MVP) are shown. A subtle gradation (cross-hatched area) exists between the normal mitral valve and valves that produce mild FMV/MVP without mitral valvular regurgitation (MVR). Progression from the level FMV/MVP–no MVR to another level may or may not occur. Most of the patients with FMV/MVP–syndrome occupy the area above the dotted line, while patients with progressive mitral valve dysfunction occupy the area below the dotted line. Right panel: The large circle represents the total number of patients with FMV/MVP. Patients with FMV/MVP may be symptomatic or asymptomatic. Symptoms may be directly related to mitral valve dysfunction (black circle), or to autonomic dysfunction (cross-hatched circle). Certain patients with symptoms directly related to mitral valve dysfunction may present and continue to have symptoms secondary to autonomic dysfunction. (Used with permission from Boudoulas H, et al.[1])

parent. It separates symptomatic patients with FMV/MVP and symptoms related to autonomic dysfunction from FMV/MVP patients whose symptoms are related to progressive mitral valve dysfunction. Further, the classification defines a group of patients with FMV/MVP and autonomic dysfunction who require consideration of antibiotic prophylaxis for infective endocarditis in addition to other forms of the treatment. Where it is likely that some patients with FMV/MVP syndrome will develop progressive mitral valve dysfunction and symptoms related to MVR later in life, failure to distinguish these two clinical entities may lead to erroneous clinical decisions.

References

1. Boudoulas H, Wooley CF (eds). Mitral Valve Prolapse and the Mitral Valve Prolapse Syndrome. Mount Kisco, NY, Futura Publishing Co., 1988.
2. Boudoulas H, Kolibash AJ, Baker P, King BD, Wooley CF. Mitral valve prolapse and the mitral valve prolapse syndrome: A diagnostic classification and pathogenesis of symptoms. Am Heart J 118:796–818, 1989.
3. Wooley CF, Sparks EA, Boudoulas H. The floppy mitral valve-mitral valve prolapse-mitral valvular regurgitation triad. ACC Current J Rev July/August 1994, pp 25–26.
4. Wooley CF, Baker PB, Kolibash AJ, Kilman JW, Sparks EA, Boudoulas H. The floppy, myxomatous mitral valve, mitral valve prolapse and mitral regurgitation. Prog Cardiovasc Dis 33:397–433, 1991.
5. Wooley CF, Boudoulas H. From irritable heart to mitral valve prolapse: World War I, the U.S. experience and the prevalence of apical systolic murmurs and mitral regurgitation in drafted men compared with present day mitral valve prolapse studies. Am J Cardiol 61:895–899, 1988.
6. Fontana ME, Sparks EA, Boudoulas H, Wooley CF. Mitral valve prolapse and the mitral valve prolapse syndrome. Curr Probl Cardiol 16:311–375, 1991.
7. Boudoulas H, Wooley CF. Mitral valve disorders. Curr Opin Cardiol 5:162–170, 1990.
8. Boudoulas H, Wooley CF. Mitral valve prolapse and the mitral valve prolapse syndrome. In Yu PN, Goodwin JF (eds): Prog Cardiovasc Dis 14:275–309, 1986.
9. Boudoulas H, King BD, Wooley CF. Mitral valve prolapse: A marker for anxiety or overlapping phenomenon? Psychopathology 17:98–106, 1984.
10. Boudoulas H. Valvular Disease. American College of Cardiology Self-Assessment Program (ACCSAP) 2000. In press.
11. Boudoulas H, Kolibash AH, Wooley CF. Mitral valve prolapse: A heterogeneous disorder. Primary Cardiol 17:29–43, 1991.
12. Boudoulas H, Kolibash AJ, Wooley CF. Mitral valve prolapse: The high-risk patient. Practical Cardiol 17:15–31, 1991.
13. Boudoulas H. Mitral valve prolapse and the mitral valve prolapse syndrome. In Toutouzas P, Boudoulas H (eds): Cardiac Diseases. Parissianos Medical and Scientific Editions, Athens, 2:135–156, 1991.
14. Freed LA, Levy D, Levine RA, Larson MG, Evans JC, Fuller DL, Lehman B, et al. Prevalence and clinical outcome of mitral valve prolapse. N Engl J Med 341: 1–7, 1999.
15. Savage DD, Garrison RJ, Devereux RB, et al. Mitral valve prolapse in the general population. In Epidemiologic Features: The Framingham study. Am Heart J 1983; 106:571–576.
16. Savage DD, Devereux RB, Garrison RJ, et al. Mitral valve prolapse in the general population. In Clinical Features: The Framingham Study. Am Heart J 106: 577–581, 1983.
17. Devereux RB, Kramer-Fox R, Brown WT, et al. Relation between clinical features of the mitral prolapse syndrome and echocardiographically documented mitral valve prolapse. J Am Coll Cardiol 8:763–772, 1986.
18. Malcolm AD. Mitral valve prolapse associated with other disorders. Casual coincidence, common link, or fundamental genetic disturbance? Br Heart J 53: 33–62, 1985.
19. Sukumaran TU, Manjooran RJ, Thomas K. A clinical profile of mitral valve prolapse syndrome. Indian J Pediatr 57:771–773, 1990.

20. Boudoulas H, Wooley CF. Chest pain associated with mitral valve prolapse. Chest Pain 5:1–8, 1979.
21. Boudoulas H, Wooley CF. Chest pain in patients with mitral valve prolapse. Primary Cardiol 11:16–25, 1985.
22. Nutter DO, Wickliffe C, Gilbert CA, Moody C, King SB. The pathophysiology of idiopathic mitral valve prolapse. Circulation 52:297–305, 1975.
23. Cannon RO, Leon MB, Watson RM, Rosing DR, Epstein SE. Chest pain and normal coronary arteries: Role of small coronary arteries. Am J Cardiol 55: 50–60B, 1985.
24. LeWinter MM, Hoffman JR, Shell WE, Karliner JS, O'Rourke RA. Phenyle-phrine-induced atypical chest pain in patients with prolapsing mitral valve leaflets. Am J Cardiol 34:12–18, 1974.
25. Spears PF, Koch K, Day FP. Chest pain associated with mitral valve prolapse. Arch Intern Med 146:796–797, 1986.
26. Engel PJ, Alpert BL, Hickman JR. The nature and prevalence of the abnormal exercise electrocardiogram in mitral valve prolapse. Am Heart J 98:716–724, 1979.
27. Wooley CF, Sparks EA, Boudoulas H. Aortic Pain. Prog Cardiovasc Dis 40: 563–589, 1998.
28. Boudoulas H, Toutouzas P, Wooley CF. Functional Abnormalities of the Aorta. Armonk, NY, Futura Publishing Co., Inc. , 1996.
29. Akasaka T, Yoshida K, Hozumi T, Takagi T, Kaji S, Kawamoto T, Ueda Y, et al. Restricted coronary flow reserve in patients with mitral regurgitation im-proves after mitral reconstructive surgery. J Am Coll Cardiol 2:1923–1930, 1998.
30. Tuzcu EM, Moodie DS, Chambers JL, et al. Congenital heart diseases associ-ated with coronary anomalies. Cleve Clin J Med 57:178–180, 1990.
31. Sanfilippo AJ, Harrigan P, Popvic AD, et al. Papillary muscle tension in mitral valve prolapse: Quantitation by two-dimensional echocardiography. J Am Coll Cardiol 19:564–571, 1992.
32. Wooley CF, Sparks EA, Boudoulas H. Aortic pain: The renaissance of cardio-vascular pain and detection of aortopathy. Herz 24:140–153, 1999.
33. Malkowski MT, Boudoulas H, Wooley CF, Guo R, Pearson AC. Abnormal elastic properties of the aorta in mitral valve prolapse. Circulation 12(Suppl I): I–357, 1995.
34. Hoffman JIE, Buckberg GO. The myocardial supply:demand ratio: A critical review. Am J Cardiol 41:327–332, 1978.
35. Boudoulas H, Dervenagas S, Fulkerson PK, Bush CA, Lewis RP. Effect of heart rate on diastolic time and left ventricular performance in patients with atrial fibrillation. In Diethrich EB (ed): Noninvasive Cardiovascular Diagnosis, sec-ond edition. Littleton, MA, PSG Publishing Company, Inc., 1981, pp 433–445.
36. Boudoulas H, Rittgers SE, Lewis RP, et al. Changes in diastolic time with var-ious pharmacologic agents: Implications for myocardial perfusion. Circula-tion 60:164–169, 1979.
37. Boudoulas H, Reynolds JC, Mazzaferri E, et al. Metabolic studies in mitral valve prolapse syndrome. Circulation 61:1200–1205, 1980.
38. Boudoulas H, Reynolds JC, Mazzaferri E, et al. Mitral valve prolapse syn-drome: The effect of adrenergic stimulation. J Am Coll Cardiol 2:638–644, 1983.
39. Davies AO, Mares A, Pool JL, et al. Mitral valve prolapse with symptoms of β-adrenergic hypersensitivity: β-2 adrenergic receptor supercoupling with desensitization of isoproterenol exposure. Am J Med 82:193–201, 1987.

40. Gaffney FA, Bastian BC, Lane LB, et al. Abnormal cardiovascular regulation in the mitral valve prolapse syndrome. Am J Cardiol 52:316–320, 1983.
41. Bashore TM, Grines C, Utlak D, Boudoulas H, Wooley CF. Postural exercise abnormalities in symptomatic patients with mitral valve prolapse. J Am Coll Cardiol 11:499–507, 1988.
42. Coghlan HC, Phares P, Crowley M, et al. Dysautonomia in mitral valve prolapse. Am J Med 67:236–244, 1979.
43. Gaffney AF, Karlsson ES, Campbell W, et al. Autonomic dysfunction in women with mitral valve prolapse syndrome. Circulation 59:894–901, 1979.
44. Davies AO, Su CJ, Balasubramanyam A, Codina J, Birnbaumer L. Abnormal guanine nucleotide regulatory protein in FMV/MVP dysautonomia: Evidence from reconstitution of Gs. J Clin Endocrinol Metab 72:867–875, 1991.
45. Balasubramanyam A, Davies AO, Codina J, Birnbaumer L. Abnormal Gs function in mitral valve prolapse dysautonomia is not associated with abnormal alpha S cDNA sequence. Life Sci 48:789–793, 1991.
46. Anwar A, Kohn SR, Dunn JF, et al. Altered β-adrenergic receptor function in subjects with symptomatic mitral valve prolapse. Am J Med Sci 302:89–97, 1991.
47. Rogers JM, Boudoulas H, Malarkey WB, Wooley CF. Mitral valve prolapse: Disordered catecholamine regulation with intravascular volume maneuvers. Circulation 6:310, 1983.
48. Coghlan HC, Carranza C, Hsiung MC, Alliende I, Mee-Nin K, Nanda NC. Abnormal left ventricular volume response during upright exercise in symptomatic mitral prolapse patients. X World Congr Cardiol Abstract book, 120, 1986.
49. Boudoulas H, Lewis RP, Kates RE, Dalamangas G. Hypersensitivity to adrenergic stimulation after propranolol withdrawal in normal subjects. Ann Intern Med 87:433–436,1977.
50. Nesse RM, Cameron OG, Buda AJ, McCann DS, Curtis GC, Huber-Smith MJ. Urinary catecholamines and mitral valve prolapse in panic-anxiety patients. Psychiatry Res 14:67–75, 1985.
51. Boudoulas H, Wooley CF. Mitral valve prolapse syndrome: Hyperresponse to adrenergic stimulation. Primary Cardiology, pp 119–129, May 1987.
52. Boudoulas H, Cobb TC, Leighton RF, Wilt SM. Myocardial lactate production in patients with angina-like chest pain and angiographically normal coronary arteries and left ventricle. Am J Cardiol 34:501–505, 1974.
53. Scabardonis G, Yang SS, Maranhao V, Goldberg H, Gooch AS. Left ventricular abnormalities in prolapsed mitral leaflet syndrome: Review of eighty-seven cases. Circulation 48:287–297, 1973.
54. Pitts FN, McClure JN. Lactate metabolism in anxiety neurosis. N Engl J Med 227:1329–1336, 1967.
55. Wooley CF, Sparks EH, Hirata K, Boudoulas H. The aortapathy of heritable cardiovascular disease. In Boudoulas H, Toutouzas PK, Wooley CF (eds): Functional Abnormalities of the Aorta. Armonk, NY, Futura Publishing Co., 1996, pp 312–313.
56. Stoddard MF, Prince CR, Dillon S, Longaker RA, Morris GT, Liddell NE. Exercise-induced mitral regurgitation is a predictor of morbid events in subjects with mitral valve prolapse. J Am Coll Cardiol 25:693–699, 1995.
57. Kerley CE. The effort syndrome in children. Arch Ped 37:449–454, 1920.
58. ZuWallack R, Sinatra S, Lahiri B, Godar RH, Liss P, Jeresaty RM. Pulmonary function studies in patients with prolapse of the mitral valve. Chest 76:17–20, 1979.

59. Devereux RB, Brown WT, Lutas EM, et al. Association of mitral valve prolapse with low body weight and low blood pressure. Lancet 2:792–795, 1982.
60. Boudoulas H, Nelson SD, Schaal SF, Lewis RP. Diagnosis and management of syncope. In Alexander RW, Schlant RC, Fuster V, O'Rourke RA, Roberts R, Sonnenblick EH (eds): Hurst's The Heart. 9th ed. New York, McGraw-Hill, 1998, pp 1059–1080.
61. Kavey REW, Blackman MS, Sondheimer HM, Byrum CJ. Ventricular arrhythmias and mitral valve prolapse in childhood. J Pediatr 105:885–890, 1984.
62. Wei JY, Bulkey BH, Schaeffer AH, et al. Mitral valve prolapse syndrome and recurrent ventricular tachyarrhythmias: A malignant variant refractory to conventional drug therapy. Ann Intern Med 89:6–9, 1978.
63. Santos AD, Mathew PK, Hilal H. Orthostatic hypotension: A commonly unrecognized cause of symptoms in mitral valve prolapse. Am J Med 71:746–750, 1981.
64. Boudoulas H, Schaal SF, Wooley CF. Floppy mitral valve/mitral valve prolapse: Cardiac arrhythmias. In Vardas PE (ed): Cardiac Arrhythmias, Pacing, and Electrophysiology. Great Britain, Kluwer Academic Publisher, 1998, pp 89–95.
65. Fontana ME, Wooley CF, Leighton RF, Lewis RP. Postural changes in left ventricular and mitral valvular dynamics in the systolic click–late systolic murmur syndrome. Circulation 51:165–173, 1975.
66. Swartz MH, Teichholz LE, Donoso E. Mitral valve prolapse: A review of associated arrhythmias. Am J Med 63:377–389, 1977.
67. Dobmeyer DJ, Stine RA, Leier CV, Schaal SF. Electrophysiologic mechanisms of provoked atrial flutter in mitral valve prolapse syndrome. Am J Cardiol 56:602–604, 1985.
68. Ritchie JL, Hammermeister KE, Kennedy JW. Refractory ventricular tachycardia and fibrillation in a patient with the prolapsing mitral leaflet syndrome: Successful control with overdrive pacing. Am J Med 37:314–316, 1976.
69. Winkle RA, Lopes MG, Popp RL, Hancock EW. Life-threatening arrhythmias in the mitral valve prolapse syndrome. Am J Med 60:961–967, 1976.
70. Campbell RWF, Godman MG, Fiddler GI, Marquis RM, Julian DG. Ventricular arrhythmias in syndrome of balloon deformity of mitral valve: Definition of possible high-risk group. Br Heart J 38:1053–1057, 1976.
71. Kafka W. Prevalence, therapeutic modification and prognostic significance of ventricular arrhythmias in the mitral valve prolapse syndrome. Z Kardiol 74(4):245–253, 1985.
72. Boudoulas H, Weissler AM, Lewis RP, Warren JV. The clinical diagnosis of syncope. In WP Harvey (ed): Current Problems in Cardiology. Chicago, Year Book Medical Publishers, 7:1–40, 1982.
73. Rogers JM, Boudoulas H, Wooley CF. Mitral valve prolapse: Evidence of baroreflex abnormality with intravascular volume maneuvers. J Am Coll Cardiol 3(2):559, 1984.
74. Costa AM, Maia IG, Cruz Filho F, Fagundes ML, Sa R, Alves P. Relationship between mitral valve prolapse and arrhythmogenic right ventricular disease. Arg Bras Cardiol 6:379–383, 1996.
75. Morady F, Shen E, Bhandari A, Schwartz A, Scheinman MM. Programmed ventricular stimulation in mitral valve prolapse: Analysis of 36 patients. Am J Cardiol 53:135–138, 1984.
76. Andre-Fouet X, Tabib A, Jean-Louis P, Didier A, Dutertre P, Gayet C, de Mahenge AH, et al. Mitral valve prolapse, Wolff-Parkinson-White syndrome, His bundle sclerosis and sudden death. Am J Cardiol 56:700, 1985.

77. Wilde AA, Duren DR, Hauer RN, deBakker JM, Bakker PF, Becker AE, Janse MJ. Mitral valve prolapse and ventricular arrhythmias: Observations in a patient with a 20-year history. J Cardiovasc Electrophysiol 3:307–316, 1997.

78. Ware JA, Magro SA, Luck JC, Mann DE, Nielsen AP, Rosen KM, Wyndham CRC. Conduction system abnormalities in symptomatic mitral valve prolapse: An electrophysiologic analysis of 60 patients. Am J Cardiol 53:1075–1078, 1984.

79. Boudoulas H, Wooley CF. The floppy mitral valve, mitral valve prolapse, and mitral valvular regurgitation. In Moss and Adams: Heart Disease in Infants, Children, and Adolescents. 6th edition, in press.

80. Brembilla-Perrot B, Beurrier D, Jacquemin L, de la Terrier CA, Suty-Selton C, Thiel B, Louis P, et al. Syncope associated with mitral valve prolapse: Mechanisms. Ann Cardiol Angeiol (Paris) 5:257–262, 1996.

81. Babuty D, Cosnay P, Breuillac JC, Charniot JC, Delhomme C, Fauchier L, Fauchier JP. Ventricular arrhythmia factors in mitral valve prolapse. PACE 6: 1090–1099, 1994.

82. Tieleman RG, Crijns HJ, Wiesfeld AC, Posma J, Hamer HP, Lie KI. Increased dispersion of refractoriness in the absence of QT prolongation in patients with mitral valve prolapse and ventricular arrhythmias. Br Heart J 1:37–40, 1995.

83. Zdrojewski TR, Wyrzykowski B, Krupa-Wojciehowska B. Renin-aldosterone regulation during upright posture in young men with mitral valve prolapse syndrome. J Heart Valve Dis 4:236–241, 1995.

84. LaVecchia L, Centofante P, Varotto L, et al. Arrhythmic profile, ventricular function, and histomorphometric findings in patients with idiopathic ventricular tachycardia and mitral valve prolapse: Clinical and prognostic evaluation. Clin Cardiol 21:731–735, 1998.

85. Rogers JM, Boudoulas H, Wooley CF. Abnormal renin-aldosterone response to volume depletion in mitral valve prolapse. Circulation 70(Suppl II):336, 1984.

86. Piraino P, Zura ML, Loureiro O, Andrade A. Mitral valve prolapse associated with Basedow's disease and active hyperthyroidism: Preliminary report. Rev Med Chil 118:649–652, 1991..

87. Kontopoulos AG, Harsoulis P, Adam K, Papadopoulos G, Polymenidis Z, Boudoulas H. Frequency of HLA antigents in Graves hyperthyroidism and mitral valve prolapse. J Heart Valve Dis 5:543–545, 1996.

88. Carney RM, Freedland KE, Ludbrook PA, Saunders RD, Jaffe AS. Major depression, panic disorder, and mitral valve prolapse in patients who complain of chest pain. Am J Med 89:757–760, 1990.

89. Hamada T, Fukui J, Koshino Y, et al. Mitral valve prolapse syndrome as an etiologic factor of anxiety disorder. Rinsho Byori 38:952–956, 1990.

90. Cordas TA, Rossi EG, Grinbert M, et al. Mitral valve prolapse and panic disorder. Arg Bras Cardiol 56:139–142, 1991.

91. Raj A, Sheehan DV. Mitral valve prolapse and panic disorder. Bull Menninger Clin 54:199–208, 1990.

92. Boudoulas H, Schmidt HS, Clark RW, Geleris P, Schaal SF, Lewis RP. Anthropometric characteristics, cardiac abnormalities and adrenergic activity in patients with primary disorders of sleep. J Med 14:223–237, 1983.

93. Kantor SJ, Zitrin CM, Zeldis SM. Mitral valve prolapse syndrome in agoraphobic patients. Am J Psychiatry 137:467–469, 1980.

94. Pariser SF, Pinta ER, Jones BA. Mitral valve prolapse syndrome and anxiety neurosis/panic disorder. Am J Psychiatry 135:246–247, 1978.

95. Crowe RR. Mitral valve prolapse and panic disorder. Psychiatric Clin N Am 8:63–71, 1985.
96. Meyers DG, Starke H, Pearson PH, Wilken MK. Mitral valve prolapse in anorexia nervosa. Ann Int Med 105:384–386, 1986.
97. Oka Y, Ito T, Sekine I, Sada T, Okabe F, Naito A, Matsumoto S, et al. Mitral valve prolapse in patients with anorexia nervosa. J Cardiol 14:483–491, 1984.
98. Marks AD, Channick BJ, Adlin EV, Kessler RK, Braitman LE, Denenberg BS. Chronic thyroiditis and mitral valve prolapse. Ann Int Med 102:479–483, 1985.
99. Brauman A, Algom M, Gilboa Y, Ramot Y, Golik A, Stryjer D. Mitral valve prolapse in hyperthyroidism of two different origins. Br Heart J 53:374–377, 1985.
100. Thase ME. Mitral valve prolapse and anxiety. Cardiovasc Pulmonary Technol J Oct/Nov:74–78, 1983.
101. Katerndahl DA. Panic and prolapse. Meta-analysis. J Nerv Ment Dis 181: 539–544, 1993.
102. Chesler E, Weir EK, Braatz GA, Francis GS. Normal catecholamine and hemodynamic responses to orthostatic tilt in subjects and mitral valve prolapse. Am J Med 78:754–760, 1985.
103. Leatham A, Brigden W. Mild mitral regurgitation and the mitral prolapse fiasco. Am Heart J 99:659–664, 1980.
104. Barlow JB, Pocock WA. Mitral leaflet billowing and prolapse. In Barlow JB (ed): Perspectives on the Mitral Valve. Philadelphia, FA Davis Company, 1987, pp 45–112.
105. Pasternac A, Tubern JF, Puddy PE, Kral RB, Champlain J. Increased plasma catecholamine levels in patients with symptomatic mitral valve prolapse. Am J Med 73:783–790, 1982.
106. Boudoulas H, Geleris P, Lewis RP, Rittgers SE. Linear relationship between electrical systole, mechanical systole and heart rate. Chest 80:613–617, 1981.
107. Boudoulas H, Sohn YH, O'Neil W, Brown R, Weissler AM. The QT QS$_2$ syndrome: A new mortality risk indicator in coronary artery disease. Am J Cardiol 50:1229–1235, 1982.
108. Zdrojewski TR, Purzycki Z, Rynkiewicz A, Kubasik A, Wyrzykowski B, Krupa-Wojciechowska B. QT/QS2 ration in mitral valve prolapse syndrome, hyperthyroidism and borderline hypertension: Possible indication of dysautonomia. Am J Noninvas Cardiol 7:19–22, 1993.
109. Franz MR, Cima R, Wang D, Proffit D, Kuntz R. Electrophysiological effects of myocardial stretch and mechanical determinants of stretch-activated arrhythmias. Circulation 86:968–978, 1992.
110. Pasternac A, Kouz S, Gutkowska J, Petitclerc R, Vellas B, deChamplain J, et al. Abnormal plasma levels of atrial natriuretic factor in patients with symptomatic mitral valve prolapse. J Am Coll Cardiol 7:169A, 1986.
111. Boudoulas H, Boudoulas D, Sparks EA, Pearson AC, Nagaraja HN, Wooley CF. Left atrial performance indices in chronic mitral valve disease. J Heart Valve Dis 4(Suppl2):S242–247, 1995.
112. Marron K, Yacoub MH, Polak JM, et al. Innervation of human atrioventricular and arterial valves. Circulation 94:368–375, 1996.
113. Pedersen HD, Olsen LH, Mow T, Christensen NJ. Neuroendocrine changes in dachshunds with mitral valve prolapse examined under different study conditions. Res Vet Sci 1:11–17, 1999.
114. Abinader EG, Shahar J. Exercise testing in mitral valve prolapse before and after beta blockade. Br Heart J 48:130–133, 1982.

115. Abinader EG. The effect of beta blockade on the abnormal exercise test in patients with mitral valve prolapse. J Cardiac Rehab 4:95–100, 1984.
116. Abinader EG. Clinical considerations in interpretation of the exercise electrocardiogram in the patient with mitral valve prolapse. Pract Cardiol 172–190, 1983.
117. Marcomichelakis J, Donaldson R, Green J, Joseph S, Kelly HB, Taggart P, Somerville W. Exercise testing after β-blockade: Improved specificity and predictive value in detecting coronary heart disease. Br Heart J 43:252–261, 1980.
118. Natarajan G, Nakhjavan FK, Kahn D, Yazdanfar S, Sahibzada W, Khawaja F. Myocardial metabolic studies in prolapsing mitral leaflet syndrome. Circulation 52:1105–1110, 1975.
119. Massie B, Botvinick EH, Shames D, Taradash M, Werner J, Schiller N. Myocardial perfusion scintigraphy in patients with mitral valve prolaspe: Its advantage over stress electrocardiography in diagnosing associated coronary artery disease and its implications for the etiology of chest pain. Circulation 57:19–26, 1978.
120. Wooley CF, Boudoulas H. Mitral valve prolapse. In Rakel RE (ed): Conn's Current Therapy. W.B. Saunders Co., 1999, pp 289–293.
121. Dobmeyer DJ, Stine RA, Leier CV, Greenberg R, Schaal SF. The arrhythmogenic effects of caffeine in human beings. N Engl J Med 308:814–816, 1983.
122. Scordo KA. Effects of aerobic exercise training on symptomatic women with mitral valve prolapse. Am J Cardiol 67:863–868, 1991.
123. Ostman I, Sjostrand NO. Effect of prolonged physical training on the catecholamine levels of the heart and the adrenals of the rat. Acta Physiol Scand 82:202–208, 1971.
124. Cannon RO, Quyyumi AA, Mincemoyer R, et al. Imipramine in patients with chest pain despite normal coronary angiograms. N Engl J Med 330:1411–1417, 1994.
125. Cox ID, Hann CM, Kaski JC. Low dose imipramine improves chest pain but not quality of life in patients with angina and normal coronary angiograms. Eur Heart J 19:250–254, 1998.
126. Gaffney FA, Lane LB, Pettinger W, Blomqvist CG. Effects of long-term clonidine administration on the hemodynamic and neuroendocrine postural responses of patients with dysautonomia. Chest 83:436–443, 1983.

Part XVI

Floppy Mitral Valve, Mitral Valve Prolapse, Mitral Valvular Regurgitation:
Special Considerations

Introduction

Floppy Mitral Valve, Mitral Valve Prolapse, Mitral Valvular Regurgitation:
Special Considerations

Harisios Boudoulas, MD, PhD,
Charles F. Wooley, MD

Floppy mitral valve (FMV)/mitral valve prolapse (MVP) is a common disorder of the mitral valve with a wide spectrum of valvular abnormalities from mild to severe. In addition, FMV/MVP may be present as an isolated mitral valve abnormality, or may be part of a well-recognized heritable connective tissue disorder such as Marfan syndrome, Ehlers-Danlos syndrome, etc. Further, FMV/MVP may be associated with other cardiovascular and noncardiovascular abnormalities.

Restrictions and recommendations for physical activities or participation in athletics will depend on the individual place within the spectrum of mitral valve abnormalities, the coexistence of other abnormalities, and the presence, severity, and significance of symptoms. While the majority of FMV/MVP patients may participate in physical activities and athletic competitions without any risk, restrictions should be applied in certain individuals in order to avoid catastrophic events.

As a general rule, pregnancy is well tolerated in patients with isolated FMV/MVP. Special care, however, should be considered in patients in whom FMV/MVP may be associated with heritable connective tissue disorders or other cardiovascular or noncardiovascular abnormalities. In addition, antibiotic prophylaxis for infective endocarditis during delivery is another consideration in this group of patients.

Aviation is part of our lives, and involvement in such activities will continue to increase during the 21st century. The stress of flying commer-

From: Boudoulas H, Wooley CF: *Mitral Valve: Floppy Mitral Valve, Mitral Valve Prolapse, Mitral Valvular Regurgitation.* Second revised edition. ©Futura Publishing Company, Armonk, NY, 2000.

cial airlines as a pilot or other professional personnel is not unusually high and there are no data to suggest that adverse effects occur in asymptomatic patients with isolated mild FMV/MVP while operating commercial aircraft.

High G stress, however, during high-performance maneuvers with military jets and spacecraft may result in significant mitral valvular regurgitation or ventricular tachycardia in asymptomatic individuals with mild FMV/MVP without mitral valvular regurgitation at rest. Because of the potential risks associated with high G stress in certain individuals with FMV/MVP, patients with FMV/MVP regardless of the severity of mitral valve abnormality and symptomatic status, as a general rule, are not considered candidates for high-intensity, high-performance aircraft.

Currently available information about individuals and patients with FMV/MVP related to childhood, adolescence, pregnancy, athletics, and aviation is presented in Chapter 24.

25

Floppy Mitral Valve/Mitral Valve Prolapse:

Childhood, Pregnancy, Athletics, and Aviation

Harisios Boudoulas, MD, PhD,
Charles F. Wooley, MD

Floppy Mitral Valve/Mitral Valve Prolapse (FMV/MVP): Childhood

Where Were the Children, Adolescents, and Young Adults with Floppy Mitral Valve/Mitral Valve Prolapse in Yesteryear?

In 1916, in World War I England, Sir James Mackenzie presented a paper on "Soldier's Heart" at a meeting of the Royal Society of Medicine in London.[1] By "soldier's heart" Mackenzie meant a form of heart trouble to which young soldiers were particularly liable, manifested in spare, thin young men with great vasomotor instability, easy fatigue, breathlessness, and pain over the region of the heart. Systolic murmurs were frequent, and the heart size was normal. Exertion produced undue rapidity of the heart, and Mackenzie noted that as a consequence of this cardiac excitability, the term "irritable heart" had been used also. This form of heart trouble in young soldiers had been described earlier by Jacob M. Da Costa

From: Boudoulas H, Wooley CF. *Mitral Valve: Floppy Mitral Valve, Mitral Valve Prolapse, Mitral Valvular Regurgitation*. Second revised edition. ©Futura Publishing Company, Armonk, NY, 2000.

during the U.S. Civil War under the title of "Irritable Heart ." During the discussion period following Mackenzie's 1916 presentation, one of the clinicians mentioned that the condition was common in civilian practice among children and adolescents, and it sometimes persisted until middle life. During the latter part of World War I, the soldier's heart terminology was changed, and Thomas Lewis introduced the term "effort syndrome" into the British literature.[1]

A small group of U.S. Army medical officers studied with Lewis in World War I England, and saw the same patients that Lewis did, however, they renamed the condition "neurocirculatory asthenia." Neurocirculatory asthenia became official terminology in the U.S. Army, and was also incorporated into the early nomenclature lists of the New York Heart Association.

Four million young men were examined in 1917–1918 as part of the mobilization of the U.S. Army. In both the British and the U.S. experience, the incidence of apical systolic murmurs was so high that the dogma was developed that apical systolic murmurs should be ignored unless a history of acute rheumatic fever or cardiac hypertrophy was present.[2] Thus, Da Costa's syndrome, irritable heart, soldier's heart, effort syndrome, and neurocirculatory asthenia entered the clinical nomenclature, and the wartime apical systolic murmur dogma was carried over into civilian clinical medicine.

In New York City in 1921, May G. Wilson,[3] adapting the graduated exercise programs developed for soldiers by Thomas Lewis and Francis Peabody during World War I, established standardized tests exercise to define exercise tolerance in normal children and children with heart disease. Thirty-six of the 58 patients with chronic valvular disease had mitral insufficiency; of these, 23 had normal exercise tolerance while 13 had only fair tolerance for standardized test exercise. The introduction of exercise testing in normal children and children with heart disease was an outgrowth of the wartime soldier's heart experiences intended to provide a scientific basis for intelligent regulation of the child's activities.

Charles E. Kerley in 1920[4] and Edith M. Lincoln in 1928[5] considered the effort syndrome in children in some detail. Kerley described "the boy or girl who may qualify for the 'effort syndrome' class, comes to us with a typical story, which condensed, means that there is an absence of capacity for sustained effort, both mental and physical." The common denominator was a lessened capacity for sustained effort. Edith Lincoln's extensive study, "The Hearts of Normal Children," included "Notes on Effort Syndrome." Lincoln was physician to the Bureau of Educational Experiments, and the publication resulted from a series of yearly examinations from 1919 to 1926 on growth in school children in New York City. Twenty-seven of a total group of 325 children had transient systolic murmurs, usually confined to the apex, which according to the thinking of the time, "were not of demonstrable significance." A small group of the children had symptoms referable to the circulatory system, with cyanosis, pallor, or dyspnea on exertion and undue fatigue. Lincoln described five children whose lack of capacity for sustained effort and circulatory symptoms fit the category of the effort syndrome. Three boys and two girls, ages 4 to 9 years, had intermittent symptoms that intensified after infections or unaccustomed physical exertion, with fatigue as the most common symptom, followed by dyspnea on slight physical exertion. Transient murmurs, a tendency to rapid heart rate with persistence of tachycardia after exercise, and blood pressure well below the average were noted. Transverse width of the heart on chest x-ray was below the average. Recognition of these children influenced Lincoln's approach: "I recognized. . .a juvenile case of effort syndrome, and a change in policy was made. Rather than being treated as potential cardiac patients, the children were encouraged to increase gradually the amount of exercise they were taking; their families and teachers were advised to ignore circulatory symptoms as far as possible and to try to instill in the minds of these children a liking for outdoor games and sports."

A rational approach to the apical systolic murmur controversy had been presented earlier by John P. Crozer Griffith, MD, from the University of Pennsylvania.[6] Griffith was Clinical Professor of Pediatrics at the University and author of *The Care of the Infant,* which went through six editions between 1895 and 1923. Earlier, Griffith had training in internal medicine as a clinical assistant to William Osler in 1886 when Osler was in Philadelphia. Griffith's 1892 article, "Mid-Systolic and Late-Systolic Mitral Murmurs," presented apical mid- and late systolic murmurs as examples of mitral regurgitant murmurs; classic graphic illustrations defined the timing of these murmurs by Griffith as derived from careful auscultation. This paper was also presented before the Association of American Physicians, the most prestigious academic meeting of the era.

It seems likely, then, that the children, adolescents, and young adults of yesteryear with FMV/MVP/MVR were classified under a variety of diagnostic categories. These diagnostic categories included individuals with "innocent" murmurs, systolic clicks or systolic gallop sounds, and apical mid- and late systolic murmurs, as well as many individuals who were categorized under the headings of irritable heart, soldier's heart, effort syndrome, neurocirculatory asthenia, mild mitral regurgitation, and of course, rheumatic valvular disease.

Floppy Mitral Valve/Mitral Valve Prolapse in Childhood: Clinical Presentation

FMV/MVP in children is frequently diagnosed as the result of a routine physical examination. It appears that the prevalence of FMV/MVP increases with age. Sakamoto,[7] in a clinical phonocardiographic study in Japan, found an incidence of FMV/MVP of 0.808% in the elementary school children and 1.283% in the middle school children. Hickey and Wilcken[8] investigated the incidence of FMV/MVP in 6,887 consecutive patients referred for echocardiography and in 206 unreferred first-degree relatives of 65 patients with MVP. MVP was detected by echocardiography in 23 patients (1.8%) and in 21 (10%) of the first-degree relatives. MVP was rare under the age of 10 years; only 1 of 1,385 patients younger than 10 referred for echocardiography had MVP. During the second decade the incidence increased but the increase was due mainly to the higher incidence between 15 to 19 years of age. The incidence of MVP from ages 0 to 19 was 0.3%, from 20 to 39 was 2.0%, from 40 to 59 was 2.7%, and from 60 to 79 was 2.3%. The incidence of MVP in the first-degree relatives group from ages 0 to 19 was 3%, from 20 to 39 was 15%, from 40 to 59 was 11%, and from 60 to 79 was 9%. Ohara et al.[9] studied the incidence of MVP by two-dimensional echocardiography in 4,328 children age from 1 day to 15 years. MVP was not seen in any of the 198 children ages 1 to 28 days; the incidence of MVP was 0.25% in 391 children ages from 6 to 18 months, 2.1% in 2,801 children ages 6 to 7 years, and 5.1% in 938 children ages 12 to 15 years. Significant MVR was present in six children (two ages 6–7 years, and four ages 12–15 years). Greenwood, in a clinical auscultatory study, evaluated 3,100 children aged 1 month to 18 years and diagnosed MVP in 154 children (4.97%). In another clinical auscultatory study, Greenwood evaluated 6,168 children age 2 months to 21 years; MVP was present in 331 (5.37%), 175 boys and 156 girls.[10,11]

FMV/MVP in children, as in adults, may occur as an isolated abnormality or as a part of a recognized inherited connective tissue disorder.[12-29] Auscultatory findings in children with FMV/MVP are similar to those described in the adults: an isolated systolic nonejection click is present in approximately two-thirds of the children, and a systolic click plus murmur in the other one-third. Silent FMV/MVP appears to be uncommon in children. The electrocardiogram may reveal nonspecific repolarization changes as in adults. The chest x-ray is usually normal but may reveal skeletal abnormalities.

Although FMV/MVP is genetically determined, its clinical manifestations do not usually become evident before adulthood.[19] Although children and adolescents with FMV/MVP may have the same symptoms as adults, the frequency of symptoms appears to be less. The prognosis in children with FMV/MVP appears to be good, although complications related to prolapse may be present. Bisset et al.[30] studied 119 children and adolescents for a mean follow-up period of 6 to 9 years. Neither progression of MVR nor deaths were reported; one patient developed infective endocarditis, one had a cerebrovascular accident, and two required antiarrhythmic therapy for supraventricular arrhythmias. Greenwood followed 331 children with MVP for 1 month to 8 years, a mean of 2.7 years. Chest pain developed in 12 children; one was treated with propranolol. MVR progressed with heart failure in one patient who developed thyrotoxicosis. Four patients had migraine headaches and one had a cerebrovascular accident without any other predisposing pathology detected.

Ohara et al.[9] studied the incidence of symptoms in 108 children with MVP. Chest pain was the most common symptom occurring in 11 children (10.2%). The chest pain was nonexertional, located in the left chest, and it was intermittent. Palpitations were present in 7.4%, dyspnea in 3.7%, and syncope in 0.9% of the children.

In maximal exercise stress tests, children with MVP usually reach the predicted maximum or submaximum level of work; exercise time is not different in MVP compared to controls. Kavey et al.[31] performed 24-hour ambulatory monitoring and exercise testing in 103 consecutive children with MVP; a group of 50 normal children served as control subjects. In the MVP group, 16 patients (16%) had exercise-induced premature ventricular beats (PVBs) and 39 (38%) had PVBs on ambulatory monitoring. Multiformed PVBs, couplets, and ventricular tachycardia were reported in four patients (4%) during exercise and in eight patients (8%) on ambulatory monitoring. No control subject had a single PVB in response to treadmill exercise, and only four (8%) had rare uniform PVBs on ambulatory monitoring. Physical findings, resting electrocardiogram, and symptoms were not correlated with PVBs in the MVP group.

Benign arrhythmias on a 24-hour Holter monitor were found in 49.1% of the 108 children with MVP studied by Ohara et al.[9]; the evidence of arrhythmia was lower in a group of 70 normal control children (21.4%). PVBs were the most common arrhythmias. The incidence of isolated PVBs was greater in MVP compared to control (27.3% versus 8.5%); the incidence of PVBs increased slightly with age. Isolated atrial premature beats were present in 23.6% of MVP children and in 10% of the controls.

There is evidence that the incidence of potentially lethal ventricular arrhythmias in patients with MVP without significant MVR is greater than in the general population.[28,29,32,33] Wei et al.[34] found 10 patients with MVP without significant MVR and similar number of patients without detectable heart disease among 60 consecutive patients referred for the management of refractory complex ventricular arrhythmias. If there is no selection bias and the incidence of MVP in the general population is approximately 4%, then the disproportionately high representation of MVP patients in this series suggests that complex ventricular arrhythmias in patients with MVP may be more frequent than in the general population without heart disease.

Rocchini et al.[35] studied 38 patients ages 1 to 20 years (mean 11.2 years) with recurrent ventricular tachycardia; 17 of the 21 patients with underlying heart disease were symptomatic compared with only 6 of the 17 patients without heart disease. Of the 21 patients with heart disease, 5 had MVP. Clinical observations suggest that children with MVP may be at higher risk of arrhythmias during anesthesia and the perioperative period.[36] Sudden death related to MVP appears to be extremely rare in children.

Progression of MVR

The progression of MVR through the spectrum from mild to moderate, and from moderate to severe in patients with FMV/MVP is gradual, and the entire process accelerates after a prolonged asymptomatic interval. Symptoms and complications in FMV/MVP related to mitral valve dysfunction include infective endocarditis, thromboembolic phenomena, cardiac arrhythmias, sudden death, progressive MVR, ruptured chordae tendineae, and congestive heart failure.[12–15] Due to the slow gradual progression, significant MVR usually occurs after the fourth or fifth decades and therefore is usually not seen in the pediatric population. Infective endocarditis, cardiac arrhythmias, and thromboembolic phenomena, however, although rare may occur in children.[12,19,36]

When FMV/MVP occurs as a part of a recognized heritable disorder of connective tissue syndrome or is associated with other cardiovascular abnormalities, the natural history is related to the coexisting abnormalities, the FMV/MVP, or the sum total of the structural defects.[19]

Diagnostic Evaluation and Management

Diagnostic evaluation and therapy are similar to those described for adults (see Chapters 13 and 24). The diagnosis of FMV/MVP in children should be based on auscultatory and well-defined echocardiographic findings.[19] It has been reported that other abnormalities may be present in patients with FMV/MVP (Chapter 13). Diagnostic studies for abnormalities associated with FMV/MVP should be undertaken if clinically indicated. Prophylaxis for infective endocarditis in children with FMV/MVP is recommended as it is in adults. It is wise to follow children with FMV/MVP with periodic evaluations even when they are not symptomatic.[37]

Floppy Mitral Valve/Mitral Valve Prolapse: Pregnancy

There are few studies dealing with pregnancy in patients with FMV/MVP.[38-46] Available data and clinical experience suggest that complications during pregnancy in patients with FMV/MVP are not anticipated, and that the frequency of intrapartum complications is not greater in FMV/MVP patients than in those with no cardiac disorder. Because of the expansion of intravascular volume during pregnancy, symptoms related to a low circulating blood volume or volume depletion responses in symptomatic patients with FMV/MVPS are less evident during pregnancy. Physical findings are modified during pregnancy for the same reasons, and thus nonejection clicks and mitral systolic murmurs may appear later in systole or may disappear. The role of estrogen in patients' symptoms and physical findings during pregnancy remains to be defined.

Rayburn and Fontana[38] studied 42 pregnancies in 25 patients who had FMV/MVP diagnosed before conception. The patient profile was similar to that of the 235 patients used as controls. None of the FMV/MVP patients required hospitalization for a cardiac complication. Propranolol was used in 11 pregnancies (seven patients) and was discontinued in all but two pregnancies during early gestation with no apparent adverse effect to the patient or fetus. The frequency of intrapartum complications was not significantly greater among patients with FMV/MVP than in controls. All but two patients received prophylactic antibiotics at delivery. Ten cesarean sections (24% of the deliveries) were performed for obstetrical reasons and all tolerated the procedures well. The incidence of spontaneous abortion or premature delivery in women with FMV/MVP was no higher than in controls.

Shapiro et al.[39] evaluated 23 patients with MVP detected before the onset of labor and demonstrated that labor and delivery were safe. A control was assigned to each patient, matched for parity, age, race, and infant birth weight. There was no evidence of cardiovascular disease in control subjects. It has been suggested that delivery may be easier in MVP patients because of joint hypermobility but this hypothesis has not gained additional support.

The diagnostic evaluation of patients with FMV/MVP during pregnancy is similar to that described for FMV/MVP in general (see Chapters 13 and 24). It should be emphasized that auscultatory findings may be altered during pregnancy due to increased intravascular volume and decreased peripheral resistance (see also Chapter 12). Family history is important since individual patients may have complications similar to their mothers. During the echocardiographic evaluation, special attention should be given to the aortic root, since certain patients with FMV/MVP may have aortic root dilatation.[47–49] Aortic root dilatation may be associated with a higher risk for aortic rupture or dissection during pregnancy.

It has been suggested that antibiotic prophylaxis is not needed for routine, uncomplicated vaginal deliveries, but should be given for any complicated delivery. Since it is difficult to predict if a delivery will be complicated, it is our view that patients with FMV/MVP should receive antibiotic prophylaxis for endocarditis before vaginal delivery.

Sympathomimetic drugs and dehydration may precipitate or initiate symptoms in patients with FMV/MVP.[50–54] Thus, sympathomimetic drugs should he used with great caution and every effort should be made to avoid dehydration and volume depletion.

Floppy Mitral Valve/Mitral Valve Prolapse: Athletics

Careful studies in athletes with FMV/MVP are lacking and thus hard data on which to base a judgment for recommendations are not yet available.[55–57] There are a few general statements that can be made.[58–70]

Despite the high prevalence of FMV/MVP in the general population, FMV/MVP is not a frequent cause of sudden death in competitive athletes. Overall, few subjects with FMV/MVP and sudden death have been reported.

There are no data to demonstrate that strenuous exercise in patients with FMV/MVP predisposes to death that otherwise would not have occurred, or the opposite, that withdrawal from competitive athletics will prolong life. Without hard data, at present, the best approach for recommendations to athletes should be based on common sense and good clinical judgment. While such decisions may be faulty, they are the best available until additional data become available. Recommendations and advice need to be balanced between restricting activity unduly and reducing chance of death or injury from the participation in athletics.

A few basic principles related to athletics and exercise will help in understanding the problem and in making better recommendations.

From the Bethesda Conference, dealing with eligibility for competition in athletes with cardiovascular abnormalities, the recommendations regarding eligibility for competition defined competitive athlete as follows:[58] "Competitive athlete is one who participates in an organized team or individual sport that requires regular competition against others as a central component, places a high premium on excellence and achievement and requires vigorous training in a systematic fashion." An important consideration when dealing with a competitive athlete is that the individual may not be able to use proper judgment in determining when to stop the competition. Warning symptoms such as fatigue and chest discomfort that may occur during competition may be difficult to distinguish from sensations caused by the physical activity itself. In addition, the athlete may not promptly terminate the physical exertion even when the need to do so is perceived, because of the circumstances and pressures of competition.

Exercise may be divided into two general types:[62] *dynamic* (isotonic) and *static* (isometric).

Dynamic exercise involves changes in muscle length and joint movement with rhythmic contractions that develop at relatively smaller force. It is performed with a large muscle mass, causes a marked increase in oxygen consumption, cardiac output, and systolic blood pressure, while diastolic and mean pressure remain relatively constant and peripheral vascular resistance decreases. Dynamic exercise causes a primary volume load on the left ventricle.

Static (isometric) exercise involves the development of a relatively larger force with little or no change in muscle length or joint movement. It usually involves a much smaller muscle mass than dynamic exercise and causes a smaller increase in oxygen consumption and cardiac output. There is a marked increase in systolic, diastolic, and mean arterial pressure while peripheral vascular resistance increases only slightly. Static exercise produces a primary pressure load on the left ventricle.

Sports may be classified according to the type and intensity of exercise performed, and according to the danger of body collision (Table 1).[62] This classification does not consider the emotional stress that a particular athlete may be exposed to during a specific athletic event, which may be an important factor in FMV/MVP patients. Thus, in a low-intensity competition (e.g., golf), during championship play the subject may be extremely anxious and the resulting catecholamine response may cause marked tachycardia or other cardiac arrhythmias.

FMV/MVP occurs in a heterogeneous group of patients with a wide spectrum of connective tissue abnormalities, mitral valve involvement, and hemodynamic abnormalities. A careful analysis of the family history for connective tissue disorders may be necessary in order to reach proper decisions in certain circumstances. Thus, it is important in each case to define where within the spectrum of connective tissue, mitral valve, and hemodynamic abnormalities the specific individual belongs (see also Chapter 13). In addition, the aortic root size, the presence of cardiac arrhythmias, and the symptomatology (if present) should be determined. Thus, recommendations should be based on the status of mitral valve function, left ventricular (LV) and left atrial (LA) structure and function, aortic root size, and in the presence or absence of symptoms.

Table 1
Classification of Sports

I. Intensity and Type of Exercise Performed
  A. High to moderate intensity
    1. High to moderate dynamic and static demands
      Boxing
      Crew/rowing
      Cross-country skiing
      Cycling
      Downhill skiing
      Fencing
      Football
      Ice hockey
      Rugby
      Running (sprint)
      Speed skating
      Water polo
      Wrestling
    2. High to moderate dynamic and low static demands
      Badminton
      Baseball
      Basketball
      Field hockey
      Lacrosse
      Orienteering
      Ping-pong
      Race walking
      Racquetball
      Running (distance)
      Soccer
      Squash
      Swimming
      Tennis
      Volleyball
    3. High to moderate static and low dynamic demands
      Archery
      Auto racing
      Diving
      Equestrian
      Field events (jumping)
      Field events (throwing)
      Gymnastics
      Karate or judo
      Motorcycling
      Rodeoing
      Sailing
      Ski jumping
      Water skiing
      Weight lifting

Table 1
(Continued)

B. Low intensity (low dynamic and low static demands)
    Bowling
    Cricket
    Curling
    Golf
    Riflery
II. Danger of Body Collision
    Auto racing*
    Bicycling
    Boxing
    Diving*
    Downhill skiing*
    Equestrian * activities
    Football
    Gymnastics*
    Ice hockey
    Karate or judo
    Lacrosse
    Motorcycling*
    Polo*
    Rodeoing*
    Rugby
    Ski jumping*
    Soccer
    Water polo*
    Water skiing*
    Weight lifting*
    Wrestling

* Increased risk if syncope occurs. From JH Mitchell et al. with permission

Floppy Mitral Valve/Mitral Valve Prolapse: Mitral Valve Status, Left Ventricular–Left Atrial Structure and Function

Patients with FMV/MVP with myxomatous and collagen changes in the mitral valve may be in danger of further prolapse and increased chordal tension by strenuous activity, but little objective information is available at present. Chronic, excessive, prolonged volume overload leads to a progressive decrease in myocardial contractility. The presence of intermittent repetitive increases in volume load may be deleterious and contribute to the progression of the disease. Static exercise increases arterial pressure and may worsen MVR and increase LA pressure. As a general rule, in patients with MVR, the LV diastolic volume and LA volume reflect the severity of MVR. Thus, as a general rule, LV size and LA volumes are used in most cases as a guide for recommendations (Table 2).

Table 2
FMV/MVP: Abnormalities and Recommendations for Participation in Competitive Sports

Severity of Mitral Valve Abnormalities	Recommendation
No or mild mitral valvular regurgitation (MVR)	No restriction
Mild to moderate MVR Normal LV size and function	No restriction
Asymptomatic, mild LV enlargement, normal LV function	Low-intensity sports (Class IB)

Symptomatic or asymptomatic moderate or
   more than moderate LV enlargement; any
   degree of LV dysfunction
	No participation in competitive
	athletics

LV = left ventricle; FMV = floppy mitral valve; MVP = mitral valve prolapse.

In general, asymptomatic patients with FMV/MVP without, or with mild, MVR with normal aortic root size, normal LV and LA structure and function, and without cardiac arrhythmias can participate in all competitive athletics. Patients with mild to moderate MVR in sinus rhythm with normal LV and LA size and function may participate in all competitive sports.[19]

Asymptomatic patients with mild LV enlargement and normal LV function may participate in sports with a low intensity.

Symptomatic or asymptomatic patients with definite LV enlargement and any degree of LV dysfunction should not participate in any competitive sport.

Floppy Mitral Valve/Mitral Valve Prolapse: Presence of Symptoms

Palpitations–Arrhythmias

Patients with a history of palpitations should be carefully evaluated to exclude any significant arrhythmia before permission to participate in competitive sports.[13,19,58,71] The prognosis of ventricular or supraventricular arrhythmias detected with exercise testing or ambulatory monitoring in patients with FMV/MVP and normal LV structure and function appears to be good, although not completely defined. Patients with suspected cardiac arrhythmias being considered for competitive athletics should have long-term ambulatory monitoring, if possible during the type of exercise the athlete performs, and an exercise test.[58] Arrhythmias may not be reproducible during a routine exercise test and exercise may need to be adapted specifically for the athlete (e.g., begin exercise at peak level in a sprinter rather than with a slowly increasing workload). Patients with arrhythmias should be reevaluated at intervals after they have been trained to determine the effect of training on arrhythmia. Recommendations for participation in athletics are related mostly to the nature and severity of the arrhythmia.

Younger patients with ventricular preexcitation or concealed atrioventricular pathways should have an in-depth evaluation before recommendation for participation in competitive athletics. Arrhythmias due to abnormal atrioventricular pathways may be abolished with radiofrequency ablation.[73]

Coelho et al.[60] studied 19 young athletes aged 14 to 32 years with documented symptomatic tachyarrhythmias; five had paroxysmal atrial fibrillation, five paroxysmal supraventricular tachycardia, eight paroxysmal ventricular tachycardia, and one ventricular fibrillation. Nine of these patients (47%) had MVP, and five (26%) had abnormal atrioventricular pathway. Tachyarrhythmias started during strenuous exercise in 13 patients (68%); tachyarrhythmia that closely resembled the spontaneous arrhythmia induced by programmed cardiac stimulation began in 13 patients (68%) and was reproducibly provoked by treadmill exercise testing in eight patients (48%). In four of the eight patients with ventricular tachycardia, tachycardia was provoked with isoproterenol infusion.

Syncope–Presyncope

Syncope may be related to or result from a life-threatening condition; thus a complete evaluation is indicated to define the cause of syncope.[73] Patients with syncope or presyncope should not participate in competitive sports until the cause of syncope has been defined and appropriately treated.[58] Patients with neurocardiogenic syncope may participate in high-intensity sports with caution and if symptoms do not occur during competition. Patients with orthostatic syncope due to dehydration or volume depletion from vigorous exercise may participate in low-intensity competitive sports if, with appropriate therapy, they remain free of symptoms for at least 6 months. Selective patients may participate in high-intensity sports. Excess fluid and sodium intake are advisable before and during the competition. Patients with arrhythmic syncope can participate in low-intensity competitive sports if, with appropriate therapy, they remain free of symptoms for at least 6 months.

Patients with a history of syncope regardless of the etiology should not participate in sports with a danger of body collision when syncope occurs.

Chest Pain

Coronary artery disease or other underlying cardiac pathology should be excluded before permission to participate in sports in patients with chest pain.[12,13] An exercise test should be performed, and if clinically indicated, further diagnostic studies including coronary arteriography should be undertaken.

It has been suggested that patients with a family history of sudden death due to FMV/MVP should not participate in competitive sports. No data are available, however, to support this thesis.

Floppy Mitral Valve/Mitral Valve Prolapse: Aviation

Specific data regarding individuals or patients with FMV/MVP related to aviation are lacking; thus, recommendations must be based on common sense and good clinical judgment.[74-81] Aviators in high-performance aircraft may operate under stressful conditions and maneuvers that produce a high positive G stress. The application of +G stress forces in either the horizontal (X axis) or the posteroanterior (Z axis) Gx and Gz, respectively) has been demonstrated to decrease LV volume and to increase systolic and diastolic pressure in the ascending aorta.

Thus, in certain cases because of the volume and pressure changes, MVR might occur under high +G acceleration forces in a person with FMV/MVP who had little or no MVR under normal conditions. In addition, +G stress may precipitate arrhythmias and produce syncope or motion sickness.

Brown et al.[77] reported in 1973 that two pilots with MVP developed ventricular tachycardia (four PVBs in a row) and multiformed PVBs while sustaining 4 to 6 +G stress during flight. The arrhythmias that occurred during the +G in these two pilots were the first significant arrhythmias encountered in over 270 in-flight hours of electrocardiographic monitoring performed in a group of 90 student aviators; they do not specify, however, whether any of the other 90 students had FMV/MVP. They recommended that persons with FMV/MVP should be evaluated for arrhythmias not only with exercise testing and ambulatory monitoring, but also during and after Valsalva maneuvers performed in the upright posture. In addition, when aviation personnel are involved, monitoring during high +G conditions should be considered if there has been any suggestion of arrhythmias.

Whinnery (1986)[78] reported his experience with 78 U.S. Air Force air crew personnel with auscultatory and/or echocardiographic evidence of MVP who were evaluated for tolerance to G stress. The MVP group was found to have a normal response to the gradual onset of +G stress, both while relaxed and when performing a protective straining maneuver. A small but statistically significant decrease in tolerance to the rapid onset of +G stress was found. During the +G stress 15% of those with MVP lost consciousness. This incidence of syncope was greater (p<0.01) than the 7% incidence of syncope in 1,126 normal individuals without MVP. The incidence of motion sickness during the +G stress was also greater in those with MVP than in the 1,126 normal individuals (17% versus 11%).

The effect of +G stress on the ascending aorta should also be taken into consideration. Persons with MVP should be carefully evaluated for possible aortic root enlargement, which may be present in certain patients with FMV/MVP.

There are no specific recommendations regarding persons or patients with FMV/MVP in civil air personnel. The FAA 1998 recommendations for a first-class airman are as follows: (A) No established medical history or clinical diagnosis of any of the following: (1) myocardial infarction; (2) angina pectoris; (3) coronary heart disease that has required treatment or, if untreated, that has been symptomatic or clinically significant; (4) cardiac valve replacement; (5) permanent cardiac pacemaker implantation; or (6) Heart replacement. (B) A person applying for first-class medical certification must demonstrate an absence of myocardial infarction and other clinically significant abnormality on electrocardiographic examination: (1) at the first application after reaching the 35th birthday; and (2) on an annual basis after reaching the 40th birthday. (C) An electrocardiogram will satisfy a requirement of paragraph B of this section if it is dated no earlier than 60 days before the date of the application it is to accompany and was performed and transmitted according to acceptable standards and techniques.

References

1. Wooley CF. Where are the diseases of yesteryear? DaCosta's syndrome, soldier's heart, the effort syndrome, neurocirculatory asthenia - and the mitral valve prolapse syndrome. Circulation 53:799–751, 1976.
2. Wooley CF, Boudoulas H. From irritable heart to mitral valve prolapse: World War I - the U.S. experience and the prevalence of apical systolic murmurs and mitral regurgitation in drafted men compared with present day mitral valve prolapse studies. Am J Cardiol 61:895–899, 1988.
3. Wilson MG. Exercise tolerance of children with heart disease as determined by standardized test exercises. JAMA 76:1629–1633, 1921.
4. Kerley CE. The effort syndrome in children. Arch Ped 37:449–454, 1920.
5. Lincoln EM. The hearts of normal children. Am J Dis Children 298–410, 1928.
6. Griffith CJP. Mid-systolic and late-systolic mitral murmurs. Am J Med Sci 10: 285–294,1892.

7. Sakamoto T. Prospective phonocardiographic study of mitral valve prolapse: Prevalence of nonejection click in schoolchildren. In Diethrich EB (ed): Noninvasive Assesment of the Cardiovascular System. John Wright, PSG, 1982, pp 153–157.

8. Hickey AJ, Wilcken DEL. Age and the clinical profile of idiopathic mitral valve prolapse. Br Heart J 55:582–586, 1986.

9. Ohara N, Mikajima T, Takagi J, Kato H. Mitral valve prolapse in childhood: The incidence of clinical presentations in different age groups. Acta Paediatr Jpn 33: 467–475, 1991.

10. Greenwood RD. Mitral valve prolapse: Incidence and clinical course in a pediatric population. Clin Pediatr 23:318–320, 1984.

11. Greenwood RD. Mitral valve prolapse in childhood. Hosp Pract August: 41–42, 1986.

12. Boudoulas H, Wooley CF (eds). Floppy Mitral Valve, Mitral Valve Prolapse, Mitral Valvular Regurgitation And The Mitral Valve Prolapse Syndrome. Mount Kisco, NY. Futura Publishing Company, Inc., 1988.

13. Boudoulas H, Kolibash AJ, Baker P, King BD, Wooley CF. Mitral valve prolapse and the mitral valve prolapse syndrome: A diagnostic classification and pathogenesis of symptoms . Am Heart J 118:796–818, 1989.

14. Wooley CF, Baker PB, Kolibash AJ, Kilman JW, Sparks EA, Boudoulas H. The floppy, myxomatous mitral valve, mitral valve prolapse and mitral regurgitation. Prog Cardiovasc Dis 33:397–433, 1991.

15. Wooley CF, Sparks EA, Boudoulas H. The floppy mitral valve-mitral valve prolapse-mitral valvular regurgitation triad. ACC Current Journal Review July/August 1994, pp 25–26.

16. Bowen J, Boudoulas H, Wooley CF. Cardiovascular disease of connective tissue origin. Am J Med 82:481–488, 1987.

17. Boudoulas H. Valvular disease. American college of Cardiology Self-assessment Program (ACCSAP) 2000, in press.

18. Boudoulas H, Kolibash AJ, Wooley CF. Mitral valve prolapse: The high-risk patient. Practical Cardiol 17:15–31, 1991.

19. Boudoulas H, Wooley CF. The floppy mitral valve, mitral valve prolapse, and mitral valvular regurgitation.

20. Barlow JB, Pocock WA. Mitral leaflet billowing and prolapse. In Barlow JB (ed): Perspectives on the Mitral Valve. Philadelphia, FA Davis Company, 1989, pp 45–112.

21. Deliagin VM, Pil'kh AD, Basenove LK. Echocardiographic study of the heart in children with mitral valve prolapse and connective tissue dysplasia. Pediatriia (1)52–58, 1990.

22. Suzuki K, Murakami Y, Mori K, Mimori S. Four boys with multiple floppy valves involving all cardiac valves and hyperextensive joints. J Cardiol 21: 161–172, 1991.

23. Malkowski MT, Boudoulas H, Wooley CF, Guo R, Pearson AC. The spectrum of structural abnormalities in the floppy mitral valve: Echocardiographic evaluation. Am Heat J 132:145–151, 1996.

24. Dhuper S, Ehlers KH, Fatica NS, Byridakis DJ, Klein AA, friedman DM, Levine DB. Incidence and risk factors for mitral valve prolapse in severe adolescent idiopathic scoliosis. Pediatr Cardiol 18:425–428, 1997.

25. Gupta R, Jain BK, Gupta HP, Ranawat SS, Sharma AK, Gupta KD. Mitral valve prolapse: Two dimensional echocardiography reveals a high prevalence in three to twelve year old children. Indian Pediatr 29(4):415–423, 1992.

26. Chandraratna PA, Vlahovich G, Kong Y, Wilson D. Incidence of mitral valve

prolapse in one-hundred clinically stable newborn baby girls: An echocardiographic study. Am Heart J 98(3):312–314, 1979.

27. Krishnan US, Welton M, Gersony MD, Berman-Rosenzweig E, Apfel HD. Late left ventricular function after surgery for children with chronic symptomatic mitral regurgitation. Circulation 96:4280–4285, 1997.

28. Babkowski W, Siwinska A, Gorzna H, Niedbalski R, Paluszak W, Maciejewski J. Dysrhythmias documented by 48-hour electrocardiographic monitoring in children with mitral valve prolapse. Pediatr Pol 71:493–497, 1996.

29. Nowak A, Czerwionka-Szaflarska M. Arrhythmias in children with mitral valve prolapse syndrome. Pediatr Pol 71:499–504, 1996.

30. Bisset GS III, Schwartz DC, Meyer RA, et al. Clinical spectrum and long-term follow-up of isolated mitral valve prolapse in 119 children. Circulation 62:423–429, 1980.

31. Kavey REW, Blackman NS, Sondheimer HM, Byrum CJ. Ventricular arrhythmias and mitral valve prolapse in childhood. J Pediatr 105:885–890, 1984.

32. Sorbo MD, Buja FF, Miorelli M, Nistri S, Perrone C, Manca S, Grasso F, et al. The prevalence of the Wolff-Parkinson-White syndrome in a population of 116,542 young males. G Ital Cardiol 25:681–688, 1995.

33. Boudoulas H, Schaal SF, Stang JM, et al. Mitral valve prolapse: Cardiac arrest with long-term survival. Int J Cardiol 26:37–44, 1990.

34. Wei JY, Bulkey BH, Schaeffer AH, et al. Mitral valve prolapse syndrome and recurrent ventricular tachyarrhythmias: A malignant variant refractory of conventional drug therapy. Ann Int Med 89:6–9, 1978.

35. Rocchini AP, Chun PO, Dick M. Ventricular tachycardia in children. Am J Cardiol 47:1091–1097, 1981.

36. Berry FA, Lake CL, Johns RA, Rogers BM. Mitral valve prolapse: Another cause of intraoperative dysrhythmias in the pediatric patient. Anesthesiology 62:662–664, 1985.

37. Dajani AS, Taubert KA, Wilson W, et al. Prevention of bacterial endocarditis. Recommendations by the American Heart Association. JAMA 277:1794–801, 1997.

38. Rayburn WF, Fontana ME. Mitral valve prolapse and pregnancy. Am J Obstetr Gynecol 141:9–11, 1981.

39. Shapiro EP, Trimble EL, Robinson JC, Estruch MT, Gottlieb SH. Safety of labor and delivery in women with mitral valve prolapse. Am J Cardiol 56:806–807, 1985.

40. Haas JM. The effect of pregnancy on the midsystolic click and murmur of the prolapsing posterior leaflet of the mitral valve. Am Heart J 902:407–408, 1976.

41. Fuenzalida CE. A selective advantage with mitral valve prolapse. Ann Int Med 98:670–671, 1983.

42. Boudoulas H, Wooley CF. Mitral valve prolapse. In Eliseev OM (ed): Cardiovascular Diseases and Pregnancy. Berlin, Springer-Verlag, 1988, pp 69–70.

43. Siu SC, Sermer M, Harrison DA, Grigoriadia E, Liu G, Sorensen S, Smallhorn JF, et al. Risk and predictors for pregnancy-related complications in women with heart disease. Circulation 96:2789–2794, 1997.

44. Chia YT, Yeoh SC, Lim MC, Viegas OA, Ratnam SS. Pregnancy outcome and mitral valve prolapse. Asia-Oceania J Ob Gyn 20(4):383–388, 1994.

45. Mishra M, Chambers JB, Jackson G. Murmurs in pregnancy: An audit of echocardiography. MBJ 304:1413–1414, 1992.

46. Wada H, Chiba Y, Murakami M, Kawaguchi H, Kobayashi H, Kanzaki T. Analysis of maternal and fetal risk in 594 pregnancies with heart disease. Nippon Sanka Fujinka Gakkai Zasshi 48(4):255–262, 1996.

47. Donnelly TJ, Wooley CF, Boudoulas H. Mitral valve prolapse: Aortic dimensions may reflect a connective tissue disorder. Am J Noninvas Cardiol 5:47–51, 1991.
48. Seliem MA, Duffy CE, Gidding SS, Berdusis K, Benson DW Jr. Echocardiographic evaluation of the aortic root and mitral valve in children and adolescents with isolated pectus excavatum: Comparison with Marfan patients. Pediatr Cardiol 13:20–23, 1992.
49. Ivy DD, Shaffer EM, Johnson AM, Kimberling WJ, Dobin AM, Gavow PA. Cardiovascular abnormalities in children with autosomal dominant polycystic kidney disease. J Am Soc Nephrol 5:2032–2036, 1995.
50. Boudoulas H, Reynolds JC, Mazzaferri E, et al. Metabolic studies in mitral valve prolapse syndrome. Circulation 61:1200–1205, 1980.
51. Boudoulas H, Reynolds JC, Mazzaferri E, et al. Mitral valve prolapse syndrome: The effect of adrenergic stimulation. J Am Coll Cardiol 2:638–644, 1983.
52. Davies AO, Mares A, Pool JL, et al. Mitral valve prolapse with symptoms of beta adrenergic hypersensitivity: Beta$_2$ adrenergic receptor supercoupling with desensitiation of isoproterenol exposure. Am J Med 82:193–201, 1987.
53. Davies AO, Su DJ, Balasubramanyam A, Codina J, Birnbaumer L. Abnormal guanine nucleotide regulatory protein in FMV/MVP dysautonomia: Evidence from reconstitution of G. J Clin Endocrinol Metab 72:867–875, 1991.
54. Anwar A, Kohn SR, Dunn JF, et al. Altered beta adrenergic receptor function in subjects with symptomatic mitral valve prolapse. Am J Med Sci 302:89–97, 1991.
55. Stoddard MF, Prince CR, Dillon S, Longaker RA, Morris GT, Liddell NE. Exercise-induced mitral regurgitation is a predictor of morbid events in subjects with mitral valve prolapse. J Am Coll Cardiol 25:693–699, 1995.
56. Jeresaty R. Mitral Valve Prolapse: Definition and Implications in Athletes. JACC 7:231–236, 1986.
57. Warth DC, King ME, Cohen JM, Tesoriero VL, Marcus E, Weyman AE. Prevalence of mitral valve prolapse in normal children. J Am Coll Cardiol 5:1173–1177, 1985.
58. Maron BJ, Mitchell JH. Revised eligibility recommendations for competitive athletes with cardiovascular abnormalities, 26th Bethesda Conference. J Am Coll Cardiol 24:845–899, 1994.
59. Maron BJ, Mitten MJ, Quandt EF, Zipes DP. Competitive athletes with cardiovascular disease: The case of Nicholas Knapp. N Engl J Med 339:1632–1635, 1998.
60. Coelho A, Palileo E, Ashley W, et al. Tachyarrhythmias in young athletes. J Am Coll Cardiol 7:237–243, 1986.
61. McLaren MJ, Hawkins DM, Lachman AS, Lakier JB, Pocock Wa, Barlow JB. Nonejection systolic clicks and mitral systolic murmurs in black school children of Soweto, Johannesburg. Br Heart J 38:718–724, 1976.
62. Mitchell JH, Blomqvist CG, Haskell WL, James FW, Miller HS, Miller WW. Classification of sports. J Am Coll Cardiol 1196–1198, 1985.
63. Glover DW, Maron BJ. Profile of Preparticipation Cardiovascular Screening for High School Athletes. JAMA 279(22):1817–1819, 1998.
64. Huston TP, Puffer JC, Rodney WM. The athletic heart syndrome. N Engl J Med 313:32, 1985.
65. George KP, Wolfe LA, Burggraf GW. The 'athletic heart syndrome.' A critical review. Sports Med 11(5):300–330, 1991.
66. Pelliccia A, Maron BJ, Spataro A, Proschan MA, Spirito P. The Upper Limit of

Physiologic Cardiac Hypertrophy in Highly Trained Elite Athletes. N Eng J Med 324:295–301, 1991.

67. Spirito P, Pelliccia A, Proschan MA, Granata M, Spataro A, Bellonep, Caselli G, et al. Morphology of the Athlete's Heart Assessed by Echocardiography in 947 Elite Athletes Representing 27 Sports. Am J Cardiol 74:802–806, 1994.

68. Henriksen E, Landelius J, Wesslen L, Arnell H, Nystrom-Rosander C, Kangro T, Jonason T, et al. Echocardiographic right and left ventricular measurements in male elite endurance athletes. Euro Heart J 17:1121–1128, 1996.

69. Maron BJ, Thompson PD, Puffer JC, McGrew CA, Strong WB, Douglas PS, Clark LT, et al. Cardiovascular Preparticipation Screening of Competitive Athletes: Addendum. Circulation 97:2294, 1998.

70. Matheson GO. Preparticipation Screening of Athletes. JAMA 279:1829–1830, 1998.

71. Boudoulas H, Schaal SF, Wooley CF. Floppy mitral valve/mitral valve prolapse: Cardiac arrhythmias. In Vardas PE (ed): Cardiac Arrhythmias, Pacing and Electrophysiology. Great Britain, Kluwer Academic Publisher, 1998, pp 89–95.

72. Bashore TM, Grines C, Utlak D, Boudoulas H, Wooley CF. Postural exercise abnormalities in symptomatic patients with mitral valve prolapse. J Am Coll Cardiol 11:499–507,1988.

73. Boudoulas H, Nelson SD, Schaal SF, Lewis RP. Diagnosis and management of syncope. In Alexander RW, Schlant RC, Fuster V, et al (eds): Hurst's The Heart, 9th ed, New York, McGraw-Hill, 1998, pp 1059–1080.

74. Whinnery FE. Acceleration tolerance of asymptomatic aircrew with mitral valve prolapse. Aviat Space Environ Med October 986–992, 1986.

75. Zakharov VP, Karlov VN, Bondareva SV, Vlasov VD. Arrhythmias and heart blocks in flying personnel with mitral valve prolapses. Aviakosm Ekolog Med 33(1):41–46, 1999.

76. Towne WD, Rahimtoola SH, Rosen KM, Casten CP, Gunnar RM. Systolic prolapse of the mitral valve: Possible aeromedical significance. Aerospace Med March: 341–344, 1971.

77. Brown DD, Stoop DR, Stanton KC. Precipitation of cardiac arrhythmias in the mid-systolic click/late-systolic murmur syndrome by in-flight +G_2 maneuvers. Aerospace Med Oct: 1169–1172, 1973.

78. Whinnery JE. Acceleration tolerance of asymptomatic aircrew with mitral valve prolapse. Aviat Space Environm Med Oct: 986–992, 1986.

79. Rayman RB. The prolapsed mitral valve syndrome and the flyer. Aviat Space Environm Med March: 287–289, 1980.

80. Engelberg AL, Gibbons HL, Doege TC. A review of the medical standards for civilian airmen. JAMA 255:1589–1599, 1986.

81. Preobrazhenskii VN, Zakharov VP. Clinico-function evaluation of the significance of mitral valve prolapse in flight personnel. Terapevticheskii Arkhiv 67(12):25–27, 1995.

Part XVII

The Floppy Mitral Valve, Mitral Valve Prolapse, Mitral Valvular Regurgitation:

Veterinary Medicine

Introduction

The Floppy Mitral Valve, Mitral Valve Prolapse, Mitral Valvular Regurgitation:
Veterinary Medicine

Charles F. Wooley, MD,
Harisios Boudoulas, MD, PhD

Clinicians are quite aware of the importance of animal models in cardiovascular research, and the molecular genetic era has seen a resurgence of interest in basic cardiovascular phenomenology in both large and small animal systems. There is less awareness among clinicians about the incidence and nature of cardiac disease in the animal kingdom, particularly in domestic animals, from household pets to the domesticated large animals.

There are many interesting genetic and pathogenetic parallels between mitral valve disease in the dog and in the human. In the next chapter, Dr. Robert Hamlin discusses mitral valvular regurgitation (MVR) in the dog, the role of mitral valve prolapse (MVP) in the genesis of the MVR, and the nature of the valvular lesions involved, including the floppy mitral valve (FMV).

Interacting with the Veterinarians

Recall, if you will, the heritage clinical cardiologists share with veterinary physicians in the area of hemodynamics and the circulation, specifically, the collaborative studies by Marey and Chauveau in 1861.

Etienne Jules Marey (1830–1904), Professor at the College de France, outstanding cardiovascular physiologist, master of the graphic method, devised air-filled manometers for registering biological phenomena. Au-

From: Boudoulas H, Wooley CF: *Mitral Valve: Floppy Mitral Valve, Mitral Valve Prolapse, Mitral Valvular Regurgitation*. Second revised edition. ©Futura Publishing Company, Armonk, NY, 2000.

guste Chaveau (1827–1917), Professor of Veterinary Medicine in Lyon, had previously performed many experiments in the horse.

Using their ingenious system of sounds, or cardiac catheters in the contemporary sense, they developed a novel, double-lumen technique to catheterize the right atrium and right ventricle in the horse via the jugular vein. They recorded chamber pressures in the right atrium, right ventricle, and pulmonary artery, and used the recorded pressure pulses to show the relation of atrial and ventricular systole to the apex beat. The carotid artery approach was used to enter the left ventricle. Chauveau also constructed a projecting kymograph at the Veterinary School at Lyon to demonstrate these events and relations to students and visitors.

Both men had extraordinary careers. Marey went on to studies of animal locomotion, in particular, the gait of horses and dogs, and in time devised methods to capture the flight of birds on film, becoming one of the founders of cinematography. Chauveau analyzed the production and mechanisms of cardiac murmurs, and later performed important research in body energetics.

The same spirit of inquiry that motivated these illustrious clinician-veterinary predecessors is alive and well at the College of Veterinary Medicine at The Ohio State University.[1] We have had the opportunity to experience this first-hand while making clinical rounds with our colleagues in the veterinary hospital. Learning the nuances of cardiac examination and auscultation in small and large animals, participating in the cardiac catheterization in the horse, and understanding the intricacies of echo Doppler studies in creatures large and small were all part of our education in this environment. These experiences impressed upon us the value of exchange with our veterinary colleagues, and the many lessons to be learned from the process.

Over the years these interactions with Dr. Robert Hamlin and his associates made us aware of the unique challenges and problems the veterinary physicians face in day-to-day diagnostics and clinical management.

The Floppy Mitral Valve/Mitral Valve Prolapse/Mitral Valvular Regurgitation Triad in Other Animals

Dr. Hamlin limits his discussion to MVR in the dog in the following chapter.

There are other references that may be of interest to our readers. The first is the description of MVP in 26 of 92 animals in a breeding colony of rhesus monkeys (*Macaca mulatta*) described in 1985.[2] The affected animals had systolic murmurs best heard over the mitral area with the animal in a sitting position; mid- to late systolic clicks were also heard, and recorded with phonocardiography. There was good auscultatory and echo correlation in this study, with necropsy confirmation of posterior and/or anterior mitral leaflet prolapse into the left atrium. Breeding records suggested that the MVP was a dominant genetic trait with an approximate birth incidence of 16% to 20% in the colony.

Severe MVR and congestive heart failure in 43 horses studied with two-dimensional echo and Doppler echocardiography was reported from the University of Pennsylvania in 1998.[3] The mean age was 7.6 ± 8.1 years, with signs of left heart enlargement; grade 3–6/6 systolic murmurs were present at cardiac auscultation; atrial fibrillation was noted in 24 horses with congestive failure at presentation. Exertional intolerance, respiratory signs, and fever were common signs. Mitral valve thickening, flail mitral leaflets with ruptured chordae, mitral valve prolapse, and large systolic regurgitant jets into the left atria were consistent findings. Postmortem examinations in 35 horses confirmed the echo findings.

Veterinarians as Patients

A few observations about veterinarians and their exposure to occupational hazards may be appropriate. Clinical awareness about the potential medical consequences of the occupational hazards that veterinary physicians face has not received a great deal of attention in the medical literature. A recent American Veterinary Medical Association survey with 995 respondents emphasizes the point. Major animal-related injuries were reported by 65%, and 17% had been hospitalized during the previous year. Hand injuries (53%), arm trauma (28%), lacerations requiring sutures (35%), scalpel injuries, and zoonotic disease were the significant findings.[4]

The infectious consequences of scratches, bites, and unusual forms of trauma are frequently the result of uncommon pathogens. Cat-scratch disease associated with *Bartonella henseae* as the causal agent, or animal bites introducing *Pasteurella multicida*, are examples.[5–10]

Thus, the veterinary physician with FMV may be at risk for the development of infective endocarditis due to unusual pathogens. We have seen two of our veterinary medicine colleagues with FMV/MVP/MVR complicated by infective endocarditis due to unusual organisms; both required informed and sophisticated laboratory and infectious disease management.

Several other veterinary physicians with auscultatory evidence of FMV/MVP have been seen in consultation; numerous scratches and cuts were present on physical examination and were casually dismissed as badges of office. In these situations, infective endocarditis prophylaxis in veterinary physicians may also involve the use of gloves and other protective measures when dealing with the spectrum of animals encountered in the office, the field, the hospital, and the zoo.

It is possible that individuals with the FMV/MVP/MVR triad who work or labor in other fields in which occupational exposure or trauma may be followed by infections may benefit from such precautions.

References

1. Pipers FS, Bonagura JD, Hamlin RI, Kittleson M. Echocardiographic abnormalities of the mitral valve associated with left-sided heart diseases in the dog. J Am Vet Med Assoc 6:580–586, 1981.
2. Swindle MM, Blum JR, Lima SD, Weiss JL. Spontaneous mitral valve prolapse in a breeding colony of rhesus monkeys. Circulation 1:146–153, 1985.
3. Reef VB, Bain FT, Spencer PA. Severe mitral regurgitation in horses: Clinical, echocardiographic and pathological findings. Equine Vet J 1:18–27, 1998.
4. Landercasper J, Cogbill TH, Strutt PJ, Landercasper BO. Trauma and the veterinarian. J Trauma 8:1255–1259, 1988.
5. Fox JG, Lipman NS. Infections transmitted by large and small laboratory animals. Infect Dis Clin North Am 1:131–163, 1991.
6. Tan JS. Human zoonotic infections transmitted by dogs and cats. Arch Intern Med 17:1933–1943, 1997.
7. Hill DJ, Langley RL, Morrow WM. Occupational injuries and illnesses reported by zoo veterinarians in the United States. J Zoo Wildl Med 4:371–385, 1998.
8. Jensen BS, Lings S. Working environment in Danish veterinary clinics. Ugeskr Laeger 3:265–269, 1999.
9. Margileth AW, Wear DJ, Hadfield TL, Schlagel CJ, Spigel GT, Muhlbauer JE. Cat-scratch disease: Bacteria in skin at the primary inoculation site. JAMA 252:928–931, 1984.
10. Burdge DR, Scheifele D, Speert DP. Serious pasteurella multocida infections from lion and tiger bites. JAMA 253:3296–3297, 1985.

26

Naturally Occurring Mitral Regurgitation in the Dog

Robert L. Hamlin, DVM, PhD, DACVIM

Incidence of Mitral Regurgitation in Dogs

Eleven percent of dogs presented to a veterinarian have some form of heart disease.[1–4] Of that 11%, 95% have a form of acquired heart disease, and approximately 80% of those with acquired heart disease have mitral regurgitation (Fig. 1). Thus, if we presume mitral regurgitation is distributed in the general canine population of over 60 million dogs as it is in the dogs presented to the veterinarian, it occurs in approximately 4.8 million dogs in the United States alone.

Mitral regurgitation occurs predominantly in older, smaller, chondrodystophic, male dogs; but it occurs most prevalently in Cavalier King Charles spaniels,[5,6] next most prevalently in whippets, and with greater than expected prevalences in cocker spaniels, dachshunds, and poodles. Because of these prevalences, it is thought that mitral regurgitation has a familial tendency, but neither the mechanics of genetic transmission nor why it is a disease most severe in relatively small dogs has been identified.

The prevalence of mitral regurgitation increases with age. It occurs in a small percentage of dogs before age 5, but increases in prevalence until approximately 40% of dogs over 10 years of age are afflicted. Of course prevalence is much higher in small, male, chondrodystophic dogs. As many as 75% of aged Cavalier King Charles spaniels have mitral regurgitation.

From: Boudoulas H, Wooley CF. *Mitral Valve: Floppy Mitral Valve, Mitral Valve Prolapse, Mitral Valvular Regurgitation.* Second revised edition. ©Futura Publishing Company, Armonk, NY, 2000.

703

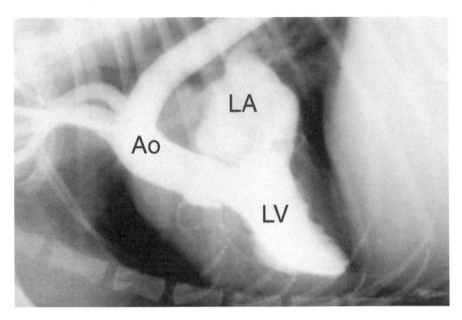

Figure 1. Lateral angiocardiogram from a dog with mitral regurgitation, viewed from the left side. Head is to the left, back is to the top. Radiopaque was injected into the left ventricle (LV), and indicator can be visualized regurgitating into the left atrium (LA) and preceding antegradely into the aorta (Ao).

It is estimated from a Scandanavian study that almost 90% of 3-year-old Cavalier King Charles Spaniels have mitral valve prolapse (Fig. 2), most without mitral regurgitation, while the prevalence is less than 10% in 3-year-old beagles in the same study.[5,6] This exceptionally high prevalence, as compared to what is reported in the US, may be an artifact of the families of dogs in Scandanavian countries or of the criteria used for identification. It is proposed, but not supported, that mitral valve prolapse may be the prodromata of endocardiosis; however, an equally appealing proposal is that both mitral valve prolapse and endocardiosis are unrelated familial lesions that happen to occur with greatest prevalence in certain breeds.

Sixty-four cases of mitral regurgitation and/or mitral valve prolapse were found when examining 306 hearts from three different institutions in Japan. This prevalence, almost 21% of dogs necropsied at random in Japan, is almost twice the prevalence expected in the US based on the presence of a murmur. The difference in prevalences may be due to the inclusion of mitral valve prolapse in the dogs in Japan, or to the fact that dogs in Japan tend to be of the smaller breeds (with the exception of Akitas) in which mitral valvular disease occurs most prevalently.[8]

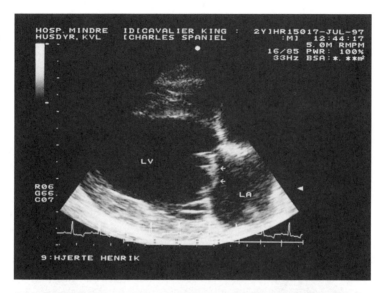

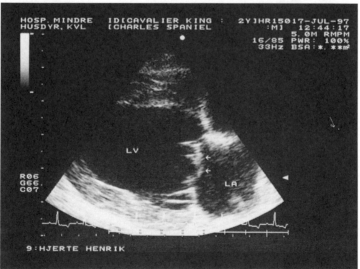

Figure 2. 2-D echocardiogram from a dog with leaflets of the mitral valve (to which the arrows are pointing) prolapsing into the left atrium (LA). Left ventricle is marked LV. (This figure was provided by Dr. H. Pedersen, The Royal Veterinary and Agricultural University, Denmark.)

Morbid Anatomy

Mitral regurgitation occurs the vast majority of the time in dogs because of chronic valvular disease, termed endocardiosis (Fig. 3) in veterinary medicine. Whereas the mitral valve alone is affected 62% of the time, the tricuspid and the mitral valves together are affected 33% of the time, and the tricuspid valve alone is affected less than 1% of the time.

The canine mitral apparatus is very similar to that of man, the valve being comprised of two major leaflets, the larger and longer septal cusp, and the mural cusp. The cusps comprise between 35% and 63% of the annular circumference; and the anterior and posterior papillary muscles are attached to the cusps by 1st and 2nd order, but seldom 3rd order, chordae tendineae. The canine cusp is comprised of the same layers as the human cusp—atrial (containing sparse smooth muscle cells) and ventricular endocardium surrounding a diffuse thin layer of collagen fibers, elastic fibers, and fibroblasts. There is little to no capillarity to the mitral cusps or to the chordae tendeneae.

As dogs age, their mitral valves normally thicken, and there is no agreement on what degree of thickening is considered either pathologic or

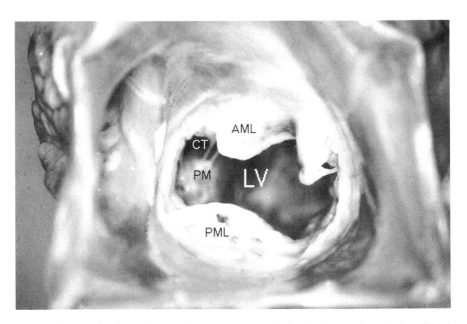

Figure 3. Mitral orifice from a dog showing anterior (AML) and posterior (PML) leaflets of the mitral valve shrunken and gnarled, characteristic of endocardiosis. The left ventricle (LV), a papillary muscle (PM) and chordae tendineae (CT) can be observed through the mitral orifice. See color appendix.

the prodromata of endocardiosis and mitral regurgitation. Mitral valve disease is often categorized into three groups by severity of valvular deformity. In group I there are small, discrete lesions with or without nodules on the valves. In group II there is extensive valvular thickening. In group III chordae tendineae become involved, valves are dramatically thickened, and they may become either contracted and gnarled or redundant and prolapse. A number of dogs with mitral regurgitation will have chordal rupture (Fig. 4) that permits flailing of a portion of a valve. After the rupture occurs, the chords shrink and become "silent" to the echocardiogram, but the valve is seen to flail into the left atrium during systole. It is not known how often observers call a flailing valve mitral valve prolapse. A study including both echocardiography and postmortem examination of dogs with mitral valve disease and normal dogs is required before the true prevalences of endocardiosis, endocardiosis with prolapse, and prolapse without endocardiosis is known for dogs.

The leaflets of the mitral valve from dogs with pure mitral regurgitation are usually only thickened and gnarled (Fig. 5) in contradistinction with the dorsal displacement of leaflets from dogs with mitral valve prolapse (Fig. 2). Often there is disruption of the chordae tendineae, which permits evulsion of a portion of a leaflet. In fact, most often one of the ini-

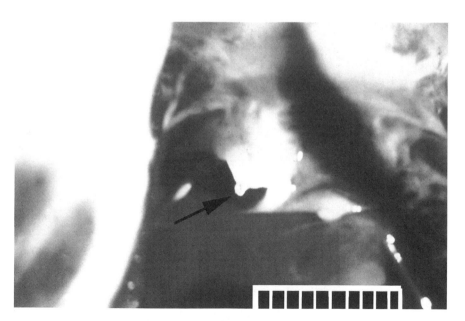

Figure 4. Mitral leaflet with torn chord (to which arrow is pointing) retracted to the edge of the leaflet. This leaflet flailed during ventricular systole. See color appendix.

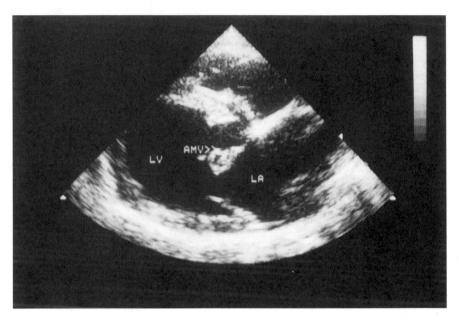

Figure 5. 2-D echocardiogram obtained during atrial systole from dog with endo-cardiosis and mitral regurgitation showing an extremely thickened anterior leaflet of the mitral valve (AMV).

tial chordal lesions is lengthening of the primary chords, which permits the free edges of the cusps to evert toward the atrium. Quite often there are hemorrhagic lesions on the atrial and less so on the ventricular faces of the leaflets (Fig. 3), and rarely vegetations are observed both echocardiographically and at postmortem examination. Most of the time "jet lesions" (Fig. 6) appear as deposits of fibrous tissue on the endocardium of the left atrium where the high-velocity regurgitant jet impacts. These lesions may also appear on the atrial surface of the valves. It is possible that jet lesions result from high shear forces that impart energy to the endocardial surfaces, and that this energy promotes growth of this fibrous tissue.

Of course dogs with mitral regurgitation have left atrial (Fig. 1) and left ventricular dilatation, which correlates quite well with the regurgitant fraction and the clinical severity of the disease.[7] This dilatation produces expansion of the mitral annulus, which makes the valve even more incompetent. Quite commonly, because they share a common etiology or because one produces the other, dogs with mitral regurgitation will have the left ventricular free wall and posterior papillary muscle riddled with fibrotic scars (Fig. 7) and with arteriolar sclerotic vessels. There has been some conjecture that myointimal proliferation of coronary arterioles, leading to diffuse microscopic myocardial infarcts, might share an etiology with infiltration of the valves with glycosaminoglycans. Some believe that both endocardiosis and arteriolarsclerosis share a common etiology in

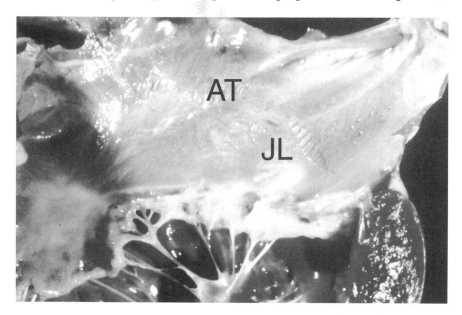

Figure 6. Fresh specimen from a dog showing fibrous tissue (JL) basilar to the thickened, gnarled leaflets of the mitral valve. A line ("railroad tracks") where the torn left atrium sutured spontaneously (AT) is also observed. See color appendix.

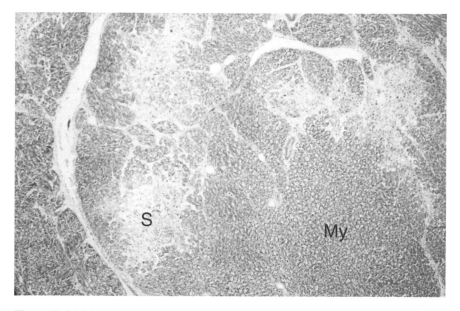

Figure 7. A histological section of the left ventricle from a dog with mitral regurgitation and myocardial fibrosis. Fibrotic tissue (S) appears grayish, while healthy myocardium (My) appears reddish. The scar in which the S appears is approximately 1 mm in diameter. See color appendix.

which promotion of cell growth is stimulated be excess angiotensin II, and therefore may be retarded by use of angiotensin-converting enzyme inhibitors.

As mentioned, in veterinary medicine, the most typical lesions on the mitral valves are called endocardiosis. They are characterized by destruction of collagen fibers with deposition of acid mucopolysaccarides, predominantly hyaluronic acid and chondroitin sulfate in the spongiosa and fibrosa lamina of the valves. The lesions originate as small nodules on the leaflets, and then grow to distort the valves. In later stages of endocardiosis, the chordae tendineae become thickened and weakened, and often rupture, with similar abnormal glycosaminoglycans. Older dogs have proliferation and occassional splitting of the atrial endocardium possibly analogous to senile valvular sclerosis in humans.[13] A number of dogs with mitral regurgitation develop tears (Fig. 6) in the left atrium, and hemorrhage into the pericardial sac. Most of these dogs die acutely, but in some there is spontaneous suturing of the tear and the dogs may live an indefinite time. Increased metabolic activity and cellular proliferation of the cusps has been suggested to support Angrist's unitary hypothesis of the origin of both endocardiosis and arteriosclerosis.[1] Endocardiosis in dogs is thought to represent a dystrophic process rather than a process of resolution of endocarditis.

Presenting Signs/Symptoms

Although the vast majority of dogs with mitral regurgitation are without symptoms, the majority of dogs that are referred to a veterinarian because they manifest symptoms are presented because of a hacking cough and/or exercise intolerance. Only a very small percentage are presented for signs/symptoms of left-sided congestive heart failure. The hacking cough comes from compression of the left mainstem bronchus (Fig. 8) but from neither pulmonary congestion nor edema. Pulmonary congestion is more likely to produce wheezing, and pulmonary edema a "half-hearted" cough. The origin of exercise intolerance is unknown, but may arise from inadequate ventilation, from adequate ventilation but requiring increased effort, from reduced cardiac output, from maldistribution of cardiac output, from primary alterations in metabolism of working muscles, or from combinations of the above.

Diagnosis

The hallmark of mitral regurgitation is the left apical systolic murmur (Fig. 9) produced by the high-velocity jet from the left ventricle into left atrium. There is considerable dispute over the relationship between the in-

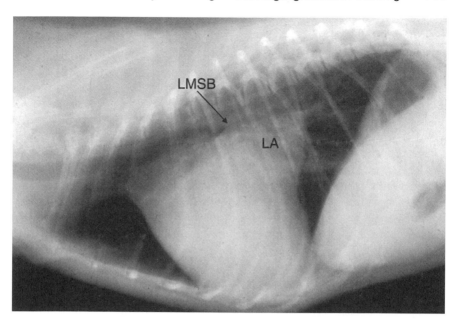

Figure 8. Left lateral radiograph of the thorax of a dog with severe mitral regurgitation. The pendulously dilated left atrium (LA) is observed to deviate dorsad and to compress the left mainstem bronchus (LMSB) to which an arrow is pointing. This dog was presented for a "hacking" cough due to heart disease, but not for heart failure. The pulmonary fields are clear.

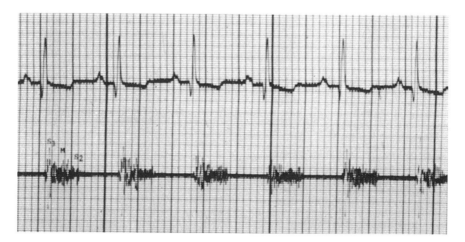

Figure 9. Noisy, holosystolic murmur classified as iii/vi and heard with maximal intensity at the left 5th intercostal space at the costochondral juncture. Notice also the broad, notched P-waves compatible with left atrial enlargement.

tensity of the murmur and the severity of the mitral valve disease in dogs. Unlike reports in humans, a study on Cavalier King Charles spaniels shows that the intensity of the murmur correlates well with the ratio of left atrial diameter to aortic diameter on the echocardiogram.[10–12] To the contrary clinical observations by others suggest that, while the murmur is very soft at the onset of the disease and becomes louder as the disease progresses, it appears to depend as much on the health of the left ventricle as on the severity of the mitral valve lesions.[14] It is possible that the intensity of the murmur appears to correlate with the severity of the regurgitation because the more severe the regurgitation, the larger the heart and the better the sounds are coupled to the thoracic wall. This is consistent with the extraordinarily loud first heart sound. Quite often, the murmur develops a musical quality resulting from rupture of the chordae tendineae (Fig. 10) and evulsion of a portion of a leaflet. Severity of the mitral regurgitation can be predicted by the degree of left atrial and left auricular enlargement observed both radiographically and echocardiographically, and finally by the presence of pulmonary venous engorgement and pulmonary edema (Fig. 11); but in certain instances, presumably when the left atrial capacity has not had time to increase, dogs may develop pulmonary edema without pendulous enlargement of the left atrium.

Dogs with mitral regurgitation and rather pendulous dilatation of the left atrium are presented most commonly with a hacking cough resulting from compression and dorsal displacement of the left mainstem bronchus. Whereas thousands of dogs each year are presented for cough due to mitral regurgitation and compression of the mainstem bronchus, many

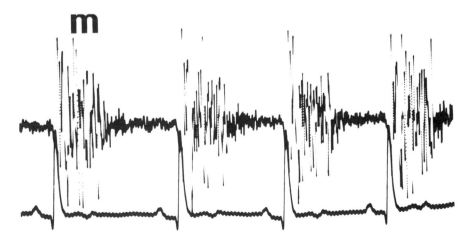

Figure 10. Loud systolic murmur with both noisy and musical components classified as v/vi. Although the baseline on this phonocardiogram appears "noisy," there was also a softer, lower-pitched early diastolic filling murmur of relative mitral stenosis.

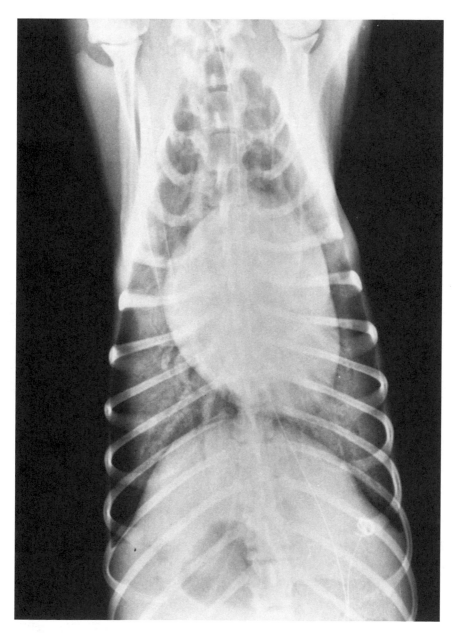

Figure 11. A dorsoventral radiograph of the thorax viewed from the ventral surface from a dog with mitral regurgitation and bilateral pulmonary edema. This dog was tachypneic and cyanotic.

fewer—actually an unknown number but possibly between 0.1% and 0.25% of the dog population—are presented with pulmonary edema obviously resulting from elevation of the pulmonary capillary pressure. Whereas the upper limit of normal for pulmonary capillary pressure is less than 8 mm Hg, many dogs with mitral regurgitation may develop enormous cv waves with mean pulmonary capillary pressures of 40 or 50 mm Hg (Fig. 12). With less severe mitral regurgitation but with engorgement of the left mainstem bronchus, dogs commonly wheeze. It is thought that such wheezing, termed "cardiac asthma," results from a bronchoconstrictory reflex initiated by engorgement of pulmonary veins.

Because of the often pendulous dilatation of the left atrium, dogs with advanced stages of mitral regurgitation often develop supraventricular arrhythmias (Fig. 13) culminating in atrial fibrillation (Fig. 14), usually with a rapid ventricular response. Ventricular rates commonly reach 260 beats/minute or even higher.

Many dogs with mitral regurgitation develop exercise incapacity. Because many of these dogs are very old and have degenerative diseases of the skeleton and skeletal muscles and also chronic bronchitis and pulmonary fibrosis, it is quite difficult, sometimes impossible, to determine if the exercise incapacity arises from the mitral regurgitation or from disease of other organ systems. Nonetheless, in many instances, dogs with mitral regurgitation do have exercise incapacity that parallels, roughly, the degree of left atrial enlargement and/or pulmonary edema. Such incapacity may arise from cough, dyspnea, or apparent fatigue of skeletal muscles.

Finally, dogs with mitral regurgitation may faint. It is thought that this syncope results from extraordinarily vigorous motion of the left ventricle, which has a large ejection fraction due to ejecting both antegradely and retrogradely. This vigorous motion activates left ventricular mechanoreceptors mediated over B_1 adrenergic fibers, and initiates both bradycardia and

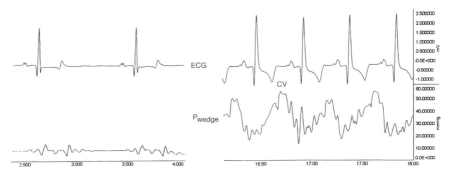

Figure 12. Recordings of ECG (top) and pulmonary wedge pressure (bottom) from a normal dog (left) and a dog with mitral regurgitation. Pressure scale appears to the right. Notice the elevated mean wedge pressure and the pronounced cv wave in the dog with mitral regurgitation.

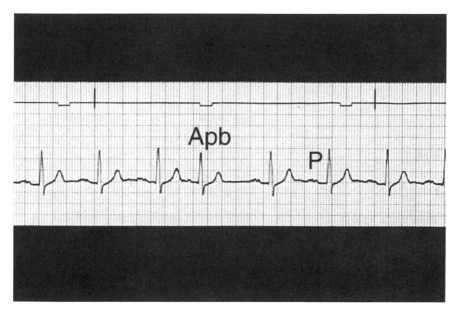

Figure 13. ECG from a dog with mitral regurgitation, demonstrating broad, notched P waves and an atrial premature depolarization.

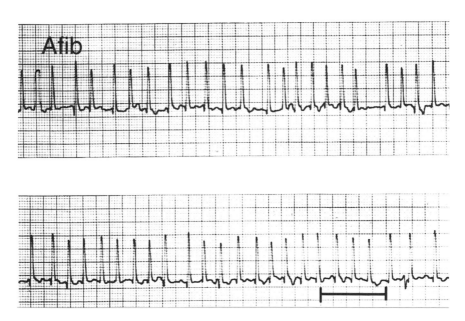

Figure 14. ECG from a dog with mitral regurgitation showing atrial fibrillation with the typically rapid ventricular response.

vasodilatation, resulting in systemic arterial hypotension. Beta blockers have been used quite successfully in treating this syncope.

An indeterminate number of small dogs of a breed prone to develop mitral regurgitation are presented with early to mid-systolic clicks (Fig. 15). In only a variable fraction of these dogs is a prolapsing mitral valve docu-

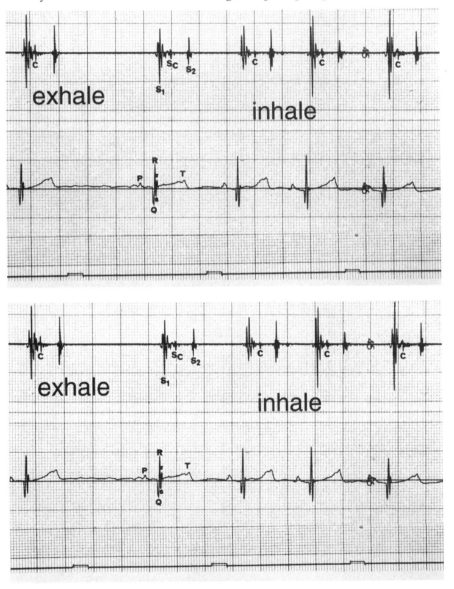

Figure 15. Phonocardiogram and electrocardiogram from a dog with respiratory sinus arrhythmia and early systolic click (c). At times a short, decrescendo systolic murmur could be heard beginning with the click.

mented echocardiographically. This lack of concordance may result from inadequate echocardiographic technique, or from the click arising from some source other than mitral prolapse.

A large number of aging cocker spaniels, the vast majority with mitral regurgitation, have pronounced respiratory sinus arrhythmias with periods of sinus arrest up to 3 seconds. Whereas the US veterinary cardiologist interprets this arrhythmia as disease of the sinoatrial node (not documented histologically, however), the feeling among European veterinary cardiologists is that the arrhythmia is analogous to the arrhythmias observed in humans with autonomic imbalance coincident with mitral valve prolapse in that species.

Management

There is good agreement among veterinary cardiologists on how to treat dogs with left-sided congestive heart failure due to mitral regurgitation. They are given enalapril (the only ACE inhibitor currently approved by the FDA for use in dogs), digoxin, and diuretics—usually furosemide. Many cardiologists also recommend theophylline to counter the bronchoconstrictory reflex generated by pulmonary venous engorgement and to strengthen the muscles of respiration. If the dog is in atrial fibrillation, usually with a ventricular rate of over 240 beats/minute, it is uncommon to slow the ventricular rate adequately with digoxin, so diltiazem is used to decrease the ventricular rate to below 130 beats/minute, although there is no agreement on what ventricular response is optimal. Many dogs with mitral regurgitation have ventricular ectopia occurring most often as single ventricular premature depolarizations, but occasionally as paroxysmal ventricular tachycardia. Occasionally dogs with mitral regurgitation die suddenly without signs of congestive heart failure, and it is presumed that these die from ventricular fibrillation. Currently most veterinary cardiologists do not treat ventricular arrhythmias unless the dog is syncopal.

Of the total number of dogs with mitral regurgitation, only a small percentage—estimated at less than 5%—are considered in functional class III or IV of the NYHA. The vast majority are in classes I or II; and there is much less agreement on treating these dogs with mitral regurgitation that may have failing hearts (i.e., reduced contractility) but are not in congestive heart failure (i.e., have pulmonary edema). The majority of veterinary cardiologists treat dogs with significant left atrial enlargement, documented either radiographically or echocardiographically, with enalapril, presuming that the afterload reduction may deter the onset of heart failure by both improving forward flow and reducing regurgitant fraction. In addition, there is some conjecture that angiotensin II may be a factor responsible, in part, for endocardiosis; therefore it is thought that enalapril may actually prevent or slow the evolution of the disease. Currently there are two multicenter trials—one in the US and one in the Scandinavian countries—addressing the potential benefit of treating dogs in NYHA classes I or II.[15]

Three surgical procedures have been used, albeit infrequently, to treat mitral regurgitation: placing a prosthetic valve, placing a purse-string suture around the mitral orifice, or plicating the redundant leaflet of the mitral valve. For financial reasons and because many dogs with mitral regurgitation have multisystemic disorders, surgical procedures are performed rarely.

Prognosis

With the rare exception of traumatic mitral regurgitation, the vast majority of dogs afflicted with mitral regurgitation progress very slowly from the initial valvular defect to pulmonary edema. It is not uncommon to examine a dog that has minimal mitral regurgitation at the age of 5 years, and then to reexamine the dog in heart failure at 16 years of age. Once heart failure develops, the life expectancy is in months. Of course the disease progresses much faster in Cavalier King Charles spaniels than in other breeds. A Cavalier spaniel in which mitral regurgitation is detected at 3 years of age may be in heart failure by 5 years.

With medical management, the life expectancy of dogs in functional class II may be prolonged, in comfort, for years; however, as mentioned previously, once heart failure is functional class IV, the life expectancy is months. Unfortunately there have been no longevity trials to provide data on the natural history of the disease or the affects of therapy on longevity.

Perspective

Mitral regurgitation that occurs naturally in dogs possesses many hemodynamic features in common with the same disease in humans. A major difference between the species is in treatment. In humans, repair or replacement of the diseased valve is the treatment of choice. Hacking cough probably occurs much more frequently in dogs with mitral regurgitation than in humans. In dogs, treatment is almost always medical. If one is convinced by data obtained by postmortem examination of dogs, mitral valve prolapse occurs much more commonly in dogs than in humans. Most echocardiographic diagnoses have been made by European colleagues, and many fewer by US veterinary cardiologists. Mitral prolapse rarely progresses to significant mitral regurgitation. Endocardiosis with mitral regurgitation appears to be a disease of the mitral valve in rather old dogs, and chordal rupture with flailing of a mitral valve occurs in a small proportion. Mitral valve prolapse usually without mitral regurgitation is observed most often in younger dogs, but in breeds with a high prevalence of endocardiosis. It is not known if mitral valve prolapse is a prodromata of endocardiosis. Iatrogenic models of mitral regurgitation in dogs differ rather dramatically from naturally occurring mitral regurgitation. Dogs with the naturally occurring disease that develops over years have more massive cardiomegaly, the pulmonary edema in naturally occurring disease is usually distributed throughout the lung, while in the iatrogenic models it may be limited to regions impacted by a regurgitant jet, and dogs with naturally occurring mitral regurgitation are more likely to have myocardial disease and ventricular ectopia secondary to coincident disease.

References

1. Angrist A. J Gerentol 19:135–143, 1964.
2. Buchanan J. Chronic valvular disease (endocardiosis) in dogs. Adv Vet Sci Comp Med 21:75–106, 1977.
3. Das K, Tashjian R. Chronic mitral valve disease in the dog. Vet Med Small Anim Clin 60:1209–1215, 1965.
4. Detweiler D, Patterson D. The prevalence and types of cardiovascular disease in dogs. Ann NY Acad Sci 127:481–516, 1965.
5. Haggstrom J, Hansson K, Kvart C, Swenson L. Chronic valvular disease in the Cavalier King Charles Spaniel. Vet Rec 131:549–553, 1992.
6. Haggstrom J, Kvart C, Hansson K. Heart sounds and murmurs: Changes related to severity of chronic valvular heart disease in the Cavalier King Charles Spaniel. J Vet Intern Med 9:75–85, 1995.
7. Kihara Y, Sasayama S, Miyazaki S, et al. Role of left atrium in adaptation of the heart to chronic mitral regurgitation in conscious dogs. Circ Res 62:543–553, 1988.
8. Kogure K. Pathology of chronic mitral valvular disease in the dog. Jpn J Vet Sci 42:323–335, 1980.
9. Oka M, Angrist A. Proc NY State Assoc Public Health Lab 41:21–23, 1961.
10. Pedersen H, Lorentzen K, Kristensen B. Observer variation in the two-dimensional echocardiographic evaluations of mitral valve prolapse in dogs. Vet Radiol Ultrasound 37:367–372, 1996.
11. Pedersen H, Kristensen B, Lorentzen K, Koch J, Jensen A, Flagstad A. Mitral valve prolapse in 3 healthy Cavalier King Charles Spaniels: An echocardiographic study. Can J Vet Res 59:294–298, 1959.
12. Pedersen H, Kristensen B, Norby B, Lorentzen K. Echocardiographic study of mitral valve prolapse in dachshunds. J Vet Med 43:103–110, 1996.
13. Pomerance A, Whitney J. Heart valve changes common to man and dog: A comparative study. Cardiovasc Res 4:61–66, 1970.
14. Whitney J. Observations on the effect of age on the severity of heart valve lesions in the dog. J Small Anim Pract 15:511–522, 1974.
15. The COVE Study Group. Controlled clinical evaluation of enalapril in dogs with heart failure: Results of the cooperative veterinary enalapril study group. J Vet Intern Med 9:243–252, 1995.

Part XVIII

Floppy Mitral Valve, Mitral Valve Prolapse:

Concluding Remarks and Projections for the Future

The Floppy Mitral Valve, Mitral Valve Prolapse, Mitral Valvular Regurgitation, and Mitral Valve Prolapse Syndrome:

Concluding Remarks and Projections for the Future

Harisios Boudoulas, MD, PhD, Charles F. Wooley, MD

Time present and time past
Are both perhaps present in time future,
And time future contained in time past.
–T.S. Eliot[1]

Introduction

The modern history of valvular heart disease in general and mitral valvular disease in particular may be traced to the early 1800s. The mitral valvular regurgitation (MVR) lineage is more complex than other forms of valvular heart disease, full of contradictions, reversals, and paradox. The

From: Boudoulas H, Wooley CF. *Mitral Valve: Floppy Mitral Valve, Mitral Valve Prolapse, Mitral Valvular Regurgitation.* Second revised edition. ©Futura Publishing Company, Armonk, NY, 2000.

earlier medical literature contained impressive insights into MVR, observations that were lost and then rediscovered, widely scattered in time and space. However, doctrine without data prevailed for prolonged intervals along with a notable absence of scientific inquiry. Certain biological and clinical concepts were prerequisites to appreciating the central role of the floppy mitral valve (FMV), in the mitral valve prolapse (MVP), MVR story.[2-4]

In this book, data from multiple sources emphasize the central role of the FMV in the FMV/MVP/MVR triad and the FMV/MVP syndrome. This chapter emphasizes current clinical diagnostic guides, the importance of individual patient analysis, the basis for clinical classification, and the role of the mitral valve complex function on circulatory homeostasis. We incorporate with some projections of thought about future lines of inquiry.

Terminology and Diagnosis

It is apparent that the FMV is the central issue of the FMV, MVP, MVR triad and the FMV/MVP syndrome. Thus, it is our view that use of the FMV/MVP/MVR terminology, with qualitative and/or quantitative terms for each segment of the FMV/MVP/MVR triad, improves clarity of expression.

For the diagnosis of FMV/MVP, the key issue is precise definition of the FMV. New technology with three-dimensional reconstruction of the mitral valve apparatus allows better definition of the mitral valve complex and the floppy mitral valve morphology and dimensions.

At present, the diagnosis of FMV/MVP/MVR is based on the auscultatory postural complex with confirmatory echophonocardiographic and Doppler findings to provide clinical coherence. The likelihood of finding FMV/MVP using echocardiography in patients with normal, carefully performed dynamic auscultation is extremely low. A confounding issue arises when patients with symptoms, negative auscultatory findings, and nonspecific echocardiographic FMV/MVP findings should be labeled as having FMV/MVP and their symptoms ascribed to FMV/MVP. We avoid labeling these patients with a diagnosis of FMV/MVP. At times, distinguishing between the normal mitral valve with its minor variants, and a mitral valve with an intrinsic structural derangement, may be difficult. In certain cases, repeat physical examination and echocardiograms over several years' time may be necessary before the matter is resolved. Family history is important in such situations since FMV/MVP may be inherited.

Individual Patient Analysis

The FMV is a common mitral valve abnormality with a broad spectrum of structural and functional changes, extending from mild to severe (Fig. 1). Physical examination and laboratory findings are directly related to the nature and extent of the valvular abnormality. As a general rule, patients with more severe disease will have more clinical and laboratory findings and vice versa. Similarly, the management and natural history obviously differ in each subgroup of patients with FMV/MVP (Fig. 1). Thus, individual patient analysis for patients with FMV/MVP, as in any other situation in clinical medicine, is extremely important.

The individual patient analysis represents a logical approach to the diagnostic and risk stratification process. Emphasis should be placed on the individual patient profile (Fig. 2). Much depends on the physician's experience, diagnostic facilities, and available technology. Diagnostic facilities vary from institution to institution, from country to country, and will continue to change dramatically in years to come. Thus, specific definition of the anatomic lesion(s), physiological or pathophysiological state, and the extent of morphological and pathophysiological abnormalities for the individual patient remain as the ultimate standards.

Floppy Mitral Valve/Mitral Valve Prolapse: Clinical Classification

Based on our clinical experience and that of our colleagues worldwide, we proposed the following classification of patients with FMV/MVP (Fig. 3).

FMV/MVP refers to patients with FMV/MVP with a wide spectrum of mitral valve abnormalities from mild to severe. The term "floppy" mitral valve comes from surgical and pathological studies and refers to the intrinsic morphological changes resulting in the expansion of the area of the mitral valve leaflets, with elongated chordae tendineae, frequently including a dilated mitral annulus. Symptoms, physical findings, diagnostic phenomena, and complications in these patients are directly related to mitral valve dysfunction and progressive MVR.

FMV/MVP syndrome refers to the occurrence of symptoms resulting from neuroendocrine or autonomic dysfunction in patients with FMV/MVP, in whom the symptoms cannot be explained on the basis of the valvular abnormality alone.

This clinically useful classification separates symptomatic patients with FMV/MVP and symptoms related primarily to neuroendocrine or autonomic nervous system dysfunction from patients whose symptoms

Severity of disease in patients with FMV.

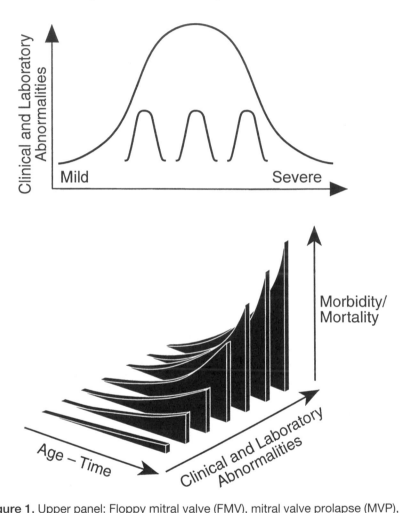

Figure 1. Upper panel: Floppy mitral valve (FMV), mitral valve prolapse (MVP), mitral valvular regurgitation (MVR). The spectrum of mitral valve abnormalities in patients with FMV/MVP. Lower panel: Relationship between the number of clinical and laboratory abnormalities and the morbidity/mortality (schematic presentation). FMV/MVP includes a wide spectrum of valvular abnormalities from mild to severe and at any particular time the number of abnormal clinical (e.g., click, click plus late systolic murmur, holosystolic murmur, gallop rhythm, cardiac arrhythmias, etc.) and laboratory findings (e.g., late systolic prolapse, thickened mitral leaflets, holosystolic prolapse, left ventricular and left atrial enlargement on echocardiogram, and mitral regurgitation on Doppler) is directly related to the severity of the disease. The natural history and complications such as infective endocarditis, MVR, etc. of patients with FMV/MVP is also directly related to the severity of mitral valve abnormalities.

Individual Patient Analysis

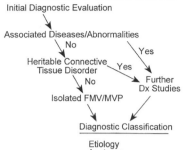

Floppy Mitral Valve / Mitral Valve Prolapse

- Isolated abnormality
  – may be heritable

- Associated with structural cardiac defects

- Cardiac manifestation of heritable disorders of connective tissue

- Cardiac manifestation of incompletely defined connective tissue disorder

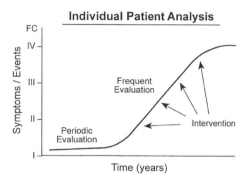

Figure 2. Individual patient analysis. Incorporates the diagnostic steps necessary to develop a diagnostic classification. Periodic evaluation is replaced by more frequent evaluation with the development of symptoms or events. Intervention indicated by multiple arrows, may involve medical therapy or surgical procedure at varying times during the course of the disease. (Used with permission from Boudoulas H, et al.[5])

are related primarily to mitral valve dysfunction. It specifies a group of patients with FMV/MVP and autonomic dysfunction who require consideration for antibiotic prophylaxis for infective endocarditis in addition to other forms of treatment. It also defines a group of symptomatic patients who need attention from physicians who are aware of newer developments in neuroendocrine and autonomic nervous system function and dysfunction.

Floppy Mitral Valve/Mitral Valve Prolapse/Mitral Valvular Regurgitation: Natural Progression

Patients with FMV/MVP who have minimal MVR may be, and remain, asymptomatic. Certain of these patients progress to more severe

FMV/MVP/MVR:
Dynamic Spectrum & Natural Progression

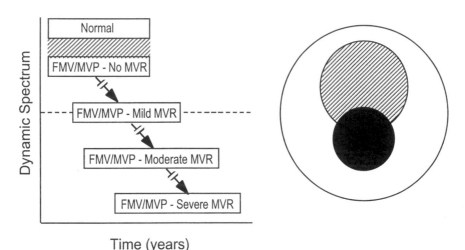

Time (years)

Figure 3. Left panel: The dynamic spectrum, time in years, and the progression of floppy mitral valve (FMV), mitral valve prolapse (MVP) are shown. A subtle grada-tion (cross-hatched area) exists between the normal mitral valve and valves that produce mild FMV/MVP without mitral valvular regurgitation (MVR). Progression from the level FMV/MVP - no MVR to another level may or may not occur. Most of the patients with FMV/MVP syndrome occupy the area above the dotted line, while patients with progressive mitral valve dysfunction occupy the area below the dotted line. Right panel. The large circle represents the total number of patients with FMV/MVP. Patients with FMV/MVP may be symptomatic or asymptomatic. Symptoms may be directly related to mitral valve dysfunction (black circle), or to autonomic dysfunction (cross-hatched circle). Certain patients with symptoms di-rectly related to mitral valve dysfunction may present and continue to have symp-toms secondary to autonomic dysfunction. (Used with permission from Boudoulas H, et al.[2])

forms of MVR. Complications directly attributable to the FMV/MVP in-clude progressive MVR, left atrial and left ventricular enlargement and dysfunction, congestive heart failure, thromboembolic phenomena, infec-tive endocarditis, progressive elongation or disruption of the valve appa-ratus associated with the rupture of abnormal chordae tendineae, the con-sequences of flail mitral leaflets, and cardiac arrhythmias.

While the conventional wisdom presented in the medical literature states that the prognosis of patients with FMV/MVP is benign in the ma-jority of patients, serious complications may and do occur. The long natu-ral history of patients with the FMV/MVP/MVR triad has served to obscure the true incidence of complications. While the prognosis is good over the short term, the same may be said for a variety of serious diseases, as for example, lipid abnormalities or arterial hypertension. While the extremely long clinical course of FMV/MVP makes the natural history difficult to define, important strides have been made in this area (see Chapter 20).

For better definition of the natural progression of the FMV/MVP/MVR triad, accurate definition of the degree of MVR at rest and during physical activities, as well as its effect on left atrial and left ventricular structure and function are necessary. At present, magnetic resonance imaging offers quantitative assessment of regurgitant volume and the regurgitant fraction in patients with MVR. This is a reproducible technique and allows follow-up of patients with FMV/MVP/MVR with quantitative analysis of all three facets of the triad over time. In addition, magnetic resonance imaging gives accurate measurements of left ventricular and left atrial structure and function. Thus, progression of the FMV morphological changes, the severity of MVR, and the effects on left atrium and left ventricle can be assessed and followed by magnetic resonance imaging.

Advances in color flow Doppler, transesophageal, and three-dimensional echocardiography will allow clinicians to better define and follow the progress of the disease. Exercise testing in patients with FMV/MVP without MVR at rest may result in significant MVR in certain patients with FMV/MVP. The dynamics of postural changes and the effect of exercise testing on the degree of MVR, left atrial and left ventricular size and function in patients with FMV/MVP, and the effect of exercise on these parameters on the natural history of the disease, requires better definition.

The long-term effect of therapeutic interventions on the natural history of patients with FMV/MVP/MVR triad remains to be defined. It has been suggested that therapy with angiotensin-converting enzyme inhibitors may prevent the progression of MVR, resulting in regression of left ventricular dilatation and hypertrophy. Further assessment of the effects of medical therapy will be of increasing importance to clinicians.

During the long natural history of the disease, certain patients with FMV/MVP/MVR will require valve surgery, either reconstructive FMV surgery or mitral valve replacement. After valve surgery, especially after reconstructive surgery, these patients may live a long productive life. The natural history of patients with FMV/MVP/MVR after valve surgery is gradually becoming clearer and for the most part, the results are most encouraging. In fact, surgical reconstruction of the FMV has become part of the natural history of many patients with the FMV/MVP/MVR triad.

Subgroups of FMV/MVP patients with a higher incidence of complications—progression to severe MVR, chordae tendineae rupture, thromboembolic phenomena, infective endocarditis, and sudden death—must be defined more effectively. Comparing the natural history of one group of patients with FMV/MVP with that of another, without further stratification results in fallacies similar to that of comparing the natural history of two groups of patients with coronary artery disease without further stratification (Fig. 1).

Floppy Mitral Valve/Mitral Valve Prolapse Syndrome

Whether a FMV/MVP syndrome exists has been a source of concern and debate for some time. It is our present opinion that certain symptomatic patients with FMV/MVP manifest a neuroendocrine-cardiovascular process resulting from a close relationship between FMV/MVP and central or peripherally mediated states of neuroendocrine or autonomic nervous system dysfunction or imbalance.[2,4]

It has been documented that the incidence of palpitations, orthostatic hypotension, low body weight, and symptoms related to positive G stress are more common in patients with FMV/MVP than in the general population. Parasympathetic abnormality, baroreflex modulation abnormality, decreased intravascular volume, decreased left ventricular volume in the upright posture, renin-aldosterone regulation abnormality, catecholamine regulation abnormality, hyperresponse to adrenergic stimulation, or abnormal β-receptor function have been demonstrated in certain patients with FMV/MVP syndrome (see Chapter 24). Just how these clinical phenomena, symptom complexes, neuroendocrine abnormalities, and autonomic nervous system alterations are interrelated in patients with FMV/MVP syndrome, and how they are genetically transmitted, will be better defined in the years to come (Fig. 4).

The coexistence of FMV/MVP with anxiety states and panic disorder has stimulated a dialogue between psychiatrists, primary care physicians, and cardiologists. While FMV/MVP and anxiety states may be transmitted independently, further clinical and genetic studies will be necessary to clarify possible associations. Many primary care physicians may be out of touch with contemporary developments in psychiatry, while psychiatrists are returning to a more active role in the care of patients with medical disorders. Both groups are using neuropharmacological agents with cardiovascular effects and toxicity. Thus, it is important to encourage mutual, interdisciplinary communication and studies in order to avoid the inappropriate diagnosis of FMV/MVP, as well as to

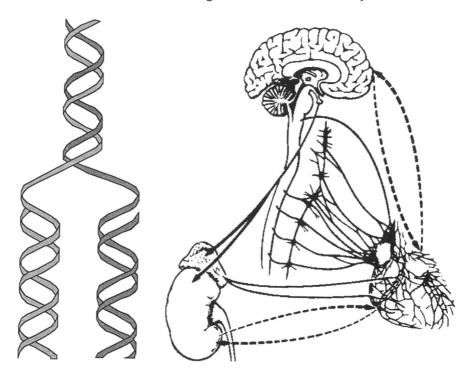

Figure 4. A possible genetic association between the floppy mitral valve/mitral valve prolapse and neuroendocrine–autonomic nervous system dysfunction remain to be defined.

avoid missing the diagnosis of basic, treatable neuropsychiatric disorders.

The management of patients with FMV/MVP syndrome requires an understanding of neuroendocrine mechanisms, autonomic nervous system function and dysfunction, and better definition of hyperresponsiveness or abnormalities in these systems. Ideally, cardiologists should treat patients with hemodynamic abnormalities after careful hemodynamic evaluation with continued hemodynamic observations during therapy. The same rules should also be applied to the management of patients with neuroendocrine dysfunction and autonomic nervous system dysfunction.

While the long-term history of patients with FMV/MVP syndrome has not been well defined, their symptoms may persist for years, and certain FMV/MVP syndrome patients may develop symptoms related to mitral valve dysfunction. Patients with FMV/MVP syndrome and significant MVR may present with, and continue to have, symptoms secondary to autonomic nervous system dysfunction following satisfactory FMV surgical reconstruction.

Floppy Mitral Valve/Mitral Valve Prolapse/Mitral Valvular Regurgitation: Effects on the Circulation

The pathophysiological consequences of mitral valve apparatus function and dysfunction in FMV/MVP are incompletely understood at present. Certainly, prolapsing mitral valve leaflet(s) resulting in left atrial space-occupying lesions, with development of a third chamber or "neutral" space between mitral annulus and prolapsing mitral valve leaflet(s), increased papillary muscle traction, and activation of papillary muscle stretch receptors, contribute significantly to the clinical picture of FMV/MVP/MVR and the FMV/MVP syndrome while influencing the natural history of the disease.

Left atrial function is an important determinant of the natural history in patients with chronic MVR. Left atrial dilatation and dysfunction resulting in left atrial myopathy may occur prior to left ventricular structural and functional changes. Monitoring indices of left atrial performance therefore provides important information for the understanding of the natural history of the disease and in our opinion is as important as assessment of left ventricular function.

Aortic function is well recognized as an important determinant of left ventricular performance and myocardial perfusion. Elastic properties of the aorta including aortic distensibility, decrease with age. Since patients with FMV/MVP/MVR have decreased aortic distensibility compared to normal subjects, we postulate that stiffening of the aorta may increase the degree of MVR and precipitate complications in the natural history in patients with FMV/MVP. Determination of the elastic properties of the aorta, which is gradually entering clinical practice, may also help us to better understand and define the natural history of the FMV/MVP/MVR disease process with the potential for new forms of therapeutic interventions.[6]

The prolapse of the FMV into the left atrium results in the development of a third left heart chamber with decreased cardiac output, and alterations in papillary muscle traction with stretch receptor stimulation that may result in myocardial ischemia and cardiac arrhythmias. Stimulation of nerve ending within the mitral valve apparatus as part of these interactions of mitral valve may result in a central nervous system phenomena yet to be defined (Fig. 5). Further, alterations of papillary muscle traction as part of the MVP process may lead to left ventricular contraction and relaxation abnormalities. Once it is recognized that FMV/MVP/MVR

Floppy Mitral Valve/Mitral Valve Prolapse: Cardiac Arrhythmias

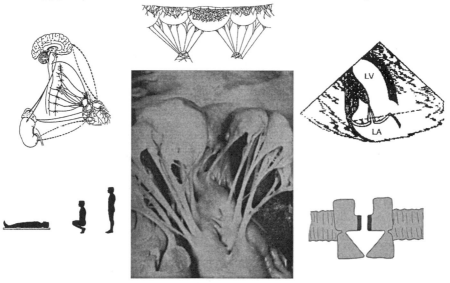

Figure 5. Floppy mitral valve is shown in the middle (from Edwards JE. Circulation 43:606–612, 1971); above the mitral valve innervation of the mitral valve is shown schematically; upper right shows papillary muscle tension during ventricular systole; lower right stretch-activated receptor is shown schematically. Left upper part shows schematically interactions between the brain-heart-kidneys and adrenals. Lower left part shows schematically orthostatic phenomena. (Used with permission from Boudoulas H, et al.[7])

may lead to left atrial and left ventricular dilatation and dysfunction and is associated with abnormal elastic properties of the aorta, the global effects of FMV/MVP/MVR on the cardiovascular system will be better appreciated (see Chapter 21).

Future research will help to better define these incompletely understood and complex phenomena related to function or dysfunction of the FMV apparatus within the cardiovascular system.

Genetics–Molecular Mechanisms

As yet, genetic diagnostic testing for FMV/MVP has not entered into clinical practice. It seems likely that patients with FMV/MVP represent a heterogeneous group in which heritable defects in protein chemistry may result in myxomatous degeneration of the mitral valve. Definition of genetic defects in patients with the FMV will allow rational classification schemes for this complex valvular abnormality (see Chapter 8). Better understanding of the molecular mechanisms that determine the progression of a mild mitral valve abnormality to floppy mitral valve (Fig. 6 A–C), and the progress to myxomatous degeneration, collagen and elastin dissolution, changes in the extracellular matrix, and FMV surface phenomena may lead to methods preventing the progress to significant mitral valve dysfunction (Fig. 7).

The genetic association between FMV/MVP and the FMV/MVP syndrome remains to be defined.

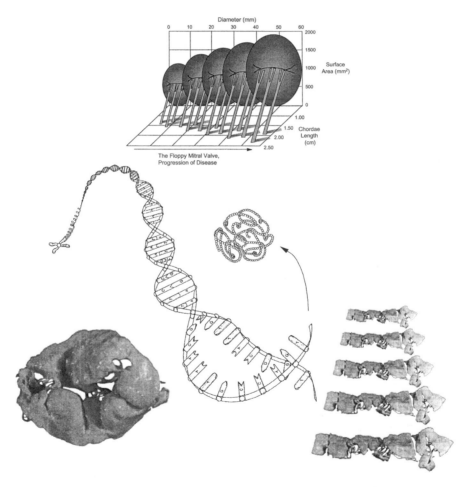

Figure 6. Gradual progression of a normal mitral valve to floppy mitral valve (top, schematic presentation). Lower left: Floppy mitral valve. Lower right. Progression of normal mitral valve to floppy mitral valve. Genetic factors determining the progression of a normal to floppy mitral valve remain to be defined.

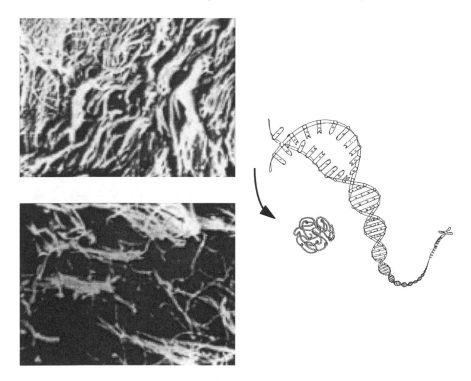

Figure 7. Collagen structure in a normal mitral valve (upper) and in a floppy mitral valve (lower). Genetic factors determining collagen dissolution remain to be defined.

Floppy Mitral Valve/Mitral Valve Prolapse: Frequency in Relation to Other Cardiovascular Abnormalities

In the future, as the etiologic causes and pathogenetic mechanisms of certain cardiovascular diseases become better understood, it is probable that true prevention will become a reality. The prevalence of FMV/MVP in the general population will either remain the same or increase in an aging population, while the prevalence of coronary artery disease, the complications of arterial hypertension, and other cardiovascular diseases will decline. Thus, in the near future, patients with FMV/MVP may constitute a greater proportion of cardiovascular abnormalities than today (Fig. 8). Further, since the MVR usually becomes significant after the age of 60, complications related to MVR will increase as the life expectancy increases.

Better understanding of molecular mechanisms of protein chemistry,

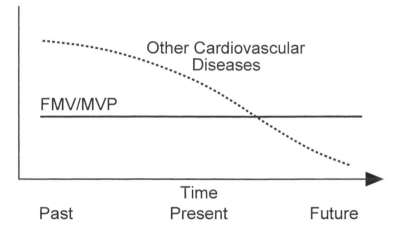

Figure 8. A projection: The frequency of floppy mitral valve (FMV) and mitral valve prolapse (MVP) will remain the same while the prevalence of other cardiovascular disorders (coronary artery disease, complications of arterial hypertension, etc. will decline.

composition of extracellular matrix, collagen and elastin synthesis and degradation will provide insights leading to interventions that will prevent the valve structure dissolution or degenerative process, and inhibit the progress of the disease.

Floppy Mitral Valve/Mitral Valve Prolapse/Mitral Valvular Regurgitation and the FMV/MVP Syndrome: An Incomplete Mosaic

We had the experience but missed the meaning.[9]

The FMV occupies the central position, the high ground, in the MVP story. FMV morphology, biochemistry, and genetics coupled with the dynamic pathophysiology of MVP are powerful extensions of our knowledge of the etiology and pathophysiology of MVR, and of valvular heart disease of connective tissue origin. The FMV odyssey reflects multicentury patterns of learning similar to those clinicians experienced with the recognition of the relationship of angina pectoris with coronary artery disease; the links between sore throats, rheumatic fever, and resultant valvular heart disease; and the recognition and classification of myocardial diseases.

Definition of the FMV, its place in the hierarchy of valvular heart disease, and awareness of disorders of connective tissue origin during the past two centuries reflect a learning process that certainly will expand in the next millennium. Cardiovascular morphologists, pathologists, auscultors, clinicians, hemodynamicists, surgeons, and imagers "had the experience but missed the meaning" of the FMV/MVP/MVR triad for prolonged time intervals. The development of clinically coherent patterns required time, multidisciplinary observations and experiences, with the development of basic concepts burnished by considerable controversy. A FMV mosaic now exists (Fig. 9).

The outlines of the FMV mosaic may be indistinct in places with missing sections; however, there is enough information, definition, and experience to form the basis for a rational approach in the next millennium, in order "to recover what has been lost and found and lost again and again."[10]

FMV/MVP/MVR: Contributions of Various Disciplines to Date

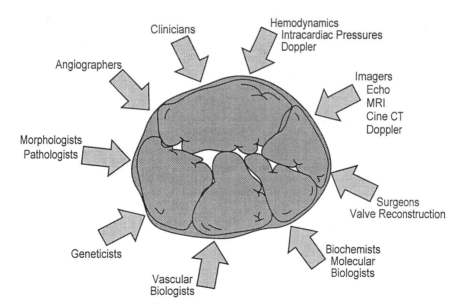

Figure 9. Floppy mitral valve mosaic. Emphasis on contributions of various disciplines to date. See text for further details.

References

1. Eliot TS. Burnt Norton, Four Quartets. A Harvest HRJ Book, Harcourt, Bruce Jovanovitch, Publishers, San Diego, New York, London, 1971, p 13.
2. Boudoulas H, Wooley CF (eds). Mitral Valve Prolapse and the Mitral Valve Prolapse Syndrome. Mount Kisco, NY, Futura Publishing Co., 1988.
3. Wooley CF, Baker PB, Kolibash AJ, Kilman JW, Sparks EA, Boudoulas H. The floppy, myxomatous mitral valve, mitral valve prolapse, and mitral regurgitation. Progr Cardiovasc Dis 33:397–433, 1991.
4. Boudoulas H, Kolibash AJ, Baker P, King BD, Wooley CF. Mitral valve prolapse and the mitral valve prolapse syndrome: A diagnostic classification and pathogenesis of symptoms. Am Heart J 118:746–818, 1989.
5. Boudoulas H, Wooley CF. Mitral valve prolapse. In Moss and Adams' Heart Diseases in Infants, Children and Adolescents. Fifth Edition, pp 1063–1086.
6. Boudoulas H, Toutouzas PK, Wooley CF, eds. Functional Abnormalities of the Aorta. Futura Publishing Company, Inc., Armonk, NY, 1996.
7. Boudoulas H, Schaal SF, Wooley CF. Floppy mitral valve/mitral valve prolapse: Cardiac arrhythmias. In Vardas PE (ed): Cardiac Arrhythmias, Pacing, and Electrophysiology. Great Britain, Kluwer Academic Publisher, 1998, pp 89–95.
8. Disse S, Abergel E, Berrebi A, Houot AM, Le Heuzey JY, et al. Mapping of a first locus for autosomal dominant myxomatous mitral valve prolapse to chromosome 16p11.2-p12.1. Am J Hum Genet 65:1242–1251, 1999.
9. Eliot TS. The Dry Salvages. Four Quartets. New York, NY, Harcourt, Brace and World, 1943, p 17.
10. Eliot TS. East Coker. Four Quartets. New York, NY, Harcourt, Brace and World, 1943, p 24.

Color Appendix

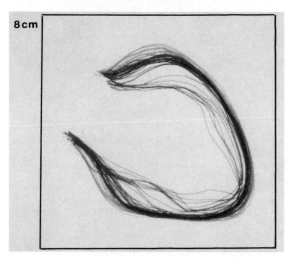

Chapter 3. Figure 4. Superimposed left ventricular cavity outlines during diastole, derived from the cineangiogram of a normal subject, at 50 frames/s. Outlines derived from early diastole and diastasis are shown in black, and those during atrial systole in red. Note that the ventricular volume increase during atrial systole is due almost entirely to an increase in long axis.

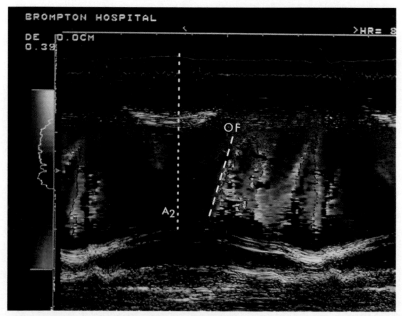

Chapter 3. Figure 9. Color M-mode with transducer at the apex, from a normal subject showing transmitral flow velocities from the level of the mitral ring to the apex of the ventricle. A2 represents aortic valve closure. OF represents the onset of flow, which is progressively delayed with respect to A2 with distance into the cavity.

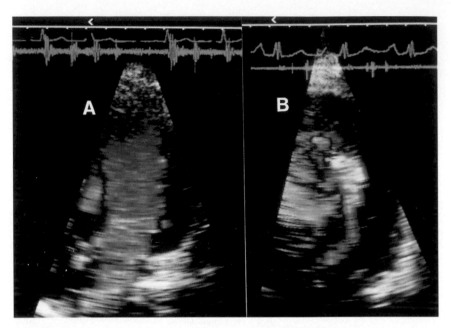

Chapter 3. Figure 12. A. Apical color flow echocardiogram, showing the normal inflow jet, recorded at the time of peak early diastolic filling velocity. Note that the jet is directed toward the ventricular free wall, and is broad, occupying the whole mitral ring. The onset of vortex development (in blue) is also apparent. B. Similar recording from a patient with a restrictive filling pattern due to dilated cardiomyopathy. Note that the jet is narrow, occupying only a small part of the mitral ring. (Used with permission from Fujimoto S, et al.[37])

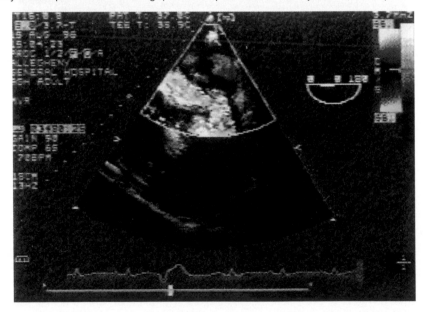

Chapter 10. Figure 6. Transesophageal two-dimensional color Doppler image demonstrating eccentric and anteriorly directed jet of mitral regurgitation caused by a floppy mitral valve with flail posterior leaflet.

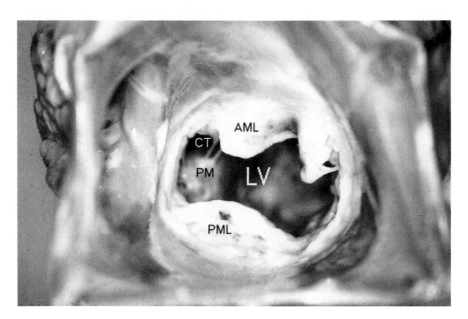

Chapter 26. Figure 3. Mitral orifice from a dog showing anterior (AML) and posterior (PML) leaflets of the mitral valve shrunken and gnarled, characteristic of endocardiosis. The left ventricle (LV), a papillary muscle (PM) and chordae tendineae (CT) can be observed through the mitral orifice.

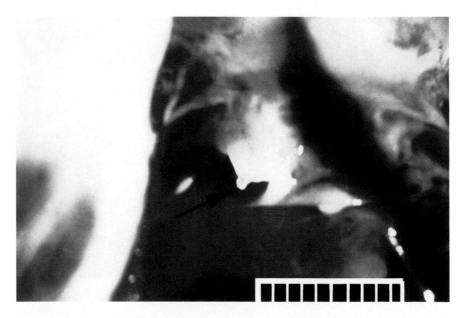

Chapter 26. Figure 4. Mitral leaflet with torn chord (to which arrow is pointing) retracted to the edge of the leaflet. This leaflet flailed during ventricular systole.

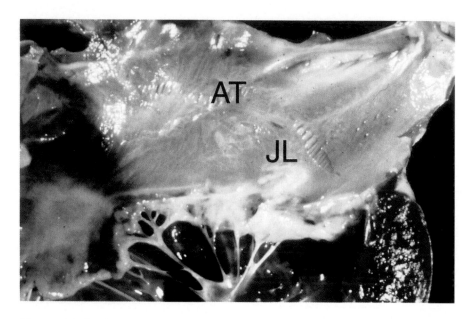

Chapter 26. Figure 6. Fresh specimen from a dog showing fibrous tissue (JL) basilar to the thickened, gnarled leaflets of the mitral valve. A line ("railroad tracks") where the torn left atrium sutured spontaneously (AT) is also observed.

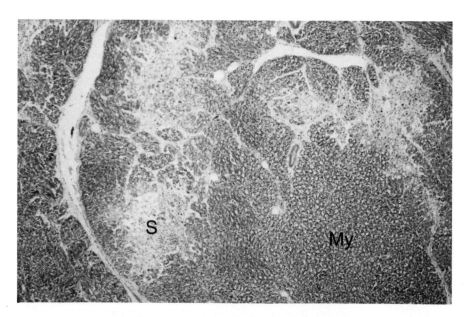

Chapter 26. Figure 7. A histological section of the left ventricle from a dog with mitral regurgitation and myocardial fibrosis. Fibrotic tissue (S) appears grayish, while healthy myocardium (My) appears reddish. The scar in which the S appears is approximately 1 mm in diameter.

Index